1999
YEAR BOOK OF
OBSTETRICS, GYNECOLOGY, AND WOMEN'S HEALTH

Statement of Purpose

The YEAR BOOK Service

The YEAR BOOK series was devised in 1901 by practicing health professionals who observed that the literature of medicine and related disciplines had become so voluminous that no one individual could read and place in perspective every potential advance in a major specialty. In the final decade of the 20th century, this recognition is more acutely true than it was in 1901.

More than merely a series of books, YEAR BOOK volumes are the tangible results of a unique service designed to accomplish the following:

- to *survey* a wide range of journals of proven value
- to *select* from those journals papers representing significant advances and statements of important clinical principles
- to provide *abstracts* of those articles that are readable, convenient summaries of their key points
- to provide *commentary* about those articles to place them in perspective

These publications grow out of a unique process that calls on the talents of outstanding authorities in clinical and fundamental disciplines, trained literature specialists, and professional writers, all supported by the resources of Mosby, the world's preeminent publisher for the health professions.

The Literature Base

Mosby and its Editors survey approximately 500 journals published worldwide, covering the full range of the health professions. On an annual basis, the publisher examines usage patterns and polls its expert authorities to add new journals to the literature base and to delete journals that are no longer useful as potential YEAR BOOK sources.

The Literature Survey

The publisher's team of literature specialists, all of whom are trained and experienced health professionals, examines every original, peer-reviewed article in each journal issue. More than 250,000 articles per year are scanned systematically, including title, text, illustrations, tables, and references. Each scan is compared, article by article, to the search strategies that the publisher has developed in consultation with the 270 outside experts who form the pool of YEAR BOOK editors. A given article may be reviewed by any number of editors, from one to a dozen or more, regardless of the discipline for which the paper was originally published. In turn, each editor who receives the article reviews it to determine whether or not the article should be included in the YEAR BOOK. This decision is based on the article's inherent quality, its probable usefulness to readers of that YEAR BOOK, and the editor's goal to represent a balanced picture of a given field in each volume of the YEAR BOOK. In addition, the editor indicates when to include figures and tables from the article to help the YEAR BOOK reader better understand the information.

Of the quarter million articles scanned each year, only 5% are selected for detailed analysis within the YEAR BOOK series, thereby assuring readers of the high value of every selection.

The Abstract

The publisher's abstracting staff is headed by a seasoned medical professional and includes individuals with training in the life sciences, medicine, and other areas, plus extensive experience in writing for the health professions and related industries. Each selected article is assigned to a specific writer on this abstracting staff. The abstracter, guided in many cases by notations supplied by the expert editor, writes a structured, condensed summary designed so that the reader can rapidly acquire the essential information contained in the article.

The Commentary

The YEAR BOOK editorial boards, sometimes assisted by guest commentators, write comments that place each article in perspective for the reader. This provides the reader with the equivalent of a personal consultation with a leading international authority—an opportunity to better understand the value of the article and to benefit from the authority's thought processes in assessing the article.

Additional Editorial Features

The editorial boards of each YEAR BOOK organize the abstracts and comments to provide a logical and satisfying sequence of information. To enhance the organization, editors also provide introductions to sections or individual chapters, comments linking a number of abstracts, citations to additional literature, and other features.

The published YEAR BOOK contains enhanced bibliographic citations for each selected article, including extended listings of multiple authors and identification of author affiliations. Each YEAR BOOK contains a Table of Contents specific to that year's volume. From year to year, the Table of Contents for a given YEAR BOOK will vary depending on developments within the field.

Every YEAR BOOK contains a list of the journals from which papers have been selected. This list represents a subset of the approximately 500 journals surveyed by the publisher and occasionally reflects a particularly pertinent article from a journal that is not surveyed on a routine basis.

Finally, each volume contains a comprehensive subject index and an index to authors of each selected paper.

The 1999 Year Book Series

Year Book of Allergy, Asthma, and Clinical Immunology: Drs. Rosenwasser, Boguniewicz, Borish, Nelson, Routes, and Spahn

Year Book of Anesthesiology and Pain Management®: Drs. Tinker, Abram, Chestnut, Roizen, Rothenberg, and Wood

Year Book of Cardiology®: Drs. Schlant, Collins, Gersh, Graham, Kaplan, and Waldo

Year Book of Chiropractic®: Dr. Lawrence

Year Book of Critical Care Medicine®: Drs. Parrillo, Balk, Calvin, Franklin, and Shapiro

Year Book of Dentistry®: Drs. Meskin, Berry, Jeffcoat, Leinfelder, Roser, Summitt, and Zakariasen

Year Book of Dermatology and Dermatologic Surgery™: Dr. Thiers and Lang

Year Book of Diagnostic Radiology®: Drs. Osborn, Dalinka, Groskin, Maynard, Pentecost, Ros, Smirniotopolous, and Young

Year Book of Emergency Medicine®: Drs. Wagner, Dronen, Davidson, King, Niemann, and Hamilton

Year Book of Endocrinology®: Drs. Bagdade, Braverman, Horton, Kannan, Landsberg, Molitch, Morley, Odell, Poehlman, Rogol, and Fitzpatrick

Year Book of Family Practice®: Drs. Berg, Bowman, Davidson, Dexter, and Scherger

Year Book of Gastroenterology®: Drs. Aliperti and Fleshman

Year Book of Hand Surgery®: Drs. Amadio and Hentz

Year Book of Medicine®: Drs. Klahr, Frishman, Malawista, Mandell, Jett, Young, Barkin, and Bagdade

Year Book of Neonatal and Perinatal Medicine®: Drs. Fanaroff, Maisels, and Stevenson

Year Book of Nephrology, Hypertension, and Mineral Metabolism: Drs. Schwab, Bennett, Emmett, Hostetter, and Moe

Year Book of Neurology and Neurosurgery®: Drs. Bradley and Gibbs

Year Book of Nuclear Medicine®: Drs. Gottschalk, Blaufox, Neumann, Strauss, and Zubal

Year Book of Obstetrics, Gynecology, and Women's Health: Drs. Mishell, Herbst, and Kirschbaum

Year Book of Oncology®: Drs. Ozols, Eisenberg, Glatstein, Loehrer, and Urba

Year Book of Ophthalmology®: Drs. Wilson, Augsburger, Cohen, Eagle, Grossman, Laibson, Maguire, Nelson, Penne, Rapuano, Sergott, Spaeth, Tipperman, Ms. Gosfield, and Ms. Salmon

Year Book of Orthopedics®: Drs. Morrey, Beauchamp, Currier, Tolo, Trigg, and Swiontkowski

Year Book of Otolaryngology–Head and Neck Surgery®: Drs. Paparella, Holt, and Otto

Year Book of Pathology and Laboratory Medicine®: Drs. Raab, Cohen, Dabbs, Olson, and Stanley

Year Book of Pediatrics®: Dr. Stockman

Year Book of Plastic, Reconstructive, and Aesthetic Surgery®: Drs. Miller, Bartlett, Garner, McKinney, Ruberg, Salisbury, and Smith

Year Book of Psychiatry and Applied Mental Health®: Drs. Talbott, Ballenger, Frances, Lydiard, Meltzer, Jensen, and Tasman

Year Book of Pulmonary Disease®: Drs. Jett, Castro, Maurer, Peters, Phillips, and Ryu

Year Book of Rheumatology, Arthritis, and Musculoskeletal Disease™: Drs. Panush, Hadler, Hellman, LeRoy, Pisetsky, and Simon

Year Book of Sports Medicine®: Drs. Shephard, Drinkwater, Eichner, Torg, Alexander, and Mr. George

Year Book of Surgery®: Drs. Copeland, Bland, Deitch, Eberlein, Howard, Luce, Seeger, Souba, and Sugarbaker

Year Book of Urology®: Drs. Andriole and Coplen

Year Book of Vascular Surgery®: Dr. Porter

1999 The Year Book of OBSTETRICS, GYNECOLOGY, AND WOMEN'S HEALTH

Editors

Daniel R. Mishell, Jr., M.D.

The Lyle G. McNeile Professor and Chairman, Department of Obstetrics and Gynecology, University of Southern California School of Medicine, Los Angeles, California

Arthur L. Herbst, M.D.

Joseph Bolivar De Lee Distinguished Service Professor and Chairman, Department of Obstetrics and Gynecology, University of Chicago Pritzer School of Medicine, Chicago, Illinois

Thomas H. Kirschbaum, M.D.

Professor of Obstetrics and Gynecology, University of Alabama at Birmingham, Alabama

Contributing Editors

Arieh Bergman, M.D.

Clinical Professor, Department of Obstetrics and Gynecology, University of Southern California School of Medicine, Los Angeles, California

William H. Hindle, M.D.

Director, Breast Diagnostic Center, Women's and Children's Hospital; Professor of Clinical Obstetrics and Gynecology, University of Southern California, Los Angeles, California

Mosby

St. Louis Baltimore Boston Carlsbad Naples New York Philadelphia Portland London Madrid Mexico City Singapore Sydney Tokyo Toronto Wiesbaden

Mosby

Dedicated to Publishing Excellence

Publisher: Cheryl A. Smart
Acquisitions Editor: Susan Patterson
Developmental Editors: Tania Banak, Colleen Cook
Manager, Periodicals Editing: Kirk Swearingen
Production Editor: Amanda Maguire
Project Supervisor, Production: Joy Moore
Project Assistant, Production: Karie House
Manager, Literature Services: Idelle Winer
Illustrations and Permissions Coordinator: Chidi C. Ukabam

1999 EDITION

Printed in the United States of America
Composition by Reed Technology and Information Services, Inc.
Printing/binding by Maple-Vail

Mosby, Inc.
11830 Westline Industrial Drive
St. Louis, MO 63146

International Standard Serial Number: 1090-798X
International Standard Book Number: 0-8151-9705-5

Table of Contents

Journals Represented

Mosby and its editors survey approximately 500 journals for its abstract and commentary publications. From these journals, the editors select the articles to be abstracted. Journals represented in this YEAR BOOK are listed below.

Acta Cytologica
Acta Obstetricia et Gynecologica Scandinavica
American Journal of Epidemiology
American Journal of Human Genetics
American Journal of Industrial Medicine
American Journal of Kidney Diseases
American Journal of Medicine
American Journal of Obstetrics and Gynecology
American Journal of Pathology
American Journal of Perinatology
American Journal of Physiology
American Journal of Public Health
American Journal of Reproductive Immunology
American Journal of Surgical Pathology
American Society of Anesthesiologists Newsletter
Anesthesiology
Annals of Internal Medicine
Archives of Disease in Childhood
Archives of Internal Medicine
Archives of Surgery
Breast Journal
British Journal of Cancer
British Journal of Obstetrics and Gynaecology
British Journal of Urology
British Medical Journal
CA: A Cancer Journal for Clinicians
Cancer
Cephalalgia
Circulation
Clinical Chemistry
Clinical Infectious Diseases
Clinical Nephrology
Contraception
Diabetes Care
Endocrinology
European Journal of Obstetrics, Gynecology and Reproductive Biology
Family Planning Perspectives
Fertility and Sterility
Gynecologic Oncology
Human Pathology
Human Reproduction
International Journal of Cancer
International Journal of Gynaecology and Obstetrics
International Journal of Gynecological Cancer
International Journal of Gynecological Pathology
International Journal of Radiation, Oncology, Biology, and Physics
International Journal of Sports Medicine

International Urogynecology Journal
Journal of Clinical Endocrinology and Metabolism
Journal of Clinical Oncology
Journal of Clinical Psychopharmacology
Journal of Hypertension
Journal of Infectious Diseases
Journal of Maternal-Fetal Investigation
Journal of Medical Genetics
Journal of Pediatric Surgery
Journal of Pediatrics
Journal of Reproductive Medicine
Journal of Urology
Journal of the American Medical Association
Journal of the National Cancer Institute
Journal of the North American Menopause Society
Journal of the Royal College of Surgeons of Edinburgh
Lancet
Maturitas
Nature Medicine
New England Journal of Medicine
Obstetrics and Gynecology
Pediatric Infectious Disease Journal
Pediatric Neurology
Pediatric Pathology & Laboratory Medicine
Pediatric Research
Pediatrics
Pharmacotherapy
Prenatal Diagnosis
Proceedings of the National Academy of Sciences
Public Health Reports
Radiology
Radiotherapy and Oncology
Science
Southern Medical Journal
The Breast
Thrombosis and Haemostatis
Ultrasound in Obstetrics and Gynecology
Urology
Western Journal of Medicine

Standard Abbreviations

The following terms are abbreviated in this edition: acquired immunodeficiency syndrome (AIDS), cardiopulmonary resuscitation (CPR), central nervous system (CNS), cerebrospinal fluid (CSF), computed tomography (CT), deoxyribonucleic acid (DNA), electrocardiography (ECG), health maintenance organization (HMO), human immunodeficiency virus (HIV), intensive care unit (ICU), intramuscular (IM), intravenous (IV), magnetic resonance (MR) imaging (MRI), and ribonucleic acid (RNA).

NOTE

The YEAR BOOK OF OBSTETRICS, GYNECOLOGY, AND WOMEN'S HEALTH is a literature survey service providing abstracts of articles published in the professional literature. Every effort is made to assure the accuracy of the information presented in these pages. Neither the editors nor the publisher of the YEAR BOOK OF OBSTETRICS, GYNECOLOGY, AND WOMEN'S HEALTH can be responsible for errors in the original materials. The editors' comments are their own opinions. Mention of specific products within this publication does not constitute endorsement.

To facilitate the use of the YEAR BOOK OF OBSTETRICS, GYNECOLOGY, AND WOMEN'S HEALTH as a reference tool, all illustrations and tables included in this publication are now identified as they appear in the original article. This change is meant to help the reader recognize that any illustration or table appearing in the YEAR BOOK OF OBSTETRICS, GYNECOLOGY, AND WOMEN'S HEALTH may be only one of many in the original article. For this reason, figure and table numbers will often appear to be out of sequence within the YEAR BOOK OF OBSTETRICS, GYNECOLOGY, AND WOMEN'S HEALTH.

Introduction

The YEAR BOOK OF OBSTETRICS, GYNECOLOGY, AND WOMEN'S HEALTH contains abstracts of the last year's most relevant scientific articles in the area of women's health, followed by editorial comments discussing the articles' relevance to the reader. Topics covered include care of the pregnant, parturient and postpartum woman and abnormalities of the female genital tract. Other areas covered include breast disease, disorders of the urinary tract, and surveillance and treatment of the post-menopausal woman.

Throughout the year, the editors of the YEAR BOOK OF OBSTETRICS, GYNECOLOGY, AND WOMEN'S HEALTH periodically review articles published in women's health journals, as well as relevant articles appearing in other medical journals. The editors select those articles that provide the most pertinent clinical information for clinicians, and write comments discussing the relevance of the findings for the reader. Once abstracts are written, they are sent to the editor who selected the article for placement in the YEAR BOOK for final review.

By reading the YEAR BOOK, Clinicians with limited time will gain knowledge of the most important articles on women's health published in the previous year.

As in the past years, Dr. Tom Kirschbaum reviewed the field of maternal fetal medicine for articles in this volume. Dr. Arthur Herbst reviewed and selected articles on gynecologic oncology and pelvic surgery, and I have reviewed and selected articles in the areas of reproductive endocrinology, infertility, menopause, contraception, and gynecologic infection. Drs. William Hindle and Arieh Bergman are contributing editors in the areas of breast disease and gynecologic urology, respectively.

During the past year, after receiving numerous scientific journals the authors selected 320 articles from 84 journals for publication in this volume of the YEAR BOOK.

The editors believe that reading this volume will enhance each clinicians' knowledge of their specialty. We welcome suggestions to assist our efforts in providing clinically relevant information to our readers.

Daniel R. Mishell, Jr., M.D.

OBSTETRICS

1 Maternal and Fetal Physiology

Local Paracrine Effects of Estradiol Are Central to Parturition in the Rhesus Monkey

Nathanielsz PW, Jenkins SL, Tame JD, et al (Cornell Univ, Ithaca, NY; NYU Med Ctr, New York)

Nature Med 4:456–459, 1998 1–1

Background.—The basic biochemical mechanisms in primate parturition have not been determined. Studies of humans and of the baboon and

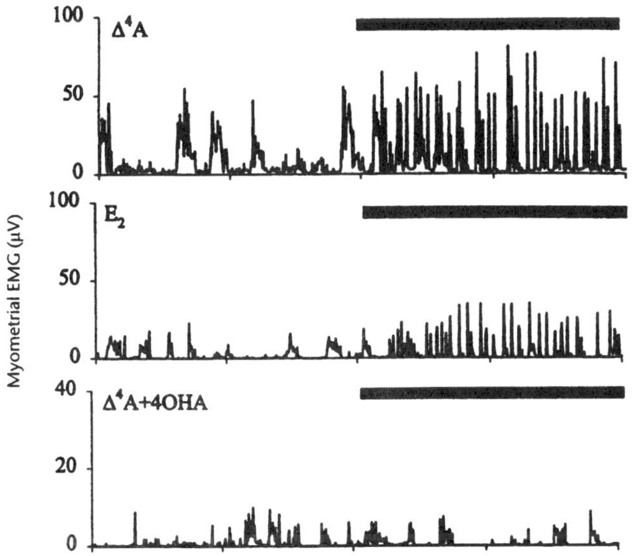

FIGURE 1.—Myometrial electromyogram records on the second night of infusion in 3 monkeys during androstenedione infusion (Δ^4A), estradiol infusion (E2), and simultaneous infusion of androstenedione and the aromatase inhibitor 4-hydroxyandrostenedione (Δ^4A + 4OHA). The *bold horizontal lines* indicate lights off in the animal's environment at 0. (Courtesy of Nathanielsz PW, Jenkins SL, Tame JD, et al: Local paracrine effects of estradiol are central to parturition in the rhesus monkey. *Nature Med* 4:456–459, 1998.)

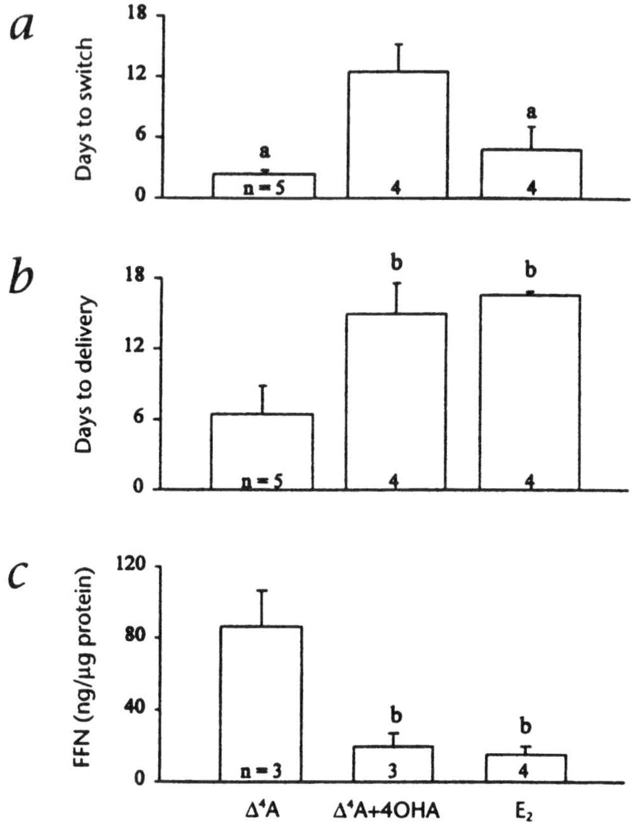

FIGURE 2.—Effect of infusion of androstenedione alone (Δ^4A) or concomitantly with the aromatase inhibitor 4-hydroxyandrostenedione (Δ^4A + 4OHA) or estrogen (E2) alone on **A**, time to the first switch from contractures to contractions; **B**, time to delivery; and **C**, amnion fetal fibronectin (*FFN*) in tissue removed at cesarean section. Mean ± SEM. **a** indicate $P < 0.05$ compared to Δ^4A + 4OHA; **b** indicate $P < 0.05$ compared to Δ^4A. (Courtesy of Nathanielsz PW, Jenkins SL, Tame JD, et al: Local paracrine effects of estradiol are central to parturition in the rhesus monkey. *Nature Med* 4:456–459, 1998.)

rhesus monkey show that there are multiple factors involved in the many interactive positive feedforward loops that promote parturition, including a change in maternal endocrinology; a nocturnal switch in myometrial activity from low-amplitude, infrequent contractures to high-amplitude, high-frequency contractions (Fig 1); cervix dilation; and biochemical changes in the fetal membrane causing rupture.

Methods.—Pregnant rhesus monkeys were used in treatment and control groups. Blood specimens were obtained from 1 to 6 hours after darkness onset. Estradiol, oxytocin, and progesterone were measured by radioimmunoassay. Amniotic fetal fibronectin was measured, and uterine electromyography (EMG) was analyzed.

Findings.—Infusion of 4-hydroxyandrostenedione (4OHA), an aromatase inhibitor, inhibited conversion of androgen to estrogen and prevented premature delivery after androgen was administered to rhesus monkeys at 0.8 of pregnancy term. Also, 4OHA inhibited androstenedione-induced biochemical changes in maternal endocrine and fetal membrane, and also inhibited changes in myometrial activity patterns. After peripheral estrogen infusion, myometrial activity increased, but preterm delivery and changes in the fetal membrane did not occur (Fig 2).

Discussion.—These findings indicate that paracrine functions of estrogen at its production site have a major role in the delivery of nonhuman primates. Although administration of exogenous estrogen caused a switch in myometrial activity patterns, perhaps partly mediated by its systemic effects on the maternal pituitary, the administration of estrogen did not reproduce an increase in fetal membrane fibronectin or hasten live delivery.

► In domesticated ruminants, fetal cortisol produced in late pregnancy induces changes in sex steroid enzymatic activities, which enhance placental estrogen production and diminish its progesterone production. These changes lead ultimately to increments in prostaglandin production that stimulate the onset of labor. In the human and other primates, the placenta lacks the capacity to regulate both progesterone and estrogen production rates by itself. Placental progesterone production relies principally on the transfer of maternal cholesterol to placental sites where the hormone is synthesized from pregnenolone, while estrogen metabolism requires use of maternal and fetal androgens (dehydroepiandrosterone sulfate) for aromatization of ring 1 of the androgen. Progesterone and estrogen metabolism are not linked in human reproduction, and maternal plasma progesterone remains unchanged in late labor while fetal androgen concentrations, the substrate for estrogen production, increase. A significant increase in plasma estradiol in maternal blood appears in late pregnancy in humans and other primates. Although increasing estradiol concentrations appear necessary for the onset of normal human labor, infusion of estradiol does not induce labor nor do estrogen antagonists inhibit it.

In a very important observation, this group demonstrates the capacity to induce preterm labor and delivery in rhesus monkeys by infusing an androgen (androstenedione) that is converted by the placenta into estrogen.[1] This demonstrates an effect of estrogen production in situ in the placenta and uterus in a paracrine mechanism which is separate and distinct from the requisite estradiol in circulating blood that functions in an endocrine fashion. Here the goal is to analyze the relative significance of endocrine and paracrine estradiol production by observing the conversion of low-frequency, low-intensity uterine contractions to conventional uterine contractions, which mark the onset of labor. The techniques used are to block placental aromatization in order to isolate the paracrine mechanism and to add estradiol to androstenedione to evaluate the endocrine role of estradiol. Although exogenous estradiol has the effect of producing uterine contractions, it does not result in labor and delivery, nor does amniotic fluid fibronectin, a biochemical indicator of labor, increase. The paracrine role for estrogen production in situ in placenta and uterus suffices to produce labor, while the systemic estrogenic effect is necessary but not sufficient for labor. In the human, fetal adrenal androgen generated by the fetal zone of the gland appears to play a role analogous to fetal cortisol, assisted by maternal androgen production, in the initiation of normal labor in primates.

T.H. Kirschbaum, M.D.

Reference

1. Mecenas CA, Cyssani J, and Oweno I, et al: The production of premature delivery in pregnant rhesus monkeys by androstenedione infusion. *Nature Med* 2:443, 1996.

Maternal Serum Dehydroepiandrosterone Sulfate Levels and Successful Labor Induction

Maciulla J, Goolsby L, Racowsky C, et al (Univ of Arizona, Tucson)
Obstet Gynecol 91:771–773, 1998 1–2

Background.—Dehydroepiandrosterone (DHEA) sulfate may be involved in cervical connective tissue function. Although it has been reported that DHEA sulfate can induce cervical ripening and labor, the effect of endogenous maternal serum DHEA sulfate levels on the outcome of labor induction has not been determined. It has been found that among young nulliparas in labor at term, these levels are significantly lower in those who need oxytocin induction of labor than in those who progress spontaneously. It was hypothesized that levels of endogenous maternal serum DHEA sulfate would affect the outcome of labor induction. It was also hypothesized that women with higher levels would have a higher rate of successful outcome of labor induction.

Methods.—Blood specimens were obtained from 155 women with singleton pregnancies at the beginning of labor induction. Serum DHEA sulfate was measured by radioimmunoassay and correlated to the outcome of labor induction. Successful induction was defined as progression to active labor. Analysis was performed using the Welch approximate *t* test, Mann-Whitney test, Fisher exact test, simple regression, and multiple regression.

Results.—In the 147 women who progressed to active labor, mean DHEA sulfate levels were higher than in women with unsuccessful induction attempts. The odds ratio of unsuccessful induction in women with DHEA sulfate levels less than 70 µg/dL was 4.46, compared with women with levels greater than 70 µg/dL. As DHEA sulfate levels decreased, the odds ratio increased.

Discussion.—These results suggest that DHEA sulfate may have a key role in the outcome of labor induction. The mechanism of the action of DHEA sulfate is unclear, although there is evidence of collagenase activation and remodeling of uterine connective tissue.

► The reader would benefit by reviewing Abstract 1–1, which describes the increasing evidence for serum androgens of both maternal and fetal origins and their paracrine conversion to estrogen at the site of the placenta in the onset of primate labor. What this study shows is that increased circulating DHEA concentrations represent a means of determining that a woman has started on the path of serum androgen increment which will eventuate in spontaneous labor with time. The closer a gravida is to spontaneous labor, the easier it is to induce her labor. This is a nice clinical confirmation of the hypothesis of Nathanielsz et al. delineated in Abstract 1–1.

T.H. Kirschbaum, M.D.

Direct Evidence to Support the Role of HLA-G in Protecting the Fetus From Maternal Uterine Natural Killer Cytolysis

Rouas-Freiss N, Gonçalves RM-B, Menier C, et al (Hôpital Saint Louis, Paris; Found Jean Dausset, Paris)

Proc Natl Acad Sci U S A 94:11520–11525, 1997 1–3

Background.—Human lymphocyte antigen (HLA)-G, a nonclassical major histocompatibility complex class I molecule, is selectively expressed on cytotrophoblasts at the fetomaternal interface. It may have an important role in maternal tolerance of the fetus. The role of HLA-G molecules expressed on the trophoblast cell surface in protecting the fetus from the lytic activity of maternal uterine natural killer (NK) cells in several combinations was demonstrated ex vivo.

Methods and Findings.—Freshly obtained first-trimester fetal and maternal tissues were used. Six semiallogeneic and 20 allogeneic combinations were tested. In all cases, the HLA-G-mediated protection was abolished by the treatment of cytotrophoblasts with an HLA-G-specific mAb. Similar protection and abolition occurs in the HLA class I-negative K562 cell line transfected with the predominant HLA-GI isoform.

Conclusions.—Extending the findings of previous research, the current study provides evidence for the role of HLA-G in maternofetal tolerance. The expression of HLA-G on cytotrophoblast target cells inhibits the lytic activities of NK cells in both maternal uterine blood and allogeneic peripheral blood. This observation supports the hypothesis that HLA-G is the public ligand for killer inhibitory receptor present in all individuals and expressed on most if not all NK cells.

► Part of the explanation for the maternal tolerance of the fetal allograft during pregnancy was proposed to stem from the production during pregnancy of a unique product of the major histocompatibility complex on chromosome 6—HLA-G.[1] This class of molecule, thought at first to have the same structure in all individuals (monomorphy) was purported to conceal other trophoblastic surface antigens of the HLAA, B and C classes that possess epitopes capable of generating activated T lymphocytes and antibody production from B lymphocytes which would have the effect of destroying fetal cells by virtue of their recognition as foreign to the host. Later, it became clear that there were 5 distinguishable forms of HLA molecules (isoforms) and this raised questions about the ability of this unique class of molecule to provide immune tolerance to fetal tissues in normal pregnancy[2] and in some pregnancy abnormalities.[3]

This study employs in vitro combinations of first trimester placental trophoblast cells and NK cells obtained in 6 cases from uterine blood of the pregnant women undergoing abortion and in 20 cases from other pregnant women. Natural killer cells are derived from large granular lymphocytes, are neither T nor B cells, and are part of the system of natural immunity not dependent on prior exposure to specific antigens. They have the capacity to recognize cell surface structure and destroy targeted cells by lysis. These were obtained from maternal blood by physical methods and HLA-G1 and G2 obtained by cell sorting using fluorescent-labeled antibodies (CD 158 a and b, CD 94). Uniformly, both HLA-G isoforms, when added to trophoblast cells, protected them from lysis by NK cells subsequently added to the cell culture. This is direct confirmation of the role of HLA-G in conferring immune tolerance of the host to allograft trophoblast and suggests that at least the HLA-G 2 isoform is just as effective as the more prevalent HLA-G1 molecule in this undertaking.

T.H. Kirschbaum, M.D.

References

1. 1995 Year Book of Obstetrics and Gynecology, pp 215–216.
2. 1996 Year Book of Obstetrics and Gynecology, pp 10–12.
3. 1997 Year Book of Obstetrics, Gynecology, and Women's Health, pp 45–46.

Regulation of Human Placental Development by Oxygen Tension

Genbacev O, Zhou Y, Ludlow JW, et al (Univ of California, San Francisco; Univ of Rochester, NY)

Science 277:1669–1672, 1997 1–4

Objective.—Differentiation of epithelial stem cells, known as cytotrophoblasts, plays an important role in the unique anatomy of the human placenta. These cells proliferate during early pregnancy, after which they differentiate into tumor-like cells. These cells establish placental blood flow through invasion of the uterus and its vasculature. For unknown reasons, the cells invade only the superficial portions of uterine venules. The effects of oxygen tension on placental development were studied.

Methods and Results.—Cytotrophoblasts were cultured in 2% oxygen, reflecting the hypoxic environment near the uterine surface before 10 weeks' gestation. Under these conditions, the cells showed continued proliferation but poor differentiation. Another group of cytotrophoblasts were cultured in 20% oxygen, chosen to resemble conditions near the uterine arterioles. Under this oxygen tension, the cells stopped proliferating and started differentiating normally.

Conclusions.—Oxygen tension has important effects on the proliferative capacity of human cytotrophoblasts. Cell differentiation occurs under conditions of relatively high oxygen tension, which may explain why the tumor-like placental cells invade only the venous side of the uterine circulation. The capacity to differentiate may be inhibited if they cannot find an adequate supply of maternal arterial blood. This could play a role in preeclampsia and other conditions of pregnancy associated with shallow cytotrophoblast invasion and inadequate differentiation.

► During the first trimester, trophoblastic epithelium appears to have the option of either differentiation of the cytotrophoblast into syncytium, which is optimal for covering placental villi surfaces and facilitating nutrient transfer, or remaining as undifferentiated cytotrophoblast. The latter retains its ability to invade maternal decidua and myometrium, protected from maternal immune rejection by HLA-G expression and pregnancy-inhibited cellular immunity. In its undifferentiated form, the cytotrophoblast serves to anchor segments of cotyledons to the decidual surface. Cytotrophoblast cells also have the capacity to enter maternal vascular lumina by acquiring the ability to express cell adhesion molecules as though they were endothelial cells.[1]

The authors propose a hypothesis that ambient endometrial Po_2, roughly 40 mm Hg before 8–10 weeks' gestational age, increases into the range of 90 to 100 mm Hg by virtue of the maternal arterial dilatation that occurs with cytotrophoblast invasion. Further, they propose that the higher oxygen activity facilitates differentiation of trophoblast into syncytium and the development of an effective placental transfer surface in contact with maternal blood. The supporting evidence is based on tissue culture of villi with attached cytotrophoblast columns and the ability of cytotrophoblast to incorporate thymidine and thymidine-related compounds at low but not high Po_2, and the failure of syncytial nuclei to show this evidence of cell growth with any level of oxygen availability. This concept has importance for the proposition that preeclampsia stems from insufficient cytotrophoblast invasion in the maternal vasculature to allow the increase in tissue Po_2 associated with that vascular ingrowth, thereby preventing differentiation of an optimal syncytial villous surface and impeding placental transfer. The fact that cytotrophoblast invades maternal arterioles more extensively than venules fits the hypothesis nicely, because venular dilatation plays no essential role in the regulation of Po_2 on the maternal exchange surface.

T.H. Kirschbaum, M.D.

Reference

1. 1998 Year Book of Obstetrics, Gynecology, and Women's Health, p 104.

Human Cytotrophoblast Differentiation/Invasion Is Abnormal in Preeclampsia

Lim K-H, Zhou Y, Janatpour M, et al (Univ of California, San Francisco)

Am J Pathol 151:1809–1818, 1997 1–5

Background.—During normal placental development in humans, cytotrophoblast stem cells differentiate, break through the syncytium, and form multilayered columns of cells that invade the uterus. At the same time, these cells modulate the expression of stage-specific antigens that mark transitions in the differentiation process and are involved in uterine invasion (integrin cell extracellular matrix receptors and matrix metalloproteinase-9) or immune interactions (human lymphocyte antigen-G). Preeclampsia is a disease occurring in pregnancy and is associated with shallow cytotrophoblast uterine invasion. Immunofluorescence localization on placental tissue has shown that in preeclampsia, invasive cytotrophoblasts do not modulate integrin properly, which indicates there may be abnormalities in the differentiation process leading to uterine invasion.

Methods.—A culture system that supports the differentiation process leading to uterine invasion was used to compare the potential for differentiation and invasion of cytotrophoblasts obtained from placentas. There were 9 women with preeclampsia at 24–38 weeks' gestation, and 8 control subjects at 22–38 weeks' gestation.

Results.—Cells from the placentas of women with preeclampsia did not properly modulate $\alpha 1$ integrin or expression of matrix metalloproteinase-9 at the protein and mRNA levels. The invasive potential of the cells was significantly decreased. The cells did not upregulate HLA-G protein or mRNA expression.

Discussion.—These findings indicate that defective cytotrophoblast differentiation and invasion can significantly affect the outcome of pregnancy. These results also suggest that by the time delivery becomes necessary, removal of the cells from the mother does not reverse the defect.

► The authors are responsible for generating 1 of 2 currently promising approaches to a study of the vascular pathology of preeclampsia. Their work concerns the role of integrins—protein receptors for extracellular matrix proteins such as laminen, collagen, and fibronectin that bind connective tissue matrix to the cytoskeleton of cells. These receptor bindings largely determine cell motility, shape, and movement, but also determine cell differentiation and function. Three classes of the integrin family include fibroblast fibronectin receptors, platelet receptors, which bind to fibronectin and fibrinogen, and leukocyte integrins, which help determine lymphocyte and macrophage functions. Integrins are heterodimers that have a common β-segment but differing α-peptide sequences.[1]

At issue in this study is the failure of expression of trophoblast integrins that normally enable trophoblast cells to attach to decidual cells and anchor the placenta in the intervillous space ($\alpha 5\ \beta 1$ integrins) and penetrate and connect with maternal myometrial connective tissue and endovascular cells (α 1 β1 integrins, matrix metalloproteinase -9), which in turn, enable intimate maternal placental vascular interrelationships. Endovascular trophoblastic invasion of maternal arterioles renders the arterioles grossly dilated with reduced resistance to maternal blood flow entering the intervillous space, a vital protective vascular feature.[2] The techniques involve cytotrophoblast mesh culture, studies of cell invasiveness into polycarbonate coated with Matrigel, immunohistochemistry, and RNA analysis by Northern blot. Adding new data to previous work,[3] the authors demonstrate the failure of trophoblastic expression of integrins necessary to maximize uterovascular invasion. This observation is consonant with earlier observations that preeclampsia is characterized by shallow placental implantation. Simultaneously, the ability of the trophoblast to produce human lymphocyte antigen-G, a largely monomorphic type of cell recognition antigen that protects trophoblast against maternal cellular immune rejection reaction, is impaired. The important remaining question is whether these changes represent a primary defect in gene content by virtue of mutational events or errors in gene transcription, or whether the changes are secondary to another chain of events. The best guess is that the latter is true.

T.H. Kirschbaum, M.D.

References

1. 1992 Year Book of Obstetrics and Gynecology, pp 18–20.
2. 1994 Year Book of Obstetrics and Gynecology, pp 59–60.
3. 1998 Year Book of Obstetrics, Gynecology, and Women's Health, pp 18–21, 50–51.

Cervical Fetal Fibronectin Correlates to Prostaglandin E_2-induced Cervical Ripening and Can Be Identified in Cervical Tissue

Sennström MS, Granström LM, Lockwood CJ, et al (Karolinska Hosp, Stockholm; Karolinska Inst, Stockholm; Univ of Lund, Sweden; et al)

Am J Obstet Gynecol 178:540–545, 1998 1–6

Introduction.—Cervical ripening during normal pregnancy becomes apparent during the last weeks of pregnancy and occurs independently of uterine contractions. Although factors inducing and regulating this final ripening process are not fully known, a key factor appears to be release of prostaglandin E_2 (PGE_2) from the amnion and the choriodecidual tissue. A study of 28 women assessed the relationship between PGE_2-induced cervical ripening and changes in fetal fibronectin (FFN) levels and sought to determine whether FFN can be detected in amniotic and cervical tissue.

Methods.—Study participants were at term and had been scheduled for labor induction for a variety of medical reasons. All had vertex presentations, intact membranes, and unfavorable cervical states. FFN levels in cervical mucus were measured before and after intracervical application of PGE_2 gel. An enzyme immunoassay determined fetal fibronectin concentrations. Cervical biopsy specimens were obtained from 3 pregnant women, 3 women after parturition, and 2 nonpregnant women.

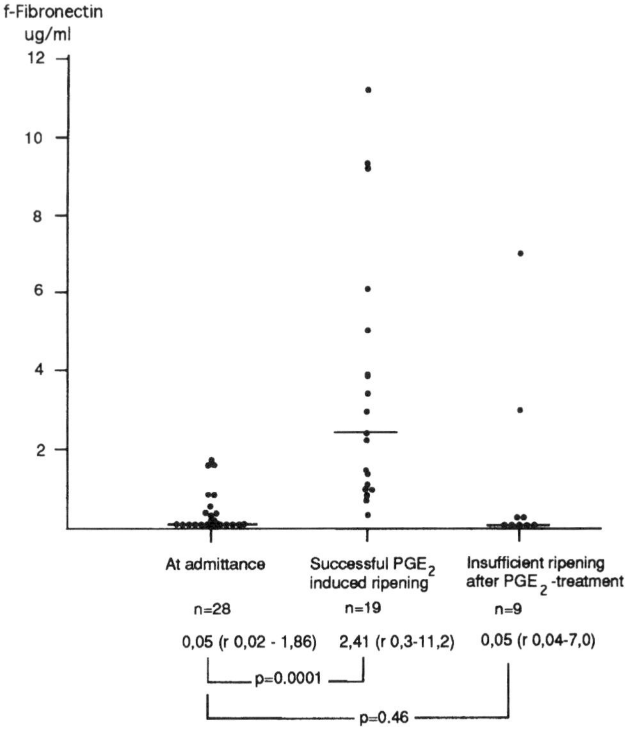

FIGURE 1.—Levels of fetal fibronectin in cervical samples in 28 term pregnant women with unripe cervices, before and after intracervical application of PGE_2, which resulted in successful cervical ripening in 19 women or insufficient ripening in 9 women, respectively. Level of fetal fibronectin expressed as micrograms per milliliter of sample buffer. Comparison of median values between groups. *Bars*, median values. *Abbreviation: PGE_2*, prostaglandin E_2. (Courtesy of Sennström MB, Granström LM, Lockwood CJ, et al: Cervical fetal fibronectin correlates to prostaglandin E_2-induced cervical ripening and can be identified in cervical tissue. *Am J Obstet Gynecol* 178:540–545, 1998.)

Results.—Levels of cervical FFN in women requiring induced labor was low in all cases (median 0.05 μg/mL buffer) before application of PGE_2. A successful cervical ripening was induced by PGE_2 in 19 women, and their cervical score increased from a median of 2.0 to a median of 6.0. Fetal fibronectin levels in these women increased significantly to a median of 2.41 μg/mL buffer. Women who did not achieve sufficient cervical ripening after PGE_2 treatment showed no significant increase in fetal fibronectin levels (Fig 1). Immunohistochemical analyses identified FFN in the epithelial cells of the cervix uteri.

Conclusion.—A significant increase in cervical fetal fibronectin levels was observed after cervical ripening was successfully induced by PGE_2 treatment. Immunohistochemical analysis can detect FFN in the pregnant human cervix.

▶ This study demonstrates that, in 28 primigravidas scheduled for labor induction with cervical PGE_2 at term, successful cervical ripening as judged by an increased Bishop score of at least 3 points was associated with increased activity of cervical FFN by enzyme immunoassay with the customary FDC-6 antiserum. Some overlap occurred, with 8 of 19 women who had successful cervical ripening showing FFN values in the same range as women who were not in labor and with 2 of 9 women with unsuccessful ripening exhibiting concentrations in the elevated range appropriate to those candidates in whom induction was successful. This is the same kind of overlap with normal that appears to have led to the 50% false-positive rate in predicting preterm labor in women at low risk from fetal fibronectin activity. A more important point, however, is a technologic advance in which these workers report successful immunohistochemical localization of FFN in cervical epithelium and amnion employing a flour-conjugated donkey anti-IgG combined with the FDC-6 FFN antibody. Histochemical confirmation of the rapid disappearance of FFN is also offered in the few cases. This advance opens the door to exploration of the role of FFN in connective tissue ground substance and its interaction with collagen, proteogylcans, and adhesion molecule receptors (integrins), which may play a role in cervical incompetence and premature cervix ripening associated with preterm labor and preterm premature rupture of membranes.

T.H. Kirschbaum, M.D.

Serum Leptin Concentrations During Pregnancy and Their Relationship to Fetal Growth

Tamura T, Goldenberg RL, Johnston KE, et al (Univ of Alabama, Birmingham)

Obstet Gynecol 91:389–395, 1998 1–7

Background.—Research has established that serum concentrations of leptin, the protein product of the obese gene, are significantly associated with percentage of body fat or body mass index (BMI). The current authors hypothesize that circulating maternal and fetal leptin concentration is an indicator of fetal growth.

Methods.—One hundred thirty-five pregnant women of low socioeconomic status who delivered infants at full term were studied. Sixty-six infants had fetal growth retardation (FGR), and 69 did not. These 2 groups were further divided into 3 subgroups based on BMI: less than 19.8%, 19.8% to 28.9%, and 29% or greater.

Findings.—Mean maternal serum leptin levels, adjusted for BMI, were highest between 22 and 27 weeks' gestation, declining thereafter until birth. Prepregnancy BMI was correlated significantly with leptin concentration. Leptin concentrations did not differ significantly between women with and without FGR infants. Maternal leptin concentrations did not correlate significantly with infant birth weight. The average cord serum leptin level was lower than maternal concentrations and was associated with birth weight (Figs 1 and 2).

Conclusion.—Maternal leptin concentration during pregnancy does not accurately predict fetal growth. Cord serum leptin levels were lower than

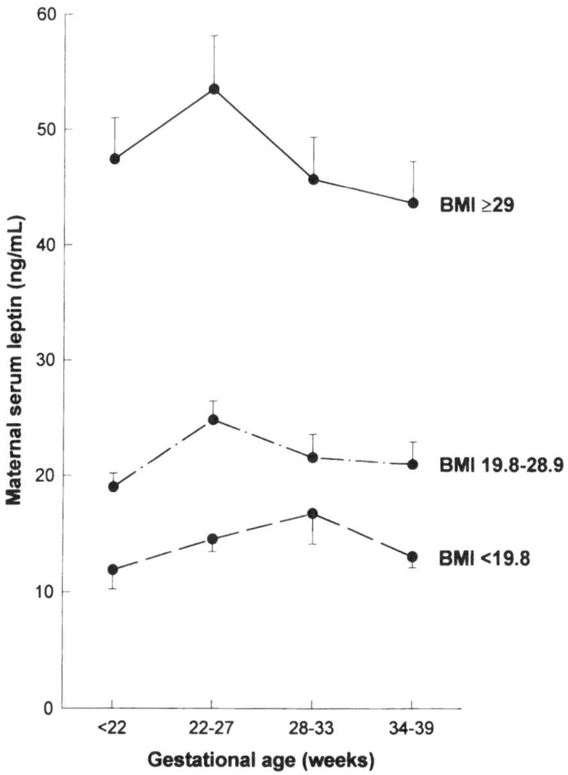

FIGURE 1.—Serum leptin concentrations during pregnancy in subjects in the 3 body mass index (*BMI*) groups. The concentrations were highest between 22 and 33 weeks' gestation and declined thereafter. The decline was significant with repeated-measures analysis of variance (*P* less than 0.001). *Error bars* indicate standard error of the mean. (Courtesy of Tamura T, Goldenberg RL, Johnston KE, et al: Serum leptin concentrations during pregnancy and their relationship to fetal growth. *Obstet Gynecol* 91:389–395, 1998. Reprinted with permission from the American College of Obstetricians and Gynecologists.)

maternal serum concentrations and were significantly associated with birth weight.

► With identification of a gene segregating with obesity in the mouse and evidence of a homologous human gene, hopes for a major impact on human obesity seem possible and are now being explored by several investigators. In the mouse, leptin concentrations correlate well with body weight, and the protein derived from lipid storage cells appears to decrease body weight by decreasing food intake and increasing energy expenditure. The effects in the human are less clear.

This article is part of the general picture of emerging knowledge of changes in leptin concentration during pregnancy. The study includes 135 gravidas providing at least 3 maternal blood samples during pregnancy. Sixty-six women who gave birth to full term infants with FGR were compared with 69 women delivered at term with infants appropriate for gesta-

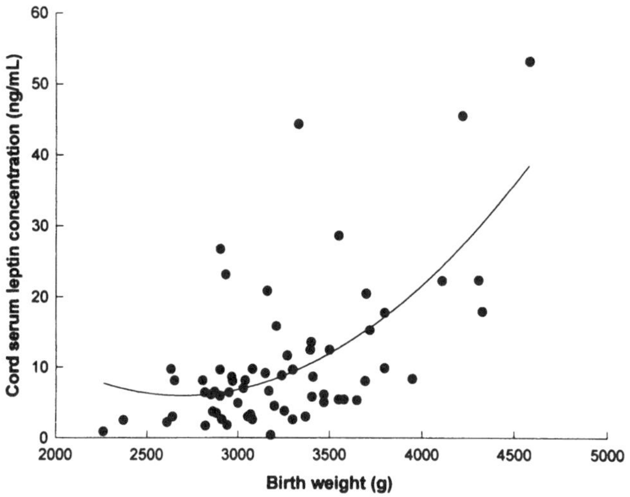

FIGURE 2.—Relationship between cord serum leptin concentrations and birth weight of 64 infants. The correlation coefficient was 0.61 (*P* less than 0.001). The equation of the regression line was as follows: serum leptin = 9.15×10^{-6}(birth weight)^2 − 0.049 × (birth weight) + 72.4. (Courtesy of Tamura T, Goldenberg RL, Johnston KE, et al: Serum leptin concentrations during pregnancy and their relationship to fetal growth. *Obstet Gynecol* 91:389–395, 1998. Reprinted with permission from the American College of Obstetricians and Gynecologists.)

tional age. Maternal serum leptin concentrations correlated well with prepregnancy BMI but with neither weight gain during pregnancy nor infant birth weight. Maternal leptin concentration cannot, therefore, be used to predict fetal weight.

Unlike other workers, these investigators were unable to find relationships between leptin concentration and smoking or alcohol consumption at 18 weeks, nor with race. Cord blood leptin concentration is correlated significantly with birth weight in a parabolic relationship. No evidence emerged of a relationship with glucose tolerance at 24–26 weeks nor with dietary intake estimated at 18 and 30 weeks' gestational age. Leptin appears to be an important determinant of birth weight, likely 1 of multiple interrelated factors. We will be hearing more about this in the future.

T.H. Kirschbaum, M.D.

Doppler Evidence of Intervillous Flow in the Embryonic Period

Simpson NAB, Nimrod CA, De Vermette R (Ottawa Gen Hosp, Canada)

J Matern Fetal Invest 8:11–16, 1998 1–8

Background.—The published evidence of intervillous flow in human and monkey embryos was reviewed and new data from Doppler imaging was provided to confirm that intervillous flow occurs early in the first trimester.

Development of the Intervillous Space.—Development of the intervillous space (IVS) is similar in humans and is the macaque and, thus, the

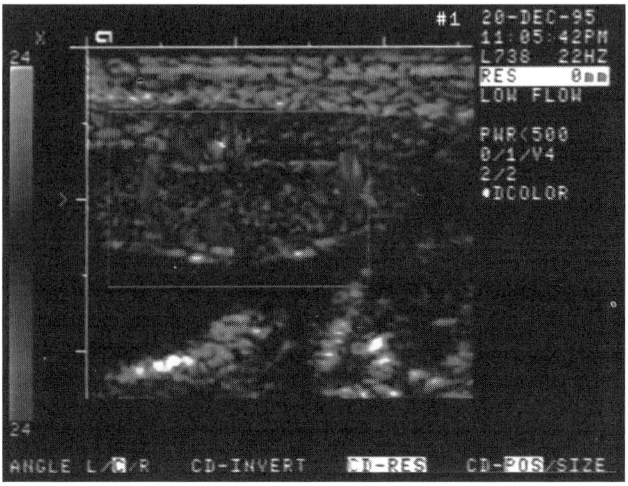

FIGURE 3.—Blood flow into 3 discrete intervillous spaces is identified using color Doppler imaging within the anterior placental disk in the monkey. (Courtesy of Simpson NAB, Nimrod CA, De Vermette R. Doppler evidence of intervillous flow in the embryonic period. *J Matern Fetal Invest* 8:11–16, 1998.)

macaque is often used to study intervillous flow. Both models provide evidence that as the trophoblastic covering of the blastocyst thickens, lacunae gradually coalesce to create the IVS. Extraembryonic mesenchyme migrates down the center of these new structures to create the primary villi; further branching of these villi creates secondary and tertiary villi.

By the third week after conception, there is a potential space around these villi. Soon after implantation, trophoblasts invade adjacent capillar-

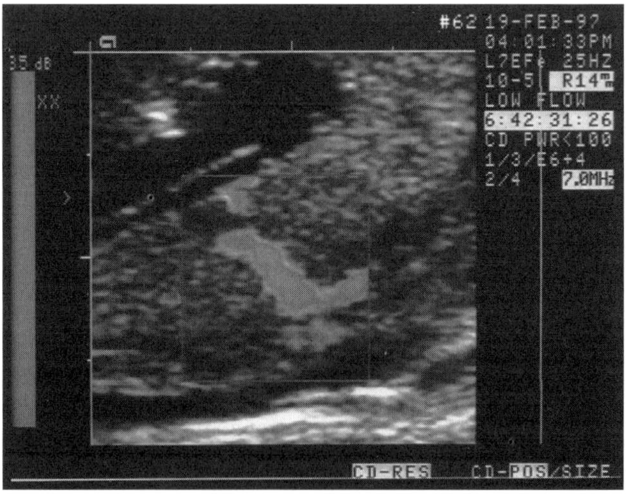

FIGURE 6.—Color amplitude obtained from the intervillous space. Note the spiral artery perfusing the intervillous space. (Courtesy of Simpson NAB, Nimrod CA, De Vermette R: Doppler evidence of intervillous flow in the embryonic period. *J Matern Fetal Invest* 8:11–16, 1998.)

ies and then decidual veins. By day 15 after conception, one can see connections between these vessels and the early IVS. Therefore, an effective runoff from the IVS is established before any direct arterial connection has developed (although some have challenged this interpretation). As pregnancy continues, the spiral arteries begin to open directly into the IVS through the intracotyledonary space (at the center of the cotyledon supplied by the spiral artery) (Fig 3). Pressure drives the blood through the villi until it arrives at the periphery of the cotyledon, at which time it exits into the venous system at the basal plate.

Intervillous Flow in the Embryonic Period.—At each gestational age, flow within the spiral arteries has low resistance and pulsatility compared with flow from the uterine arteries. There is no evidence to indicate that any arteriovenous anastomoses are present and, thus, there is no shunting of blood away from the pregnancy. As early as 8 weeks after conception in humans, flow-velocity waveforms reveal a nonpulsatile or venous type of flow that is generally unidirectional. And as early as 5 weeks after conception in humans, Doppler imaging reveals intervillous flow within the chorion. Doppler imaging in the macaque as early as 18 days after conception also reveals that intervillous flow is pulsatile (but weakly so), unidirectional, and not shunted away from the placenta. Studies in macaques show that flow within the IVS is discharged at the intracotyledonary space (Fig 6).

Conclusion.—Blood flow through the IVS is a normal and consistent finding during the early first trimester of pregnancy. It can be characterized by its unidirectional, weakly pulsatile flow, and it can be seen at the openings of the spiral arteries into the intracotyledonary space. Further application of Doppler technology—especially echo enhancement agents and color amplitude imaging—will, hopefully, shed more light on IVS flow in the embryologic period.

► In the years between 1950 and 1966, Dr. Elizabeth Ramsey, working in the Department of Embryology at the Carnegie Institution in Washington, D.C., was able to construct a model of maternal uteroplacental circulation using primate histologic and dye contrast fluoroscopic techniques as well as India ink vasodilator infusions in intact section hysterectomy specimens.[1] Designed in part to explore a contrary view that intervillous circulation does not begin in the human until the second trimester, this careful Doppler study of early human placentas refutes that contrary view and supports Dr. Ramsey's model, limited only by the limitation of Doppler shift ultrasound.

Maternal blood appears to flow with less impedance as it leaves spiral arterioles to enter the IVS than it had proximally. This is understandable because the IVS is lined not with endothelium but only with decidua and trophoblastic epithelium and lacks vasoregulation. Arterial blood is not shunted into uterine vein orifices within the IVS but passes through bodies of cotyledons, losing its pulsatile characteristics as it leaves arteriolar restructures and flowing without pulsation through uterine vein orifices. Blood flow begins as early as 5 to 8 weeks of gestational age, and arterial inflow proceeds through a limited number of discrete inflow sites before some mixing in the IVS. Dr. Ramsey would be proud of the extent to which these physical methods have confirmed her work, much of it completed 30 years ago.

T.H. Kirschbaum, M.D.

Reference

1. Harris JWS, Ramsey EM: The morphology of human utero-placental vasculature. *Contributions to Embryology*, No. 260. Carnegie Institution of Washington, 1966.

Renal and Amniotic Fluid Responses to Umbilicoplacental Embolization for 20 Days in Fetal Sheep

Cock ML, Harding R (Monash Univ, Melbourne, Australia)
Am J Physiol 273:R1094–R1102, 1997 1–9

Background.—Placental insufficiency in human pregnancy is often associated with intrauterine growth restriction and oligohydramnios. Because fetal urine production is the major contributor to amniotic fluid, oligohydramnios may result from alterations in urine production during fetal hypoxemia. Experiments in sheep, however, suggest that factors other than hypoxemia may lead to reduced urine production in chronically hypoxemic or growth-restricted fetuses. Fetal sheep were used in this study, which was designed to determine the effects of placental insufficiency induced by umbilicoplacental embolization on fetal renal function and amniotic fluid.

Methods.—Fetal vascular, bladder, and amniotic sac catheters were implanted in anesthetized pregnant ewes at a mean of 115 days after mating (term, 145 to 147 days). Five fetuses were studied for 1 day of normoxemia followed by 20 days (from 120 to 140 days' gestation) during umbilicoplacental embolization. Six animals served as controls. Fetal plasma, urine, and amniotic fluid samples were obtained periodically for analysis.

Results.—At post mortem (140 days), the mean body weight of embolized fetuses (3.45 kg) was significantly lower than that of control fetuses (4.32 kg). Mean brain weight was significantly greater in embolized fetuses after adjustment for body weight. Except for the ponderal index, other indices of growth were reduced in embolized fetuses. Umbilicoplacental embolization reduced the mean fetal arterial partial pressure of oxygen from 24.1 mm Hg pretreatment to 14.6 mm Hg. At 135 days of gestation, both urine production and the glomerular filtration rate were significantly lower in treated fetuses than in controls. The 2 groups did not differ, however, in amniotic fluid volume or (after adjustment for body weight) in fetal urine production. Amniotic fluid volume was unchanged over the study period in both control and embolized fetuses.

Conclusion.—Embolized, growth-restricted fetal sheep had reduced net urine production compared with control fetal sheep, but the 2 groups did not differ in urine production after adjustment for body weight. Findings indicate that fetal urine production is influenced by the reduced size of the kidneys rather than by placental insufficiency and fetal hypoxemia per se.

▶ This experimental study, done of necessity in experimental animals, attacks 2 hypotheses simultaneously: that fetal growth retardation or fetal hypoxemia, with or without reduced cardiac output, results in oligohydramnios. The experimental approach required repeated embolization of the umbilical circulation for 20 days beginning at 120 days' gestational age in pregnant sheep to the point where umbilical artery partial pressure of oxygen was at least 8 mm of mercury below control levels.

With delivery, mean fetal weight reduction to 80% of the control values was noted. Modest metabolic acidosis resulted, and there was a transient interval of fetal hypertension and increased urine production, together with more sodium and chloride excretion lasting no more than 10 days after the beginning of embolization. Urine production and fetal glomerular filtration rate measured with tritiated inulin infusion and bladder catheterization remained unchanged per unit fetal weight as did amniotic fluid volume and osmolality during the 20-day course of the experiments.

All findings can be explained by reduction in fetal kidney size as part of the general growth retardation noted in the fetuses. It is well to remember that fetal embolization of the placenta perturbs both the potential fetal production of amniotic fluid volume and the placental interface for maternal-fetal exchange of water, as well as nutrients and excretory products. However, this work makes it clear that assuming that growth retardation caused by impaired nutrient access or chronic fetal hypoxemia results in oligohydramnios is simplistic and probably incorrect.

T.H. Kirschbaum, M.D.

Apoptosis and Fas Expression in Human Fetal Membranes

Runić R, Lockwood CJ, LaChapelle L, et al (New York Univ)

J Clin Endocrinol Metab 83:660–666, 1998 1–10

Introduction.—Reproductive function in the ovary, mammary glands, prostate, uterus, and testis is partially governed by apoptosis, or programmed cell death. The cell surface receptor Fas (CD95) mediates apoptosis of target cells after binding of Fas ligand. Whether human fetal membrane cells undergo apoptosis and express Fas was determined using biochemical and morphological parameters.

Methods.—Studies were performed in amnion epithelial, chorionic trophoblast, and decidua parietalis cell layers of human fetal membranes. The terminal deoxynucleotidyl transferase deoxy-UTP-nick end labeling immunohistochemical technique was used to identify apoptotic nuclei. The apoptotic index was calculated as the percentage of terminal deoxynucleotidyl transferase deoxy-UTP-nick end labeling–positive nuclei. Electron microscopy was performed to look for ultrastructural characteristics of

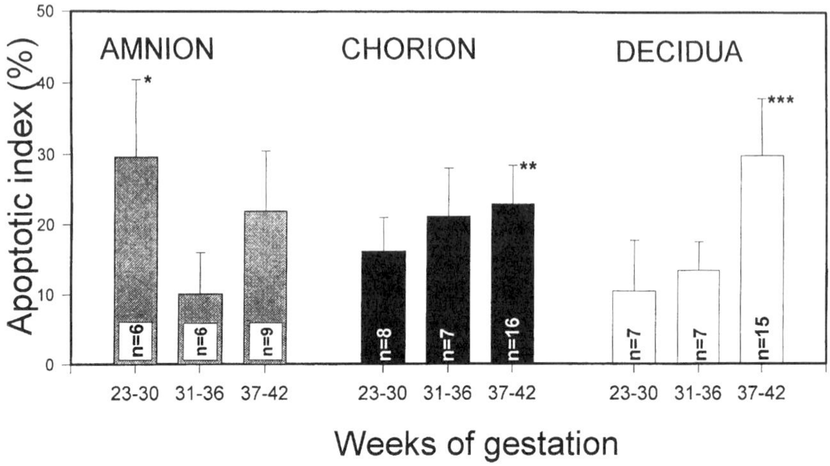

FIGURE 3.—Effect of gestational age on apoptotic index of amnionic, chorionic, and decidual cell layers of human fetal membranes. The apoptotic indexes (apoptotic nuclei/total nuclei × 100) in amnionic, chorionic, and decidual cell layers at the indicated gestational age were calculated and expressed as the mean ± SE. Statistical analyses were performed using analysis of variance (ANOVA). *Numbers within the bars* reflect the number of independent samples obtained for each tissue. *Asterisk*, statistical difference ($P < 0.05$) between 23–30 and 31–36 week groups; *double asterisk*, statistical differences ($P < 0.05$) between 37–42 and 23–30 week groups; *triple asterisk*, statistical difference ($P < 0.01$) for the 37–42 week group compared to 23–30 and 31–36 week groups. (Courtesy of Runić R, Lockwood CJ, LaChapelle L, et al: Apoptosis and Fas expression in human fetal membranes. *J Clin Endocrinol Metab* 83(2):660–666. Copyright 1998, The Endocrine Society.)

apoptosis. Immunohistochemistry, reverse transcription–polymerase chain reaction, and Northern blotting studies for Fas were performed as well.

Results.—Ultrastructural signs of apoptosis were noted in the amnion epithelium and chorion trophoblast cell layers, including chromatin condensation along the nuclear periphery and nuclear shrinkage. In various types of tissues from women at 23–30, 31–36, and 37–42 weeks' gestation, the apoptotic index ranged from 8% to 29%. In the chorionic trophoblast and decidual cell layers, the apoptotic index was significantly greater in 37–42-week tissues than in 23–30-week tissues. In the amnion epithelial cell layer, the apoptotic index was greater in 23–30-week tissues than in 31–36-week tissues (Fig 3). Thus apoptosis appeared to be regulated separately in the different tissue types. Immunohistochemical studies using Fas antibody localized Fas in all 3 cell layers. Reverse transcription–polymerase chain reaction identified a 266-bp band corresponding to the cytoplasmic domain of Fas in amnion, chorion, decidua, and placental tissues. Northern blotting of amniotic tissue demonstrated a molecular weight of approximately 1.9 kb for Fas messenger RNA.

Conclusions.—The presence of apoptosis and Fas was demonstrated in human fetal membranes. The results indicate that apoptosis and Fas signaling play a role in remodeling the fetal membrane architecture throughout gestation. Future research will clarify the role of Fas signaling in association with childbirth.

▶ Apoptosis is an important mechanism widely displayed in reproductive tissues of both genders, and this is a convincing body of evidence of its probable role in the human placenta. The process is initiated by receptor coupling to a cell surface receptor (Fas), which binds to a family of ligands characterized most often by the inclusion of tumor necrosis factors (TNF) and nerve growth factors (NGF). The postreceptor process consists of consecutive enzymatic transections of DNA, leading ultimately to segments of roughly 180 base pairs each. Morphologically apoptosis is characterized by nuclear fragmentation, condensation of chromatin at the nuclear membrane, loss of some cellular organelles, cytoplasmic shrinkage, but preservation of mitochrondia. Inflammatory and immunologic host responses do not occur. In placental tissue, the implications are for possible roles in premature rupture of membranes and decidual degeneration, leading to the release of precursors for prostaglandin production by the placenta. Abnormal Fas receptor development is one mechanism that allows autoimmune disease development through failure of Fas-mediated apoptosis of cells recognized by the immune system as nonself or foreign to the host. Apoptosis has been identified in animal placentas as well.[1]

In this study, electron microscopy is used for morphological identification of apoptosis and immunohistochemistry using antibody to the Fas-Fas ligand complex to identify and quantify apoptosis and its corresponding receptor activators. Both are seen in the chorion increasingly in late pregnancy, in amnion in early pregnancy, and in the decidua at and past term. Apoptosis then exists in the human placenta and may well play a role in development, aging, and abnormalities in placentation, as well as in premature rupture of membranes and the onset of normal or abnormal labor.

T.H. Kirschbaum, M.D.

Reference

1. 1998 Year Book of Obstetrics, Gynecology, and Women's Health, pp 34–35.

Maternal Growth Hormone Treatment Increases Placental Diffusion Capacity But Not Fetal or Placental Growth in Sheep

Harding JE, Evans PC, Gluckman PD (Univ of Auckland, New Zealand)

Endocrinology 138:5352–5358, 1997 1–11

Background.—Growth hormone (GH) and placental lactogen, which induce relative insulin resistance in the mother, may influence fetal growth by increasing maternal glucose levels and the substrate supply available to the fetus, influencing fetal growth. However, previous research on maternal GH administration has yielded conflicting results on its effects on fetal growth. The hypothesis that chronic maternal GH administration would increase fetal substrate supply as well as maternal and fetal insulin-like growth factor I levels, thereby enhancing growth in late gestation, was tested in fetal sheep.

Methods.—Eleven ewes were given bovine GH, 0.1 mg/kg, twice a day for 10 days. Another 10 ewes, comprising a control group, were given saline.

Findings.—Treatment with GH increased placental capacity for simple diffusion, with a trend toward increased placental capacity for facilitated diffusion. Treatment with GH also reduced maternal and fetal blood urea levels. There was a trend toward increased fetal protein oxidation. Maternal insulin-like growth factor I and insulin concentrations increased, though fetal concentrations did not. Growth hormone treatment did not affect fetal or placental growth. Maternal food intake significantly affected maternal and fetal metabolic status.

Conclusions.—In a sheep model, maternal GH treatment increased placental transport capacity. However, anabolic effects in the mother may limit fetal substrate supply, preventing increases in fetal growth.

► Slowly, the factors responsible for fetal growth regulation are becoming clear, at least in animal subjects. Growth hormone acts often through insulin-like growth factor I (IGF-I), which is in turn influenced by a series of 6 binding proteins, some facilitative and others inhibitory of fetal growth. The binding factors are distributed in a complex way differentially among organs and among various tissues within organs.[1] Insulin and the distribution and density of its receptors play an important role.[2] Glucose availability is in turn influenced by the gene expression of several isoforms of glucose transporter proteins that serve as the basis for facilitative glucose transport by the placenta.[3]

In an effort to create a model of growth regulation in fetal sheep, these investigators have proposed that GH acts in ewes by increasing IGF-I and insulin concentration, the former serving to increase maternal blood glucose and fatty acid concentrations. Insulin-like growth factor I administered to the fetus stimulates placental amino acid production and increases fetal uptake while inhibiting protein catabolism as a requisite for growth.[4] This comprehensive study explored that proposition in an analysis of 21 gravid ewes employing GH and untreated controls in which fetal growth was measured by in utero catheters. Fetal and maternal blood nutrients were measured, uteroplacental and umbilical blood flow rates were estimated by the steady-state tritiated antipyrine method of Meschia, and uteroplacenta and fetal consumptions of oxygen, glucose, and lactate were calculated after Fick. Carbon-14–labeled urea placental clearance and tritiated glucose clearance were calculated to estimate simple and facilitated diffusion capacity of the placenta, respectively.

Although maternal GH had the expected effect in increasing maternal IGF-I and insulin concentration, no differences were noted in fetal or placental growth nor in fetal IGF-I. Maternal and fetal urea concentrations were halved during GH administration, denoting decreased protein catabolism, but no other changes in blood nutrient concentration or uteroplacental nutrient uptake were noted. Umbilical blood flow, lactate, and oxygen consumption increased over the 10 days of experimentation as normal fetal growth continued. There were no changes in glucose diffusion capacity, but there was increased placental simple diffusion capacity facilitating respiratory gas and small molecular weight lipid soluble transport. In a sense, the experiment was flawed by pregnancy-induced resistance to GH, which prevented the investigators from demonstrating the expected increase in maternal glucose concentration. Secondly, reduced fetal protein oxidation induced by IGF-I may have deprived the fetuses of an important energy source. We may expect more work from this talented group as they strive to improve our understanding of the regulation of normal fetal growth.

T.H. Kirschbaum, M.D.

References

1. 1996 Year Book of Obstetrics and Gynecology, pp 17–19.
2. 1995 Year Book of Obstetrics and Gynecology, pp 87–88.
3. 1995 Year Book of Obstetrics and Gynecology, pp 16–19, 88–90.
4. 1996 Year Book of Obstetrics and Gynecology, pp 20–21.

Expression of Superoxide Dismutase and Xanthine Oxidase in Myometrium, Fetal Membranes and Placenta During Normal Human Pregnancy and Parturition

Telfer JF, Thomson AJ, Cameron IT, et al (Univ of Glasgow, Scotland)
Hum Reprod 12:2306–2312, 1997 1–12

Background.—Much recent research has focused on the role of nitric oxide in human parturition. Superoxide attenuates the half-life of nitric oxide (NO). Whether the onset of human parturition is correlated with changes in the expression of copper/zinc superoxide dismutase (Cu/Zn SOD), manganese superoxide dismutase (Mn SOD), and xanthine oxidase in the uterus was investigated.

Methods.—Samples of myometrium, placenta, decidua, and fetal membranes were acquired from women before and after labor onset at term. Immunocytochemistry was used to localize Cu/Zn SOD, Mn SOD, and xanthine oxidase and measure SOD enzyme activity.

Findings.—Copper/zinc and Mn SOD-like immunoreactivity was found in syncytiotrophoblast cells, villous stromal cells, and endothelial cells of blood vessels in the placenta. Copper/zinc and Mn SOD in the myometrium were localized to myocytes and endothelial cells as well as some vascular smooth muscle cells. Staining for Cu/Zn SOD and Mn SOD in fetal membranes was noted in the amnion, chorion, extravillous trophoblast, and decidua. Superoxide dismutase enzyme activity and SOD staining intensity did not differ between cell types before and during labor. Xanthine oxidase immunoreactivity did not differ in tissues obtained from women delivered before and after labor onset.

Conclusions.—The pregnant uterus can both synthesize and degrade superoxide. Superoxide dismutase and xanthine oxidase may play a role in maintaining uterine quiescence during pregnancy but not in initiating parturition.

► The capacity of NO, derived from arginine by means of NO synthetase, to produce vasodilatation, inhibit platelet aggregation, and produce uterine contractile quiescence makes it an interesting candidate for a role in the initiation of labor and of pregnancy-induced hypertension. Thus far, the evidence suggests increasing endothelial production rates are important in maintaining vasodilatation and low vascular resistance in normal pregnancy.[1] As noted here earlier, a role in pregnancy-induced hypertension appears unlikely in view of evidence of its increased production rates in preeclampsia[2] where a reduced production rate for NO was anticipated. The reduction in NO production rates appears to play a role in the onset of labor in rodents and rabbits, but no such decrease has been documented during the onset of human labor.

This immunocytochemical study of the human uterus and placenta explores the possibility that increased inactivation of NO, not decreased production, may be at work. Superoxide anion inactivates NO and superoxide dismutase, by inactivating superoxide anions, tends to prolong the activity of superoxide anion. Xanthine oxidase is an important enzymatic facilitator of endothelial nitric oxide production. None of these, including 3 isoforms of superoxide dismutase, show any changes in apparent activity in myometrium, decidua, the placenta, or its membranes during pregnancy. This is a further negative vote for the role of NO in the onset of human labor.

T.H. Kirschbaum, M.D.

References

1. 1995 Year Book of Obstetrics and Gynecology, pp 25–26.
2. 1997 Year Book of Obstetrics, Gynecology, and Women's Health, pp 22–26.

Brain Lipid Peroxidation and Antioxidant Levels in Fetal Lambs 72 Hours After Asphyxia by Partial Umbilical Cord Occlusion

Ikeda T, Murata Y, Quilligan EJ, et al (Univ of California, Irvine)

Am J Obstet Gynecol 178:474–478, 1998 1–13

Introduction.—Antepartum and intrapartum asphyxia may account for about 90% of cases of perinatal hypoxic-ischemic encephalopathy, a major cause of childhood neurologic disability. An animal model of near-term fetal lamb asphyxia was used to examine the role of oxidative stress in the pathogenesis of brain damage caused by intrauterine fetal asphyxia.

Methods.—The experimental group included 6 asphyxiated and 6 control near-term fetal lambs. Asphyxia was achieved by partial umbilical cord occlusion for approximately 60 minutes. The chronically instrumented fetuses were killed after 72 hours, and their brains were removed. Eight different regions were dissected from the left half of the brain and assayed for thiobarbituric acid–reactive substances, glutathione, and superoxide dismutase, indicators of oxidative stress.

Results.—The sham-asphyxia control and asphyxiated fetal lambs were similar in gestational age at time of harvest, mean weight, and mean brain weight. Compared with control animals, asphyxiated fetal lambs had elevated thiobarbituric acid–reactive substance levels in frontal and parietal white matter, basal ganglia, and thalamus. Concentrations of superoxide dismutase were also higher in frontal and parietal white matter, basal ganglia, and cerebellum of asphyxiated animals. The study and control animals did not differ significantly in glutathione concentrations. Brains of sham-asphyxia control lambs showed no consistent histologic changes, whereas the brains of asphyxiated fetal lambs demonstrated highly variable neuropathologic changes. There were no apparent correlations between severity of brain damage and assay values.

Conclusion.—In this fetal lamb model, oxidative stress appeared to be a major factor contributing to the development of brain damage after intrauterine asphyxia.

▶ Knowledge of the pathophysiology of asphyxial brain injury has been expanded over the past 10 years by the work of Peter Glucksman and his colleagues at the University of Auckland, New Zealand.[1–4] Those investigators have employed brain histopathology, cortical impedance measurements, magnetic resonance spectroscopy, and near-infrared spectroscopy to provide a clear picture of cell energetics, biochemistry, vasoregulation, and structural neuronal injury as they follow total cerebral ischemia of 30 minutes' duration. Their findings differ from those depicted here. An initial period of 60–80 minutes of occlusion is followed by a second interval of 60–70 hours, during which little permanent structural injury or reduction of available adenosine triphosphate activity takes place in the brain. Since cord occlusion as done here allows fetal blood shunting to preserve fetal brain oxidative metabolism longer than does carotid occlusion with the vertebral arteries ligated, it is likely that measurements in these sheep fetuses were made during the latter of the two intervals. Glutamate activity is known to be present but declining at that time, and oxygen-free radicals are maximally present. After 60–70 hours in the second phase of injury, oxygen free radical activity is diminished a great deal and irreversible brain injury begins in force. Superoxide dismutase, a free radical inactivator, has proved useless in prophylaxis or rescue therapy of ischemic brain injury in such fetuses, and the deleterious influences of macrocyte infiltration and apoptosis begin after the point at which these observations were made and result in permanent cataclysmic brain injury. In timing their observations as they have, these investigators appear to focus on an early, relatively preliminary phase of the development of a neuropathology and one that excessively emphasizes the role of oxygen free radicals.

T.H. Kirschbaum, M.D.

References

1. 1990 YEAR BOOK OF OBSTETRICS AND GYNECOLOGY, pp 206–207.
2. 1992 YEAR BOOK OF OBSTETRICS AND GYNECOLOGY, pp 189–191.
3. 1993 YEAR BOOK OF OBSTETRICS AND GYNECOLOGY, pp 123–124.
4. 1998 YEAR BOOK OF OBSTETRICS AND GYNECOLOGY, AND WOMEN'S HEALTH, pp 137–139 and 150–153.

Respiratory and Metabolic Responses to Endurance Cycle Exercise in Pregnant and Postpartum Women

Lotgering FK, Spinnewijn WEM, Struijk PC, et al (Erasmus Univ, Rotterdam, The Netherlands)

Int J Sports Med 19:193–198, 1998 1–14

Background.—The physiologic effects of strenuous endurance exercise in pregnancy have not been well investigated. Whether women can perform a strenuous endurance task in pregnancy and have similar physiologic responses to such exercise in pregnant and postpartum states was determined.

Methods.—Sixteen women were assessed at about 32 weeks' gestation and at about 10 weeks after delivery. Measures were obtained at rest, during maximal testing, and during 35–40 minutes of cycling at 70% to 75% peak oxygen uptake ($\dot{V}O_{2peak}$).

Findings.—During pregnancy, mean endurance exercise time was 37.6 minutes and power, 124 W. These values were similar to those obtained after delivery. Heart rate and respiratory responses near the end of endurance exercise were also comparable during and after pregnancy. Minute

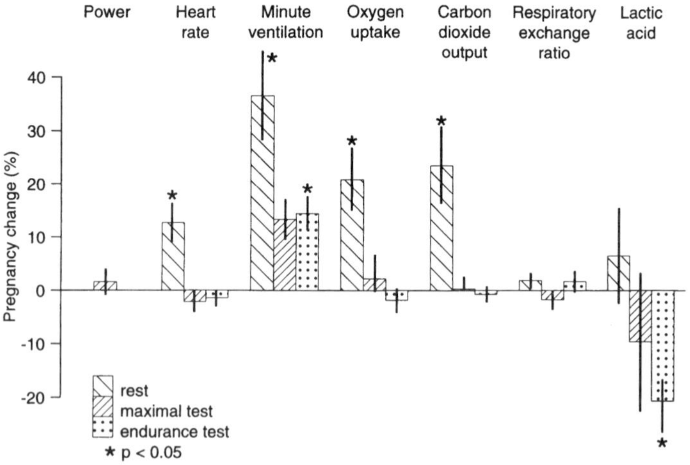

FIGURE 2.—Pregnancy-induced changes of selected variables, expressed as mean percent changes ± SE. *Asterisk*, $P < 0.05$ compared with postpartum control values. (Courtesy of Lotgering FK, Spinnewijn WEM, Struijk PC, et al: Respiratory and metabolic responses to endurance cycle exercise in pregnant and postpartum women. *Int J Sports Med* 19:193–198, 1998 Georg Thieme Verlag.)

ventilation of 70 L/min was 14% higher during pregnancy than after delivery. Plasma concentrations of free fatty acids, glucose, and lactic acid were lower during pregnancy than postpartum by 9%, 24%, and 19%, respectively. Catecholamine levels did not differ from those determined after delivery (Fig 2).

Conclusions.—Pregnant women can perform about 40 minutes of cycling at 70% to 75% $\dot{V}O_{2peak}$ at levels equal to those of women postpartum. The physiologic responses to endurance exercise appear to be largely independent of gestation.

► Experiments in exercise physiology require an estimate of work performed by experimental subjects measured in watts (joules of energy expended per second) to standardize the intensity of work among individual subjects. A common approach is to measure oxygen consumption ($\dot{V}O_2$) as a function of increased work expenditure until $\dot{V}O_2$ reaches a maximum; that is, it cannot be further increased with additional work. After that point is determined, exercise is commonly conducted at 70% to 75% of the maximum $\dot{V}O_2$.[1–4] For fear of compromising pregnant women, their exercise loads are commonly held at 30%–50% of maximum $\dot{V}O_2$.[1–4] This study of 22 hearty, normal Dutch gravidas raises the exercise load to 75% $\dot{V}O_2$, and the results are somewhat surprising.

Each of 19 women at 30–34 weeks of pregnancy were subjected to a maximum cycle test in which power requirement was increased by 20 W each minute to the point where $\dot{V}O_2$ failed to increase by as much as 5% with the next power increment. This experience was used to define maximum $\dot{V}O_2$ and a power equivalent to 70% to 75% $\dot{V}O_2$ maximum was used for 40 minutes in endurance studies that followed. Studies of the same women were conducted at 8–12 weeks postpartum to serve as internal controls. At rest, the pregnant women exhibited the effects of increased respiratory sensitivity to PCO_2 and the demands for increased cardiac output by exhibiting tachycardia, increased resting $\dot{V}O_2$, increased CO_2 production, and an elevated minute volume of respiration. At 75% $\dot{V}O_2$, pregnant and nonpregnant women behaved similarly except for increased hypoglycemia and a tendency to elevated blood free fatty acid content in pregnancy. These findings suggest the presence of a reduced respiratory quotient and an increased lipid metabolism during severe exercise during pregnancy in comparison with the nonpregnant state. In no case was there short- or long-term evidence of adverse fetal effects of exercise. This work attests both to the ability of healthy pregnant women to manage periods of high work output and the comparability of exercise studies done in pregnant and nonpregnant women.

T.H. Kirschbaum, M.D.

References

1. 1990 Year Book of Obstetrics and Gynecology, pp 26–28, 91–92.
2. 1992 Year Book of Obstetrics and Gynecology, pp 10–11, 20–21.
3. 1994 Year Book of Obstetrics and Gynecology, pp 22–23.
4. 1996 Year Book of Obstetrics and Gynecology, pp 32–34.

Massive Decline in Lung Liquid Before Vaginal Delivery at Term in the Fetal Lamb

Berger PJ, Kyriakides MA, Smolich JJ, et al (Monash Univ, Clayton, Australia)

Am J Obstet Gynecol 178:223–227, 1998 1–15

Background.—An excess of liquid in the air spaces may contribute to the respiratory morbidity associated with elective cesarean delivery. The volume of liquid remaining in the lungs of the fetal lamb just before a normal vaginal delivery at term was determined.

Methods.—In 8 fetal lambs, liquid volume in the future air space of the lungs was determined at the end of labor from the dilution of an impermeable tracer mixed into the liquid. For comparison, a second group of 10 fetal lambs was assessed 7 days before the expected date of delivery.

Findings.—Mean lung liquid volume at the end of labor was 6.8 mL/kg. In the second group, studied before labor onset at 140 days' gestation, mean lung liquid volume was 28.2 mL/kg. (Fig 1).

Conclusion.—More than three fourths of the liquid that fills fetal lamb lungs at 140 days' gestation is cleared before term. Thus, the adverse respiratory effect of elective cesarean delivery may be largely explained by denying the fetus the opportunity for this important adaptive mechanism.

► Clearly, the incidence of complications in the initiation of air breathing during the transition from fetal to neonatal life is greater in infants born abdominally than in those delivered vaginally, almost without regard to

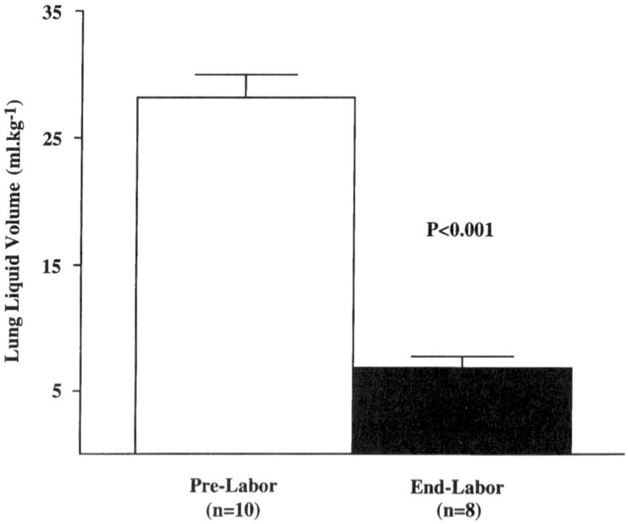

FIGURE 1.—Lung liquid volume in late gestation and in labor. Note that the volume of liquid in the air spaces of a group of 10 fetuses at 140 days of gestation (*Pre-Labor*) is significantly less than the volume measured in 8 fetuses at the end of labor (*End Labor*). (Courtesy of Berger PJ, Kyriakides MA, Smolich JJ, et al: Massive decline in lung before vaginal delivery at term in the fetal lamb. *Am J Obstet Gynecol* 178:223–227, 1998.)

gestational age. The effect is commonly attributed to thoracic compression in the birth canal, but this study—done of the necessity in experimental animals—indicates that there may be more to the advantage of vaginal birth than that.

In 8 fetal lambs in the process of vaginal birth at term, the trachea was occluded prior to the first breath and the neonate removed after the ewe received a lethal anesthetic overdose. Fluid volume filling the fetal airway was carefully measured by dilution of ^{125}I-labeled albumin suspension and compared with the same measurements made in 10 fetal lambs not subject to labor 4 days before term. Then, parenchymal alveoli fluid at the end of labor was calculated by subtracting the weight of air space liquid from total lung weight plus the expected wet weight obtained at term by multiplying the weight of dry lung by the wet-to-dry lung ratio measured from fetal lungs without alveoli fluid.

The results showed a 76% reduction in fluid in the bronchiolar apparatus during the 4 days before the onset of labor. Estimations of parenchymal fluid at delivery indicated that the reduction of an average of 21.4 mL/kg fetal weight was transferred to the parenchyma of the lung to the extent of 10% of the reduction of bronchiolar fluid (that is, 2.0 mL/kg) with the rest (19 mL/kg) absorbed into the fetal circulation during the 4-day interval before labor. This in utero removal of bronchiolar fluid—whether because of activation of sodium absorption channels by epinephrine or arginine vasopressin, or of the behavioral reduction in fetal breathing and an increase in sighing fetal exhalations in utero before the onset of labor—is uncertain. It is clear from animal data that this reduction in intrapulmonary fluid at the beginning of neonatal life enhances the efficacy of air breathing at the time of birth. Perhaps the same is true in the human neonate.

T.H. Kirschbaum, M.D.

2 Maternal Complications in Pregnancy

Shedding of Syncytiotrophoblast Microvilli Into the Maternal Circulation in Pre-eclamptic Pregnancies

Knight M, Redman CWG, Linton EA, et al (John Radcliffe Hosp, Oxford, England)

Br J Obstet Gynaecol 105:632–640, 1998 2–1

Background.—The endothelial damage that occurs in preeclampsia may result from the shedding of higher than normal levels of syncytiotrophoblast microvilli (STBM) into the circulation. Increased shedding of STBM as a possible cause of maternal vascular endothelial dysfunction was investigated.

Methods.—Twenty women with established preeclampsia and 20 with normal pregnancies, matched for age, gestation, and parity, were studied. In addition, 10 nonpregnant women of reproductive age were studied. Paired uterine and peripheral venous plasma were obtained at cesarean section from 10 women with preeclampsia and 10 with normal pregnancies. A time-resolved fluoroimmunoassay was developed to measure STBM levels in the peripheral and uterine venous plasma. Three-color flow cytometry was used to evaluate the microparticulate nature of the STBM.

Findings.—Both flow cytometry and time-resolved fluoroimmunoassay demonstrated STBM in the plasma of pregnant women. Women with preeclampsia had significantly higher levels of STBM. Concentrations of STBM were greater in the uterine than in the peripheral venous plasma, confirming that the origin of STBM is the placenta. The amount of STBM in the plasma was significantly correlated with endothelial cell inhibitory activity (Figs 1 and 3).

Conclusions.—Syncytiotrophoblast microvilli are shed into the maternal circulation. In preeclamptic women, STBM are shed in increased amounts and may contribute to the endothelial dysfunction underlying this disorder.

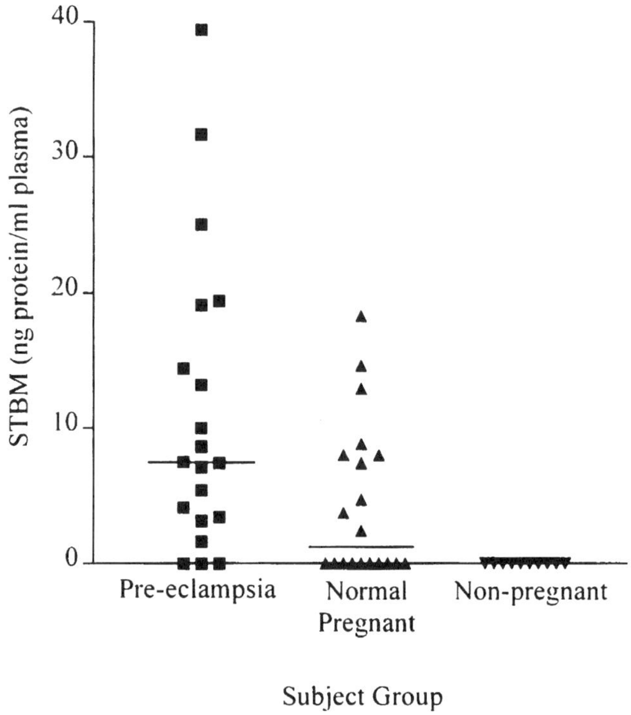

FIGURE 1.—Syncytiotrophoblast microvilli (*STBM*) detected in peripheral plasma from normal and preeclamptic women. *Bars* indicate median values. (Courtesy of Knight M, Redman CWG, Linton EA, et al: Shedding of syncytiotrophoblast microvilli into the maternal circulation in preeclamptic pregnancies. *Br J Obstet Gynaecol* 105:632–640. Copyright 1998, Blackwell Science Ltd.)

▶ Investigators from the Nuffield Department of the John Radcliffe Hospital have provided us with a considerable body of qualitative data regarding the potential role of plasma trophoblastic microvilli in inducing endothelial injury in preeclampsia, and here they report some inferences based on quantitative data.[1] Microvillus preparations in maternal plasma but not serum inhibit endothelial cell growth in cell culture, inhibit endothelial cell relaxation factor activity in small arterioles in vitro, and are shed into the maternal circulation in apparently higher density in preeclampsia than in normotensive pregnant women. Morphologic study of the trophoblast in preeclamptic placentas has shown microvilli on the trophoblastic surface to be reduced in number as though partially shed into the maternal circulation, and to be abnormal in structure compared to fragments isolated from normotensives.[2]

Syncytiotrophoblast microvilli were assayed by fluorescent-activated cell sorting using 2 antibodies to STBM chosen for their specificity. Cross-reactivity of one of the antibodies to placental alkaline phosphatases was controlled, and additional fluorescent antibody labels were used in fluorescent immunoassay to exclude fragments of platelets and red blood cell membrane from inadvertent analysis. Standardization curves were prepared,

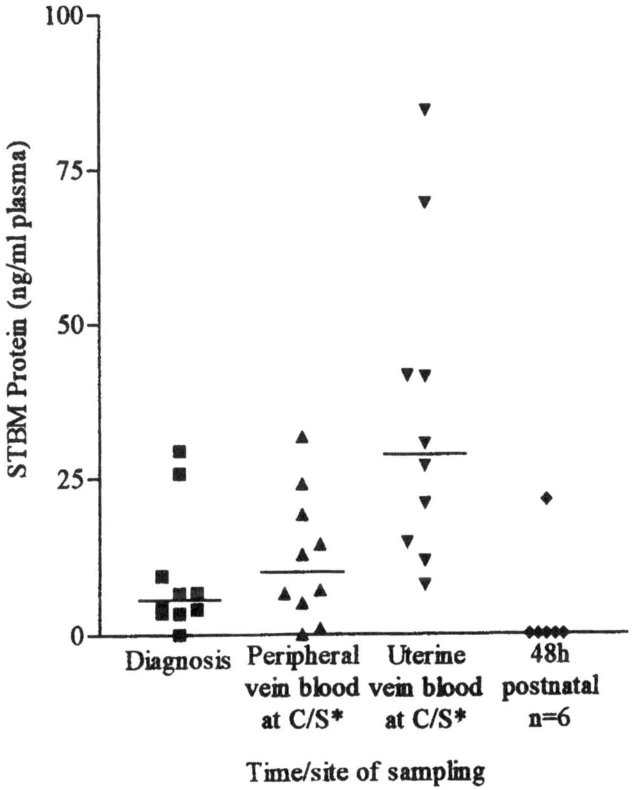

FIGURE 3.—Longitudinal detection of syncytiotrophoblast microvilli (*STBM*) in plasma of women with preeclampsia; $n = 10$ unless otherwise indicated. *Bars* indicate median values. *Abbreviation: C/S*, delivery by cesarean section. (Courtesy of Knight M, Redman CWG, Linton EA, et al: Shedding of syncytiotrophoblast microvilli into the maternal circulation in preeclamptic pregnancies. *Br J Obstet Gynaecol* 105:632–640. Copyright 1998, Blackwell Science Ltd.)

a linear range from .05 to 5 µg/mL demonstrated, and sensitivity of the assay set at less than 2 µg of protein per milliliter of plasma.

Syncytiotrophoblast microvilli were found in all pregnant women, but were found more often and in higher concentrations in the plasma of preeclamptics than from normotensive controls. No STBM were found in nonpregnant blood. Uterine vein plasma concentrations were higher than those in peripheral plasma, and no relationship between the severity of preeclamptic symptoms and findings and the concentration of STBM could be noted. Evidence that STBM may be deported from placental sites by the formation of complexes with maternal white blood cells, red blood cells, or macrophages, and thereby distributed to the general circulation is cited. Whether the effect is direct or indirect, STBM fragments appear to have some role in the endothelial dysfunction that seems to be an important part of the preeclamptic syndrome.

T.H. Kirschbaum, M.D.

References

1. 1997 Year Book of Obstetrics, Gynecology, and Women's Health, pp 37–39.
2. Jones CJP, Fox H: An ultrastructural and ultrahistochemical study of the human placenta in maternal preeclampsia. *Placenta* 1:61–76, 1980.

Preterm Premature Rupture of Membranes: Aggressive Tocolysis Versus Expectant Management

How HY, Cook CR, Cook VD, et al (Univ of Louisville, Ky; Marshall Univ, Huntington, W VA)

J Matern Fetal Invest 7:8–12, 1998 2–2

Introduction.—Up to 40% of all preterm deliveries occur after preterm premature rupture of membranes (PPROM). The optimal management of PPROM remains controversial. A randomized study sought to determine whether aggressive tocolysis can improve outcome in patients between 24 and 34 weeks of gestation.

Methods.—Patients eligible for the study had no evidence of chorioamnionitis, fetal stress, or advanced active labor, and were free of obstetrical indications for expedient delivery. The women were prospectively randomized either to aggressive tocolysis (AT, 78 patients) or to no tocolysis (NT, 67 patients). The AT regimen consisted of IV magnesium sulfate (6-g loading dose), initiated when uterine contractions were 6 or more per hour. Doses were increased to a maximum of 5 g/hour as required to reduce contractions to 3 or fewer per hour. The lecithin/sphingomyelin (L/S) ratio was determined at admission and every 48 to 96 hours until delivery. Patients were delivered promptly at the first signs of chorioamnionitis, fetal stress, or an L/S of 2 or more.

Results.—The AT and NT groups did not differ significantly in mean maternal age, gravity, racial distribution, or gestational age at enrollment. Also comparable were the latency period (time between PPROM and delivery), the mode of and indications for delivery, number of days in the neonatal ICU, days on oxygen or ventilatory support, neonatal mortality, and the frequency of hyaline membrane disease, necrotizing enterocolitis, intraventricular hemorrhage, and neonatal sepsis.

Conclusion.—Patients with PPROM are given tocolytics to prolong gestation and reduce perinatal morbidity. A number of studies, however, have questioned the benefits of tocolytic treatment. Findings in this series of patients with PPROM also suggest that tocolysis does not significantly improve perinatal outcome compared with expectant management.

▶ This study is narrowly and specifically focused on the role of tocolytics when premature preterm rupture of membranes occurs at 24 to 34 weeks of gestation. Tocolytic use seldom appears as a dependent variable where the merits of expectant management[1] or antibiotic therapies are the variables of particular interest.[2-4] The experiment is well designed, with women randomly assigned to receive large doses of intravenous magnesium sulfate, up to 5 g per hour, until uterine contractions occur less often than 3 per hour and then the dose is progressively diminished. All women were cultured, the women treated for cervical pathogens and received antenatal corticoids and prophylactic ampicillin or clindomycin. Amniotic fluid LS ratio determination was done by a vaginal collection; the patients delivered spontaneously or labor was induced with evidence of chorioamnionitis, LS ratio greater than 2, or evidence of fetal concerns on monitoring. The latency interval (median 3–4 days) was somewhat shorter than average, but cesarean section rates, need for respiratory support, and length of nursery stay were average and fetal morbidity and mortality rates were low. The treated and control groups were comparable, and there was no apparent advantage to the use of tocolytics. Women with pregnancy-induced hypertension, cervices greater than 3 cm, uterine bleeding, or chorioamnionitis were excluded. The data do not allow a rigorous test of the effect of short-term tocolytic therapy but no differences in outcome were seen in infants born less than 24 hours after tocolytic therapy with presumably less than optimal adrenal steroid effect on pulmonary maturity. This is a nice confirmation of the failure of tocolysis to make much difference in the treatment of preterm rupture of membranes.

T.H. Kirschbaum, M.D.

References

1. 1997 Year Book of Obstetrics, Gynecology, and Women's Health, pp 107–108; 191–192.
2. 1992 Year Book of Obstetrics and Gynecology, pp 117–118.
3. 1993 Year Book of Obstetrics and Gynecology, pp 31–33.
4. 1995 Year Book of Obstetrics and Gynecology, pp 185–186.

The Preterm Prediction Study: Patterns of Cervicovaginal Fetal Fibronectin as Predictors of Spontaneous Preterm Delivery

Goldenberg RL, and the (Natl Inst of Child Health and Human Development Maternal-Fetal Medicine Units Network) (Univ of Alabama at Birmingham)

Am J Obstet Gynecol 177:8–12, 1997 2–3

Background.—The presence of fetal fibronectin in the cervix or vagina at 20–34 weeks' gestation is a strong predictor of preterm delivery after spontaneous labor and premature rupture of the membranes. The presence of fetal fibronectin in the cervix or vagina at 24 or 26 weeks' gestation in asymptomatic women was shown to be linked with a high relative risk for prediction of spontaneous preterm birth; a weaker relationship was seen at 28 and 30 weeks' gestation.

Methods.—Vaginal and cervical fetal fibronectin tests were performed in 2,929 women at least once between 24 and 30 weeks; 1,870 of those women had testing done each time at 24, 26, 28 and 30 weeks. A fetal fibronectin value of 50 ng/mL or greater was considered a positive result. Various patterns of positive and negative test results were analyzed for the ability to predict if the next fetal fibronectin test would be positive or negative, and for the ability to predict the percentage of women who would have spontaneous preterm delivery at 4 weeks or more after the last fetal fibronectin test at less than 30, 32, 35, and 37 weeks' gestational age.

Results.—Women with a previous negative test result had a 3% chance of a later positive test result; if the last test result was positive, 29% of the next tests would be positive. Among the 1,870 women who were tested at 24, 26, 28 and 30 weeks, 89.0% had all negative test results, 8.4% had 1 positive result, 1.8% had 2 positive test results, and 0.8% had 3 or 4 positive test results. The higher the percentage of positive test results at 24–26 weeks, 28–30 weeks, or 24–30 weeks, the greater the risk of spontaneous preterm delivery. For example, the risk of spontaneous preterm delivery at less than 30 weeks was 0.3% for women with 2 negative results of fetal fibronectin tests at 24 and 26 weeks and 16.0% for women with 2 positive results of tests at 24 and 26 weeks.

Discussion.—These findings show that a positive result on a cervical or vaginal fetal fibronectin test predicts fetal fibronectin positivity in later tests and spontaneous preterm delivery. The risk of spontaneous preterm birth increases as the percentage of positive test results increases. After a positive test result, 2 negative test results are needed before the risk of spontaneous preterm delivery returns to baseline values.

▶ This is a continuation of the National Institute of Child Health and Human Development-sponsored Maternal-Fetal Medicine Network study of cervicovaginal fetal fibronectin (FFN) as a predictor of preterm delivery defined as birth before 35 weeks of gestation. The earlier publication of results[1] reported results of FFN assays done every 2 weeks from 20–30 weeks' gestation in 2,929 women initially enrolled. In that report, preterm birth was defined as birth at or before 34 weeks. Asymptomatic women were enrolled independent of medical or socioeconomic status, though women with fetal anomalies, placenta previa, cervical cerclage, or multiple pregnancies were excluded. With an incidence of preterm birth of 10.3% overall, positive assays for FFN measured with a monoclonal antibody occurred in 3%–4% of women at each exposure. Expressed in intervals of 2 weeks, sensitivity values were roughly 20% at each interval with an incidence of false positive assays varying from 68% to 87%. Sensitivity of a positive assay declined with advancing gestational age. Although overall sensitivity for delivery at 24–36 weeks was only 10%, for the interval 24–27 weeks when somewhere between 6% and 9% of preterm births occurred, sensitivity was 63%.

Here, the intent is to see what can be learned from patterns of changes in FFN status with time in relation to preterm birth in the same 24–30 weeks interval. What emerges is that the more positive test results, the more likely is preterm birth, and the last test performed is the best predictor. A single positive test result loses its predictive strength for preterm birth only after 2 subsequent negative results and 60% of women with 1 positive test result later reverted to negative status. The authors infer, reasonably, that these are instances of decidual trophoblastic ground substance suffering inflammatory and/or infectious injury from which there is recovery as a result of inflammatory repair and natural and/or acquired immunity. Perhaps this, in addition to reaction to the FDC-6 monoclonal antibody to plasma fibronectin[2] helps explain the false positive rates that have dogged this assay and decreased its usefulness.

T.H. Kirschbaum, M.D.

References

1. 1997 YEAR BOOK OF OBSTETRICS, GYNECOLOGY, AND WOMEN'S HEALTH, pp 146–148.
2. 1996 YEAR BOOK OF OBSTETRICS AND GYNECOLOGY, pp 61–63.

Management Options in Women With Preterm Uterine Contractions: A Randomized Clinical Trial

Guinn DA, Goepfert AR, Owen J, et al (Univ of Alabama, Birmingham)
Am J Obstet Gynecol 177:814–818, 1997 2–4

Introduction.—Management of women with preterm uterine contractions is controversial because up to 45% respond to bed rest alone. In an attempt to arrest uterine contractions, many therapies have been administered, including bed rest, sedation, intravenous hydration, subcutaneous terbutaline sulfate, or parenteral tocolysis. Little is known about the benefit from any of these therapies. In women with preterm uterine contractions, 3 management strategies and the resultant pregnancy outcomes were prospectively evaluated.

Methods.—There were 179 women with a singleton gestation between 20 and 34 weeks, intact membranes, more than 3 contractions in 30 minutes, and a cervical dilatation of less than or equal to 1 cm and effacement of more than 80%. They were divided into 3 groups: 56 were observed, 62 received hydration, and 61 received terbutaline. Intravenous tocolysis was administered to women who had progressive cervical change at less than 34 weeks, and women with recurrent preterm uterine activity remained in their assigned group when they had follow-up triage visits. The women were similar in their mean cervical dilatation, contraction frequency, gestational age at randomization, prior preterm births, parity, maternal age, and race.

Results.—In the mean days to delivery, there were no intergroup differences, nor were there differences in the frequency of preterm deliveries at less than 34 weeks and less than 37 weeks, in the incidence of preterm labor at less than 34 weeks, or in the frequency of preterm deliveries at less than 34 weeks. There was an earlier discharge with women assigned to terbutaline who had their contractions stopped. The terbutaline group was 4.1 ± 5.1 hours, the hydration group was 6.0 ± 5.7 hours, and the observation group was 5.2 ± 5.3 hours. There was no evidence of complications of therapy.

Conclusion.—There was no benefit in the use of intravenous hydration in the management of preterm contractions. Pregnancy outcome was not affected by the use of 1 dose of subcutaneous terbutaline, but it resulted in the shortest length of triage stay.

► This prospective, randomized, controlled trial attempts to rationalize the management of women at 20–34 weeks' gestational age who had uterine contractions at least every ten minutes and had intact membranes and closed cervixes. The authors test the value of significant intravenous hydration and a single dose of a beta adrenergic agent in preventing preterm labor. The women proved in retrospect to be at increased risk of preterm delivery with 24% of them delivering prior to 37 weeks. The average gestational age at admission to the study was 30 weeks, and the interval between entry and the onset of labor averaged 58 days with a very large range of variability. Compared to simple observation, neither intravenous hydration nor terbutaline influenced either the prematurity rate, gestational age at delivery, or the latency period which followed. Despite this, costs derived from management by hydration ranged 40% to 50% higher than those for observation in the control group or following terbutaline use, with total charges for simple observation averaging about $35,000. Fifteen percent of these women received a diagnosis of preterm labor based on cervical change and were admitted for intravenous tocolysis. Because the apparent effectiveness of tocolysis was 100%—that is, none promptly proceeded into labor—those instances probably represented errors in evaluation or an inappropriate willingness to accept cervical effacement as evidence of labor without dilatation. This study points up our inability to recognize the subset of such women destined for preterm labor and the costliness either of hydration or terbutaline dosage unbalanced by apparent benefit.

T.H. Kirschbaum, M.D.

Impact of Metronidazole Therapy on Preterm Birth in Women With Bacterial Vaginosis Flora (Gardnerella Vaginalis): A Randomised, Placebo Controlled Trial

McDonald HM, O'Loughlin JA, Vigneswaran R, et al (Women's and Children's Hosp. Adelaide, Australia; Queen Elizabeth Hosp, Adelaide, Australia; Lyell McEwin Health Service, Adelaide, Australia; et al)
Br J Obstet Gynaecol 104:1391–1397, 1997 2–5

Objective.—Genital tract infections are suspected of causing one third of the spontaneous preterm births. Antibiotic treatment of women with asymptomatic bacterial infections may reduce the risk of preterm labor by 50%. A randomized, multicenter, double-blind, placebo-controlled trial examined the effects of systemic antibiotic treatment with oral metronidazole for pregnant women with a heavy growth of *Gardnerella vaginalis* or bacterial vaginosis.

Methods.—Either placebo (440 patients) or oral metronidazole (439 patients given 400 mg) was administered twice daily for 2 days to 879 women with a heavy growth of *G. vaginalis* at 24 weeks' gestation and at

29 weeks if *G. vaginalis* was found in test-of-cure swabs 4 weeks after treatment. Swabs were also taken at 32 and 36 weeks' gestation. Outcomes measured were spontaneous preterm births before 37 weeks' gestation and preterm prelabor membrane rupture.

Results.—Compliances in the treatment and placebo groups were 81.3% and 83.1% respectively. After a positive test-of-cure swab at 28 weeks' gestation, 189 women in the treatment group and 236 in the placebo group received a second course of allocated treatment. Of the 11 treatment patients and 16 placebo patients that later became symptomatic, all received 7 days of metronidazole but remained in their original groups. After 4 weeks of therapy, the efficacy of metronidazole was 75%. Preterm births of less than 37 weeks' gestation were similar in the treatment and placebo groups (7.2% and 7.5%, respectively). Spontaneous preterm births were similar in the treatment and placebo groups (4.7% and 5.6%, respectively). Preterm birth rates were similar in 480 women with bacterial vaginosis whether treated with metronidazole or placebo (6.6% and 7.6%, respectively). In 46 women with a previous preterm birth, patients receiving metronidazole had a significant reduction in spontaneous preterm births (9.1% and 41.7%, respectively). In 34 women with a previous preterm birth and bacterial vaginosis, patients receiving metronidazole had a significant reduction in spontaneous preterm births (5.9% and 35.3%, respectively). There were no significant differences between groups in incidence and type of side effects or discontinuation of treatment.

Conclusion.—Metronidazole significantly reduced the incidence of spontaneous preterm births in women with previous preterm births and in women with vaginosis and previous preterm births. Metronidazole did not reduce the preterm birth rate of women with a heavy growth of *G. vaginalis*.

▶ Readers might wish to review the 1997 YEAR BOOK, pages 31–33, for a similar study done by J.C. Hauth at the University of Alabama at Birmingham, who reached somewhat different conclusions. Here, 879 women were randomized between placebo and metronidazole, 1.6 grams given over 48 hours. Women were accepted into the trial either with heavy *G. vaginalis* culture findings (43.8%), vaginal smear positive for bacterial vaginosis (4.2%), or both (52%) after screening at 18 weeks of pregnancy. Therapy was begun at 24 weeks.

Repeat culture indicated cure in 84% of women at 28 weeks' gestation and women persistently testing positive were retreated. Although the incidences of preterm birth and premature rupture of membranes were both smaller in the treated groups, they failed a test of statistical significance among the 44 cases of preterm birth. When a subset of women with prior preterm birth was isolated and compared, 2 of 22 (9.1%) receiving metronidazole and 10 of 24 controls (41.7%) had preterm births, a significant difference. There was no apparent effect on the incidence of premature rupture of membranes.

In contrast, the University of Alabama study used 1 week of metronidazole and 2 weeks of erythromycin in a population that was 72% black, compared with the 84% Caucasion composition of this study. References to 6 earlier prospective, randomized, controlled studies showing no benefit of prophylactic antibiotics in preventing preterm labor are included in the review referred to above. The usefulness of this approach remains debatable, and the bulk of evidence is negative. Nonetheless, the prospect of reducing the incidence of preterm birth by treating latent infection is compelling and deserving of a large, multicenter trial.

Fortunately, the Medical Research Council is undertaking a study entitled Oracle and has more than 4,000 women already recruited. Perhaps, Oracle will help clarify this important issue of latent infection as a cause of preterm birth.

T.H. Kirschbaum, M.D.

Prolonged Pregnancy: Evaluating Gestation-specific Risks of Fetal and Infant Mortality

Hilder L, Costeloe K, Thilaganathan B (Queen Mary Westfield College, London; Homerton Hosp, London)

Br J Obstet Gynaecol 105:169–173, 1998 2–6

Background.—The risks of prolonged pregnancy include meconium aspiration, birth injury, and hypoxia, and fetal loss. The risk of stillbirth can be calculated as a proportion of ongoing pregnancies at a specific gestation because only women who are still pregnant have a risk of stillbirth. The number of live births should be used as the denominator in determining neonatal mortality because a neonate is at risk of dying only after it is liveborn. The rates of stillbirth and infant mortality per 1,000 total or live births and ongoing pregnancies at each specific gestation were determined.

Methods.—A retrospective analysis was performed of 171,527 births and of infant survival at 1 year. The incidence of births, stillbirths, and neonatal and postneonatal deaths at each gestation after 28 weeks was determined. Mortality per 1,000 total or live births and per 1,000 ongoing pregnancies at each gestation was also determined.

Results.—No significant differences were seen between stillbirth rates at term and post-term. When the rate of stillbirth was calculated per 1,000 ongoing pregnancies, the rate increased sixfold from 0.35 per 1,000 ongoing pregnancies at 37 weeks of gestation to 2.12 per 1,000 ongoing pregnancies at 43 weeks. With advancing gestation, neonatal and postneonatal mortality decreased significantly, from 151.4 neonatal deaths and 31.7 postneonatal deaths per 1,000 live births at 28 weeks, to 0.7 neonatal deaths and 1.3 postneonatal deaths per 1,000 live births at 41 weeks of gestation. However, neonatal and postneonatal mortality increased thereafter to 1.6 neonatal deaths and 2.1 postneonatal deaths per 1,000 live births at 43 weeks of gestation. When the overall risk of pregnancy loss (stillbirth plus infant mortality) was calculated per 1,000 ongoing pregnancies, the risk increased eightfold from 0.7 per 1,000 ongoing pregnan-

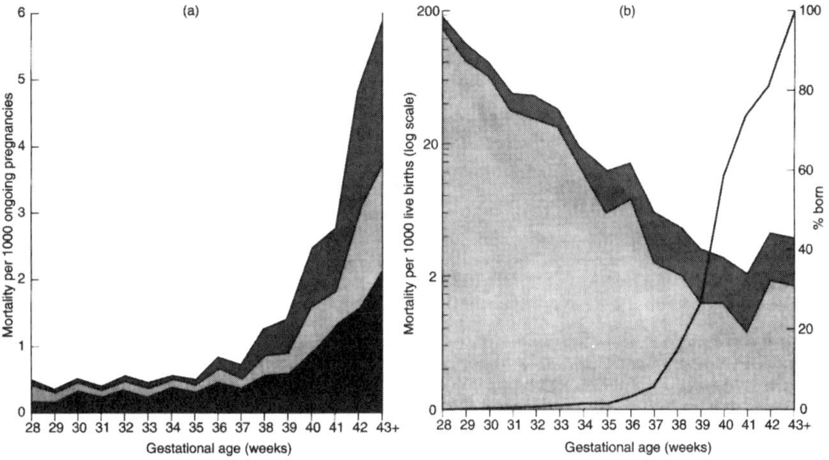

FIGURE 1.—The summed mortality at each gestation for the rate of stillbirth (*black shaded area*), neonatal death (*light shaded area*), and postneonatal death (*dark gray shaded area*) expressed per 1,000 ongoing pregnancies (**A**), and per 1,000 live births (**B**). In (**B**), the likelihood of delivery at each gestation is also shown (*dark solid line*). (Courtesy of Hilder L, Costeloe K, Thilaganathan B: Prolonged pregnancy: Evaluating gestation-specific risks of fetal and infant mortality. *Br J Obstet Gynaecol* 105:169–173. Copyright 1998, Blackwell Science Ltd.)

cies at 37 weeks of gestation to 5.8 per 1,000 ongoing pregnancies at 43 weeks (Fig 1).

Discussion.—A more accurate method of determining the risks of prolonged gestation on pregnancy is by calculating fetal and infant loss per 1,000 ongoing pregnancies. In prolonged pregnancy, the risk of stillbirth and neonatal and postneonatal mortality are significantly higher. These data may help pregnant women and health care providers make decisions about obstetric intervention.

► Whether perinatal mortality is increased after either 41 or 42 completed weeks of gestation remains controversial in our literature, and this study of births registered from 18 regional hospitals in London helps explain some of the confusion. Bear in mind that registry data do not allow evaluation of approaches to the clinical management of "postdatism," nor how often induction of labor was used for postdate pregnancy, if at all. Clinical management is a major unspecified and therefore uncontrolled variable. So too is the availability of skilled newborn care including neonatal intubation. If one calculates the risk of perinatal and early neonatal death in the total of 171,527 births reported here as a function of deaths per 1,000 births, there are no significant rate increases as one goes sequentially from 38 to 43 weeks' gestation or beyond. The same lack of surplus postdates mortality appears in the Oxford University Database when one goes from 40 to 42 weeks' gestation.[1] The same result is seen in data derived from the Dublin National Mortality Center.[2] If, however, one uses as the denominator the number of women with ongoing pregnancies after 41 weeks, that number being consecutively reduced by continuing births from 23% at 41 weeks to

6% at 42 weeks to 1% at 43 weeks, total perinatal and neonatal mortality rates calculated in that way increase sequentially past 41 weeks. Much of that increase is the augmented impact of perinatal deaths divided by an increasingly small denominator. When the same approach is applied to stillbirth rates, the primary concern in managing postdate pregnancy, no significant increase is seen after 40 weeks using as the denominator the number of still ongoing pregnancies. Which statistic is appropriate depends on whether one's point of view is with the entire population of parturients, or only with those still pregnant after 42 weeks' gestation. Remember that attempts to improve survival in postdate pregnancy, regardless of the estimated risk, has never been demonstrated uniformly failed by controlled study. This experience helps support the contention that the risk of stillbirth is not increased in postdate pregnancy.

T.H. Kirschbaum, M.D.

References

1. Bakketieg LS, Bergso P: Post-term pregnancy: Magnitude of the problem, in Chalmers I, Enkin M, Keirse MJNC (eds): *Effective Care in Pregnancy and Childbirth*, vol 1. Oxford, Oxford University Press, 1989, pp 765–775.
2. Crowley P: Post-term pregnancy: Induction or surveillance? in Chalmers I, Enkin M, Keirse MJNC (eds): *Effective Care in Pregnancy and Childbirth*, vol 1. Oxford, Oxford University Press, 1989, pp 776–791.

Intrapartum Mucosal Exposure to Human Immunodeficiency Virus Type 1 (HIV-1) of Infants Born to HIV-1–Infected Mothers Correlates With Maternal Plasma Virus Burden

Ait-Khaled M, Lyall EGH, Stainsby C, et al (Imperial College School of Medicine at St Mary's, London)
J Infect Dis 177:1097–1100, 1998 2–7

Background.—Most vertical infections with HIV type 1 (HIV-1) occur at or near delivery, which strongly suggests a mucosal route of transmission. The frequency and level of intrapartum mucosal exposure to HIV-1 of infants born to infected mothers was determined.

Methods.—Twenty-two infants were studied. Maternal plasma HIV-1 RNA and CD4 cell count were measured at delivery. Reverse transcription–polymerase chain reaction and qualitative nucleic acid sequence-based amplification were used to determine the presence of HIV-1 RNA infant oropharyngeal aspirates taken at birth.

Findings.—Forty-one percent of the infants had detectable levels of HIV-1 RNA. In 3 of these 9 infants, the levels were quantifiable, with a mean of 3,000 copies/mL. However, mucosal exposure during delivery did not result in infection in any of the infants. Cesarean delivery did not decrease mucosal exposure to HIV-1. Mucosal exposure was unassociated with maternal CD4 cell count but was correlated with maternal plasma virus load and was decreased by antiviral treatment.

Conclusion.—About 40% of the infants in this series had virus in oropharyngeal aspirates. Intrapartum exposure to a detectable level was correlated with maternal plasma HIV burden. Perinatal antiretroviral treatment was significantly correlated with a decreased incidence of oral exposure to HIV-1.

▶ This pilot study involving 22 infants born to HIV-1–positive women serves to confirm the role of the fetal oropharyngeal route in maternal-to-fetal transmission of the virus. Among these women (median age, 28 years), there was only a single case of AIDS; maternal diagnosis was made by viral culture and polymerase chain reaction for blood HIV RNA. Included were 7 women with proven prior maternal-to-fetal infection experiences. Twelve women had received azidothymidine in accordance with the AIDS Clinical Trial Group 076 protocol.[1] Nine of 22 newborns shows HIV-1 virus present in oropharyngeal aspirates obtained immediately after birth, and in 7 of those cases, delivery was by cesarean section.

If confirmed in larger numbers of patients, this observation weighs against the use of cesarean section to avoid contact with vaginal secretions in HIV-1–positive gravidas, and suggests maternal hematogenous seeding of amniotic fluid before delivery or indirectly through contact with maternal blood at the time of surgery. Although the oropharyngeal route has been proven to cause infection in newborn rhesus monkeys, the viral dosage in that case was very large, and in these human infants, the oropharyngeal viral load was small. No cases of newborn infection occurred in these infants. As expected, 12 of 13 women being treated on the azidothymidine protocol 076 were delivered of infants without evidence of HIV RNA and benefited by a roughly 85% reduction in the maternal plasma viral load at the time of delivery.

T.H. Kirschbaum, M.D.

Reference

1. 1995 Year Book of Obstetrics and Gynecology, pp 76–77.

Acceptability and Impact of Zidovudine for Prevention of Mother-to-Child Human Immunodeficiency Virus-1 Transmission in France

Mayaux M-J, Teglas J-P, Mandelbrot L, et al (INSERM, Hôpital Bicêtre, Le Kremlin Bicêtre, France; Hôpital Necker Enfants Malades, Paris)

J Pediatr 131:857–862, 1997 2–8

Objective.—Whereas the ACTG076 (zidovudine) trial established a two-thirds reduction in the transmission rate of HIV-1 from mother to child, efficacy in routine practice has not been proven. The acceptability and impact of zidovudine prophylaxis on prevention of HIV transmission in a nationwide cohort of infants born to HIV-seropositive mothers was studied prospectively in France.

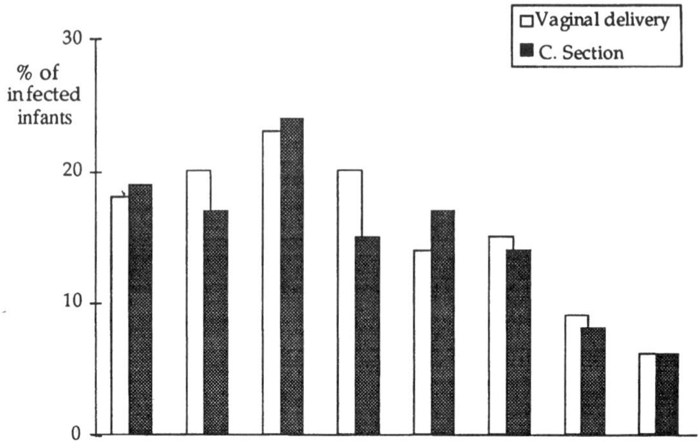

FIGURE.—Percentage of infected infants delivered vaginally or by cesarean procedure in the French prospective cohort from 1986 through 1995. (Courtesy of Mayaux M-J, Teglas J-P, Mandelbrot L, et al: Acceptability and impact of zidovudine for prevention of mother-to-child human immunodeficiency virus-1 transmission in France. *J Pediatr* 131:857–862, 1997.)

Methods.—From 1986 through 1995, the transmission rate among treated and untreated women was compared. Children were followed up at 3-month intervals from birth to 18 months, and then at 6-month intervals if infected. Women's clinical and biological characteristics, mode of delivery, and use of zidovudine therapy before pregnancy were recorded.

Results.—From 1986 through 1989, no women were treated with zidovudine. From 1990 through 1993, 9% of women were treated. During 1994 and 1995, 501 women received zidovudine therapy, and 154 did not. Only 6 mothers refused treatment. The percentage of children born infected was 5% in treated mothers and 14% in untreated mothers. Women who received zidovudine before pregnancy had a 20% transmission rate despite prevention therapy, whereas women who were not pretreated had a transmission rate of 5%. The difference was significant and remained significant after adjusting for maternal CD4+ cell count and p24 antigenemia. The transmission rate in untreated women declined from 18% during the period between 1986 and 1993 to 14% during 1994 and 1995, regardless of mode of delivery (Fig).

Conclusions.—Prophylactic zidovudine therapy for pregnant women significantly lowers the transmission rate of HIV-1, and justifies offering HIV screening to all pregnant women.

► It is 1 thing to demonstrate the usefulness of AZT in preventing maternal-to-fetal newborn transmission in a study population,[1–3] but another to demonstrate actual drug utility in the longitudinal study of HIV-positive women. This report is part of the continuing work of the French Pediatric HIV Infection Study Group,[4] and it shows extremely rapid utilization by the population and prompt effectiveness.

The cohort began to be assembled in 1986 and consists of one-third African-born women, yielding data from about 250 pairs of pregnant women and their infants each year. When results of the ACTC 076 study were released in February 1994, AZT was being used by only 24% of pregnant women. By the last 4 months of 1994, that rate had risen to about 90% where it has remained since. Eighty-three percent of gravidas receiving AZT received dosages during pregnancy, the intrapartum period, and the neonatal interval. Using as concurrent controls women not taking AZT with comparable severity of disease judged by CD4/CD8 counts and P24 antigenemia, infant transmission fell from 13%–17% to 5%. Despite data suggesting lower transmission with abdominal vs. vaginal birth by other centers,[5, 6] no difference in transmission rate by route of delivery was seen in this study. That same observation was previously reported by the French Study Group. Neither CD4 counts nor P24 antigenemia were in greater evidence in cases of infant transmission. This matches the observation that virus load, i.e., the amount of circulating HIV-RNA, is a better measure of the potential for transmission from maternal blood.[7] This sort of cohort study needs to be repeated using HIV-RNA assay as an independent variable.

T.H. Kirschbaum, M.D.

References

1. 1995 Year Book of Obstetrics and Gynecology, pp 76–77.
2. 1996 Year Book of Obstetrics and Gynecology, pp 84–85.
3. 1997 Year Book of Obstetrics, Gynecology, and Women's Health, pp 84–86.
4. 1996 Year Book of Obstetrics and Gynecology, pp 79–80.
5. 1996 Year Book of Obstetrics and Gynecology, pp 77–79.
6. 1997 Year Book of Obstetrics, Gynecology, and Women's Health, pp 86–87.
7. 1997 Year Book of Obstetrics, Gynecology, and Women's Health, pp 82–84.

Prospective Evaluation of 618 Pregnant Women Exposed to Parvovirus B19: Risks and Symptoms

Harger JH, Adler SP, Koch WC, et al (Univ of Pittsburgh, Pa; Med College of Virginia/Virginia Commonwealth Univ, Richmond)
Obstet Gynecol 91:413–420, 1998 2–9

Background.—The exact risk of fetal death in pregnant women with parvovirus B19 infection is unknown. The risk of fetal morbidity from such maternal infection was determined, together with the risk of maternal parvovirus B19 infection from exposure to various sources.

Methods.—Demographic and occupational data were obtained on pregnant women exposed to sources of B19 and on the nature and duration of the exposures. Serologic testing was performed 10 to 14 days after exposure, using an indirect capture enzyme-linked immunosorbent assay. Women with IgM were assessed by US weekly until 12 weeks after exposure. Pregnancy outcomes were documented.

Findings.—Half of the 618 women exposed were immune to B19. Fifty women (16.7% of all susceptible) contracted B19 infection. None of the fetuses of these infected women experienced nonimmune hydrops. No fetal deaths were attributable to B19 in this group. If the source of infection was a related child living in the household, the relative risk of maternal B19 infection was 2.8. Occupation did not affect infection rates. Symptoms of polyarthralgia occurred in 46% of the women, fever in 19%, and non-specific rash in 38%. These symptoms were significantly more common in immunoglobulin (Ig)M-positive patients than in uninfected women. Thirty-three percent of the IgM-positive women were completely asymptomatic.

Conclusion.—The fetal risk of nonimmune hydrops after maternal B19 infection appears to be very low. Excluding pregnant women from the workplace during endemic periods with seasonal clusters of cases is unwarranted. Weekly fetal US assessment in this population has a low yield.

► Although it has been known that parvovirus B19 can infect fetuses and cause hydrops and fetal death, it has never been clear what the prospective risks are following a significant maternal exposure. In these 618 gravidas with likely exposure to erythema infectiosum collected during an endemic episode in Pittsburgh, the results are comforting. Of those women exposed, 50% bore IgG to parvovirus B19 and were immune. Of those 311 women who were susceptible, 52, or 16.7%, were shown to have IgM without IgG, suggesting recent infection.

The risk of infection was greater (29.4%) among women exposed to a child in their own residence but was less (8.4%) for all other contacts. This means that the risk of infection varies in this group from 4.2% to 14.7% depending on the site of contact. No cases of fetal hydrops or perinatal death occurred, but the 95% confidence interval based on sample size is 0 to 8.6%. This means that the maximum risk of hydrops and fetal death varies between 0.4% and 1.2% based on this report. Remember that not all cases of hydrops are fatal and that fetal transfusion can effectively treat some hydropic fetuses and sustain them into the third trimester, at which point the effects of the fetal infection are ameliorated.[1, 2]

T.H. Kirschbaum, M.D.

References

1. 1993 Year Book of Obstetrics and Gynecology, p 239.
2. 1996 Year Book of Obstetrics and Gynecology, p 133.

Detection of Parvovirus B19 Infection in First and Second Trimester Fetal Loss

de Krijger RR, van Elsacker-Niele A-MW, Mulder-Stapel A, et al (Erasmus Univ, Rotterdam, The Netherlands; State Univ, Leiden, The Netherlands)

Pediatr Pathol Lab Med 18:23–34, 1998 2–10

Background.—More research is needed to determine the potential developmental effect of parvovirus B19 on the human fetus. The frequency of parvovirus B19 infection was established in a large series of first and second trimester fetal losses.

Methods.—Fetal and placental tissue and maternal sera were obtained from 273 women experiencing first and second trimester fetal loss. Fetal tissues were assessed for the presence of congenital anomalies. The presence of parvovirus B19 infection was detected by serology of maternal sera, histology of fetal tissue and placenta, polymerase chain reaction (PCR), in situ hybridization, and immunohistochemistry. Serum samples were assessed for B19-specific immunoglobulin M (IgM) and/or IgG using an enzyme-linked immunosorbent assay method.

Findings.—Serology indicated that 149 cases were not related to B19 infection. These cases were excluded from the final analysis. Overall, 0.7% of the cases had parvovirus B19-specific IgM and IgG at the time of abortion. Histology revealed 10 cases of nuclear vacuolization in fetal erythroid progenitor cells in fetal or placental tissue in 10 patients. However, this vacuolization was judged to be a fixation artifact. Parvovirus B19 DNA was detected in placental tissue by PCR in only 1 of these 10 cases. No congenital anomalies were found in any of the 41 patients in whom fetal tissue was available.

Conclusion.—The frequency of maternal parvovirus B19 infection in this series was only 0.8%. This low frequency does not permit conclusions regarding the occurrence of congenital anomalies resulting from parvovirus B19 infection. The use of nuclear histology to detect fetal parvovirus B19 infection is a nonspecific parameter requiring PCR confirmation.

► This study of 273 first-and second-trimester fetal deaths is useful in establishing an incidence figure for lethal fetal parvovirus infections in unselected cases and confirms the superiority of PCR using primers specific to a known segment of viral DNA for the diagnosis.[1] In only 2 of the cases studied was the development of maternal IgM to parvovirus antigen useful in making the diagnosis of maternal infection (0.7 % incidence) and in 1 case, placental PCR was positive, proving coincident fetal infection. The authors believe that histologic diagnosis based on intranuclear vacuole formation is relatively useless because of the large number of false positives. This article sets a far lower incidence estimate for fetal infection than the 18% estimate found in archival specimens of cases of lethal nonimmune hydrops reported earlier[2] and gives a more realistic estimate of occurrence than that derived from sporadic endemic outbreaks of erythema infectiosum.

T.H. Kirschbaum, M.D.

References

1. 1994 Year Book of Obstetrics and Gynecology, pp 131–132.
2. 1997 Year Book of Obstetrics, Gynecology, and Women's Health, pp 195–196.

Concomitant Use of Glucocorticoids: A Comparison of Two Metaanalyses on Antibiotic Treatment in Preterm Premature Rupture of Membranes

Leitich H, Egarter C, Reisenberger K, et al (Univ of Vienna)

Am J Obstet Gynecol 178:899–908, 1998 2–11

Background.—Preterm birth occurs in 8% to 10% of pregnancies, and about 35% of preterm births are preceded by premature rupture of membranes. There is evidence that infections are involved in preterm birth and in preterm premature rupture of membranes. Three meta-analyses have shown that antibiotic treatment in such cases can be beneficial. Glucocorticoids are recommended in preterm premature rupture of membranes because they have a protective effect on neonatal mortality, respiratory distress syndrome, and intraventricular hemorrhage. In a meta-analysis, it was determined whether the beneficial effect of antibiotics on maternal and neonatal morbidity is changed when glucocorticoids are included in the treatment of preterm premature rupture of membranes.

Methods.—A meta-analysis was conducted of 5 randomized trials of antibiotic treatment for preterm premature rupture of membranes, in which treatment glucocorticoids were also used. The results were compared to the results of a previous meta-analysis of antibiotic treatment in which glucocorticoids were not used. Outcome measures were chorioamnionitis, postpartum endometritis, neonatal sepsis, respiratory distress syndrome, intraventricular hemorrhage, necrotizing enterocolitis, and neonatal mortality. The effect of glucocorticoids on antibiotic treatment was determined by logistic regression analysis.

Results.—The 5 previously published trials of antibiotic treatment and use of glucocorticoids analyzed 509 patients (Table 4). No significant effect of antibiotic treatment was seen on the outcomes analyzed was seen. However, antibiotic treatment without use of glucocorticoids reduced the odds of chorioamnionitis by 62%, postpartum endometritis by 50%, neonatal sepsis by 68%, and intraventricular hemorrhage by 50% (Table 6). Logistic regression analysis revealed that glucocorticoids significantly decreased the effect of antibiotics on chorioamnionitis and neonatal sepsis (Table 7).

Discussion.—These findings indicate that glucocorticoids decrease the benefits of antibiotic treatment in preterm premature rupture of mem-

TABLE 4.—Neonatal Outcome of Antibiotic Plus Glucocorticoid Treatment vs. Glucocorticoid Treatment

	Mortality		*Sepsis*		*RDS*		*IVH*		*NEC*	
Study	*Antibiotics*	*Control*	*Antibiotics*	*Control*	*Antibiotics*	*Control*	*Antibiotics*	*Control*	*Antibiotics*	*Control*
Dunlop et al.	4/24	1/24	5/24	1/24	8/24	7/24	3/24	7/24	1/24	1/24
Amon et al.	2/43	6/39	1/42	6/36	—	—	4/42	6/36	5/42	4/36
Morales et al.	2/44	5/43	3/44	3/43	9/44	14/43	7/44	6/43	1/44	0/43
Mercer et al.	9/109*	10/114*	14/109*	15/107*	27/109*	24/107*	11/109*	14/107*	8/109*	12/107*
Lockwood et al.	3/37†	3/35†	2/36†	3/34†	23/36†	20/34†	5/36†	7/34†	2/36†	0/34†
TOTAL	20/257	25/255	25/255	28/244	67/213	65/208	30/255	40/244	17/255	17/244
Percent	7.8	9.8	9.8	11.5	31.5	31.3	11.8	16.4	6.7	7.0
OR	0.78		0.84		1.00		0.68		0.94	
95% CI	0.42–1.43, NS		0.48–1.49, NS		0.65–1.54, NS		0.41–1.13, NS		0.47–1.90, NS	

*Including 6 sets of twins.
†Three patients without results.
Abbreviations: IVH, intraventricular hemorrhage; *NEC*, necrotizing enterocolitis; *NS*, not significant; *RDS*, respiratory distress syndrome.
(Courtesy of Leitich H, Egarter C, Reisenberger K, et al: Concomitant use of glucocorticoids: A comparison of two metaanalyses on antibiotic treatment in preterm premature rupture of membranes. *Am J Obstet Gynecol* 178:899–908, 1998.)

TABLE 6.—Neonatal Outcome of Antibiotic Treatment vs. No Treatment (Results From Our Previous Meta-analysis)

	Mortality		*Sepsis*		*RDS*		*IVH*		*NEC*	
Study	*Antibiotics*	*Control*	*Antibiotics*	*Control*	*Antibiotics*	*Control*	*Antibiotics*	*Control*	*Antibiotics*	*Control*
TOTAL	17/212	19/217	8/254	27/254	94/251	105/258	19/210	37/217	17/210	14/217
Percent	8.0	8.8	3.1	10.6	37.5	40.7	9.0	17.1	8.1	6.5
OR	0.92		0.32		0.84		0.50		1.27	
95% CI	0.46–1.81, NS		0.16–0.65, $p=0.001$		0.58–1.22, NS		0.28–0.89, $p=0.019$		0.61–2.62, NS	

Abbreviations: CI, confidence interval; *IVH*, intraventricular hemorrhage; *NEC*, necrotizing enterocolitis; *NS*, not significant; *OR*, odds ratio; *RDS*, respiratory distress syndrome.

(Courtesy of Leitich H, Egarter C, Reisenberger K, et al: Concomitant use of glucocorticoids: A comparison of two metaanalyses on antibiotic treatment in preterm premature rupture of membranes. *Am J Obstet Gynecol* 178:899–908, 1998.)

TABLE 7.—Results of Logistic Regression Analyses

	Chorioamnionitis	*Endometritis*	*Neonatal sepsis*	*IVH*
Univariate analyses				
Effect of antibiotic treatment in all studies	OR = 0.53, $p = 0.0001$	OR = 0.64, $p = 0.048$	OR = 0.56, $p = 0.01$	OR = 0.59, $p = 0.007$
Effect of antibiotic treatment in studies *without* concomitant glucocorticoid treatment	OR = 0.37, $p = 0.0001$	OR = 0.47, $p = 0.03$	OR = 0.27, $p = 0.002$	OR = 0.48, $p = 0.02$
Effect of antibiotic treatment in studies *with* concomitant glucocorticoid treatment	OR = 0.88, $p = 0.57$	OR = 0.83, $p = 0.56$	OR = 0.84, $p = 0.55$	OR = 0.68, $p = 0.14$
Multivariate analyses				
Test of interaction between antibiotic and glucocorticoid treatment	$p = 0.006$	$p = 0.22$	$p = 0.03$	$p = 0.39$
OR of antibiotic plus glucocorticoid treatment versus antibiotic treatment	OR = 1.32	OR = 1.89	OR = 3.34	OR = 1.34

Abbreviations: IVH, intraventricular hemorrhage; *OR*, odds ratio.

(Courtesy of Leitich H, Egarter C, Reisenberger K, et al: Concomitant use of glucocorticoids: A comparison of two metaanalyses on antibiotic treatment in preterm premature rupture of membranes. *Am J Obstet Gynecol* 178:899–908, 1998.)

branes. It is recommended that patients who may benefit from these treatment protocols be selected carefully.

► As discussed here often before,[1] meta-analyses, adapted from the social and behavioral sciences, group similar studies with the same research aim in the hope of obtaining evidence of statistical significance, not previously established, by increasing the number of cases available for study. Its problems are not computational, nor with claims of statistical significance, but, rather, with the meaning of those claims, in view of the inevitable differences among aggregated studies de facto. These investigators are careful, thoughtful statisticians, who freely list the possibilities for heterogeneity in data aggregates and the possible confounding variables. Patients studied here had premature preterm rupture of membranes as early as 20–26 weeks of pregnancy. In an early meta-analysis of neonatal outcome of 7 clinical trials comparing results of antibiotic therapy with those with no therapy, the authors were able to establish the value of antibiotic therapy quite convincingly.[2] Here, in a group of 5 studies of such patients treated with glucocorticoids with and without antibiotics, the authors attempt to estimate the impact of glucocorticoids added to antibiotic therapy in these cases. All 5 studies are randomized and controlled including a total of 509 women. The studies differ among themselves with respect to the inclusion of patients between 20 and 26 weeks of gestational age, the presence of chorioamnionitis, the inclusion of twins, the absence of observer blinding, the method of randomization, the antibiotic and glucocorticoid types, the dosages, and the use of tocolytics. As before, the authors were able to demonstrate improved outcome with antibiotics in preterm premature rupture of membranes, in treating chorioamnionitis, preventing endometritis, and reducing the likelihood of neonatal sepsis or newborn infant ventricular hemorrhage with or without steroids. In examining the differences between women on antibiotics with and without steroids, no beneficial effects of added steroids could be proven. Women on antibiotics without steroids had odds ratios suggesting a more favorable benefit among the outcome variables than women on antibiotics with steroids. No impact on infant mortality was discerned with any treatment combination of drugs aimed at this problem. This is an interesting set of observations which would justify a well-constructed prospective controlled study. One cannot exclude nor estimate the likelihood that these results are caused by a lack of uniformity in gestational age, type and dose of antibiotics, use of tocolytics, and inclusion of twin pregnancies, which all act as confounding variables in producing what may be a spurious conclusion.

T.H. Kirschbaum, M.D.

References

1. 1997 Year Book of Obstetrics, Gynecology, and Women's Health, pp 33–37.
2. 1997 Year Book of Obstetrics, Gynecology, and Women's Health, pp 36–37.

Effect of Maternal Carbohydrate Metabolism on Fetal Growth

Caruso A, Paradisi G, Ferrazzani S, et al (Catholic Univ, Rome; Indiana Univ, Indianapolis)

Obstet Gynecol 92:8–12, 1998 2–12

Background.—Identifying the causes of fetal growth restriction (FGR) is essential for designing effective preventive and treatment strategies. The effects of maternal carbohydrate metabolism and anthropometric characteristics on fetal growth were investigated.

Methods.—Eight women in their third trimester of pregnancy with unexplained FGR and 11 women in the third trimester with normally developing fetuses were studied. Maternal carbohydrate metabolism was assessed using oral glucose tolerance tests and hyperinsulinemic-euglycemic clamps.

Findings.—Compared with the control group, the women with FGR fetuses were more sensitive to insulin and had lower insulin and glucose areas under the curve (Fig 1). The 2 groups did not differ in fasting plasma glucose, insulin, and human placental lactogen samples, age, height, pregravid weight, weight gain, and parity. Overall, maternal insulin sensitivity and weight gain were associated with relative birth weight. Analyzed separately, insulin sensitivity was strongly negatively correlated with relative birth weight in women with FGR pregnancies but not in control subjects. In the control group, the best correlation between relative birth weight and other variables was in maternal weight gain.

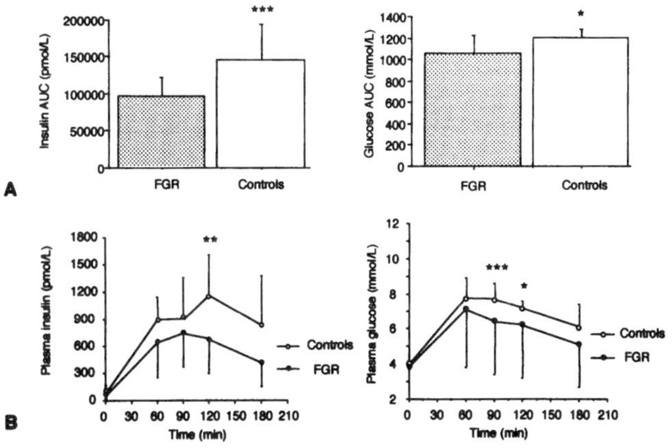

FIGURE 1.—Mean insulin and glucose areas under the curve (AUC) (**A**) and plasma levels (**B**) after glucose tolerance test in pregnancies with normal fetal growth (controls, n = 11) and pregnancies with fetal growth restriction (*FGR*, n = 8). *$P < 0.05$, **$P < 0.04$; ***$P < 0.03$ compared with other group. *Error bars*, standard deviation of the mean. (Courtesy of Caruso A, Paradisi G, Ferrazzani S, et al: Effect of maternal carbohydrate metabolism on fetal growth. *Obstet Gynecol* 92:8–12, 1998. Reprinted with permission from the American College of Obstetricians and Gynecologists.)

Conclusions.—Glucose metabolic patterns differ between women with unexplained FGR and women with normal pregnancies. Increased insulin sensitivity may lead to a decrease in metabolic substrates for fetal growth.

▶ Although this study of 8 pregnant women in the third trimester of pregnancy with unexplained fetal growth retardation and of 11 controls needs to be extended to provide additional data, the work is well done and the inference provocative. The usual maternal pregnancy metabolic adaptations include hyperlipidemia, insulin resistance, and postprandial hyperglycemia—all apparently designed to ensure sufficient maternal blood nutrient concentration to guarantee the presence of a sharp concentration gradient between maternal and fetal blood. Such a gradient is necessary to provide adequate fetal nutrient supply acquired by either simple or facilitated diffusion, both of which depend on that concentration gradient. In aggregate, these 8 women bearing growth-retarded fetuses verified by newborn examination failed to show the decreased insulin sensitivity of normal pregnancy. Insulin sensitivity was measured as a function of the quantity of infused 20% glucose required to maintain normoglycemia in the face of a constant insulin infusion of 40 mU per square meter of maternal surface area—the hyperinsulinemic-euglycemic clamp technique. Human placental lactogen, a prominent factor in reducing insulin sensitivity during pregnancy, was also found to be lower in concentration in women bearing growth-retarded infants than in controls. This evidence strongly suggests that among the causes of fetal growth retardation is failure to develop the insulin resistance and the tendency to hyperglycemia of normal pregnancy. The mechanisms by which this comes about are uncertain, but this is an important observation.

T.H. Kirschbaum, M.D.

Elevated Levels of Lipoprotein(a) in Women With Preeclampsia

Wang J, Mimuro S, Lahoud R, et al (Univ of Sydney, Australia; Univ of New South Wales, Westmead, Australia)

Am J Obstet Gynecol 178:146–149, 1998 2–13

Objective.—Preeclampsia is a serious complication of the second half of pregnancy that reduces placental perfusion and can lead to growth retardation, morbidity, and mortality. Because altered coagulability may be involved in the pathogenesis of preeclampsia, levels of lipoprotein(a), a blood coagulation enhancer, may be a marker of the severity of preeclampsia. The associations between circulating lipoprotein(a) and the presence of mild and severe preeclampsia in 50 pregnant women was investigated.

Methods.—Plasma lipoprotein(a) levels were measured using enzyme-linked immunosorbent assay in 24 normal pregnant women and in 26 women with preeclampsia (18 mild and 8 severe). Lipoprotein(a) levels were compared statistically between groups.

Results.—Plasma lipoprotein(a) levels were significantly higher in women with severe preeclampsia than in women with mild preeclampsia

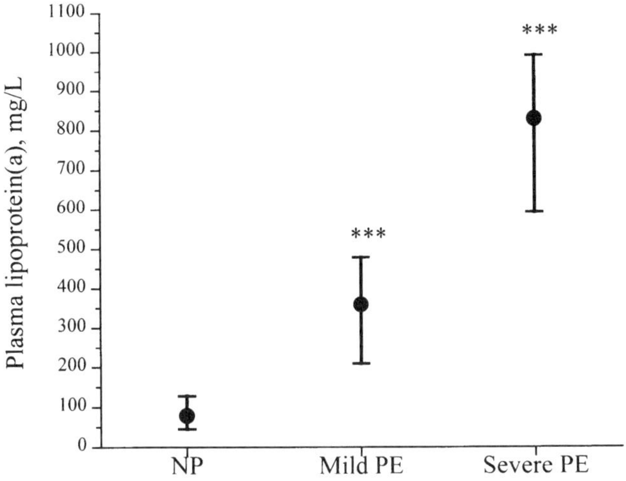

FIGURE 1.—Plasma lipoprotein(a) in normal pregnant (*NP*), mild preeclamptic (*mild PE*), and severe pereclamptic (*severe PE*), women. Data are median and interquartile range. *Three asterisks*, *P* less than 0.001 mild PE versus NP or severe PE versus mild PE. (Courtesy of Wang J, Mimuro S, Lahoud R, et al: Elevated levels of lipoprotein(a) in women with preeclampsia. *Am J Obstet Gynecol* 178:146–149, 1998).

and in women with normal pregnancies (Fig 1). The difference in lipoprotein(a) levels between women with mild preeclampsia and women with normal pregnancies was also significant.

Conclusion.—The plasma lipoprotein(a) level is a marker for severity of preeclampsia.

▶ This group of investigators demonstrates an extremely strong relationship between plasma lipoprotein(a) concentration measured by enzyme-linked immunosorbent assay and the severity of pregnancy hypertension in 26 women with preeclampsia compared with 24 normotensive gravidas. The observation is particularly interesting because the role of this bifid molecule, with covalent binding between a lipid portion rendering it active in cell membrane physiology and a protein portion serving as conduit for lipid transport and deposition, nicely fits the pathology of pregnancy-induced hypertension (PIH). The protein portion is structurally similar to plasminogen and competitively inhibits plasminogen binding to fibrin and damaged endothelium. Normally, plasminogen bound to fibrin is activated through interaction with a series of plasminogen activators and inhibitors, generating plasmin and initiating fibrinolysis. Lipoprotein (a), therefore, impedes fibrinolysis and facilitates clot formation. At the same time, the protein transport part of the molecule facilitates lipid deposition and atherosis at sites of damaged vascular endothelium and platelet aggregation.

If it is correct that PIH is characterized by endothelial injury, this helps explain the exaggerated atherosclerosis seen in maternal decidual vessels at the side of placental implantation, which is especially marked in primigravid PIH or preeclampsia. Both coagulation and atherosclerosis may well play a role in the vascular occlusion and resistance to blood flow characteristic of

PIH. This cohesive story makes lipoprotein(a) potentially a very important maternal marker of the severity of vascular injury in PIH.

T.H. Kirschbaum, M.D.

Is Tocolytic Magnesium Sulphate Associated With Increased Total Paediatric Mortality?

Mittendorf R, Covert R, Boman J, et al (Univ of Chicago)

Lancet 350:1517–1518, 1997 2–14

Introduction.—Previous retrospective studies suggest that antenatal magnesium sulfate may reduce the frequency of cerebral palsy among very preterm infants. This intervention was tested in a randomized, controlled trial, including tocolytic and preventive arms.

Methods.—The tocolytic arm of the study included women in preterm labor at less than 34 weeks' gestation and 4 cm or less dilation. The women were randomized in unblinded fashion to receive either magnesium sulfate in a 4 g bolus or other tocolytic therapy. The preventive arm included women in preterm labor with advanced cervical dilation who were not eligible for tocolysis. They were randomized in double-blind fashion to receive either magnesium sulfate, 4 g, or saline.

Results.—Among the patients randomized and exposed to magnesium sulfate, there were 9 deaths: 1 fetal, 4 neonatal, and 4 postneonatal. One pediatric death occurred in a woman randomized but not exposed to tocolytic magnesium sulfate, and another in a woman randomized but not exposed to saline. All deaths in the tocolytic arm occurred among patients initially randomized to magnesium sulfate. Overall, there were 10 pediatric deaths among 75 maternal randomizations to magnesium sulfate, and 1 pediatric death among 75 randomizations to other tocolytic agents or saline solution. In the tocolytic arm, there were 8 pediatric deaths in 46 randomizations to magnesium sulfate, and no pediatric deaths in 47 randomizations to other tocolytics, a risk difference of 15%.

Conclusions.—When used in women with very premature labor—particularly when used as a tocolytic—magnesium sulfate appears to be associated with increased pediatric deaths. For preeclamptic women at term, the safety and efficacy of magnesium sulfate are well documented.

▶ When 2 retrospective studies suggest a negative association between magnesium sulphate for tocolysis and cerebral palsy in preterm infants, a prospective randomized study is clearly warranted.[1, 2] These investigators from the Pritzker School of Medicine, funded by the United Cerebral Palsy Research and Education Foundation, undertook such a study. Preterm pregnancies were enrolled in a tocolytic arm (less than 34 weeks' gestational age, cervix equal to or less than 4 cm) and a preventive arm (cervix greater than 4 cm) with pregnancy-induced hypertension an exclusion variable. In the former study, magnesium sulphate was compared with any other tocolytic, and in the preventive arm, it was compared with saline administration.

This study, known as MAGnet, was terminated when a cluster of 1 fetal, 4 neonatal, and 4 perinatal deaths occurred, 7 in the tocolytic trial. No single pattern of pediatric mortality appeared. In one twin pregnancy at 26 weeks, complicated by twin-twin transfusion, the donor twin died in utero while the recipient twin, weighing 692 g at birth, died at 3 days. Both received magnesium sulphate. One neonatal twin died of apnea at 16 days (birth weight 1825 g) and another died at 24 days (1585 g) of congenital anomalies. Most suggestive were 3 cases of sudden infant death syndrome at greater than 30 days, and an infant death at 280 days due to respiratory apnea. Since these constituted a statistically significant increased incidence of pediatric mortality, compared to controls not given magnesium sulfate, the trial was terminated. The case numbers are small, frequency distributions by gestational age are not provided, and it is not clear that the same prolonged follow-up, extending as long as 9 months, was carried out in the control group as it was in the magnesium-treated group. There is more work that needs to be done on this observation. We should, however, be warned that magnesium tocolysis in preterm fetuses carries the potential for increased mortality, as these investigators showed. But the level of proof required for the discontinuance of this relatively common approach to the management of preterm labor is greater than the level required to terminate a study for which patient benefit is not assured.

T.H. Kirschbaum, M.D.

References

1. 1996 Year Book of Obstetrics and Gynecology, pp 126–128.
2. 1998 Year Book of Obstetrics, Gynecology, and Women's Health, pp 235–237.

Do Prostacyclin and Thromboxane Contribute to the "Protective Effect" of Pregnancies With Chronic Hypertension? A Preliminary Prospective Longitudinal Study

Moutquin J-M, Lindsay C, Arial N, et al (Laval Univ, Quebec City)
Am J Obstet Gynecol 177:1483–1490, 1997 2–15

Background.—Systemic production of thromboxane A_2 (TxA_2) and prostacyclin (PGI_2) can now be measured reliably through assessment of their major vascular metabolites. Nonpregnant patients with essential hypertension have been found to have reduced urinary concentrations of renal and systemic metabolites of these prostanoids compared to normotensive persons. The urinary excretion of the renal and systemic metabolites of TxA_2 and PGI_2 during normotensive and chronic hypertensive pregnancies was assessed prospectively.

Methods.—Pregnant hospital employees participated in the study. They collected 24-hour urine samples weekly from the seventh week to delivery. Renal metabolite concentrations were measured by radioimmunoassay

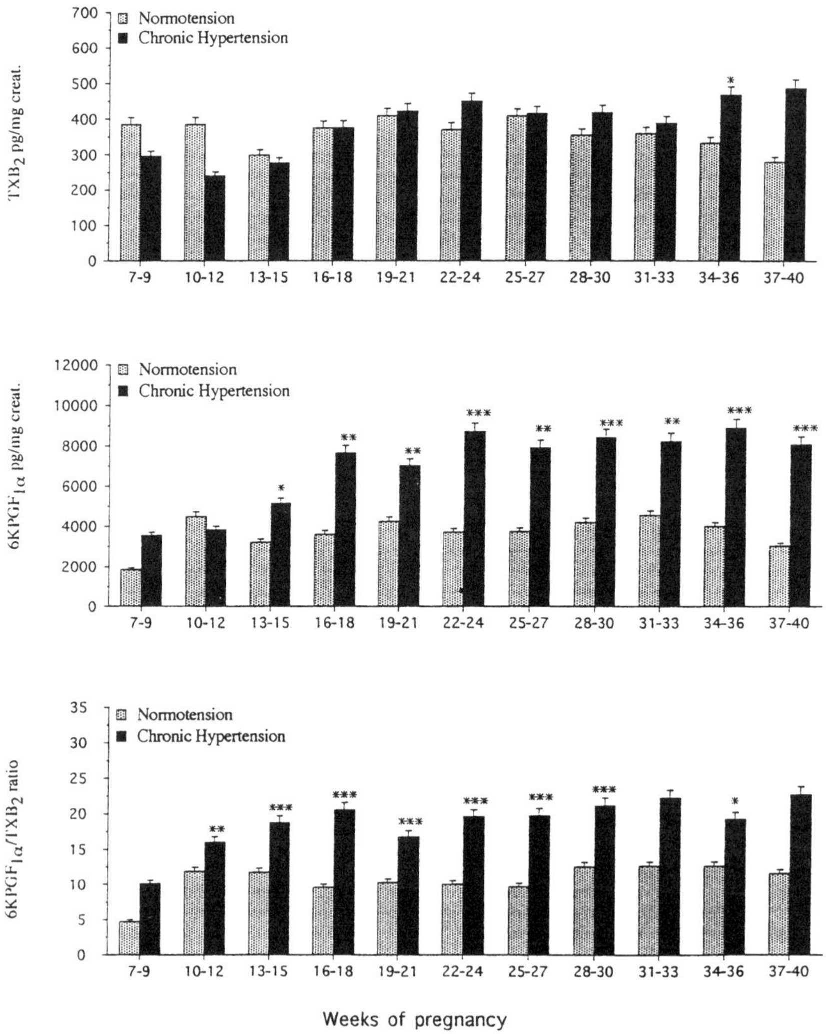

FIGURE 1.—Weekly 24-hour urinary excretion (mean ± SEM) of 2,3-dinor-thromboxane B_2 (TxB_2 (**upper panel**), 6-keto-prostaglandin$_{1\alpha}$ ($6KPGF_{1\alpha}$, **middle panel**), and ratios 6-keto-$PGF_{1\alpha/TXB_2}$ (**lower panel**) grouped in 3-week periods in normotensive and chronic hypertensive pregnancies. * $P < 0.05$; ** $P < 0.01$; *** $P < 0.001$. (Courtesy of Moutquin J-M, Lindsay C, Arial N, et al: Do prostacyclin and thromboxane contribute to the "protective effect" of pregnancies with chronic hypertension? A preliminary prospective longitudinal study. *Am J Obstet Gynecol* 177:1483–1490, 1997.)

after extraction, and systemic metabolites were measured by enzyme immunoassay after extraction and high-pressure liquid chromatographic separation.

Findings.—Normotensive and hypertensive pregnant women had similar thromboxane B_2 excretion. Compared to the normotensive women, however, hypertensive women had a 2-fold increase in 6-keto-prostaglan-

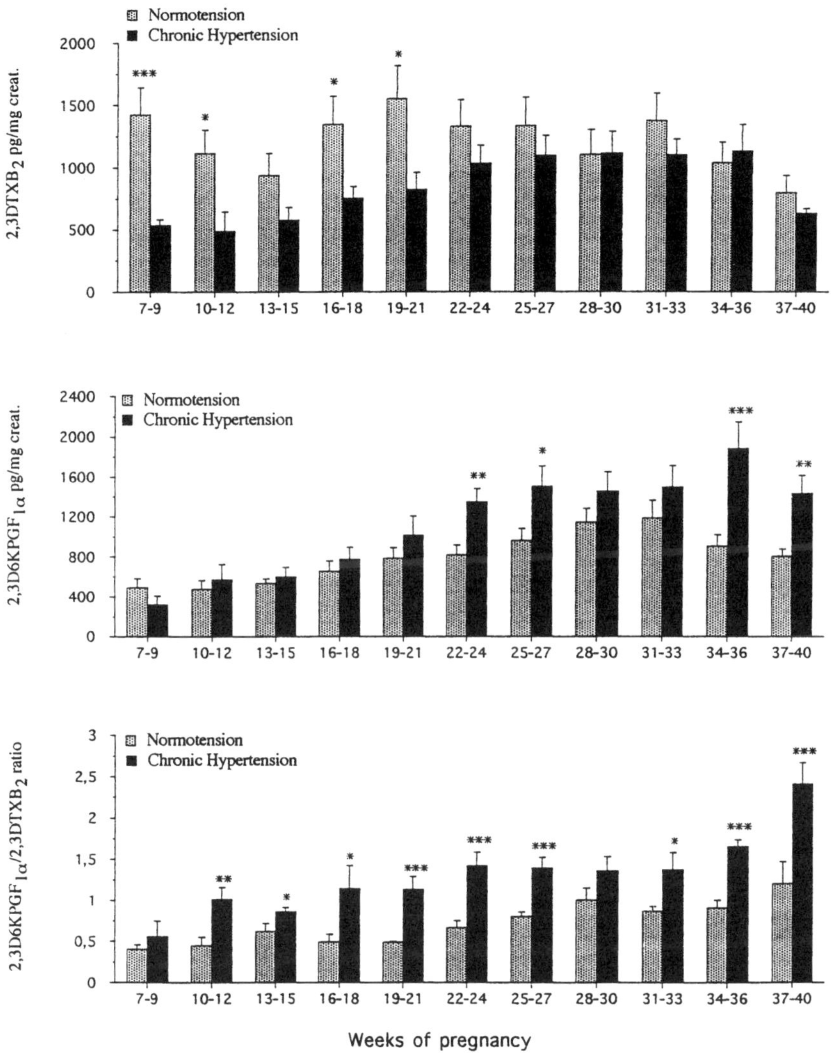

FIGURE 2.—Weekly 24-hour urinary excretion (mean ± SEM) of 2,3-dinor-thromboxane TxB_2 ($2,3DTXB_2$, upper panel), 2,3-prostaglandin$_{1\alpha}$ ($2,3D6KPGF1_{\alpha}$, (**middle panel**), and ratio 2,3-dinor-TxB_2/ 2,3-dinor-6-keto-$PGF_{1\alpha}$ (**lower panel**) grouped in 3-week periods in normotensive and chronic hypertensive pregnancies. * $P < 0.05$; ** $P < 0.01$; *** $P < 0.001$. (Courtesy of Moutquin J-M, Lindsay C, Arial N, et al: Do prostacyclin and thromboxane contribute to the "protective effect" of pregnancies with chronic hypertension? A preliminary prospective longitudinal study. *Am J Obstet Gynecol* 177:1483–1490, 1997.)

din $F_{1\alpha}$. Both groups had uniform excretion of thromboxane B_2 with progressively increased levels of 6-keto-prostaglandin $F_{1\alpha}$ in chronic hypertension. Mean 2,3-dinor-thromboxane B_2 was 1,208 pg/mg creatinine in the normotensive group and 898 pg/mg creatinine in the hypertensive group. This difference was mainly caused by significantly reduced concentrations in hypertension in the first half of the pregnancy. Conversely, mean

2,3-dinor-6-keto-prostaglandin $F_{1\alpha}$ levels were 845 and 1,226 pg/mg creatinine, respectively, primarily because of significantly increased production in hypertensive patients from 22 weeks and after. The ratios of renal and systemic metabolites favored increased PGI_2 production in chronically hypertensive women (Figs 1 and 2).

Conclusions.—Unlike preeclampsia, uncomplicated mild to moderate chronic hypertensive pregnancies are characterized by an excess of PGI_2 production with unchanged or even reduced concentrations of TxA_2. This may contribute to the generally favorable outcome of this hypertensive condition.

► Walsh and colleagues[1] suggested that a deficit of PGI_2 activity and a surplus of TxA_2 in preeclamptic women could account for the increase in the normally low peripheral vascular resistance of pregnancy and an enhanced capacity for vasoconstriction, platelet activation, and thrombopenia with release of platelet products underlying preeclampsia. This is a remarkable study of weekly urinary excretion of the metabolites of TxA_2 and PGI_2, including the 2, 3 dinor-metabolites thought to represent production rates of these prostanoids. Both sets of assays reveal women with chronic hypertension have reduced TxB_2 compared to normotensive women at from 7 to 13 weeks of gestational age but elevated PGI_2 metabolites thereafter to term. Two points are of special interest. Evidence of increased production and metabolism of PGI_2 coincides in gestation with the interval during which 40% to 50% of pregnant hypertensive women show a significant decrease in resting blood pressure. Second, increasing production of PGI_2 may be responsible for the generally benign course in women with chronic hypertension not complicated by renal insufficiency or superimposed pregnancy-induced hypertension and the normal survival rates in their infants. The authors plan to explore cases of superimposed pregnancy-induced hypertension and growth retardation in chronic hypertensive pregnancies as well. The results will be of great interest to all of us.

T.H. Kirschbaum, M.D.

Reference

1. 1993 Year Book of Obstetrics and Gynecology, pp 48–50.

The Obstetric Implications of Teenage Pregnancy

Lao TT, Ho LF (Univ of Hong Kong; Tsan Yuk Hosp, Hong Kong)

Hum Reprod 12:2303–2305, 1997 2–16

Background.—Teenage pregnancy is usually considered a high-risk category, as it has been associated with an increased risk of adverse pregnancy outcomes. However, previous studies that established such risk have generally involved teenagers who were socially and economically disadvantaged, whose pregnancies were unplanned, and who sought prenatal care

TABLE 2.—Labor and Delivery in Teenage and Nonteenage Mothers

	Teenage (n = 194)	Nonteenage (n = 4914)	Overall % (n = 67 925)
Labour			
spontaneous	166 (85.5)	4078 (83.0)	51 351 (75.6)
induced	23 (11.9)	674 (13.7)	8491 (12.5)
Delivery			
Vaginal, total	186 (95.9)	4350 (87.5)	52 642 (77.5)
spontaneous	154 (79.4)	3350 (67.8)	41 163 (60.6)
instrumental	30 (15.5)	902 (18.2)	10 800 (15.9)
breech	2 (1.0)	98 (2.0)	475 (0.7)
Cesarean section	8 (4.1)*	621 (12.6)	15 283 (22.5)
elective	5 (2.6)	162 (3.3)	7879 (11.6)
emergency	3 (1.6)	459 (9.3)	7401 (10.9)

Note: Results are expected in number (%) unless stated.
*Significantly different from nonteenage value: $P < 0.001$.
(Reprinted by permission of Oxford University Press, from Lao TT, Ho LF: The obstetric implications of teenage pregnancy. *Hum Reprod* 12:2303–2305, 1997, copyright European Society for Human Reproduction and Embryology.)

late in the pregnancy if at all. In recent years, care for teenaged mothers in Hong Kong has been improved. The effect of improved care on obstetric outcomes in this population was assessed.

Methods.—The outcomes of 194 teenage pregnancies resulting in births at 1 center in a 1-year period were reviewed retrospectively. Outcomes were compared with those of other obstetric populations at the same hospital that year.

Findings.—Compared to nonteenaged mothers, the teenaged mothers had an increased incidence of sexually transmitted diseases (1% and 5.2%, respectively) and preterm labor (7% and 13%, respectively). However, the incidence of gestational glucose intolerance was 3.1% in the teenaged mothers, compared to 11.4% among nonteenaged mothers. Types of labor did not differ between groups. The incidence of cesarean delivery was 4.1% in the teenaged group and 12.6% in the nonteenaged group, a significant difference. No differences were found in mean birth weight, gestation at delivery, incidence of total preterm delivery, or perinatal mortality or morbidity (Table 2).

Conclusions.—The major risk associated with pregnancy in teenagers is preterm labor. However, perinatal outcomes are favorable. The good outcomes achieved in this center may be because prenatal care is free and readily available and because of the quality of support provided by the teenaged mothers' families or welfare agencies.

► Teenage pregnancy has long been associated with increased risks of preterm birth, small-for-gestational age infants, perinatal morbidity, operative birth, and perinatal mortality.[1] This interesting comparison of pregnancy outcome in Hong Kong teenagers compared to about 5,000 nonteen gravidas suggests all those differences are related to teen adjustment problems and inadequate support. Citing improved support in community acceptance of teen pregnancy, this University of Hong Kong unit reports no surplus of adverse outcomes in 194 teen pregnancies and also records an expected reduction in the incidence of glucose intolerance and a cesarean section rate of only 4.1%. Unchanged is a significantly greater incidence of preterm labor and of delivery of infants weighing 2.5 kg not reflected either in increased perinatal mortality, impaired Apgar scores or NICU admission. There seems then to be little in teen pregnancy that constitutionally mitigates against successful pregnancy given effort toward community acceptance and support.

T.H. Kirschbaum, M.D.

Reference

1. 1989 YEAR BOOK OF OBSTETRICS AND GYNECOLOGY, pp 68–69.

Changes in Size of the Functional Cyst on Ultrasonography During Early Pregnancy

Kobayashi H, Yoshida A, Kobayashi M, et al (Natl Defense Med College, Tokorozawa, Saitama, Japan)

Am J Perinatol 14:1–4, 1997 2–17

Introduction.—Despite the advent of ultrasonic technology, it is still difficult to distinguish functional cysts from other anechoic adnexal cystic masses in early pregnancy. Some doctors recommend exploring masses surgically if they are present after 14 weeks or are greater than 6 cm in diameter, however, it is unknown whether operative intervention is necessary. This study reviews ultrasonic records of functional cysts to avoid unnecessary surgical intervention.

Methods.—There were 250 pregnant women with adnexal masses; of these, 58 were confirmed by ultrasonography at term. The masses were

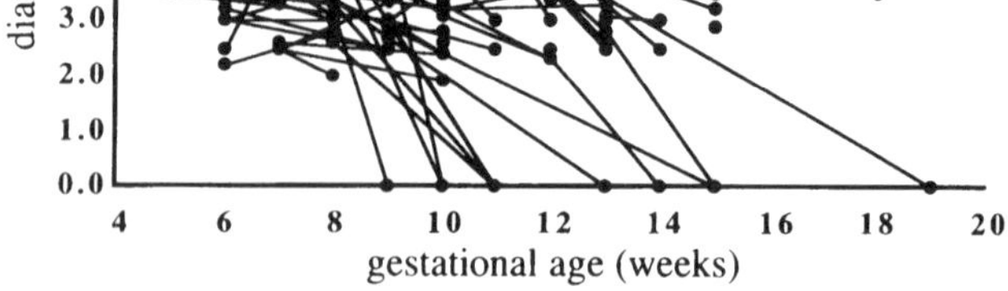

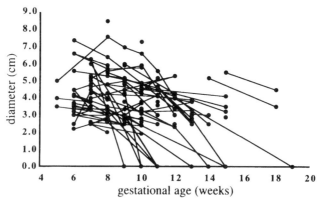

FIGURE 2.—Changes in the diameter of the functional cyst during the first 20 weeks of gestation (a total of 58 cases). The antepartum absence of all cysts was confirmed by ultrasonography at term. This absence on the term scans is not shown in the figure. (Reprinted with permission from *American Journal of Perinatology* Kobayashi H, Yoshida A, Kobayashi M, et al: Changes in size of the functional cyst on ultrasonography during early pregnancy. *Am J Perinatol* 14:1–4, 1997 Thieme Medical Publishers, Inc.)

smooth, round, and thin-walled with no evidence of internal echoes or nodularity on ultrasound and were considered to be functional cysts. Changes in size of the cysts were calculated, regression and disappearance were monitored throughout pregnancy, and the clinical behaviors of the cysts were more clearly defined. The cysts had their percent changes calculated from diameters of all the patients. Percent changes were divided into 4 groups of 5–7 weeks, 7–9 weeks, 9–12 weeks, and 12–15 weeks.

Results.—There were 58 sonolucent ovarian cysts, and of these 7 were functional cysts of more than 6 cm in diameter and 5 were seen after 15 weeks. The largest diameter was 8.6 cm (Fig 2). There was a tendency for the cyst size to increase from 5–7 weeks, but after 7 weeks the size diminished. As the gestation advanced, the cyst began tended to decrease in size by 8.3% at 7–98 weeks, 11.7% at 9–12 weeks and 15.2% at 12–15 weeks.

Conclusion.—At about 7 weeks, the maximum cyst size is reached, and there is gradual diminution afterward. Even if it is large or persists after 14 weeks, the sonolucent ovarian cyst may be followed as a functional cyst.

▶ With longitudinal ultrasound measurements in 58 women, these investigators describe the natural history of functional ovarian cysts in pregnancy and make some recommendations for management. Products of follicular events, most such cysts are probably derived from corpora lutea of pregnancy. All were smooth, devoid of internal echoes or surface excrescences and had thin walls. In 20 cases, 3 or more scans were performed in each patient. In aggregate, such cysts tended to enlarge to a maximum at 7–8 weeks of pregnancy, and then decreased in size for the first half of the second trimester. Cyst diameter exceeded 6 cm in 12% of cases, and 8% persisted beyond 15 weeks of gestation. If the cystic lesion meets the inclusion criteria for this study, the authors suggest temporization independent of cyst size, past the 7th week of pregnancy with repeat scans after the 12th week of gestation to verify the expected size regression. They warn against repeat scans around the 7–8 week gestational age mark when variability in the cyst size is greatest and may motivate unnecessary surgical action. The presence or suggestion of potential neoplasia-internal cyst structure, nodularity and surface excrescences, should lead to excision.

T.H. Kirschbaum, M.D.

Fetal Carriers of the Factor V Leiden Mutation Are Prone to Miscarriage and Placental Infarction

Dizon-Townson DS, Meline L, Nelson LM, et al (Univ of Utah, Salt Lake City)
Am J Obstet Gynecol 177:402–405, 1997 2–18

Introduction.—The factor V Leiden mutation, recently identified as the most common genetic predisposition to thrombosis, is reported to have a carrier frequency of 3%–4% in the white population. A case-control study examined the hypothesis that the factor V Leiden mutation may cause miscarriage or placental thrombosis and infarction. A second cohort study evaluated placental infarction in fetuses carrying the mutation.

Methods.—Samples for the case-control study were collected consecutively from women with a spontaneous miscarriage. Maternal blood from 176 women was obtained for DNA extraction; fetal DNA was extracted from 139 abortus specimens. Of the 396 placentas examined in the cohort study, 85 were from normal uncomplicated deliveries and 311 from high-risk pregnancies. Hypertensive disorders were present in 104 high-risk pregnancies.

Results.—The mean estimated gestational age at miscarriage in the case-control study was 12 weeks. Carrier frequency of the factor V Leiden mutation was 4.2% in the control group vs. 8.6% in the miscarriage group. Data from the 102 cases in which both maternal and fetal genotypes were determined showed a tendency for both mother and fetus to carry the same mutated gene, indicating maternal inheritance. In 3 of the 25 cases (12%) of recurrent miscarriage, either maternal or fetal DNA was positive for the factor V Leiden mutation. The overall factor V Leiden carrier frequency was 4.3% in the placentas studied. There was a tenfold increase, however, in the fetal carrier frequency in placentas with greater than 10% placental infarction compared with placentas with less than 10% placental infarction (10 of 24, or 42%, vs. 7 of 372, or 1.9%, respectively).

Discussion.—Circulatory disturbances at the fetoplacental interface may result in placental infarction and spontaneous miscarriage. This is the first report to suggest that the thrombogenic factor V Leiden mutation predisposes to this adverse pregnancy outcome. The fetal carrier frequency of the mutation in miscarried fetuses is more than twice that of the general population, and it appears with a tenfold increase in placentas showing greater than 10% placental infarction.

► In 1994, a point mutation—that is, mutational exchange of a single base for another in the gene for factor V located on the long arm of chromosome 1—was associated with increased thrombotic tendencies.[1] Factor V is a kinogen which, when activated by thrombin, facilitates the activation of factor X and the conversion of prothrombin to thrombin. Normally, factor V_a is held in check by protein C and its cofactor protein S, themselves activated by thrombin/thrombomodulin complexes. Protein C cleaves factor V_a and reduces its activity. The point mutation lies in the cleavage site and the presence of the mutation named the Leiden V mutation shifts the checks and balances in coagulation in the procoagulant direction.

The mutation is inherited as an autosomal dominant and exists in a gene frequency in whites in the range of 10% to 20%. Search for its presence should be part of the work-up with thrombotic disease in pregnancy. This study points to an increased risk ratio for spontaneous abortion in women who carry the mutation, and in a cohort study links the presence of the Leiden mutation in maternal and/or fetal blood to an increased risk for placental infarction at delivery.

This is the first suggestion that this mutation may be associated with placental infarction from either the uterine or umbilical circulation. This provocative suggestion warrants exploration in instances of placental infarction of significant size, that is otherwise not explained. The potentially wide implications of this relatively common mutation have attracted the interest of the Maternal Fetal Network of the National Institutes of Child Health and Human Development, and an expanded study is in the offing.

T.H. Kirschbaum, M.D.

Reference

1. Bertina RM, Koelman BPC, Koster T, et al: Mutation in blood coagulation factor V associated with resistance to activated protein C. *Nature* 369:64–67, 1994.

Effect of Long-term Cocaine Administration to Pregnant Ewes on Fetal Hemodynamics, Oxygenation, and Growth

Arbeille P, Maulik D, Salihagic A, et al (Natl de la Santé et de ka Recherche Médicale, Tours, France; Winthrop Univ, Mineola, NY; Station INRAPRMD, Nouzilly, Monnaie, France; et al)

Obstet Gynecol 90:795–802, 1997 2–19

Introduction.—In the United States, there are 100,000 infants born who were exposed to cocaine prenatally. There are multiple and interrelated adverse cocaine effects on the mother and the fetus. The effect of repeated administration of cocaine to pregnant ewes was evaluated on the uterine and fetal blood flows, oxygenation and fetal growth. Observations were made to determine uteroplacental flow reduction, prolonged fetal hypoxia and cerebral vasoconstriction and fetal growth restriction. The fetal heart rate and cerebral blood flow responses were assessed during 2 acute hypoxic tests to determine if long-term exposure to cocaine induces mod-

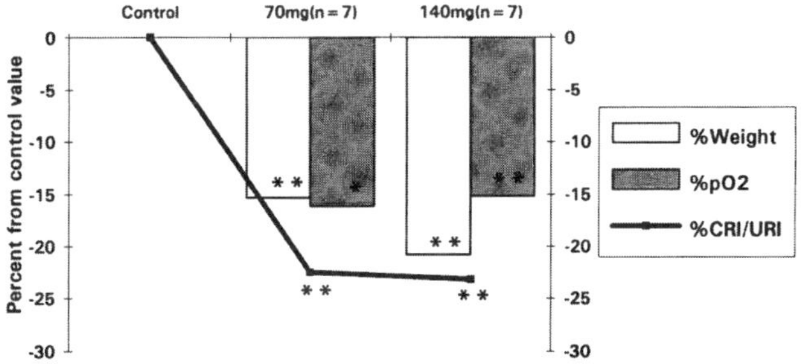

FIGURE 2.—Fetal weight, oxygenation (PO2), and cerebral-umbilical ratio (CRI/URI) at delivery. Variations between the cocaine groups and control group are expressed in percentage of the control group values. *P < .05; **P < .01. (Courtesy of Arbeille P, Maulik D, Salihagic A, et al: Effect of long-term cocaine administration to pregnant ewes on fetal hemodynamics, oxygenation, and growth. *Obstet Gynecol* 90:795–802, 1997. Reprinted with permission from The American College of Obstetricians and Gynecologists.)

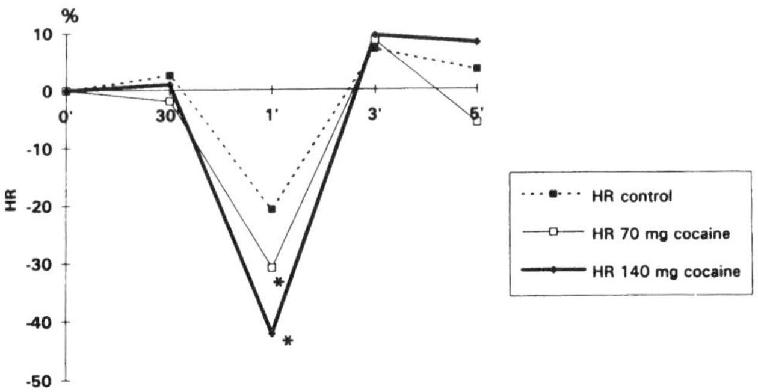

FIGURE 5.—Variation of the heart rate (HR) during the aorta compression test in the 3 groups. Changes are expressed in percentage of the pretest value. *$P < .05$. (Courtesy of Arbeille P, Maulik D, Salihagic A, et al: Effect of long-term cocaine administration to pregnant ewes on fetal hemodynamics, oxygenation, and growth. *Obstet Gynecol* 90:795–802, 1997. Reprinted with permission from The American College of Obstetricians and Gynecologists.)

erate hypoxia and whether an increase of the brain perfusion can induce brain edema.

Methods.—Seven pregnant ewes received 70 mg of cocaine and seven received 140 mg of cocaine, whereas 7 controls received placebo injected intramuscularly every day on days 60 to 134. On day 134, at cesarean delivery, hemodynamic data were measured at rest and during 2 acute hypoxic tests.

Results.—In the cocaine groups, the fetal heart rate and umbilical and uterine resistance indices (RIs) were higher when compared to the control group. The fetal heart rate was 9% to 11% higher than in controls; the umbilical resistance indices were 11% to 17% higher in the cocaine group than in the controls; and the uterine resistance indices were 13% to 35% higher in the cocaine group. At delivery on day 134, fetal weight in the cocaine group was 15% to 21% lower than in the controls; partial pressure of oxygen 15% to 16% lower in the cocaine group; umbilical resistance index was 11% to 17% higher in the cocaine group; cerebral resistance index was 9% to 15% lower in the cocaine group, and the cerebral-umbilical ratio was 22% to 23% lower in the cocaine group (Fig 2). In the 2 cocaine groups, the cerebral resistance index and the cerebral-umbilical ratio decreased significantly less. In the 2 cocaine groups, the fetal heart rate response was reduced significantly (Fig 5).

Conclusion.—Hypoxia, fetal growth restriction, and uterine and fetal blood flow disorders are induced by long-term exposure to cocaine. Cerebral vessels are less able to vasodilate and the heart rate is less able to increase during acute hypoxia because of exposure to cocaine.

► The effects of chronic cocaine use in causing fetal growth retardation are difficult to evaluate because of the behavioral and social concomitants of addiction, including poverty, malnutrition, substandard housing, and altered sleep cycles. Therein lies the value of this chronic study done in pregnant sheep in which cocaine dosage and administration to gravid ewes were unknown to those making maternal and fetal observations. Doses of 1 and 2 mg/kg per day for 9½ weeks (exempting weekends) corresponded roughly to doses employed by addicts. For a 70 kg woman, dosage of 70–140 mg of cocaine per day is a modest one since addicts have been reported to employ up to 10 g per day, their habituation protecting them from the usual lethal effects of a single dose of 1–1.2 g. No behavioral effects were noted in ewes. Primary results of this study are the 15%–20% fetal weight reduction noted at 134 days of gestational age (term is 145 days), and the 15%–16% reduction in fetal femoral artery partial pressure of oxygen. Note this level of hypoxemia does not mean the fetus was hypoxic since it could merely represent increased oxygen extraction sufficient to widen the umbilical arteriovenous oxygen content difference in the face of reduction in umbilical vein blood flow rate. Regrettably, the authors used Doppler velocimetry to evaluate both blood flow rates; all the related assumptions they make are incorrect. Cerebral and umbilical RI's are not equivalent to impedance in measurements since neither bulk blood pressure nor blood flow rates are employed. Doppler frequency shifts cannot be used to represent changes in volumetric flow. Angles of insonation vary by 20–30 degrees and cannot be assumed to be constant. Carotid and umbilical arteries do not maintain a constant diameter during the cardiac cycle and changes in vessel radius contribute to blood flow in proportion to the fourth power in accordance with Poiseuille's law. For those reasons, none of the conclusions based on Doppler velocimetry before or after birth are valid. During aortic compression, fetal bradycardia was more profound in cocaine exposed fetuses than in controls. It is safe to assume cocaine exposure produced vasoconstriction in interplacental vessels and reduced oxygen transfer to the fetus. Fetal cerebral vasoconstriction may have occurred but hypercardia may have resulted in cerebral vasodilatation explaining changes in ratios of cerebral to umbilical RI noted here. Fetal hypoxemia may or may not have occurred but surely increases in umbilical blood O_2 extraction took place. Fetal blood partial pressure of oxygen was measured but not reported. What is most important is that cocaine use similar to that in the human adult did result in fetal growth retardation as a result of increased catecholamine activity independent of the social and environmental implications of addiction.

T.H. Kirschbaum, M.D.

Decision Making in Multifetal Pregnancy Reduction for Triplets

Souter I, Goodwin TM (Univ of Southern California, Los Angeles)

Am J Perinatol 15:63–71, 1998 2–20

Introduction.—With advances in infertility treatment has come a dramatic rise in the incidence of multifetal gestation. In women with higher-order multiple gestation—triplets or more—multifetal pregnancy reduction (MFPR) may be done to reduce the complications of such gestations. The validity of this approach cannot be tested formally; it must be deduced indirectly from the literature, which makes it difficult to counsel the

TABLE 4.—Summary Data on Pregnancies That Either Underwent MFPR or Continued With Triplets

Author/ Year	*No. of Pregnancies*	**Preg. Loss Rate (%)*	*GA at Birth*	*Average BW (g)*	*% NICU Admit*	*NICU Days*	*PMR (%)*	*NMR (%)*
Lipitz et al	Tripl NR (106)	20.7	33.5	1780	—	—	10.9	4.6
1994	Twin R (34)	8.7	36.7	2350	—	—	4.8	0.0
Macones et al	Tripl NR (14)	—	31.2	1593	84.6	—	21.0†	—
1993	Twin R (47)	0.0	35.6	2279	36.2	—	3.0	—
Melgar et al	Tripl NR (20)	0.0	33.1	1924	—	21	3.3	3.3
1991	Twin R (14)	7.2	32.6	1842	—	14	3.4	0.0
Porreco et al	Tripl NR (11)	0.0	35.7	2239	—	12	3.0	3.0
1991	Twin R (13)	7.7	35.5	2227	—	13	0.0	0.0
Thorp et al	Tripl (11)	—	31.1	1537	96.9	37	12.1	9.9
1994	Twin (26)	—	34.7	2170	44.2	15	3.8‡	3.8
Muhieddine and Seoud	Tripl (26)	10.3	31.8	1666	22.7	17	0.0	0.0
1992	Twin (65)	7.7	35.5	2473	64.1	12	3.4	—
Sassoon et al	Tripl (15)	—	33.0	1720	—	29	9.5	—
1990	Twin (15)	—	36.6	2475	—	9	10.0	—

*Loss of entire pregnancy before viability.
†Excluding one set of triplets delivered at 22 weeks, the PMR is 15.3%.
‡Including one control infant who died at 100 days of life from complications of necrotizing enterocolitis, the NMR is 5.8%.
Abbreviations: GA, gestational age; *BW*, birthweight; *PMR*, perinatal mortality rate; *NMR*, neonatal mortality rate; *NR* nonreduced; *R*, reduced.
(Courtesy of Souter I, Goodwin TM: Decision making in multifetal pregnancy reduction for triplets. *Am J Perinatol* 15:63–71, 1998. Reprinted with permission from *American Journal of Perinatology*, Thieme Medical Publishers.)

patients. The authors reviewed the literature on expectant management or MFPR, focusing on triplets.

Methods and Findings.—The analysis included 83 studies on the natural history, management, and outcomes of multifetal pregnancies. Ultrasound studies suggest that some gestational sacs are spontaneously lost in multiple gestations. However, once fetal cardiac activity is observed, the likelihood of spontaneous loss drops substantially. Reported pregnancy loss rates in women undergoing MFPR range from 0% to 17%. In most triplet pregnancies, MFPR is usually done to reduce the pregnancy to twins; reduction to a singleton pregnancy is usually done only if the mother has medical complications. With expectant management, perinatal mortality for triplets and quadruplets ranges from 0% to 15%. The average gestational age at delivery in these pregnancies has remained stable at 32–33 weeks. These infants have frequent neonatal ICU admissions and long hospital stays. The link between prematurity and long-term morbidity is difficult to determine. Four studies have compared the outcomes of triplet or quadruplet pregnancies managed with MFPR vs. expectant management, and 4 have compared the results of twins resulting from MFPR vs. nonreduced twins (Table 4). Some of these studies have shown improved pregnancy and perinatal outcomes in reduced pregnancies, but others have not. The financial impact of higher-order multiple pregnancies has been little studied, but such pregnancies clearly lead to increased costs and antenatal complications. The psychological and emotional issues for the couple must be considered as well. The decision to perform MFPR must consider not only the burden of lifestyle changes for a family with triplets, but also the psychological cost of the procedure. Some parents report guilt and sadness, with some having more severe reactions. Most patients view this decision as a major life crisis.

Conclusions.—The available data permit no conclusions whether the parents with higher-order multiple gestations are more likely to take home a healthy baby after MFPR than with expectant management. There are significant secondary benefits of reducing triplet pregnancies to twin or singleton pregnancies, including reduced costs, hospital days, and morbidity associated with prolonged hospitalized and preterm delivery for both mother and infant. When MFPR is considered, the couple should receive counseling from clinicians with broad experience in this area. The authors emphasize the need for an extensive database on the outcomes of MFPR for higher-order multiple gestations. Until these data are available in usable form, couples must make a critical life decision on the basis of inadequate information.

► This is a scholarly attempt to rationalize and provide summarized data to facilitate decision making in the often agonizing options faced by increasing numbers of patients, largely as a result of new infertility procedures. It should be no surprise that the effort is only partially successful. Answers to 3 questions are discussed.

There is little support for the proposition that reduction of triplet to twin pregnancy changes the reported incidence of spontaneous loss of triplets, currently estimated at 5%–8%, compared to the 6%–8% loss following reduction to twins. Two studies purport to show reduced perinatal and neonatal mortality rates, comparing nonreduced triplets to triplets reduced to twins. But in one case, the difference was not significant. (See references 40 and 11 in original article). In the other, the apparently significant difference rested on an anomously high mortality figure for the nonreduced triplets. Secondly, several studies show reduction in preterm delivery, low and very low birthweight rates, but 2 authors refute this observation. Fairly clearly, triplet reduction decreases hospital costs and days of NICU care. Thirdly, the issues remain totally unresolved in the difficult to evaluate, but crucial domain of affective behavior. It is difficult to evaluate beyond retrospective patient interview how to balance the relief from the personal and emotional exhaustion, financial and interpersonal stresses of caring for 3 or more newborns with the potential feelings of grief, guilt, mourning, and regret that sometimes follow. Even if such data could be amassed, there is no way to quantitate it or use it to predict outcome for a prospective patient pair facing the same decisions. In brief, triplet reduction may improve perinatal mortality, likely reduces the incidence of premature and immature birth and their attendant costs in patient emotional and financial encumbrances, but the critical matter of assuring that the procedure leaves the woman and her consort with more positive than negative emotions is one that rests with the experience of those who counsel and perform the procedures, and to some extent, to luck.

T.H. Kirschbaum, M.D.

Prophylactic Cerclage in Pregnancy: Effect in Women With a History of Conization

Zeisler H, Joura EA, Bancher-Todesca D, et al (Univ of Vienna)
J Reprod Med 42:390–392, 1997 2–21

Introduction.—The number of pregnant women who have undergone previous cervical conization can be expected to increase. Studies disagree as to how a history of conization affects subsequent pregnancies. Some authors suggest that prophylactic cerclage should be performed in all pregnant women who have undergone extensive cone biopsy, whereas others have found that cerclage does not reduce the risk of preterm delivery. The effects of prophylactic cerclage in pregnant women with a history of conization were reviewed.

Methods.—The observational study included 69 pregnant women who had previously undergone cervical conization and were hospitalized before 37 weeks' gestation because of possible preterm labor and delivery. Thirty women underwent prophylactic cerclage and 39 did not. The difference resulted from a change in departmental policy, in which cerclage was performed only in women with cervical incompetence diagnosed by palpation or visualization of a dilated cervix with bulging membranes in the absence of uterine contractions.

Results.—Preterm delivery occurred in approximately 22% of women in the cerclage group and 21% in the noncerclage group. Two thirds of women undergoing cerclage were hospitalized because of threatened premature labor, compared to one third of those without cerclage.

Conclusions.—This experience suggests that prophylactic cerclage does not prevent premature delivery in women with a history of conization. There is some evidence that cerclage induces preterm uterine contractions in this group of patients. Greater circumspection in deciding to use cerclage in women with previous conization is needed.

▶ The European collaborative study of cervical cerclage sponsored by the Royal College of Obstetricians and Gynecologists (RCOG) and the Medical Research Council (MRC) has made it clear that, when cerclage is done in women without clear evidence of cervical connective tissue abnormality, the results are seldom beneficial in retrospect.[1] Indeed, uncertainty of diagnosis seems to be almost generally true of women in whom cerclage is performed. This comparison of results of 69 women in whom prophylactic cerclage was performed after cold knife conization for intraepithelial squamous lesions compared with 39 women who did not receive cerclage after conization proves that the MRC/RCOG conclusion can be generalized to include prophylactic use. Indeed, cerclage was associated with more management problems in subsequent pregnancies than in those women not operated upon, perhaps because of the relationship of the prolonged cervical foreign body and infectious disease to the onset of uterine contractile events. It would have been comforting to know the relative numbers of first and second trimester cerclages done and their relative outcomes because of the increased probability of risk of infection in preterm birth among women operated upon in the second trimester.

T.H. Kirschbaum, M.D.

Reference

1. 1995 Year Book of Obstetrics and Gynecology, pp 52–54.

Risk Factors for Pregnancy Associated Venous Thromboembolism

McColl MD, Ramsay JE, Tait RC, et al (Royal Infirmary, Glasgow, Scotland; Glasgow Royal Maternity Hosp, Scotland; Southern Gen NHS Trust, Glasgow, Scotland)

Thromb Haemost 78:1183–1188, 1997 2–22

Introduction.—The leading cause of maternal death is venous thromboembolism. The estimated incidence of pregnancy-associated venous thromboembolism is 1 in 1,000–2,000. There has been increasing evidence to support a genetic predisposition to thromboembolic disease, such as the factor V Leidin mutation. It is unclear what the role of factor V Leidin mutation is in the etiology of pregnancy-associated venous thromboem-

TABLE 1.—Thrombotic Events, Incidence of Events Per 1000 Deliveries, and Events Per 100 Women Years at Risk Based Upon a Total Number of 72,201 Deliveries During the Study Period

	DVT	Pulmonary embolism
Number	51	11
antenatal	36	5
puerperium	15	6
Median age (range)	28 years (19–41)	31 years (22–39)
Events/1000 deliveries (total)	0.71 (95% CI 0.5–0.9)	0.15 (95% CI 0.06–0.24)
Events/1000 deliveries (antenatal)	0.50 (95% CI 0.34–0.66)	0.07 (95% CI 0.01–0.13)
Events/1000 deliveries (puerperium)	0.21 (95% CI 0.11–0.31)	0.08 (95% CI 0.02–0.14)
Estimated events/100 women years (antenatal)	0.065	0.009
Estimated events/100 women years (puerperal)	0.18	0.07

(Courtesy of McColl MD, Ramsay JE, Tait RC, et al: Risk Factors for Pregnancy Associated Venous Thromboembolism. *Thromb Haemost* 78:1183–1188, 1997.)

bolism. To determine if women should be screened for factor V^{Leiden} mutation during early pregnancy to reduce the incidence of pregnancy-associated venous thromboembolism, a retrospective study was conducted.

Methods.—There were 72,201 deliveries, of which 62 resulted in objective confirmed venous thrombotic events. Fifty of the 62 attended for follow-up and thrombophilia screening.

Results.—There was a 0.71 per 1,000 incidence of deep vein thrombosis with 0.50 occurring in the antenatal period and 0.21 occurring in the puerperium (Table 1). There was a 0.15 per 1,000 deliveries incidence of pulmonary embolism with 0.07 occurring in the antenatal period and 0.08 occurring in the puerperium. No clinical risk factor for thrombosis or an identifiable thrombophilic abnormality was seen in 28% of all episodes of pregnancy-associated venous thromboembolism. In 12% of individuals, deficiency of antithrombin was identified, and in 8% the factor V Leidin mutation was seen. The thrombotic risk for a woman during pregnancy or the puerperium with the defect is about 1 in 400–500 based on estimates of the prevalence of the factor V Leiden mutation in the population.

Conclusion.—The idea of random screening for the mutation of V Leiden in early pregnancy is not supported by these results. There was a lower than expected prevalence of the factor V Leidin mutation in this study of thrombotic events occurring during pregnancy or puerperium.

▶ Evidence of factor V resistance to activated protein C conferred by a substitution (Leiden) mutation in case control studies of women with venous thromboembolism have been reported to occur in as many as 25% to 60% of women in their reproductive age range.[1] It seems likely these estimates are falsely high because of accession bias, but the true incidence figure is important not only in clinical practice but also in evaluation of the merits of routine screening for the mutated factor V, important in pregnancy thromboembolic disease and possibly related to pregnancy hypertension, recurrent abortion, and fetal death as well as some forms of growth retardation. Prospective studies are on the way, but in the interim this carefully done cohort study based on both inpatient obstetrical records and postpartum admissions for heparin therapy for puerperal thrombotic disease is of genuine interest. Records of the Scottish National Health Service for Glasgow where 99% of deliveries occur in hospitals provides the basis for the analysis. Based on 72,201 records, 50 of 62 women with evidence of pregnancy related thromboembolic disease were available for detailed coagulation assays, and 8% of these proved to exhibit the factor V Leiden mutation. Though pregnancy-related deep vein thromboses were more commonly identified antepartum than postpartum, with adjustment for the relative duration of exposure to risk during pregnancy and during the puerperium, the occurrence of deep vein thrombosis (DVT) per woman years of exposure is three times more likely a puerperal event than an antepartum event. For pulmonary embolus, the occurrence is 6 times more likely to occur after delivery. In terms of thrombotic risk, abnormalities in antithrombin III were more likely than those of factor V in this population. Note that these incidence figures are different from the carrier frequencies for the Leiden mutation reported by Ridker et al.[2] They found the carrier state to be present in 4.85% of caucasian women and to be highest among all American ethnic groups in the Caucasian subset. The difference between that study and this 1 pertains to the chances that pregnancy-related thrombotic episodes are due to the Leiden mutation. Some have estimated that figure at 30%.[3] Here the risk value of 8% makes screening impractical. It is important for future use that we have a clearer estimate, derived from prospective analysis, of that likelihood to clarify the merits of routine screening for the Leiden mutation.

T.H. Kirschbaum, M.D.

References

1. 1998 Year Book of Ostetrics, Gynecology, and Women's Health, pp 179–182.
2. Ridker PM, Miletich JP, Hennekens CH, et al. Ethnic distribution of factor V Leiden in 4,047 men and women. *JAMA* 277:1305, 1997.
3. Sneusson PJ, Dahlback BD. Resistance of activated protein C as the basis for venous thrombosis. *N Engl J Med* 330:517, 1994.

3 Medical Complications of Pregnancy

Perinatal HIV-1 Transmission: Interaction Between Zidovudine Prophylaxis and Mode of Delivery in the French Perinatal Cohort
Madelbrot L, for the French Perinatal Cohort (INSERM U149, Paris; INSERM U292, Kremlin-Bicêtre, France; Hôpital de La Grave, Toulouse, France; et al)
JAMA 280:55–60, 1998 3–1

Background.—Evidence suggests that transmission of HIV-1 from mother to child occurs primarily in late pregnancy and intrapartum. It is not known whether elective cesarean delivery protects against the transmission of HIV-1. The effect of mode of delivery in conjunction with zidovudine prophylaxis on perinatal transmission of HIV-1 was determined.

Methods.—A prospective cohort study involving 85 perinatal centers investigated 2,834 singleton children born to mothers with HIV-1 infection. The HIV infection status of the children, obstetric factors, including mode of delivery, and use of zidovudine prophylaxis were examined.

Results.—Zidovudine prophylaxis was not used in 1,917 pregnancies and was used in 902 pregnancies. The rate of cesarean delivery was 10.9% on an emergency basis and 8.3% on an elective basis (before labor or rupture of membranes). Information on mode of delivery was available for 1,877 of the 1,917 mothers who did not receive zidovudine. Of these, 17.2% transmitted HIV-1 to their child. Risk factors that were significantly associated with transmission were maternal p24 antigenemia, cervicovaginal infections during pregnancy, amniotic fluid color, and rupture of membranes at least 4 hours before delivery. Mode of delivery was not associated with transmission. Information on mode of delivery was available for 872 of the 902 mothers who had zidovudine prophylaxis. Of these, 6.4% transmitted HIV-1 to their child. In this group, elective cesarean delivery (133 mothers) was associated with a lower rate of transmission than was emergency cesarean or vaginal delivery. Multivariate analysis of all mother-child pairs, obstetric risk factors, maternal p24 antigenemia, and zidovudine prophylaxis showed that the interaction between mode of delivery and zidovudine prophylaxis was significant. Multivariate analysis of pregnancies in which zidovudine prophylaxis was used showed that maternal p24 antigenemia, amniotic fluid color, and mode of delivery were related to transmission. The adjusted odds ratio was 1.6 for emergency cesarean delivery and 0.2 for elective cesarean delivery compared with vaginal delivery.

Discussion.—An interaction between zidovudine prophylaxis and elective cesarean delivery decreased perinatal transmission of HIV-1. The mechanism of the protective effect of obstetric factors and antiretroviral therapy and of their interaction needs further investigation. This information may help in the development of new strategies for preventing perinatal transmission of HIV.

▶ It is reasonably clear that the bulk of maternal-to-infant transmission of the virus, maybe as much as 70% to 80%, occurs during late pregnancy, labor, and delivery. In view of the ease of obtaining virus from the reproductive tracts of laboring HIV-positive women, interest in the possibility of reducing the fetal transmission rate by performing cesarean delivery has often arisen. Results of cohort studies to date have been unclear, with some studies suggesting benefit[1] and others not.[2] Among those studies showing no reduction in infant transmission rate resulting from cesarean section was an earlier publication from this French Perinatal Cohort.[3] These data have been collected over the past 11 years from a series of 85 French obstetric services all operating under a common protocol. A total of 2,834 HIV-positive women and their infants are reported here; 1,986 of the cases had been published earlier. As before, infants were judged congenitally infected if they were HIV antibody positive past 18 months of life and were positive on RNA–polymerase chain reaction (PCR) for HIV-1 or were HIV culture positive. What's new in this report emerges from stratification of data based on pregnancy exposure to zidovudine (AZT). Introduced into practice in March 1994, AZT prophylaxis was rapidly adopted by French obstetricians, who achieved a 90% utilization rate in HIV-positive pregnant women by the end of 1994 (see Abstract 2–8).

As expected, AZT reduced the rate of maternal-to-infant transmission compared with untreated women from 17.2% to 6.4%. Univariate analysis of 1,917 untreated women showed rupture of membranes for more than 4 hours before delivery, cervicovaginal infection, blood- or meconium-stained amniotic fluid, and a maternal temperature greater than 38°C were associated with increased risks of viral transmission to the infant. For the 902 HIV-positive women receiving AZT, only the mode of delivery and discolored amniotic fluid were associated with increased transmission rates on univariate analysis, and multivariate analysis demonstrated a relationship only between transmission rates and mode of delivery. For vaginal births in women receiving AZT, the transmission rate was 6.6%; for those in whom cesarean section followed the onset of labor or rupture of membranes the rate was 11.4%; following elective cesarean section the transmission rate was 0.8%.

Like all cohort studies, the unresolvable question of comparability among subsets of women is a problem that can only be settled by a prospective randomized study with observer blinding. However, it is entirely possible that AZT reduces the viral RNA load to the point where prevention of cervicovaginal contact becomes a discernable benefit compared with the vertical and horizontal transmission routes that affect ultimate perinatal infection rates. The evidence presented here is strongly suggestive of the value of cesarean section in HIV-positive women receiving AZT in minimizing the risk of infant infection. Of 133 such women who delivered abdominally in this experience, only 1 infant proved to be infected past 18 months of age. Obstetric units need seriously to consider the merits of adopting this policy.

T.H. Kirschbaum, M.D.

References

1. 1993 Year Book of Obstetrics and Gynecology, pp 50–51, 78–79.
2. 1997 Year Book of Obstetrics, Gynecology, and Women's Health, pp 86–87.
3. 1998 Year Book of Obstetrics, Gynecology, and Women's Health, pp 100–101.

CCR5 Chemokine Receptor Variant in HIV-1 Mother-to-Child Transmission and Disease Progression in Children

Blanche S, for the French Pediatric HIV Infection Study Group (Hôpital Necker Enfants Malades, Paris)

JAMA 279:277–280, 1998 3–2

Objective.—Whereas adults with a deletion of 32 base pairs (δ32)in the *CCR* gene have a substantial resistance to HIV infection, the effect of the mutation in children is not known. The effect of the *CCR5* chemokine receptor variant on mother-to-child transmission of HIV type 1 (HIV-1) and subsequent disease progression in infected children was investigated in a multicenter, prospective study of infants born to HIV-positive mothers.

Methods.—Polymerase chain reaction amplification of the *CCR5* alleles of 276 non-African children born to HIV-1-infected mothers and 236 age-matched non-African controls born between 1983 and 1996 was performed on genomic DNA isolated from frozen peripheral blood mononuclear cells. The *CCR5* genotype distribution, mother-to-child transmission, and disease progression in children were determined in children followed since birth.

Results.—The frequency of the mutated allele in the entire study group was 5%. One child, homozygous for the deletion, was not infected. There were 49 heterozygous children (9.6%), including 27 children (9.8%) in the infected group and 22 children (9.3%) in the uninfected group. There were 126 infected wild type homozygotes and 26 infected heterozygotes. Heterozygotes were significantly less likely than homozygotes to have stage C symptoms at 36 months (9% vs. 28%). At 8 years, 40% of heterozygotes and 11% of homozygotes had no stage B or C symptoms. Heterozygous children had a lower risk for HIV and progressive symptoms than did children homozygous for the wild type allele.

Conclusion.—Whereas heterozygous children are not protected from infection with maternal HIV-1, the mutation does significantly slow progress of the disease in infected children.

▶ The analysis of adults found to be HIV-1 negative despite repeated exposures to the virus has led to the recognition that a 32–base pair deletion in a gene for a chemokine receptor (*CCR5*) appears to be protective in its homozygous state against HIV-1 infection.[1] The mechanism by which this protection is conferred is unknown, and whether protection is afforded in the heterozygous state is uncertain. The report from the French Pediatric HIV cohort,[2, 3] seeks to clarify the prevalence of that mutation in a study of 512 infants born of HIV-1 positive gravidas; 54% of the infants were affected through maternal transmission. African infants were excluded in this study because of the low prevalence of the *CCR5* mutation in that population.

Among all infants, the frequency of the mutation was about 5%, with only 1 infant—an uninfected 1—homozygous. The 0.4% incidence rate is based on too few cases to be taken seriously, but what does emerge clearly is that the heterozygous state appears to slow the progression of the disease, as measured either by the attainment of AIDS Class B or C or of Class III immune deficiency (less than 15% of normal CD4 counts). Clearly, it is important to learn whether the *CCR5* receptor does play a role in receptor coupling of immune cells with the HIV-1 virus, and whether pharmacologic blockade of that receptor might be useful in the prevention or treatment of HIV infection in both adults and infants.

T.H. Kirschbaum, M.D.

References

1. Huang Y, Paxton WA, Wilinsky SM, et al: The role of a mutant CCR5 allele in HIV-1 transmission. *Nature Med* 11:1240, 1996.
2. 1996 Year Book of Obstetrics and Gynecology , pp 79–80.
3. 1998 Year Book of Obstetrics, Gynecology, and Women's Health, pp 122–125.

Genetic Evaluation of Suspected Cases of Transient HIV-1 Infection of Infants

Frenkel LM, Mullins JI, Learn GH, et al (Univ of Rochester, NY; Univ of Washington, Seattle; Centers for Disease Control and Prevention, Atlanta, Ga; et al)

Science 280:1073–1076, 1998 3–3

Background.—Previous reports have described cases of transient HIV-1 infection, based on virologic or immunologic criteria. However, genetic analyses have never been performed to supply unambiguous confirmation of this finding. A large series of infants with apparent transient HIV-1 infection was reanalyzed using genetic analyses.

Methods and Findings.—The analysis included 43 cases of apparent transient HIV-1 viremia: 42 infants of HIV-1-infected mothers and 1 mother. In each case, the finding of transient viremia was ruled out by genetic criteria. In 20 cases, the presence of virus in specimens could not be confirmed by polymerase chain reaction. In another 6 cases, typing of somatic loci showed lack of concordance between the genotypes of the positive and negative specimens, suggesting that the specimens had been mislabeled. In the remaining 17 cases, phylogenetic analysis did not show the expected linkage between the mother's and infant's virus. In 29 of 29 cases, testing for a homozygous deletion within the *CCR5* gene excluded the finding of resistance to HIV-1 infection.

Conclusions.—Genetic analyses do not confirm these suspected cases of transient HIV-1 viremia in the infants of infected mothers. All cases tested appeared to be the result of sample mislabeling or laboratory contamination. If transient HIV-1 infection does exist, it will be very difficult to obtain satisfactory confirmation.

▶ This diverse group of collaborators investigated in detail 43 cases of apparently spontaneous cures, or at least of transient viremia clearance without treatment; 42 of the cases involved infants reported in 5 studies of maternal-to-fetal HIV-1 virus transmission.[1, 2] Many reported cases were based on viral culture polymerase chain reaction (PCR) assay positivity or serologic criteria. These investigators used a variety of techniques based on molecular genetic analysis of HIV material itself obtained from the mothers and infants. Mislabeling was investigated by searching for evidence of rare segments of the genotype present in nonviral material from both mother and infant. As genes mutate, they accumulate evidence of changing base sequences with time, and these changes may be used to plot the evolutionary change in the virus. Here the evolutionary tree of the *env* gene, responsible for production of the glycoprotein viral capsid, was used to search for similarity of the gene in fetal and maternal viral specimens. In 16 cases, reanalysis of blood samples failed to demonstrate the purportedly positive fetal samples. Contamination during PCR was noted by failure of appearance of *env* gene sequences along with the adjacent *gag* gene, responsible for capsular proteins and protease production. In other cases, carry-over contamination from PCR was elucidated in this way. In some cases, mislabeling was denoted through HLA typing of fetal leukocyte antigens in comparison with maternal antigens. In summary, all reported incidences of transient HIV infections proved spurious and were the result of sample mislabeling of laboratory contamination or false-positive test results.

T.H. Kirschbaum, M.D.

References

1. 1996 Year Book of Obstetrics and Gynecology, pp 84–85.
2. 1998 Year Book of Obstetrics, Gynecology, and Women's Health, pp 112–113.

Mother-Child Class I HLA Concordance Increases Perinatal Human Immunodeficiency Virus Type 1 Transmission

MacDonald KS, Embree J, Njenga S, et al (Univ of Nairobi, Kenya; Univ of Manitoba, Winnipeg, Canada; Univ of Toronto; et al)

J Infect Dis 177:551–556, 1998 3–4

Purpose.—Although the relative importance of various modes of transmission is unclear, growing evidence suggests that fetuses of HIV-infected mothers are exposed to maternal blood—and thus to free virus and infected cells—during gestation and delivery. Infected cells express major histocompatibility complex (MHC) gene products, which are incorporated into the lipid envelope of HIV virions. In monkeys, immunization with human MHC gene products confers protection against simian immunodeficiency virus grown in cells expressing the same MHC alleles. The effects of HLA concordance between mother and infant on the risk of HIV-1 transmission were examined.

Methods.—A total of 160 children born to 125 HIV-infected mothers enrolled in an African study of HIV-1 perinatal transmission and pediatric AIDS were studied. All patients underwent class I HLA typing by standard methods, and HLA matching between the mothers and children was assessed. The effects of HLA matching on the children's risk of HIV-1 infection were assessed.

Results.—Increasing class I HLA concordance was a risk factor for intrauterine, intrapartum, or early breast milk transmission of HIV-1 (Table 2). Each additional concordant allele increased the risk of perinatal HIV-1 transmission in stepwise fashion—odds ratio 2.63, 95% confidence interval 1.36–5.07.

Conclusions.—Major histocompatibility complex discordance between the mother and child appears to protect against perinatal HIV-1 transmission. The findings support the results of animal experiments suggesting that anti MHC responses can offer protection against viral challenge. An anti HLA strategy may be useful in the development of an effective HIV-1 vaccine.

TABLE 2.—Class I HLA Concordance (A, B, and C Loci) and Risk of Perinatal HIV-1 Transmission

A, B, C locus match	HIV-1–uninfected at birth (n = 141)	HIV-1 perinatal infection (n = 19)	% transmission
3 of 6 alleles	30	1	3.3
4 of 6 alleles	65	7	9.7
5 of 6 alleles	37	7	15.9
6 of 6 alleles	9	4	30.8

Note: P_t = 0.008 (Mantel-Haenszel trend test, 2-tailed).

(Courtesy of MacDonald KS, Embree J, Njenga S, et al: Mother-child class I HLA concordance increases perinatal human immunodeficiency virus type 1 transmission. *J Infect Dis* 177:551–556.)

▶ Maternal-to-fetal transmission of HIV-1 infection may occur as a result of a direct transfer of virus, of infected maternal phagocytic cells, of ingested breast milk, or any combination of those routes. The ubiquity, albeit in small numbers, of maternal cells present in fetal blood makes it remarkable that so few fetuses are regularly infected by contact with HIV-1–positive gravidas. There is direct evidence that infected infants are capable of clearing HIV-1 organisms from their blood, and antibody-negative infants have been reported to show virus-specific cytotoxic cells, evidence of prior successful immunologic clearance of the virus.

In this study of 160 infants born of infected Nairobi gravidas from 1986 to 1996, the possible role of human leukocytic antigen (HLA) discordance in protecting against fetal infection was explored. The incidence of perinatal transmission was 11.9%, with 25% transmission by 16 months of age; the incremental 13% incidence due to postnatal breast milk transfer.[1] When tested for concordance for 6 alleles in the class 1 HLA locus, evidence of discordance between mother and fetus was associated with a reduced rate of maternal-to-fetal transfer, indicating a role for recognition of nonself in the destruction of infected maternal cells . This suggests the possible role for the recognition of nonself based on HLA type in the destruction of infected maternal cells. The effect does not appear large, but it raises the possibility that anti-HLA immunization might be useful in decreasing the rate of fetal infection even further and without increasing drug resistance, as does the use of maternal AZT.[2]

T.H. Kirschbaum, M.D.

References

1. 1998 Year Book of Obstetrics, Gynecology, and Women's Health, pp 73–74.
2. 1996 Year Book of Obstetrics and Gynecology, pp 84–87.

Low-dose Aspirin to Prevent Preeclampsia in Women at High Risk

Caritis S, and the National Institute of Child Health and Human Development Network of Maternal-Fetal Medicine Units (Univ of Pittsburgh, Pa; Univ of Tennessee, Memphis; Univ of Alabama, Birmingham; et al)

N Engl J Med 338:701–705, 1998 3–5

Objective.—Whereas prophylaxis with low-dose aspirin has been recommended to prevent preeclampsia, a large trial failed to detect any major benefit of low-dose aspirin, possibly because of the inclusion of women at low-risk of preeclampsia. Whether aspirin therapy reduces the incidence of preeclampsia in women at increased risk was examined in a double-blind, randomized, placebo-controlled trial.

Methods.—Between weeks 13 and 26 of pregnancy, 2,539 women at high risk for preeclampsia, because of pregestational insulin-treated diabetes mellitus, chronic hypertension, multifetal gestations, or previous preeclampsia, received 60 mg/day of aspirin (n = 1,273) or placebo (n = 1,266) until delivery or development of preeclampsia. Patients were

TABLE 5.—Results of Preeclampsia-Prevention Trials

Outcome	Incidence		Relative Risk (95% Confidence Limits)
	Aspirin	Placebo	
	no./no. at risk (%)		
Preeclampsia			
Small trials*	10/319	50/284	0.2 (0.1, 0.4)
Large trials†	949/13,928	1032/13,765	0.9 (0.8, 1.0)
Total	959/14,247 (6.7)	1082/14,049 (7.7)	0.9 (0.8, 1.0)
Preterm delivery	2404/13,729 (17.5)	2540/13,645 (18.6)	0.9 (0.9, 1.0)
Preinatal death	418/14,407 (2.9)	450/14,253 (3.2)	0.9 (0.8, 1.0)

*Data are from Viinikka et al.[16] and Collins.[17]
†Data are from the Estudo Colaborativo para Prevenção da Préeclampsia com Aspirina,[9] Rotchell et al.,[10] and Collins.[17]
(Courtesy of Caritis S, and the National Institute of Child Health and Human Development Network of Maternal-Fetal Medicine Units. *N Engl J Med* 338:701–705. Copyright 1998, Massachusetts Medical Society. Reprinted by permission of *The New England Journal of Medicine*.)

followed up every 4 weeks until week 28, every 2 weeks until week 36, and then weekly thereafter. The primary outcome variable was preeclampsia, and the secondary outcome variables were abruptio placentae, preterm birth, infants small for gestational age, neonatal intraventricular hemorrhage, postpartum hemorrhage, and neonatal bleeding.

Results.—There were no outcome data on 19 patients receiving aspirin and 17 patients receiving placebo. The incidence of preeclampsia was similar for both groups. The results of studies of the effect of antiplatelet therapy on the incidence of preeclampsia, preterm birth, and perinatal death were different for small and large trials (Table 5). This difference is possibly attributable to publication bias; small trials with positive results are more likely to be submitted for publication than small trials with negative results.

Conclusions.—Low-dose aspirin did not reduce the incidence of preeclampsia in women at high-risk for preeclampsia.

▶ Trials of 60 mg of aspirin per day to prevent preeclampsia have yielded generally negative results,[1, 2] but this product of the collaborative Maternal-Fetal Medicine Network (MFMN) sponsored by the National Institute of Child Health and Development (NICHD) offers 2 new features to the study of the issue. The first is an attempt to seek possible benefit of prophylaxis by aspirin among women at particularly high risk for the development of pregnancy-induced hypertension—diabetics, chronic hypertensives, women with multiple pregnancies and women with a prior history of pregnancy-induced hypertension. Through the 13 centers comprising the MFMN, 2,539 women are enrolled in this randomized, double-blind, control study with 1,249 controls. Because only 5.4% of the study subjects were primigravid, this is clearly not a study of preeclamptics but of women with pregnancy-induced hypertension. Women beginning pregnancy with proteinuria were judged to have preeclampsia based on the development of thrombopenia, elevated liver enzymes, headache, abdominal pain, or increased levels of proteinuria. For other subsets, the criteria for preeclampsia were equally complex. What emerged was no evidence of benefit, nor of increased complications of pregnancy, resulting from aspirin use at this dosage.

The second feature is a well-executed summary of data from 5 other studies comprising a total of 28,000 women. In aggregate, these data reveal a reduction in "preeclampsia" from 7.7% to 6.7%, and of preterm birth from 18.6% to 17.5%, both changes statistically but not biologically significantly. The only claims for substantive benefit of prophylactic aspirin come from 2 trials, each with fewer than 200 enrollees. This study adds considerable weight to the proposition that aspirin is without benefit in the prevention of pregnancy-induced hypertension.

T.H. Kirschbaum, M.D.

References

1. 1994 YEAR BOOK OF OBSTETRICS AND GYNECOLOGY, pp 61–63.
2. 1995 YEAR BOOK OF OBSTETRICS AND GYNECOLOGY, pp 64–66, 71–76.

Hyperemesis Gravidarum Associated With *Helicobacter pylori* Seropositivity

Frigo P, Lang C, Reisenberger K, et al (Univ Hosp of Vienna)

Obstet Gynecol 91:615–617, 1998 3–6

Background.—Hyperemesis gravidarum, a severe form of morning sickness, is characterized by weight loss, ketonemia, and electrolyte imbalance. Increased serum steroid hormone and human chorionic gonadotropin levels are thought to have a role in this condition. An increased accumulation of fluid caused by increased steroid hormones in pregnant women may lead to a shift in pH, which may result in subclinical *Helicobacter pylori* infection. The possible relationship between *H. pylori* infection and hyperemesis gravidarum was explored.

Methods.—One hundred five patients with hyperemesis gravidarum were enrolled in a prospective study. Concentrations of *Helicobacter* serum IgG in this group were compared with those in asymptomatic gravidas matched by gestational week.

Findings.—Serum IgG concentrations were positive in 90.5% of the patients with hyperemesis and in 46.5% of the control subjects. This difference was significant. The mean index percentages of the IgG titers were 74.2% and 24.3% in the hyperemesis and control groups, respectively.

Conclusion.—Infection with *H. pylori* appears to be associated with hyperemesis gravidarum. However, treatment to eradicate *H. pylori* at the time of organogenesis is problematic.

▶ *Helicobacter pylori* appears to predispose to the development of duodenal and possibly gastric ulcer, and is found in nearly all cases of active duodenal ulcer. Its presence is not sufficient to cause gastrointestinal ulceration, but there is evidence that, when the organism is present, successfully eliminating it with therapy reduces the risk of recurrent ulcer disease. Little is known about the status of *Helicobacter* in normal or pathologic pregnancy.

In this group of 105 women complaining of hyperemesis gravidarum, the incidence of serum immunoglobulin antibody to the organism was significantly greater than in normal controls; all were studied in the first trimester. The presence of antibody is pathognomic of neither acute nor chronic infection, however, and culture, gastroscopy, and occasional biopsy are necessary to establish the diagnosis of infection. Effective drug therapy is not easy and evidence of recurrent infection often becomes apparent. Recommended therapy is metronidazole and bismuth preparations, sometimes supplemented with tetracyclines. Use of either antibiotic in the first trimester of pregnancy is associated with hazards. Nonetheless, despite the low incidence of peptic ulcer disease in pregnancy, this is an observation that deserves further, more definitive study.

T.H. Kirschbaum, M.D.

Vertical Transmission of Hepatitis C Virus Infection: Usefulness of Viremia Detection in HIV-Seronegative Hepatitis C Virus–Seropositive Mothers

Giacchino R, Tasso L, Timitilli A, et al ("G Gaslini" Children's Hosp, Genoa Italy; Univ of Genova, Genoa, Italy; San Martino Hosp, Genoa, Italy; et al)
J Pediatr 132:167–169, 1998 3–7

Background.—The risk of vertical transmission of hepatitis C virus (HCV) is reported to be highly variable. High levels of maternal viremia or HIV co-infection have been associated with the highest rates of transmission.

Methods.—Screening for anti-HCV antibodies was performed in 7,023 pregnant women during a 3-year period. Women who tested positive for hepatitis B virus (HBV) and HIV infection were excluded. Serologic markers of HBV, anti-HIV, and anti-HCV were determined.

Results.—Of 82 women who tested anti-HCV–positive, but HIV- and HBV-negative, 70 mother-infant pairs were enrolled in the study. The mothers and infants were examined for hepatitis C viremia to determine

TABLE.—Hepatitis C Virus–RNA in 70 Anti-Hepatitis C Virus–Positive Mothers and Their Children

	HCV-RNA$^+$ mothers		HCV-RNA$^-$ mothers
	HCV-RNA$^+$	HCV-RNA$^-$	HCV-RNA$^-$
No. of children at birth	9	36	25
No. of children during follow-up	3*	35†	21‡

*Another child was not tested for hepatitis C virus (*HCV*)–RNA, but had hepatitis.
†Six HCV-RNA$^-$ children were lost to follow-up soon after enrollment.
‡Four children (RN negative at birth) were lost to follow-up soon after enrollment.
(Courtesy of Giacchino R, Tasso L, Timitilli A, et al: Vertical transmission of hepatitis C virus infection: Usefulness of viremia detection in HIV-seronegative hepatitis C virus–seropositive mothers. *J Pediatr* 132:167–169, 1998.)

the risk of vertical transmission of HCV from mothers who tested HIV-negative. There were 45 mothers who tested HCV-RNA–positive. Four of the 45 children of these women tested positive at birth and at follow-up (Table).

Conclusion.—These findings indicate that vertical transmission is possible from mothers who test anti-HCV–positive and anti-HIV–negative and occurs at a low rate. The level of viremia is an important factor in vertical transmission. The detection of viremia is a valuable predictive risk factor.

► Because hepatitis C is associated with a high incidence of chronic hepatitis, cirrhosis, and hepatic carcinoma, its been good news that its maternal-to-fetal transmission rates are low.[1] These investigators are exploring the suggestion that the transmission rate may be higher in the presence of maternal HIV infection based on identification of HCV-RNA in infant blood. Though the numbers are small,[2] this study indicates that in a group of 70 HIV antibody–positive women compared with 50 HIV antibody–negative women, the only incidences of fetal virion transfer occurred in those women with HIV antibody who also had evidence of HCV viral fragments in their circulating blood. There is then reason for concern regarding fetal infection from HCV antibody–positive gravidas who are also HIV antibody–positive or show evidence of HCV-RNA fragments in circulating blood. The hepatitis C virus is apparently not transferred in breast milk.

T.H. Kirschbaum, M.D.

References

1. 1994 Year Book of Obstetrics and Gynecology, pp 97–98; 115–116.
2. 1996 Year Book of Obstetrics and Gynecology, pp 877–88.

Fetuses From Preeclamptic Mothers Show Reduced Hepatic Erythropoiesis

Stallmach T, Karolyi L, Lichtlen P, et al (Univ of Zürich-Irchel, Switzerland)
Pediatr Res 43:349–354, 1998 3–8

Objective.—Preeclampsia can lead to changes during pregnancy that can result in fetal death. Hematopoietic alterations in the liver of affected fetuses were examined morphologically to determine whether these alterations might be a consequence of preeclampsia rather than intrauterine growth retardation.

Methods.—The average number of hematopoietic cells per mm^2 was determined within 36 hours of death in 28 human fetuses, 23–34 weeks' gestational age. Eighteen of the mothers had preeclampsia diagnosed. Enzyme immunoassays for erythropoietin (Epo) and cytokines were performed in a second group of 12 control and 13 growth-retarded fetuses born by cesarean section.

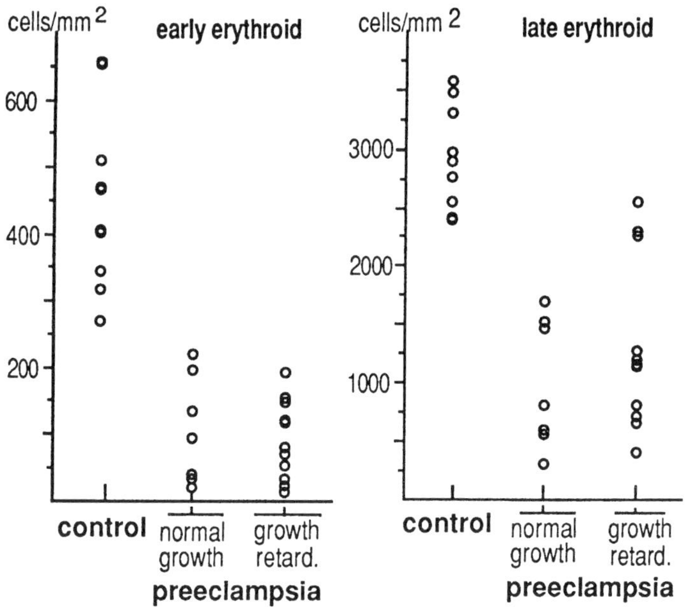

FIGURE 3.—Reduction of erythroid cells in the livers of fetuses from preeclamptic mothers; early and late erythroid cells are compared in 10 control fetuses as well as 11 fetuses with and 7 fetuses without growth retardation; elements of erythroid lineage are less numerous per mm^2 of liver tissue with preeclampsia irrespective of the intrauterine growth stage. (Courtesy of Stallmach T, Karolyi L, Lichtlen P, et al: Fetuses from preeclamptic mothers show reduced hepatic erythropoiesis. *Pediatr Res* 43:349–354, 1998).

Results.—In the first group, the number of erythroid cells in fetal livers was significantly reduced in all fetuses of preeclamptic mothers whether growth retardation was present or not (Fig 3). The number of erythropoietic cells was reduced by 80% in the early stage of differentiation and by 50% in the later stages. When Epo concentration in umbilical cord blood and levels of cytokines in amniotic fluid were compared for 12 premature newborn controls and 13 growth-retarded fetuses, levels of Epo and interleukin-3 (IL-3) were elevated by 50% and 800%, respectively, in growth-retarded fetuses of preeclamptic mothers. Granulocyte-macrophage colony-stimulating factor (GM-CSF), granulocyte-CSF (G-CSF), and IL-1β levels were reduced by factors of 1.7–3.4 in fetuses of preeclamptic mothers. Concentrations of IL-6 and IL-8 were similar in both groups. Concentrations of IL-2 and interferon-γ were below the levels of detection.

Conclusions.—Livers of fetuses of preeclamptic mothers show a severe reduction of erythroid cells. Whereas levels of Epo and IL-3 were elevated, concentrations of GM-CSF, G-CSF, and IL-1β levels were reduced. Quantitation of cytokines can possibly be used to determine the time point of therapeutic intervention for mothers with preeclampsia.

▶ In an earlier study,[1] the authors showed that granulocytes increased with amnionitis and decreased in preeclampsia. In this study, the authors compared 18 fetuses coming to autopsy between 24 and 36 weeks' gestation with a group of 10 fetuses at 23–31 weeks' gestation who came from normotensive pregnancies. Histochemistry was used to differentiate granulocytic cells from erythroid precursors in fetal liver, and lymphocytic cells were very uncommon at this gestational age. In specimens derived from preeclamptic women, erythroid precursors were decreased by 60% compared with controls, and morphologic evidence of apoptosis was abundant. The same decrease was seen in growth-retarded fetuses as in fetuses exhibiting normal weight at specified gestational age.

In a second study, growth-retarded infants from 13 preeclamptic pregnancies showed elevated EPO and IL3 levels compared with those of preterm infants from normotensive pregnancies. Both EPO and IL-3 act to increase erythropoiesis by inhibiting red blood cell apoptosis, and IL-3 also serves as a colony stimulator. Because elevated IL-3 and EPO failed to stimulate fetal erythropoiesis in maternal preeclampsia, it follows that erythroid production is neither a byproduct of fetal growth retardation nor is EPO, often stimulated to gene expression by hypoxemia, able to prevent the increased erythroid apoptosis associated here with preeclampsia. Although inferences from fetal cardiovascular response in hypertensive pregnancies have often been drawn from the study of fetal tissue, this is the first convincing of evidence that some maternal product of hypertensive pregnancy has a measurable effect on fetal tissues, specifically on hepatic red blood cell production, and provides some justification for studying pregnancy-induces hypertension in the fetus and newborn involved as a passive participant to the maternal cardiovascular disorder.

T.H. Kirschbaum, M.D.

Reference

1. Stallmach T, Kardyi L: Augmentation of fetal granulopoiesis with chorioamnionitis during the second trimester of gestation. *Hum Pathol* 25:244–247, 1993.

Methylenetetrahydrofolate Reductase Polymorphism and Pre-eclampsia

Sohda S, Arinami T, Hamada H, et al (Univ of Tsukuba, Japan)

J Med Genet 34:525–526, 1997 3–9

Introduction.—Preeclampsia is a common and serious complication of pregnancy. There is evidence that genetic factors are involved in the genesis of preeclampsia. A common missense mutation in the methylenetetrahydrofolate reductase (MTHFR) gene, a C to T substitution at nucleotide 677, causes reduced MTHFR activity and is associated with slightly elevated plasma homocysteine levels. Because pregnant women with underlying vascular disease have a higher risk of preeclampsia, it was hypothesized that the frequency of T677 alleles would be higher in patients with preeclampsia than in control subjects.

Methods.—The polymerase chain reaction restriction fragment length polymorphism method was used to determine the MTHFR genotypes in 67 pregnant women with preeclampsia, 98 normal pregnant women, and 260 healthy adults.

Results.—A significant increase in the T677 allele and genotype homozygous for the T677 allele was seen in pregnant women with preeclampsia compared to control subjects.

Discussion.—These findings suggest that the T677 variant of the MTHFR gene is a genetic risk factor for preeclampsia. These findings need to be confirmed in studies of larger and more ethnically diverse populations.

▶ Since the introduction of the working hypothesis that preeclampsia is primarily a disturbance of vascular endothelium of uncertain origin,[1] a largely fruitless search for the responsible agent has been pursued by many investigators. Plasma homocysteine has been linked by epidemiologic data to an increased risk of endothelial damage leading to occlusive coronary artery disease and stroke. Further, preeclamptic women, given excess methionine, show elevated serum homocysteine concentrations compared to controls, and women with placental abruption have demonstrated similar elevated serum levels.[2] Homocysteine is a sulfur-bearing amino acid involved in folate metabolism that is important in methylation reactions producing methionine and, with adenosine triphosphate activation, s-adenosyl methionine, a methyl donor in the production of nucleic acids, neurotransmitters, phospholipids, and hormones. The investigators have taken advantage of a common simple replacement mutation in the gene located on the long arm of chromosome 1, which results in reduced activity of the reductase and increased homocysteine serum concentrations. Searching for this mutation (T677) using restriction fragment polymorphisms shown on gel electrophoresis, they find significantly increased risk ratios for both the homozygous and heterozygous mutations in preeclamptic vs. normal pregnant women. This is a long way from proving homocysteine is the agent responsible for endothelial injury in preeclampsia, but certainly supports the need for its further study.

T.H. Kirschbaum, M.D.

References

1. 1990 Year Book of Obstetrics and Gynecology, pp 29–31.
2. Steegers-Theunissen RPM, Boers GHJ, Blom HJ, et al: Hyperhomocysteinemia and recurrent spontaneous abortion or abruptio placentae. *Lancet* 339:1122, 1992.

Ambulatory Blood Pressure Monitoring in Pregnancy Induced Hypertension

Biswas A, Choolani MA, Anandakumar C, et al (National Univ, Singapore)
Acta Obstet Gynecol Scand 76:829–833, 1997 3–10

Background.—Ambulatory blood pressure (ABP) monitoring has been found to be useful in adults. However, its role in pregnant women has not been well defined. The role of ABP monitoring in diagnosing pregnancy-induced hypertension in women with hypertension diagnosed in the clinic by the conventional method was studied.

Methods.—One hundred twenty-eight women participated in the observational study. All were 28–37 weeks pregnant and had nonproteinuric pregnancy-induced hypertension diagnosed in the clinic. Ambulatory blood pressure was monitored for 24 hours.

Findings.—Recordings were valid for 120 women. Only 38.3% were hypertensive on ABP monitoring, using a mean diastolic pressure cutoff of 85 mm Hg. The "white coat effect" (blood pressure increases only in the clinic) occurred in both hypertensive and normotensive women. The magnitude of this effect was poorly correlated with the clinic diastolic blood pressure (Fig 1). A cutoff value for diastolic load of 20% could detect all hypertensive women correctly, with a false positive rate of only 17.5% (Fig 5).

Conclusions.—"White-coat" hypertension appears to be common among pregnant women. Ambulatory blood pressure monitoring would be useful for identifying true hypertension in this population. Such monitoring would reduce unnecessary hospitalizations.

► Ambulatory intermittent blood pressure monitoring devices originally developed for aviation and space medicine surveillance have improved in time

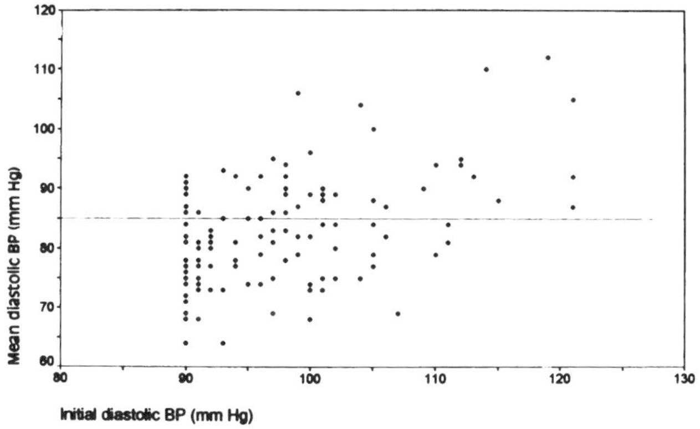

FIGURE 1.—Scattergram showing the relationship between initial diastolic blood pressure (BP) recorded in the clinic and the mean diastolic BP found on 24-hour ambulatory blood pressure monitoring. (Courtesy of Biswas A, Choolani MA, Anandakumar C, et al: Ambulatory blood pressure monitoring in pregnancy-induced hypertension. *Acta Obstet Gynecol Scand* 76:829-833, Copyright 1997 Munksgaard International Publishers Ltd, Copenhagen, Denmark.)

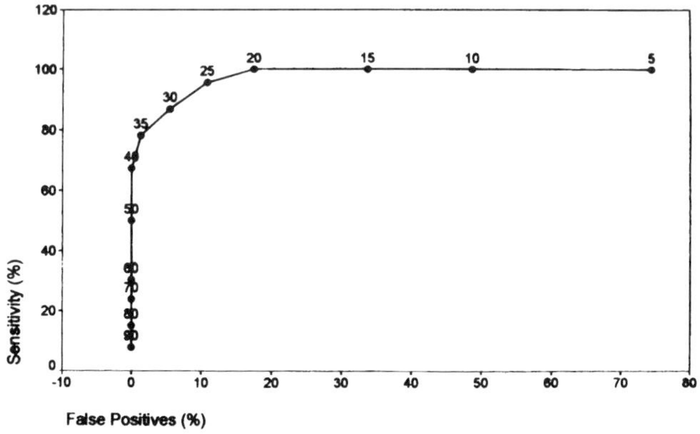

FIGURE 5.—Receiver-operator characteristics curve for using the diastolic load to detect a mean diastolic blood pressure of 85 mm Hg or higher. The graph shows the sensitivities and the false positive rates of diagnosing true hypertension at different cutoff values of diastolic load. (Courtesy of Biswas A, Choolani MA, Anandakumar C, et al: Ambulatory blood pressure monitoring in pregnancy-induced hypertension. *Acta Obstet Gynecol Scand* 76:829–833, Copyright 1997 Munksgaard International Publisher Ltd, Copenhagen, Denmark.)

and cost to the point of potential usefulness in monitoring the 24-hour course of blood pressure in women with pregnancy-induced hypertension. The results are useful both in evaluating the tendency for transient blood pressure elevations to occur in medical settings based on patient anxiety, and to evaluate changes in the normal circadian cycle of blood pressure in hypertensive disease. The device uses a pump for arterial occlusion and then senses the onset (systolic blood pressure) and disappearance (diastolic blood pressure) of blood pressure oscillations as pressure is reduced. Data are stored electronically and readily retrieved.

In this study of 120 women with pregnancy-induced hypertension from 28 to 37 weeks' gestation, all selected for auscultatory diastolic blood pressures equal to or greater than 90 mm Hg, roughly 62% proved to be normotensive on ambulatory monitoring done 36 times over 24 hours. Regularly, ABP monitoring yielded blood pressure values lower than auscultatory monitoring results, but with increasing levels of hypertension, the differences diminished. Extended monitoring allows estimation of the fraction of a 24-hour interval during which the diastolic blood pressure equals or exceeds 90 mm Hg—here called the diastolic load. In essence, load is a measure of the integral of blood pressure against time and measures the relative extent of sustained compared to transient hypertension to which the woman is subject. The authors find that, with diastolic load at or above 20% chosen as a predictive criterion for the diagnosis of hypertension, all cases of hypertension were accurately predicted with a 17.5% incidence of false positive results. This is a vast improvement over the 62% false positive rate with conventional auscultatory methods. Their data confirm the tendency during hypertension for reversal of the circadian blood pressure cycle with higher values nocturnally than during the day, but they do not provide those data in this publication. The authors demonstrate our tendency to overdiagnose hypertension at levels of marginal elevation with resultant excesses in hospital and drug utilization and with increases in related patient anxiety and operative obstetrics based on the false diagnosis of hypertension prevalent in modern obstetrics.

T.H. Kirschbaum, M.D.

Pregnancy Outcomes in Women With Gestational Diabetes Compared With the General Obstetric Population

Casey BM, Lucas MJ, Mcintire DD, et al (Univ of Texas, Dallas)

Obstet Gynecol 90:869–873, 1997 3–11

Background.—Gestational diabetes complicates 1% to 3% of all pregnancies. Authorities disagree about the significance of gestational diabetes in women without concomitant fasting hyperglycemia. Pregnancy outcomes in a homogeneous group of women with glucose intolerance were compared with those of women without this disorder.

Methods.—Data on all women with singleton cephalic-presenting pregnancies giving birth at 1 center between 1991 and 1995 were retrospectively analyzed. Of 61,209 nondiabetic women, 874 received diagnoses of class A_1 gestational diabetes.

Findings.—Women with class A_1 gestational diabetes were significantly older, heavier, of greater parity, and more often Hispanic than those without class A_1. Hypertension was present in 17% and 12%, respectively. Thirty percent of the women with gestational diabetes and 17% of those without it had cesarean deliveries. Also significant was the between-group

TABLE 3.—Infant Outcomes Among Women With Gestational Diabetes and Among the General Population

Outcome	Class A_1 gestational diabetes (n = 874)	General obstetric population (n = 61,209)	P
Birth weight			
Mean ± SD (g)	3581 ± 616	3290 ± 546	<.001
4001–4500 g	155 (18)	4141 (7)	<.001
4501–5000 g	35 (4)	572 (0.9)	<.001
≥5001 g	11 (1)	73 (0.1)	<.001
Large for gestational age*	310 (35)	8723 (14)	<.001
Admission to special care nursery	47 (5)	3214 (5)	NS
5-min Apgar score ≤3	0	120 (0.2)	NS
Umbilical artery blood pH ≤7.0	4 (0.5)	259 (0.4)	NS
Erb's palsy	3 (0.3)	114 (0.2)	NS
Fractured clavicle	15 (2)	544 (0.9)	.017
Stillbirth	4 (0.5)	259 (0.4)	NS
Neonatal death	1 (0.1)	153 (0.2)	NS

Note: Data are presented as mean ± standard deviation or n (%).

*Defined as birth weight at 90th percentile or higher for gestational age.

Abbreviation: NS, not significant.

(Reprinted with permission from the American College of Obstetricians and Gynecologists, from Casey BM, Lucas MJ, McIntire DD, et al: Pregnancy outcomes in women with gestational diabetes compared with the general obstetric population. *Obstet Gynecol* 90:869–873, 1997.)

difference in the incidence of shoulder dystocia—3% and 1%, respectively. Infants born to women with gestational diabetes were significantly larger, which explained the increase in dystocia. A 12% attributable risk for large-for-gestational age infants in women with class A_1 gestational diabetes was recorded (Table 3).

Conclusions.—Excessive fetal size is the main effect of class A_1 gestational diabetes. Large size can increase the risk of difficult labor and delivery. About 1 in 8 women with class A_1 gestational diabetes mellitus will give birth to a large-for-gestational-age infant because of glucose intolerance.

► In seeking objective evidence supporting case finding and treatment of gestational diabetes (GDM), these authors compared 874 women with class A_1 GDM and singlet vertex pregnancies recruited through outreach affiliated clinics with control nondiabetic women matched for maternal age, weight, ethnicity, and parity. The dependent variables observed were birth weight, evidence of dystocia, incidence of operative delivery, and birth trauma. The authors' reported 1.2% incidence of GDM compares well with that reported by others. The principal finding was a significant increase in the incidence of macrosomia, whether defined as greater than 4.0 or 4.5 Kg, among women with GDM. Not unexpectedly, there was an elevated incidence of pregnancy-induced hypertension (17%) among the diabetic women, perhaps a reflection of their greater mean age, parity, and weight than the controls. Induction of labor, often mandated by pregnancy-induced hypertension, was also more common. Although clavicular fracture occurred more often among infants of mothers with GDM, the incidence was still far below the incidence of 2.9% reported in normal uncomplicated vaginal births on routine survey.[1] It is intriguing to wonder as Naylor et al.[2] have recently, whether the increased diagnosis of dystocia and cesarean section might not be preconditioned by the diagnosis of diabetes mellitus because they found an increased incidence of cesarean section for dystocia among women with GDM delivering nonmacrosomic infants.

The authors' analysis suggests that benefit from identification and treatment of GDM may depend on whether reducing the incidence of macrosomia reduces the incidence of birth trauma. In their experience, there is no evidence that it does.

T.H. Kirschbaum, M.D.

References

1. 1991 Year Book of Obstetrics and Gynecology, pp 192–193.
2. Naylor CD, Sermer M, Chen E, et al: Cesarean delivery in relation to birth weight and gestational glucose tolerance: Pathophysiology or practice style? *JAMA* 275:1165–1170, 1996.

Selective Screening for Gestational Diabetes Mellitus

Naylor CD, for the Toronto Trihospital Gestational Diabetes Project Investigators (Sunnybrook Health Science Centre, North York, Ont, Canada; Univ of Toronto; Toronto Hosp; et al)

N Engl J Med 337:1591–1596, 1997 3–12

Objective.—Screening all pregnant women for gestational diabetes mellitus is expensive, time-consuming, and uncomfortable for patients. Furthermore, the merits of detecting and treating this condition are difficult to demonstrate. Results of a prospective study, evaluating if the efficiency of screening could be enhanced by considering the patients' risk of gestational diabetes based on their clinical characteristics were presented.

Methods.—The 3,131 pregnant women in the study were randomly allocated to the derivation or validation group. Risk factors of the derivation group-age, race, body mass index, parity, family history of diabetes, and adverse obstetrical history—were used to establish new screening strategies based on clinical scores that divided women into 3 risk groups: low, intermediate, and high. Low-risk women would not be screened and intermediate-risk women would receive the usual care. Women with plasma glucose levels of 130 mg/dL or high-risk women with plasma glucose levels of 128 mg/dL would receive universal screening. The strategies were evaluated by using the validation group.

Results.—According to multivariate analysis, age, race, and body mass index were independent predictors of gestational diabetes mellitus. The new strategy allowed 34.7% of women to avoid screening, and detected between 81.2% and 82.6% of women with gestational diabetes, with false-positive rates of 15.4 and 16.0%. Usual care detected 78.3% of women with gestational diabetes, with a false-positive rate of 17.9%.

Conclusion.—The new strategies taking women's clinical characteristics into account allow efficient and accurate screening for gestational diabetes mellitus in pregnant women.

► The dominant pattern of screening for gestational diabetes (GDM), a single blood sugar done after a 50 g load of glucose followed by an oral glucose tolerance test for confirmation, involves time, anxiety, expense, and effort on behalf of an estimated 3% to 4% of all pregnant women in North America. The diagnosis of GDM confers some benefit in predicting eventual fixed diabetes, but it has been hard to demonstrate other benefits to either gravidas or their infants on long-term follow-up, save the reduction in incidence of macrosomia. As a result, an expert committee on diagnosis and classification of diabetes has recommended selective screening in pregnancy.[1] This prospective bifid study, which antedated that recommendation by at least 5 years, uses roughly half of its subjects to establish criteria for selective screening and the other half to evaluate use of those criteria. Data were collected from 1989–1992. Data from the derivation group established criteria based on age, body mass index, and race, producing a 7-point scale. The authors demonstrate that by deleting glucose tolerance testing for women with scores of 0 or 1 in the scale, values of sensitivity (60% to 65%) and predictive value of a positive finding (85%) not significantly different from women receiving conventional care evolved. There was a roughly 35% decrease in the number of women screened. Arguments will continue over the items needed to be included in such a risk estimate. However, few can argue with an approach that seems to back away from universal GDM screening as long as the resultant detection rates remain unchanged.

T.H. Kirschbaum, M.D.

Reference

1. Report of the Expert Committee on the Diagnosis and Classification of Diabetes Mellitus. *Diabetes Care* 20:1183–1197, 1997.

A Randomized Controlled Trial of Strict Glycemic Control and Tertiary Level Obstetric Care Versus Routine Obstetric Care in the Management of Gestational Diabetes: A Pilot Study

Garner P, Okun N, Keely E, et al (Univ of Ottawa, Ont, Canada; Univ of Alberta, Ont, Canada)

Am J Obstet Gynecol 177:190–195, 1997 3–13

Background.—About 3% of pregnant women are affected by gestational diabetes mellitus. The extent of fetal and neonatal morbidity resulting from gestational diabetes mellitus is unclear. Several obstetric and diabetic societies and workshops have recommended universal screening of all pregnant women to identify women with a higher risk of macrosomia, operative delivery, and neonatal morbidity. Results of clinical trials of the effect of management of maternal glucose levels on maternal and fetal outcome in cases of gestational diabetes mellitus have been inconsistent.

Methods.—In a prospective, randomized, controlled trial, maternal and fetal-neonatal outcomes were compared in 300 women with gestational diabetes mellitus. Women received either strict glycemic control and tertiary level obstetric care or routine obstetric care.

Results.—The mean birth weight was 3,437 g in the treatment group and 3,544 g in the control group; this difference was not significant. The rates of macrosomia were similar in both groups. No birth trauma occurred in either group. The treatment and control groups had similar rates of neonatal hypoglycemia and other metabolic complications and similar mode of delivery patterns. Significantly lower preprandial and postprandial glucose levels by 32 weeks' gestation were seen in the treatment group; these levels continued to term.

Discussion.—These results indicate that intensive treatment of gestational diabetes mellitus has little clinical effect on birth weight, birth trauma, operative delivery rates, and neonatal metabolic disorders. These results also indicate that it is safe to proceed to a multicenter trial with a sufficient sample size to confirm the findings of this pilot study.

► Questions of the merits, and lately the cost-effectiveness, of routine screening and diabetic management for gestational diabetes mellitus (GDM) have been growing in number and intensity within the last few years. The first effective argument questioning screening for GDM came in 1989 with the recommendation of the Oxford National Perinatal Epidemiology Unit, as reflected in data then available, that "thus far improvement in neonatal outcome has not been demonstrated from insulin therapy for gestational diabetes" and that "there is, however, a great potential to do more harm than good."[1] Close scrutiny of health care costs has added to this concern. Even those who feel strongly that diabetic care for GDM reduces the incidence of macrosomia concede that there is little consequent reduction in fetal morbidity.

This is a well-planned and executed pilot study designed to test feasibility and sharpen data organization and storage systems before the major undertaking necessary to argue convincingly that GDM screening is unnecessary. Three hundred low-risk women at 24–28 weeks' gestation found to have GDM after glucose screening and a glucose tolerance test were randomly divided into special and routine care groups. Routine care consisted of unrestricted diet, 2 blood glucose finger sticks per week, and no fetal testing unless otherwise indicated. The special care group received intensive dietary management, and in 24% of the cases, insulin. The incidence of failed control in this special treatment group (fasting glucose level greater than 140 mg/dL, 1-hour postprandial glucose level greater than 200 mg/dL) was 10.6%. The 2 groups did not differ significantly regarding patient age, weight, weight increase, duration of gestation, incidence of smoking, previous obstetric history, and results of glucose screening. No differences in mean birth weight, neonatal hypoglycemia, hypocalcemia, or hyperbilirubinemia were seen. Neither were there instances of birth trauma, intracranial hemorrhage, and fetal or neonatal death in either group. Abdominal birth frequency was the same in both groups and insulin treatment of A^2 diabetic patients showed no difference in outcome compared to the A1 GDM groups in either the special or controlled group. This study will certainly be of special interest to all of us.

T.H. Kirschbaum, M.D.

Reference

1. Hunter DJS, Keirse MJNC, Chalmers I, et al: Gestational Diabetes, in *Effective Care in Pregnancy and Childbirth*. Oxford, Oxford University Press, 1989, pp 403–410.

A Change From Stimulatory to Blocking Antibody Activity in Graves' Disease During Pregnancy

Kung AWC, Jones BM (Univ of Hong Kong, Republic of China)

J Clin Endocrinol Metab 83:514–518, 1998 3–14

Background.—Remission of Graves' disease during pregnancy with recurrence after delivery is a common occurrence. Decreased activity in thyroid-stimulating antibody (TSAb) alone does not explain this remission because pregnancy is associated with type 2, not type 1, cytokine production. The authors hypothesized that a change in antibody characteristics might occur with advancing pregnancy. To investigate possible causes of remission of Graves' disease during pregnancy, the clinical course of pregnant women with Graves' disease was studied, together with their lymphocyte subset populations.

Methods.—In a prospective study, thyrotropin (TSH) receptor antibodies were determined in 15 pregnant women with Graves' disease and 14 healthy pregnant women during the first, second, and third trimesters and at 4 months postpartum. Ten nonpregnant women with Graves' disease receiving antithyroid drug treatment were also studied. Human thyroid cell cultures were used to determine TSH receptor antibodies, and flow cytometry was used to measure lymphocyte subsets.

Results.—During pregnancy, median TSAb decreased from 280% to 130% (Fig 3), but there was no significant change in TSH-binding inhibitory immunoglobulin (TBII). An increase from 16% to 43% was seen in thyroid stimulation–blocking antibody (TSBAb) (Fig 2); this increase was even seen in women who were in remission before pregnancy. During

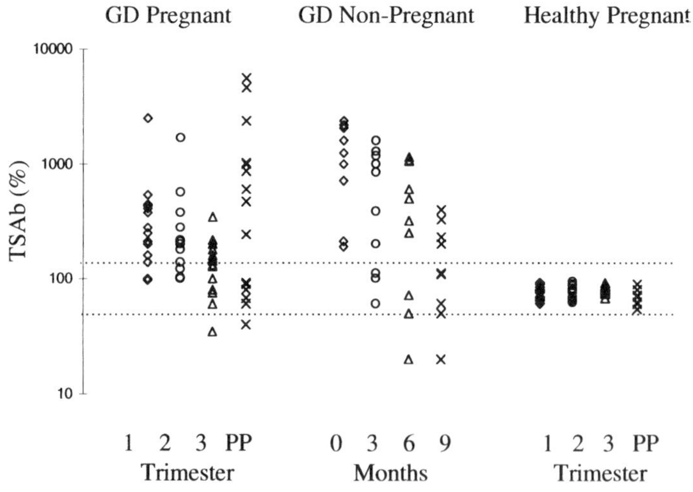

FIGURE 3.—Serial changes in thyroid stimulation–blocking antibody (*TSAb*) in pregnant patients with Graves' disease (*GD*) nonpregnant patients with GD, and healthy pregnant control subjects. *Abbreviation: PP*, postpartum. (Courtesy of Kung AWC, Jones BM: A change from stimulatory to blocking antibody activity in Graves' disease during pregnancy. *J Clin Endocrinol Metab* 83(2):514–518, copyright 1998, The Endocrine Society.)

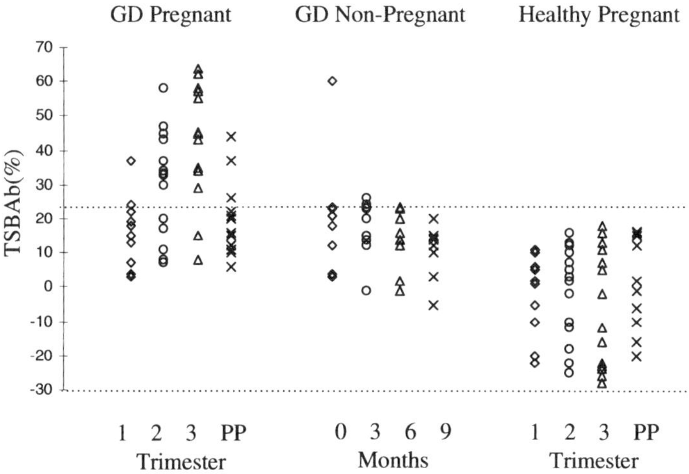

FIGURE 2.—Serial changes in thyroid stimulation–blocking antibody (*TSBAb*) in pregnant patients with Graves' disease (*GD*), nonpregnant patients with GD, and healthy pregnant control subjects. *Abbreviation*: *PP*, postpartum. (Courtesy of Kung AWC, Jones BM: A change from stimulatory to blocking antibody activity in Graves' disease during pregnancy. *J Clin Endocrinol Metab* 83(2):514–518, copyright 1998, The Endocrine Society.)

pregnancy, there was a negative correlation between TSBAb activity and free thyroxine levels. In the 7 patients who had a relapse after birth, reciprocal changes in TSAb, TBII, and TSBAb levels were seen. The healthy pregnant women tested negative for TSAb, TBII, and TSBAb during their pregnancies. In women with Graves' disease and in healthy women, the absolute number of T lymphocytes, T-helper cells, and natural killer cells—but not B cells—decreased significantly during pregnancy. Significantly more CD5+ B cells were seen at all stages of pregnancy in patients with Graves' disease than in control subjects.

Discussion.—In women with Graves' disease, a change in specificity from stimulatory to blocking antibodies was seen during pregnancy. This change may be involved in the remission of Graves' disease during pregnancy. Further studies of antibody isotype and cytokine production may help determine the mechanism of this change and help develop immunotherapy for inducing natural remission of Graves' disease.

▶ Those who treat Graves' disease during pregnancy with medication are often gratified to find that their patients become easier to manage and are often euthyroid by the late third trimester. This study, building on what is known about autoimmune factors in Graves' disease from earlier work,[1] offers some explanations for the tendency for the decline of free thyroxine in such women in late pregnancy. Many of the changes noted are reflections of the tendency for reduced cellular immunity, indicated by reductions in T lymphocytes and T-helper/suppresser cells, as well as type 1 cytokines. These changes occur early in pregnancy and are, apparently, part of the immune tolerance afforded the fetal trophoblast.

This study finds humoral immunity mediated by B lymphocytes unchanged during pregnancy but rendered relatively more important as cellular immunity declines in immunoreactivity. Among the changes in B cell–mediated antibody production are reductions in TSAbs as well as increases in TSBAb, which serves to decrease the biologic activity at the antibody of thyroid receptor sites. Late in pregnancy, both cellular and humoral immunity—as well as natural immunity associated with natural killer cells—appear suppressed. Thyrotropin-binding inhibitory immunoglobulin, an antibody to thyroglobulin and microsomal antigens important in autoimmune thyroiditis appear unchanged during pregnancy.

The tendency for remission late in pregnancy for women with Graves' disease appears to be part of a complex and incompletely understood series of changes in what now appears to be a heterogeneous array of thyroid antibody receptors and B cell products. It is now important to understand the mechanisms involved in more detail with the hope of preventing their reversal and the tendency to rebound to increased free thyroxine and thyrotoxicosis immediately after birth.

T.H. Kirschbaum, M.D.

Reference

1. 1989 Year Book of Obstetrics and Gynecology, pp 77–78.

Outcome of Differentiated Thyroid Cancer Diagnosed in Pregnant Women

Moosa M, Mazzaferri EL (Ohio State Univ, Columbus)
J Clin Endocrinol Metab 82:2862–2866, 1997 3–15

Introduction.—Thyroid cancer occurs more commonly in women, particularly during the child-bearing years, and some studies suggest that the risk of thyroid cancer is increased during pregnancy and in the first year after giving birth. A large cohort of women who were pregnant when thyroid cancer was discovered was studied to determine the effect of pregnancy on prognosis.

Methods.—Study participants were identified through the United States Air Force Central Tumor Registry and the records of The Ohio State University Hospitals. Sixty-four items were recorded for each patient, including demographic information, tumor features, treatment, and outcome. Sixty-one pregnant women with thyroid cancer were compared with 528 age-matched women with thyroid cancer who were not pregnant.

Results.—The pregnant group had a mean age of 26.0 years and a median follow-up of 22.4 years; nonpregnant controls had a mean age of 26.3 years and a median follow-up of 19.5 years. Identification of the nodule occurred in the first trimester in 30% of pregnant patients, in the second trimester in 43%, and in the third trimester in 28%. Tumors were found by a physician in 57% of pregnant women and in 22% of women

TABLE 6.—Outcome

Outcome	Pregnant*	Not pregnant
Recurrence (yr)		
10	8 (15%)	85 (21%)
20	1 (17%)	13 (26%)
30	0 (17%)	8 (31%)
40	0 (17%)	1 (33%)
Distant recurrence (yr)†		
10	1 (2%)	9 (2%)
20	0 (2%)	1 (3%)
30	0 (2%)	2 (4%)
Cancer death (yr)		
10	0	0
20	0	2 (1%)
30	0	4 (3%)

*P = nonsignificance for all recurrences, distant recurrence, and cancer death comparing women who were and were not pregnant (log-rank test for Kaplan Meier life-table events at 10, 20, and 30 years).

†Distant recurrence sites: lungs, 8 patients; bone, 1 patient; lungs and bone, 2 patients; lungs and brain, 1 patient; lungs, bone, and brain, 1 patient.

(Courtesy of Moosa M, Mazzaferri EL: Outcome of differentiated thyroid cancer diagnosed in pregnant women. *J Clin Endocrinol Metab* 82(9):2862–2866, 1997. Copyright, The Endocrine Society.)

who were not pregnant. The mean time lapse from discovery of the tumor to initial therapy did not differ significantly in the pregnant and control groups (12.7 and 10.8 months, respectively), nor did the 2 groups differ significantly in the surgical and medical therapies they received. Rates of cancer recurrence were 15% in pregnant woman and 23% in controls, not a significant difference. There were 6 deaths, all in the control group (Table 6). Women operated after delivery had outcomes similar to those who underwent surgery during pregnancy (Table 7).

Conclusion.—There is reason to believe that certain reproductive and hormonal changes that occur around the time of pregnancy may contribute to more aggressive behavior of well-differentiated thyroid cancer.

TABLE 7.—Outcome in Patients Operated on During Pregnancy

Variable	Surgery during pregnancy	Surgery after delivery	*P*
Age (yr)	23.7 ± 4.7*	26.7 ± 6.1	NS
Time (months)†	1.1 ± 1.0*	16.1 ± 19.7	0.001
Tumor diameter (cm)	2.0 ± 1.2*	2.6 ± 1.6	NS
Nodal metastases [n (%)]			
None	10 (71%)	26 (55%)	NS
Unilateral	2 (14%)	16 (34%)	NS
Bilateral	2 (14%)	4 (9%)	NS
Mediastinal	0	1 (2%)	NS
Recurrence [n (%)]	2 (14%)	7 (15%)	NS
Distant recurrences [n (%)]	0	1 (2%)	NS

*Mean ± standard deviation.

†Time from discovery of a thyroid nodule to first treatment.

(Courtesy of Moosa M, Mazzaferri EL: Outcome of differentiated thyroid cancer diagnosed in pregnant women. *J Clin Endocrinol Metab* 82(9):2862–2866, 1997. Copyright, The Endocrine Society.)

Findings in this series of patients, however, suggest that diagnostic studies and initial therapy may usually be delayed until after delivery.

► Thyroid nodules are found in 1% to 2% of gravidas and of those, 5% to 10% prove, subsequently, to be malignant. Tumors in young women tend to be well differentiated and generally not as aggressive as the less-differentiated tumors that tend to be distributed largely in postmenopausal women. The indolent nature of the malignancy and its tendency for late recurrence has led to recommendations that surgical therapy be delayed until after delivery, but that conclusion rests on relatively small numbers of reported cases.[1]

The value of this collection of experience beginning in 1962 and held in the United States Air Force Central Tumor Registry rests in the large number of patients reported. The outcomes of 61 women found to have a thyroid nodule during pregnancy, with diagnosis of malignancy made during or after pregnancy, were compared with 528 age-matched women in whom pregnancy played no coincident role in diagnosis and treatment. Many patients were seen before needle biopsy was generally available during pregnancy, but this served only to lengthen the time to therapy for the pregnant group.

In both pregnant and nonpregnant women, three fourths exhibited a single asymptomatic nodule, about 80% of which were papillary and 15% follicular. The mean time, between diagnosis and treatment was 12.7 months for pregnant and 10.8 months for nonpregnant patients. Ten-year follow-up was obtained from 77% of the women. No significant differences in outcome were noted between pregnant and nonpregnant women, nor between the 14 pregnant women treated surgically during pregnancy and the 47 women treated after delivery.

Among the 61 pregnant women, 41% had distant metastases and 10% had bilateral cervical nodes. Nonetheless, 30-year cancer mortality rates were 1.1% (6 women) among the nonpregnant women. There were no cancer fatalities in the pregnancy group. This is the strongest evidence to date in support of awaiting delivery before performing thyroidectomy on pregnant women with a malignant nodule.

T.H. Kirschbaum, M.D.

Reference

1. 1996 Year Book of Obstetrics and Gynecology, pp 64–67.

The Acquisition of Herpes Simplex Virus During Pregnancy

Brown ZA, Selke S, Zeh J, et al (Univ of Washington, Seattle; Madigan Army Med Ctr, Tacoma, Wash)

N Engl J Med 337:509–515, 1997 3–16

Background.—Women who acquire genital herpes during pregnancy are at elevated risk for spontaneous abortion, prematurity, and congenital and neonatal herpes. Few prospective studies have examined either the frequency with which herpes simplex virus (HSV) is acquired during pregnancy or the impact of its timing. A longitudinal study of the acquisition of HSV infection among pregnant women is reported.

Methods.—The study included 7,046 pregnant women at risk for HSV infection. Serum samples were taken at the first prenatal visit, at 16 to 24 weeks' gestation, and during labor for Western blot testing for antibodies to HSV types 1 and 2 (HSV-1 and HSV-2). The study definition of seroconversion was the appearance of antibody at labor that was not present at the initial visit. The time of acquisition was established as the date of the first reported genital lesions or, for subclinical cases, the midpoint between the time of the last negative and the first positive antibody test.

Results.—Seroconversion occurred during pregnancy in 94 women, 34 of whom were symptomatic. For women who were seronegative for both HSV-1 and HSV-2 at their initial visit, the risk of seroconversion was only about 4%. Patients who were initially seropositive for HSV-1 had a 2% risk of acquiring HSV-2, whereas those who were initially seropositive for HSV-2 had an estimated 0 risk of acquiring HSV-1. The timing of HSV acquisition was known in 60 cases: the first trimester in 30%, the second trimester in 30%, and the third trimester in 40%. As long as HSV seroconversion was completed by the time the woman went into labor, there was no increase in neonatal morbidity and no problems with congenital herpes infection. Nine women acquired HSV shortly before labor. Four of their babies had neonatal HSV infection, and 1 died.

Conclusions.—At least 2% of women who are at risk will acquire HSV during pregnancy. As long as HSV seroconversion is completed by the time of labor, the outcome of pregnancy does not seem to be affected. However, if the infection is acquired around the time of labor, there is a danger of neonatal herpes and perinatal morbidity. Preventive efforts should focus on avoiding maternal acquisition of HSV during the latter part of pregnancy.

► This excellent longitudinal study of HSV acquisition in pregnancy helps answer some of the questions regarding primary vs. recurrent herpes infection raised by earlier studies[1], as well as providing interesting information regarding the risks of maternal to fetal transmission of this virulent agent. The study population of 8,538 gravidas represents 55% of those who delivered over a 3–5 year interval in 2 Seattle–Tacoma area hospitals. Serum antibody determinations at the first prenatal visit and at admission in labor were entry requirements for the study, and determinations done in the second and early third trimesters of pregnancy provided some information about the time of seroconversion seen in 94 women. Those women represented 1.3% of all patients entering pregnancy who are seronegative. Primary HSV infection is defined in women seropositive at delivery but seronegative at initial contact. Women seropositive at initial examination who developed symptoms and lesions of HSV during pregnancy were deemed to have recurrent herpes. Two thirds of all women who seroconverted during the first trimester of pregnancy had subclinical infections, two thirds of them developing antibody solely to HSV-2. The average rate of seroconversion during pregnancy was 2.1%, and the time of seroconversion was roughly equally distributed among all 3 trimesters of pregnancy. No cases of neonatal herpes were noted among seroconverted women. This information allowed the probabilistic estimate of the risk of maternal to fetal transmission where primary infection occurs early enough in pregnancy to allow the 4–6 week interval needed for the development of antibody. The estimate of transmission in primary maternal herpes is less than 3.2%. Only in 9 cases in which infection without antibody development by the time of labor did 4 cases of neonatal herpes occur, 2 with late pregnancy first trimester HSV-1 infection and 2 with nonprimary late recurrent HSV-2 infection. HSV-2 antibody development appears to offer some protection against HSV-1 infection. These data indicate that when HSV primary or recurrent infection takes place in the first or second trimester, or more than 6 weeks before delivery, acyclovir may well be unnecessary to prevent transmission to the fetus. When infection occurs in a seronegative woman within 4–6 weeks before the onset of labor, chemotherapy for HSV is probably indicated to prevent fetal infection. The risk of newborn infection from maternal HSV infection is generally low.

T.H. Kirschbaum, M.D.

Reference

1. 1998 Year Book of Obstetrics, Gynecology, and Women's Health, pp 127–129.

Registry of Pregnancy in Dialysis Patients

Okundaye I, Abrinko P, Hou S (Rush Presbyterian-St Luke's Med Ctr, Chicago)

Am J Kidney Dis 31:766–773, 1998 3–17

Background.—Pregnancy is rare in women with end-stage renal disease receiving dialysis. There are few recommendations about contraception for such women, and few guidelines for the care of the women who do become pregnant. Studies of a large number of pregnancies in patients treated with dialysis have not included details about the course of pregnancy or about medical and obstetric management. The registry described in this study collects data on pregnancies in patients in the United States who are receiving dialysis.

Methods.—A survey was conducted of 2,299 dialysis centers. Responses were received from 930 centers treating 6,230 female patients aged 14–44. The frequency and course of pregnancies in these women were determined.

Results.—Of the 6,230 women, 1,699 received peritoneal dialysis and 4,531 received hemodialysis. Of women of childbearing age, 2% (1.1% of those receiving peritoneal dialysis and 2.4% of those receiving hemodialysis) became pregnant during a 4-year period. The duration of dialysis treatment was known in 128 patients (Fig 4). Among the 184 pregnancies

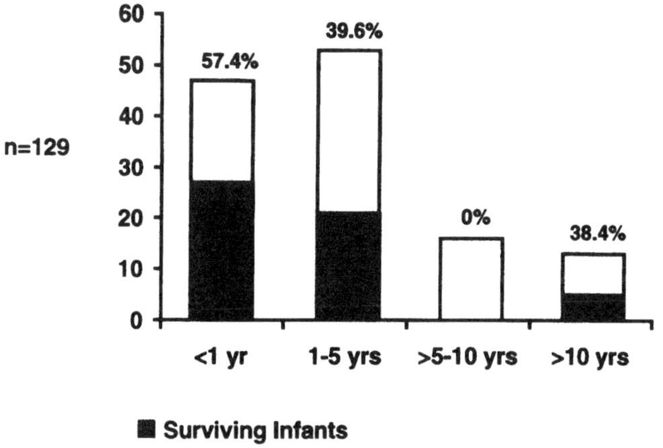

FIGURE 4.—Pregnancy outcome vs. number of years on dialysis. The shaded part of the bar represents surviving infants. (Courtesy of Okundaye I, Abrinko P, Hou S: Registry of pregnancy in dialysis patients. *Am J Kidney Dis* 31:766–773, 1998.)

in women who conceived after starting dialysis, the infant survival rate was 40.2%. Among the 57 pregnancies in women who were pregnant before starting dialysis, the infant survival rate was 73.6%. In a subset of women with a known dialysis modality, infant survival among patients receiving peritoneal dialysis and hemodialysis was similar. Infant survival was somewhat better in women who had dialysis 20 hours a week or more. There was a weak correlation between number of hours of dialysis and gestational age. There were 2 maternal deaths and 5 intensive care unit admissions for hypertensive crisis. Some degree of hypertension was present in 79% of women; 32 women had blood pressure higher than 170/110 mm Hg. A hematocrit greater than 30% was seen in only 5.9% of women throughout their pregnancy. Transfusion was needed in 26% of women treated with erythropoietin and in 77% of women not treated with erythropoietin. Eleven infants had congenital anomalies and 11 infants had long-term medical problems. Among infants conceived after the mothers started dialysis, 84% were premature.

Conclusion.—The chance that a woman who becomes pregnant during dialysis treatment will have an infant who survives is higher than previously reported. Though there is no preferred dialysis modality, more hours on dialysis may improve outcome. Prematurity is the major cause of morbidity in surviving infants, and may increase the risk of long-term medical problems.

▶ Though pregnancy is rare in women with end-stage renal disease, it did occur in uremic women, with an incidence of 2.2% from 1992–1995, in this collection of registry data. The data were derived by queries addressed to directors of Dialysis and Transplant Services, sponsored by the Federal Health Care Financing Administration. The authors describe 344 pregnancies in 318 women on dialysis, with results from 40% of the dialysis units representing 48% of women treated during the 4-year interval. Perinatal outcome was known in 320 cases, with a perinatal death rate of 13.5%, infant survival in 42%, spontaneous abortion in 32%, and therapeutic abortion in 10.5%. Infant survival, prematurity, and growth retardation rates were not measurably affected by the mode of dialysis, but for an undetermined reason, conception was rare in women on chronic ambulant peritoneal dialysis. The duration of dialysis during pregnancy also was not clearly related to infant survival. Survival was, however, clearly best among women who became pregnant with renal impairment, but who required dialysis initially only during pregnancy. This observation is consonant with the inverse relationship between infant survival and duration of dialysis, which the authors report. Erythropoetin use was clearly beneficial in dealing with the inevitable trend toward maternal anemia through pregnancy. There were 2 cases of maternal mortality, 1 apparently related to pregnancy in a woman with end-stage renal disease of 12 years' duration. An important datum is the 90% to 91% incidence of 1-year survival for these gravidas. This is the largest number of women with this hazardous complication of pregnancy reported to date, and it seems to indicate a somewhat better prognosis for surviving pregnancy, especially for those women newly requiring dialysis, than has been reported earlier.

T.H. Kirschbaum, M.D.

Pregnancy in Women With Impaired Renal Function
Jungers P, Chauveau D, Choukroun G, et al (Necker Hosp, Paris)
Clin Nephrol 47:281–288, 1997 3–18

Introduction.—Although pregnancy is usually successful and causes no adverse effects in women with renal disease and normal or near normal renal function, both maternal and fetal outcome are considered to be at risk when renal function is significantly impaired at conception. In a retrospective analysis of 43 pregnancies in women with moderate-to-severe chronic renal failure, investigators assessed the benefit of recent advances in coordinated obstetric and nephrologic management.

Patients and Methods.—Included in the study were 30 women followed in a nephrology department during a 20-year period (1975–1994). The patients had various types of well-defined primary renal disease and impaired renal function. There were 16 cases of reflux nephropathy, 5 of chronic interstitial nephritis, 5 of autosomal-dominant polycystic kidney disease, and 4 of chronic glomerulonephritis. Serum creatinine concentration (Scr) ranged from 0.11 to 0.49 mmol/L. Eighteen patients had 1 pregnancy (including 2 twin pregnancies), 9 had 2, and 1 had 3 pregnancies after Scr was more than 0.11 mmol/L. Parameters recorded for each pregnancy included Scr, blood pressure, 24-hour urinary protein excretion, and creatinine clearance. Maternal and fetal outcome were assessed in terms of potential prognostic factors.

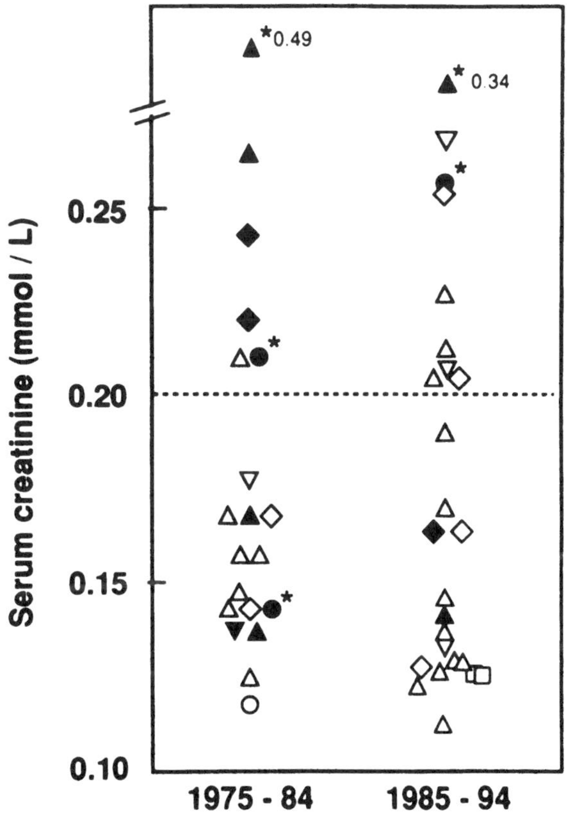

FIGURE 2.—Compared fetal outcome in the 1975–1984 (period I) and 1985–1994 (period II) decades, with respect to the serum creatinine level at conception and the primary renal disease. *Open symbols* denote live births; *closed symbols* denote fetal deaths; *asterisks* indicate first-trimester abortions. Renal disease is represented as follows: *diamond*, polycystic kidney disease; *upright triangle*, reflux nephropathy; *inverted triangle*, chronic interstitial nephritis; *circle*, IgA glomerulonephritis; and *square*, membranous nephropathy. (Courtesy of Jungers P, Chauveau D, Choukroun G, et al: Pregnancy in women with impaired renal function. *Clin Nephrol* 47:281–288, 1997.)

Results.—There were 13 fetal deaths (5 in the first trimester, including 1 therapeutic abortion, and 8 between gestational weeks 21 and 34) and 32 live births. Eighteen deliveries were preterm and 13 patients underwent cesarean section. The mean birth weight of living neonates was 2,383 grams. When the 2 decades of the study period were compared, significantly more pregnancies were successful in the last decade (Fig 2). The live birth rate was higher in pregnancies started with an Scr of less than 0.20 mmol/L (80%) than in those with an Scr of more than 0.20 mmol/L (53%). Hypertension was the most important factor influencing fetal outcome. In 7 patients, all with severe hypertension and heavy proteinuria at conception, pregnancy was associated with an accelerated deterioration in renal function.

Conclusion.—Advances in obstetrics and neonatology, together with improved blood pressure control, have led to a better maternal and fetal outcome in patients with impaired renal function. The overall success rate in this series was 82% not considering first trimester abortions. Hypertension and an Scr of more than 0.27 mmol/L increase the risk of fetal loss.

► This thorough review of 30 women with 45 pregnancies—all of the patients with significant chronic renal disease—provides the basis for cautious optimism, largely on the basis of the improved fetal survival noted during the years 1985–1994 compared with prior years. Patients were divided on the basis of Scr in early pregnancy into group 1, with values from 1.25 to 2.25 mg percent and group 2, with values of 2.25 to 5.5 mg percent. The overall incidence of fetal survival at birth was 71%—80% in group 1 and 53% in group 2—with both figures including spontaneous and induced abortions.

In general, more recent data disclosed an increased incidence of preterm labor and very low birth rate infants, but with 7 of 9 infants born to women in group 2 surviving. Figure 2 shows improved survival, a reflection of improved perinatal care; pharmacologic blood pressure regulation; and administration of synthetic erythropoetin, which has rendered anemia no longer an effective predictor of bad pregnancy outcome.

The presence of co-existing hypertension was the only major risk factor for reproductive failure discernable in this experience. The incidence of accelerated decline of creatinine clearance in 16% of the gravidas—all of them with hypertension and severe proteinuria—is a hazard that couples must weigh carefully in deciding to undertake pregnancy. Women with reflux nephropathy, a common cause of renal insufficiency in that gender, seem somewhat less prone to decompensation in pregnancy than those with other forms of renal pathology.

T.H. Kirschbaum, M.D.

4 Fetal Complications of Pregnancy

Screening of Maternal Serum for Fetal Down's Syndrome in the First Trimester

Haddow JE, Palomaki GE, Knight GJ, et al (Found for Blood Research, Scarborough, Me; Prenatal Diagnostic Ctr, Lexington, Mass)

N Engl J Med 338:955–961, 1998 4–1

Introduction.—Nearly all testing of pregnant women for Down's syndrome takes place in the second trimester. The finding that maternal serum alpha-fetoprotein concentrations were relatively low at 9–12 weeks of gestation in the presence of Down's syndrome led to studies of other potential serum markers that could be measured in the first trimester. A prospective study examined the value of serum alpha-fetoprotein, unconjugated estriol, human chorionic gonadotropin (hCG), the free beta unit of hCG, and pregnancy-associated protein A in screening for Down's syndrome in the first trimester.

Methods.—Study participants were 4,412 women with singleton pregnancies who were referred for chorionic villus sampling or amniocentesis. The women ranged in age from 15 to 51; 85% were 35 or older. Blood samples were obtained at 16 centers and sent to a single center for biochemical analysis. Also reported were US measurements of fetal nuchal translucency.

Results.—The results of fetal chromosomal analysis were available for all pregnancies. Before 14 weeks of gestation, 48 pregnancies affected by Down's syndrome and 3,169 unaffected pregnancies were identified. Rates of detection of Down's syndrome were highest for pregnancy-associated protein A (42%), hCG (29%), and the free beta subunit of hCG and lowest for unconjugated estriol (4%) and alpha-fetoprotein (17%). There was a high correlation between the results of measurements of serum hCG and its free beta subunit. Used in combination with the serum concentration of pregnancy-associated protein A and maternal age (Table 2), hCG achieved a 63% detection rate and its free beta subunit a 60% detection rate for Down's syndrome (at false-positive rates of 5%). Nuchal-translucency measurements were obtained in an average of 83% of pregnancies at the different centers. There was considerable variability in this factor among

TABLE 2.—Detection of Down's Syndrome With Two Combinations of Maternal Serum Markers at 9 Through 13 Weeks' Gestation

False Positive Rate	Detection Rate (95% CI)*	
	Maternal Age, Serum hCG, and PAP-A	Maternal Age, Serum hCG Free Beta Subunit, and PAP-A
	percent	
5	63 (47–76)	60 (45–74)
10	71 (56–83)	65 (49–78)
15	77 (63–88)	73 (58–85)
20	83 (70–93)	83 (70–93)
25	85 (72–94)	85 (72–94)

*The detection rate is the percentage of the 48 cases of Down's syndrome detected with use of the combination of markers. CI denotes confidence interval, hCG human chorionic gonadotropin, and PAP-A pregnancy-associated protein A.

(Reprinted by permission of *The New England Journal of Medicine* Haddow JE, Palomaki GE, Knight GJ, et al: Screening of maternal serum for fetal Down's syndrome in the first trimester. *N Engl J Med* 338:955–961, 1998.)

centers, and measurements could not be reliably incorporated into calculations.

Conclusion.—Measurements of pregnancy-associated protein A and either hCG or its free beta subunit in maternal serum may allow screening for Down's syndrome to be carried out in the first trimester. There are psychological advantages to early identification of the syndrome, and early termination of pregnancy involves less risk to the mother.

▶ The bulk of "triple screening" employing alpha-fetoprotein, hCG, and urinary estriol determinations for the prenatal diagnosis of Down syndrome is done in the second trimester. Timing complicates decisions for pregnancy termination in the event that is deemed desirable. This work, done by an important contributor to antenatal Down syndrome screening, explores the feasibility of screening in the first trimester to minimize patient anxiety and facilitate pregnancy termination at the reduced level of patient risk that applies then. The approach results from measurement of pregnancy-associated protein A (PAP-A), a protein that achieves discrimination between affected and unaffected pregnancies during the first but not the second trimester of pregnancy. Because of relatively rapid rates of increase of PAP-A values, ultrasonic dating of early pregnancy becomes a necessity in the first trimester, and the authors find use of menstrual dating reduces the detection rate (percentage of affected pregnancies detected at a specified cutoff value) by 3% to 5%. As before,[1] data are derived from patients submitting to chorion villus sampling or amniocentesis at any of 16 centers in the United States. Serum samples were drawn before the invasive procedures, and biochemical studies done and correlated with karyotypes. Since alpha-fetoprotein and urine estriol values are poorly discriminatory before the second trimester, and because beta hCG values cross-correlate so well, only PAP-A and beta hCG values were employed in prediction. Ultrasonic examination of nuchal lucency has a detection rate of 31% at a 5% false-positive level, but intercenter variability was deemed too large to make it useful. Calculation of age-specific risk ratios was done after the method of Cuckle et al (see *Year Book 1993*, pages 138–40). Statistical analysis of the 48 cases of Down's syndrome seen in 3,169 women in the first trimester demonstrates a detection rate of 63% (CI 47 - 76) with a false-positive rate set at 5%; that is about the same as the rate that is obtainable in second-trimester analysis. The approach seems feasible in the hands of these investigators without reduced efficacy. The disadvantages here pertain to difficulty in obtaining first-trimester chorion villus biopsy material and amniocentesis, the 20% spontaneous abortion rate that applies to efforts at 10–16 weeks of gestation, and differences in ultrasonic screening for neural tube defects, which are more effective in the second than in the first trimester. Nonetheless, this study carefully describes the biochemical approaches that are appropriate to first-trimester screening for this important genetic abnormality.

T.H. Kirschbaum, M.D.

Reference

1. 1995 Year Book of Obstetrics and Gynecology, pp 222–223.

Inhibition of Erythroid Progenitor Cells by Anti-Kell Antibodies in Fetal Alloimmune Anemia

Vaughan JI, Manning M, Warwick RM, et al (Queen Charlotte's Hosp, London; Royal Postgraduate Med School, London)

N Engl J Med 338:798–803, 1998 4–2

Background.—In infants with alloimmune anemia, more hemolysis is caused by antibodies to antigens of the Kell blood-group system than by antibodies to the D antigen of the Rh blood-group system. For the degree of anemia present, these infants have inappropriately low numbers of reticulocytes and normoblasts. Thus, sensitization to Kell antigens could lead not only to hemolysis but also to suppression of fetal erythropoiesis. Whether inhibition of erythroid progenitor cell growth is partly responsible for fetal anemia caused by anti-Kell antibodies was determined.

Methods and Findings.—The in vitro study compared the growth of Kell-positive and Kell-negative hematopoietic progenitor cells from cord blood in the presence of human monoclonal anti-Kell antibodies, anti-D antibodies, and serum from women with anti-Kell antibodies. Monoclonal immunoglobulin (Ig)G and IgM anti-Kell antibodies inhibited the growth of Kell-positive erythroid progenitor cells from cord blood in dose-dependent fashion. No inhibitory effect was noted with monoclonal anti-D antibodies. None of the 3 antibodies altered the growth of erythroid progenitor cells from Kell-negative cord blood. Growth of granulocyte or megakaryocyte progenitor cells from cord blood was unaffected by monoclonal anti-Kell antibodies or monoclonal anti-D antibodies (Fig 1, B).

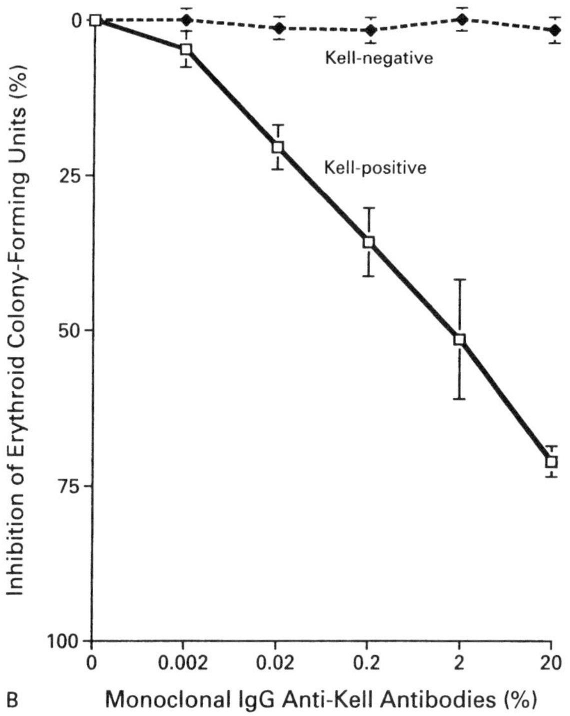

FIGURE 1, B.—Effect of monoclonal anti-Kell antibodies on the growth of cord-blood erythroid progenitor cells. Anti-Kell antibodies inhibited the growth of erythroid colony-forming units from Kell-positive cord blood ($r = -0.96$, $P < 0.001$) but not Kell-negative cord blood. Results are expressed as the mean (±SE) percentage of inhibition in experiments with 3 Kell-positive and 3 Kell-negative samples of cord blood. (Courtesy of Vaughan JI, Manning M, Warwick RM, et al: Inhibition of erythroid progenitor cells by anti-Kell antibodies in fetal alloimmune anemia. *N Engl J Med* 338:798–803. Copyright 1998, Massachusetts Medical Society. Reprinted by permission of *The New England Journal of Medicine*.)

Growth of Kell-positive erythroid burst-forming units and colony-forming units was inhibited by serum from 22 women with anti-Kell antibodies; growth of Kell-negative erythroid burst-forming units and colony-forming units was unaffected. The mothers' anti-Kell antibodies had no effect on cord blood granulocyte-macrophage or megakaryocyte progenitor cells.

Conclusions.—Growth of Kell-positive erythroid burst-forming units and colony-forming units is specifically inhibited by both monoclonal and naturally occurring anti-Kell antibodies. The results add to the evidence that anti-Kell antibodies contribute to fetal anemia by suppressing erythropoiesis at the level of the progenitor cell. The findings have important implications for the clinical management of pregnancies identified as having Kell alloimmunization.

► Although fetal Kell alloimmunization is often described as resulting in fetal hemolytic anemia, the failure of increase in circulating fetal normoblasts and reticulocytes and the lack of the same strong correlation between the severity of fetal anemia and fetal serum bilirubin concentrations as in Rh alloimmunization have been lingering problems. This study, using cell culture techniques based on cord blood mononuclear cell growth, demonstrates the capacity of IgG Kell antibody preparations to inhibit growth of Kell-positive but not Kell-negative cells in vitro in concentrations as small as 0.02%. The potentially lethal effects of anti-Kell alloimmunization seem, in terms of this study, to be a hypoplastic fetal anemia apparently without the accelerated destruction of antibody-coated red blood cells seen in Rh alloimmunization. If true, this renders amniotic fluid spectrophotometry useless in predicting the severity of the process, and means cordocentesis with intrauterine blood transfusion is the procedure of choice in dealing with this problem in its most severe stage. Kell alloimmunization has been rendered increasingly significant in the management of erythroblastosis because prophylaxis has reduced the incidence of Rh-based erythroblastosis fetalis.

T.H. Kirschbaum, M.D.

Immediate and Long Term Outcome of Human Parvovirus B19 Infection in Pregnancy

Miller E, Fairley CK, Cohen BJ, et al (Public Health Lab Service, London; Alfred Hosp, Prahran, Victoria, Australia)

Br J Obstet Gynaecol 105:174–178, 1998 4–3

Background.—In 1984, parvovirus was identified as a fetal pathogen. Since then, various studies and case reports have documented cases of fetal B19 infection, including increased risk of spontaneous abortion. However, there is inconsistent information on the risk of fetal loss and hydrops

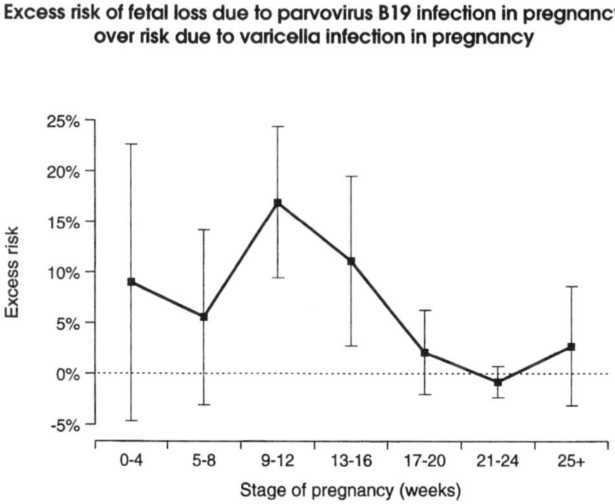

FIGURE 1.—Excess risk of fetal loss (95% confidence intervals) in women with parvovirus B19 infection compared with women with varicella by gestational stage at maternal infection. (Courtesy of Miller E, Fairley CK, Cohen BJ, et al: Immediate and long term outcome of human parvovirus B19 infection in pregnancy. *Br J Obstet Gynaecol* 105:174–178. Copyright 1998, Blackwell Science Ltd.)

TABLE 2.—Risk of Fetal Hydrops According to Stage of Gestation of Maternal B19 Infection: 1992–1995 and 1985–1988 Cohorts Combined

Stage (WLMP)	Followed up	Fetal hydrops
0–8	132	0
9–12	115	3 (2·6)
13–16	79	3 (3·8)
17–20	47	1 (2·1)
21–28	35	0

Note: Values are given as *n* and *n* (%).
Abbreviation: *WLMP*, weeks from last menstrual period.
(Courtesy of Miller E, Fairley CK, Cohen BJ, et al: Immediate and long term outcome of human parvovirus B19 infection in pregnancy. *Br J Obstet Gynaecol* 105:174–178. Copyright 1998, Blackwell Science Ltd.)

fetalis after maternal B19 infection, and little information on the long-term outcome of surviving infants. In a prospective cohort study, the risk of fetal loss and congenital abnormalities after maternal parvovirus B19 infection was determined, as well as the long-term outcome for surviving infants.

Methods.—Evaluations were performed in 427 pregnant women with B19 infection and 367 surviving infants. The rate of fetal loss in these women was compared with that in pregnant women with varicella. Of the 367 surviving infants, 129 had a follow-up evaluation at 7–10 years of age. Obstetricians and general practitioners completed a questionnaire on the outcome of pregnancy and health of surviving infants.

Results.—The average excess rate of fetal loss in women with B19 infection was 9% and was confined to the first 20 weeks of gestation. Women with B19 infection in pregnancy had a greater risk of adverse fetal outcome than did women with varicella who continued their pregnancy to term and whose fetus did not have varicella damage (Fig 1). Between 9 and 20 weeks' gestation, 7 cases of fetal hydrops occurred after maternal

TABLE 3.—Number and Percentage of Infants Positive for Parvovirus B19 IgG at a Year According to Stage of Maternal Infection: 1992–1995 and 1985–1988 Cohorts Combined

Stage of gestation (WLMP)	Tested	IgG positive
0–4	15	0 (0)
5–8	44	7 (16)
9–12	54	5 (9)
13–16	35	7 (14)
17–20	25	6 (24)
21–24	10	5 (50)
25–28	12	7 (58)
29–32	6	4 (67)
≥33	8	5 (63)
TOTAL	209	46 (22)

Note: Values are given as *n* and *n* (%).
Abbreviation: *WLMP*, weeks from last menstrual period.
(Courtesy of Miller E, Fairley CK, Cohen BJ, et al: Immediate and long term outcome of human parvovirus B19 infection in pregnancy. *Br J Obstet Gynaecol* 105:174–178. Copyright 1998, Blackwell Science Ltd.)

infection (Table 2). In surviving infants at birth, there were no abnormalities attributable to B19 infection (Table 3), and no late effects observed at 7–10 years of age.

Discussion.—About 1 in 10 women infected before 20 weeks' gestation will have a fetal loss from parvovirus B19 infection. The maximum possible risk of a congenital abnormality resulting from B19 infection is less than 1%, and long-term development is normal.

► The Public Health Laboratory Service in London has performed the first prospective study of the consequences of parvovirus B19 infection (erythema infectiosum) in pregnancy with sufficient cases to discriminate risks by weeks of gestational age. A first study consisted of 190 cases that were reported in 1985–1988, beginning the year after the first report of fetal parvovirus infection.[1] Here they add an additional 255 cases identified during the period from 1992–1995. Study entry was based solely on maternal symptoms, and cases were identified by the presence of immunoglobubin M or immunoglobin G seroconversion to the virus. Women whose disease was identified by abnormal fetal or newborn findings were excluded, so as to allow prospective estimates for gravidas showing only evidence of acute infection. In the data from 1992–1995, the risk of abortion or fetal death in utero was 12%, and when both studies are pooled, the risk becomes 15%. When compared with fetal losses caused by maternal varicella infection—an infection not known to impose an additional fetal hazard other than that occasioned by the exanthem—the surplus fetal loss of 9% was confined to the first 20 weeks of pregnancy. Fetal hydrops occurred in 30% of infected women and was seen only from 11–18 weeks of gestational age. The incidence of congenital fetal infection at 1 year of age was 20%, but no surplus infant impairment was seen on follow-up at 7–10 years of age. With a reported case attack rate for parvovirus infection in pregnancy of 0.25% and correcting for hydrops tendency to occur only between 9 and 20 weeks' gestational age, the risk of fetal hydrops caused by parvovirus B19 occurring during pregnancy is approximately 2 per 100,000.

T.H. Kirschbaum, M.D

Reference

1. Public Health Laboratory Service Working Party on Fifth Disease. Prospective study of human parvovirus (B19) infection in pregnancy. *BMJ* 300:1166–1170, 1990.

Prenatal Diagnosis of Fetal Varicella-Zoster Virus Infection With Polymerase Chain Reaction of Amniotic Fluid in 107 Cases

Mouly F, Mirlesse V, Méritet JF, et al (Université René Descartes, Paris; Institut de Puériculture, Paris; Hôpital Saint Vincent de Paul, Paris)

Am J Obstet Gynecol 177:894–898, 1997 4–4

Introduction.—Primary infection by varicella zoster virus results in varicella, and up to 7 per 10,000 pregnancies are complicated by varicella. Multiple fetal malformations can result when varicella occurs during the first 6 months of pregnancy. Manifestations of congenital varicella include distal malposition, cutaneous scars, multiorgan damage including encephalitis and chorioretinitis and segmental involvement with limb hypoplasia. Cell culture is the reference method for the detection of varicella zoster virus in pathologic samples, but polymerase chain reaction has been found to be more sensitive. Polymerase chain reaction (PCR) and cell culture were compared in women who had varicella zoster virus before 24 weeks of pregnancy.

Methods.—Clinical varicella was contracted by 107 women before 24 weeks of pregnancy in a 6-year period. All women had amniocentesis performed, and 82 had simultaneous fetal blood sampling. Cell culture inoculation and (PCR) were used to detect virus in amniotic fluid. To detect antivaricella zoster virus immunoglobulin M (IgM), fetal blood was tested.

Results.—Polymerase chain reaction resulted in 9 positive samples (8.4%) of 107 amniotic fluid samples tested, yet only 2 (1.8%) were found to be positive in cell culture. For specific anti-varicella zoster virus IgM, none of the blood samples from infected fetuses were positive.

Conclusion.—There was an 8.4% risk of transplacental passage before 24 weeks of pregnancy. There was a risk of 3.8% of isolated postnatal varicella zoster infection and a 2.8% risk of congenital varicella. For the detection of varicella zoster virus in amniotic fluid, PCR was more sensitive than cell culture.

► This fine piece of work by the renowned Parisian Institute for Research in Viral Infection nicely complements the work done earlier by the Communicable Disease Surveillance Centre of Manchester, England.[1] Here, amniotic fluid was obtained in 107 women with varicella in the first 24 weeks of pregnancy and was subjected both to viral cell culture and PCR using primers specific to the varicella zoster genome. The results showed an 8.4% incidence of maternal to fetal viral transmission, roughly 4 and a half times more than that disclosed by culture of this fastidious virus. In 82 cases, simultaneous cordocentesis was done along with amniocentesis yielding fetal blood uniformly negative at 21–26 weeks for varicella zoster IgM and interferon alpha. The incidence of fetal malformations was 2.8%; 1 patient came from a pregnancy negative on antenatal evaluation for varicella and the other 2 positive. Postnatal varicella zoster occurred in 3.8% of neonates, all of them with amniotic fluid positive on PCR prior to the 24th week of pregnancy. PCR proved far more sensitive in the diagnosis of fetal viral transmission than did viral culture, accounting in part for the rate roughly 3 times that noted in the Manchester study. IgM evaluation of fetal blood proved useless in predicting cases of fetal and/or neonatal infection noted here. Though more sensitive, PCR suffers in that it discloses only presence of viral genomic material and not viral infection, but in only 1 case of therapeutic abortion at 25 weeks was virus found without pathologic evidence of infection. As before, maternal-to-fetal transmission of varicella was confined to cases where maternal infection occurred before the 20th week of gestation. Other investigators have noted that neonatal zoster sometimes occurs where maternal infection occurs past that time in pregnancy.

T.H. Kirschbaum, M.D.

Reference

1. 1996 Year Book of Obstetrics and Gynecology, pp 35–36.

The Effect of Indomethacin Tocolysis on Fetal Ductus Arteriosus Constriction With Advancing Gestational Age

Vermillion ST, Scardo JA, Lashus AG, et al (Med Univ of South Carolina, Charleston)

Am J Obstet Gynecol 177:256–261, 1997 4–5

Objective.—The use of indomethacin as a tocolytic agent for preterm labor is limited by reports of fetal and neonatal complications, particularly fetal ductus arteriosus constriction leading to pulmonary hypertension. Based on a single clinical trial, the use of indomethacin is generally limited to gestational ages of less than 32 weeks, because the incidence of ductal constriction increases thereafter. This retrospective study sought to determine whether long-term tocolytic therapy with indomethacin leads to an increased incidence of ductal constriction with advancing gestational age.

Methods.—The review included fetal echocardiograms of 61 pregnant women treated with indomethacin, 25 mg orally every 6 hours, for preterm labor. In all, 193 echocardiograms of 72 fetuses were reviewed. The impact of indomethacin on ductal constriction with advancing gestational age was determined by density function analysis and regression analysis. Systolic and diastolic ductal flow velocities were determined in fetuses with and without constriction, and differences between singleton and multiple gestations were determined.

Results.—In half of the fetuses, constriction of the ductus arteriosus was observed between 25 and 35 weeks' gestation. Increase in systolic flow velocity with advancing age was greater in fetuses with ductal constriction than it was in those without this complication. The gestational age at which constriction was detected was 31 weeks. The diagnosis was made an average of 5 days after the start of indomethacin therapy. In 70% of cases, ductal constriction occurred within 31 weeks of gestation (Fig 1). Once

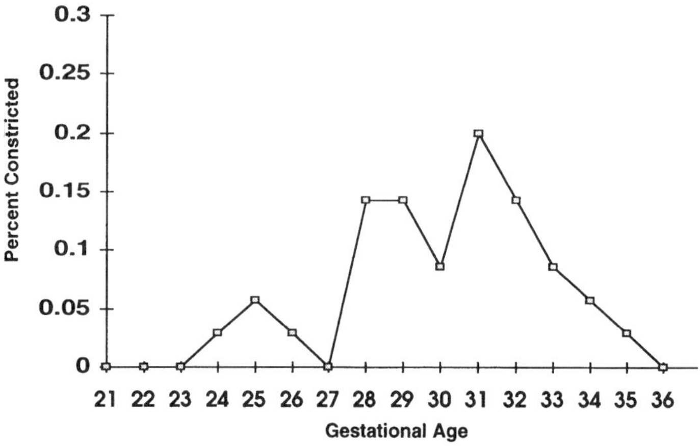

FIGURE 1.—Percent with constriction by gestational age. (Courtesy of Vermillion ST, Scardo JA, Lashus AG, et al: The effect of indomethacin tocolysis on fetal ductus arteriosus constriction with advancing gestational age. *Am J Obstet Gynecol* 177:256–261, 1997.)

indomethacin treatment was stopped, ductal flow velocities returned to their nonconstricted levels. Indomethacin caused no apparent adverse neonatal outcomes.

Conclusions.—In women receiving indomethacin for tocolysis, there is a strikingly high incidence of fetal ductus arteriosus constriction at 31 weeks' gestation. Constriction can occur at any time during pregnancy, however. It is reversible with withdrawal of indomethacin. Women receiving indomethacin as a tocolytic agent for preterm labor should be monitored with weekly fetal echocardiography throughout therapy.

► The ductus arteriosus carries blood from the pulmonary artery to the aorta, conveying the bulk of right ventricular output of relatively low oxygen content fetal blood diverted from the fetal lungs. Pulmonary vasoconstriction is maintained in fetal life by the relatively low partial pressure of oxygen of blood perfusing the lungs and traversing the ductus until air replaces amniotic fluid in the bronchiolar parenchyma when pulmonary vasodilatation decreases vascular resistance and the ductus arteriosus becomes functionally useless. It then constricts as a result of inhibition of prostaglandin production by the shunt. The presence of the foramen ovale, the ductus arteriosis, and intense pulmonary vascular resistance in fetal life means that effective fetal cardiac output is the sum of the blood flow rates of both ventricles minus the fetal pulmonary blood flow rate. In this way, the ventricles work in parallel, helping to raise cardiac output per kg of body weight to a value roughly 4 times that for adults where the 2 ventricles are connected in series by the pulmonary circulation. In adult life, cardiac output is equal to the output of a single ventricle. The high rate of fetal cardiac output compensates for the low nutrient content of even arterialized fetal blood leaving the left ventricle. Indomethacin, by inhibiting prostaglandin production in the ductus, causes vasoconstriction, raising blood pressure in the pulmonary artery and the right ventricle and induces tricuspid sufficiency. Chronic fetal pulmonary hypertension causes secondary structural vascular changes in the lung with prolonged indomethacin use and results in neonatal pulmonary hypertension. Constriction of the ductus disrupts the parallel arrangement of the ventricles and reduces net cardiac output by forcing more blood flow through the constricted lung bed. The resulting decrease in cardiac output results in decreasing urine production, decreased mesenteric blood flow and, by altering blood flow through the foramen ovale and increasing the quantity of low oxygen content blood leaving the left ventricle, decreases fetal defenses against intraventricular hemorrhage. Here the diagnosis of ductus constriction is made by observing increased blood velocity through the ductus as Bernoulli's principal comes into play while the ductus constricts. Doppler enthusiasts should note the increased flow velocity means decreased, not increased, bulk flow through the constricted ductus. This study indicates that considerable ductus constriction is noted primarily in the third trimester in as many as 30% of fetuses at 31 weeks' gestational age but is seen in the second trimester as well. In 90% of fetuses with ductus constriction, the phenomenon regresses within 8 days after discontinuation of indomethacin. This agent reduces the capacity of the fetus to maintain normal cardiovascular function and, coupled with the inability to prove its usefulness as a tocolytic and the hazards associated with its use in polyhydramnios, has little to recommend its use in pregnancy.

T.H. Kirschbaum, M.D.

The Collaborative Randomised Amnioinfusion for Meconium Project (CRAMP): 1. South Africa

Hofmeyr GJ, Gülmezoğlu AM, Buchmann E, et al (Univ of Witwatersrand, South Africa; Univ of Pretoria, South Africa; Univ of Orange Free State, South Africa; et al)

Br J Obstet Gynaecol 105:304–308, 1998 4–6

Background.—The reported incidence of meconium passage in utero is 7% to 22%, and may be higher in certain populations. Meconium aspiration syndrome has not been eliminated by the practice of suctioning the infant's airway at delivery. Amnioinfusion has been used in women with meconium staining of the amniotic fluid, and may reduce the incidence of cesarean section, meconium below the vocal cords, and meconium aspiration syndrome. The effect of amnioinfusion for meconium-stained amniotic fluid on perinatal outcome was investigated.

Methods.—In a multicenter, randomized, controlled trial, 352 women with moderate or thick meconium staining of amniotic fluid and in labor at term participated. Study patients were given transcervical amnioinfusion of 800 mL of saline at 15 mL/min, then maintenance infusion at 3 mL/min. Control patients were given routine care. The study was not blinded. Outcome measures included cesarean section, meconium aspiration syndrome, and perinatal mortality.

TABLE 4.—Meta-analysis of the Effects of Amnioinfusion for Meconium-stained Amniotic Fluid on the Rate of Meconium Aspiration Syndrome in Previous and the Current Randomized Trials, Expressed as Relative Risk and 95% Confidence Interval

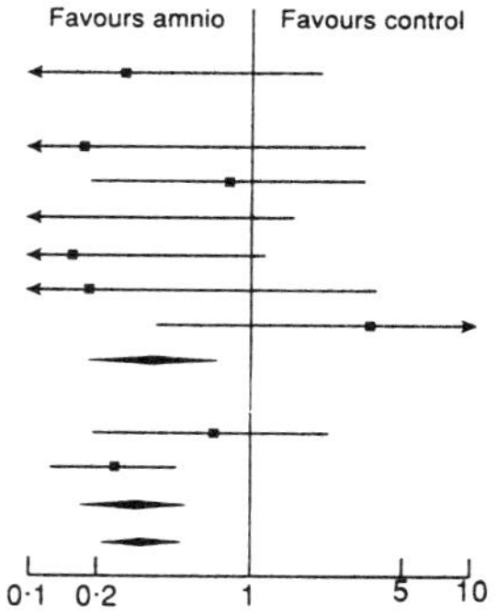

Study	Amnio	Controls	RR [95% CI fixed]
Previous trials			
Adam *et al.*[14]	1/17	4/18	0·26 [0·03–2·14]
Sadovsky *et al.*[15]	0/19	0/21	Not estimable
Wenstrom & Parsons[16]	0/36	3/44	0·17 [0·01–3·26]
Ilagan *et al.*[17]	3/38	4/40	0·79 [0·19–3·30]
Macri *et al.*[18]	0/85	5/85	0·09 [0·01–1·62]
Cialone *et al.*[19]	1/47	8/58	0·15 [0·02–1·19]
Eriksen *et al.*[21]	0/65	2/59	0·18 [0·01–3·71]
Spong *et al.*[20]	3/43	1/50	3·49 [0·38–32·32]
Total	8/350	27/375	0·37 [0·18–0·75]
Current trial (CRAMP 1, 2)			
1 (South Africa)	4/162	6/163	0·67 [0·19–2·33]
2 (Zimbabwe)	10/323	42/329	0·24 [0·12–0·48]
Total	14/485	48/492	0·30 [0·17–0·53]
TOTAL	22/835	75/867	0·32 [0·21–0·51]

Note: Values are given as number affected/number treated, unless otherwise indicated.
Abbreviations: Amnio, experimental (amnioinfusion) group; *CI*, confidence interval; *RR*, relative risk.
(Courtesy of Hofmeyr GJ, Gülmezoğlu AM, Buchmann E, et al: The Collaborative Randomised Amnioinfusion for Meconium Project (CRAMP): 1. South Africa. *Br J Obstet Gynaecol* 105:304–308. Copyright 1998, Blackwell Science Ltd.)

Results.—The rate of cesarean section was similar in both study and control patients. The incidence of meconium aspiration syndrome was lower than what was expected from previous studies (Table 4). No perinatal deaths occurred. There were no significant differences in subsidiary outcomes between groups. Most results were consistent with results of previous studies.

Discussion.—Amnioinfusion for meconium-stained amniotic fluid has no effect on the rate of cesarean section. However, pooled data from all identified trials to date indicate a significant decrease in the rate of cesarean section. In this study alone, findings regarding meconium aspiration syndrome were inconclusive because so few infants were affected, although the point estimate of the relative risk was consistent with a significant decrease as reported by previous studies and the Zimbabwe arm of this study. Pooled data support the use of amnioinfusion in women with meconium staining of the amniotic fluid to lower the incidence of meconium aspiration syndrome.

The Collaborative Randomised Amnioinfusion for Meconium Project (CRAMP): 2. Zimbabwe

Mahomed K, Mulambo T, Woelk G, et al (Univ of Zimbabwe; Univ of Witwatersrand, South Africa)

Br J Obstet Gynaecol 105:309–313, 1998 4–7

Background.—The presence of meconium in amniotic fluid is associated with higher perinatal morbidity and mortality. Passage of meconium in utero has been reported in 7% to 22% of live births. The assumption that meconium aspiration usually occurs during and immediately after delivery has led to the practice of suctioning of the infant's trachea at delivery. However, this practice has not eliminated meconium aspiration syndrome. It is possible that meconium aspiration syndrome results from intrauterine aspiration, although this has been difficult to predict or prevent. Amnioinfusion has been used in women with meconium staining of the amniotic fluid, and appears to reduce the incidence of cesarean section, meconium below the vocal cords, and meconium aspiration syndrome. The effect of amnioinfusion for meconium-stained amniotic fluid on perinatal outcome was examined in a setting with limited peripartum facilities.

Methods.—In a multicenter, randomized, controlled trial, 661 women with moderate or thick meconium staining of amniotic fluid and at term labor participated. Study patients received transcervical amnioinfusion of 500 mL of saline over 30 minutes, then 500 mL at 30 drops per minute. Control patients received routine care. The study was not blinded. Outcome measures were cesarean section, meconium aspiration syndrome, and perinatal mortality.

Results.—No difference in risk of cesarean section was noted between the 2 groups. Among patients who had amnioinfusion, a significantly

TABLE 2.—Outcomes of Women Randomly Allocated to Receive Amnioinfusion (n = 325) or to Serve as Control Subjects (n = 336)

	Amnioinfusion		Control		RR (95% CI)
Primary outcomes					
Caesarean section	317	30 (9·5)	328	37 (12·3)	0·84 (0·53–1·32)
Clinical MAS	323	10 (3·1)	329	42 (12·8)	0·24 (0·12–0·48)
Perinatal death	324	4 (1·2)	335	12 (3·6)	0·34 (0·11–1·06)
Subsidiary outcomes					
Fetal heart rate abnormality	320	30 (9·4)	334	34 (10·2)	0·92 (0·58–1·47)
Contractions ≥ 40 s at 1 h	323	206 (64)	324	211 (65)	0·98 (0·87–1·1)
Caesarean section for fetal distress	321	7 (2·2)	334	12 (3·6)	0·61 (0·24–1·52)
Assisted delivery	320	13 (4·1)	333	11 (3·3)	1·23 (0·56–2·7)
1 min Apgar < 4	324	8 (2·5)	336	18 (5·3)	0·46 (0·2–1·05)
5 min Apgar < 7	324	9 (2·8)	336	27 (8·0)	0·35 (0·17–0·73)
NICU admission	321	41 (12·8)	332	76 (22·9)	0·56 (0·39–0·79)
Ventilation	320	10 (3·1)	332	34 (10·2)	0·31 (0·15–0·61)
X-ray findings MAS	319	2 (0·6)	330	9 (2·7)	0·23 (0·05–1·06)
Pneumothorax	320	0 (0)	329	3 (0·9)	
Hypoxic ischaemic encephalopathy	320	1 (0·3)	329	14 (4·3)	0·07 (0·01–0·56)
> 4 days in NICU	320	5 (1·6)	329	10 (3·0)	0·51 (0·18–1·49)
Maternal pyrexia					
In labour ward	323	3 (0·9)	335	10 (3·0)	0·31 (0·09–1·12)
In postnatal ward	321	2 (0·6)	336	1 (0·3)	2·09 (0·19–23)

Note: Values are given as total n with n (%).
Abbreviations: MAS, meconium aspiration syndrome; *NICU,* neonatal intensive care unit.
(Courtesy of Mahomed K, Mulambo T, Woelk G, et al: The Collaborative Randomised Amnioinfusion for Meconium Project (CRAMP): 2. Zimbabwe. *Br J Obstet Gynaecol* 105:309–313. Copyright 1998, Blackwell Science Ltd.)

lower rate of meconium aspiration syndrome was noted, as well as somewhat fewer perinatal deaths (Table 2).

Discussion.—In these patients, amnioinfusion for meconium-stained amniotic fluid was associated with significantly better perinatal outcome. These results show that amnioinfusion is technically feasible in settings with limited intrapartum facilities, such as in developing countries.

► Amnioinfusion is of proven value in reducing the incidence of cesarean section due to physician interpretation of oligohydramnios and related variable fetal heart rate decelerations. These 2 articles (Abstracts 4–6 and 4–7) attempt to deal with a possible additional value that might come from diluting meconium-stained amniotic fluid in the prevention of meconium aspiration syndrome (MAS) of the newborn. The analysis is complicated by the multiple etiologic factors that contribute to MAS of the newborn, only one of which is meconium concentration in amniotic fluid, and many of which pertain to the general nature of immediate perinatal care. Eight previous randomized trials of amniocentesis have failed to show evidence of reduction of MAS, although when they are grouped in meta-analysis, a significant reduction in MAS associated with amnioinfusion is claimed (Table 2). The diagnosis is often subjectively defined and observer bias is commonplace. However, these 2 studies represent the largest patient population collected for this purpose and must be carefully considered.

Originally designed as a collaborative study between 2 institutions, the results from South Africa with a MAS incidence of 3% are reported separately from those from Zimbabwe where the incidence of MAS was 8%. Except for the 42% incidence of cesarean section in the South African population, obstetric management there is similar to that in this country. In Zimbabwe, electronic fetal heart rate monitoring is not used, midwives conducting the deliveries usually lack equipment for immediate newborn airway aspiration, and a pediatrician is never present at delivery. In the South African subset, a relationship between amnioinfusion and a reduced MAS incidence could not be established. In the Zimbabwe study, the risk ratio expressing the decreased incidence of MAS associated with amnioinfusion was 0.24 based on clinical diagnosis, but in terms of radiographic findings of MAS, no significant improvement could be documented. The incidence of neonatal ICU (NICU) admission, need for artificial ventilation, and the incidence of a hypoxic-ischemic encephalopathy with unspecified diagnostic criteria was lower in those who had amnioinfusion. No evidence of a causal relationship between amnioinfusion in these outcomes is available. The incidence of actual meconium staining of amniotic fluid in either subset is not provided and makes interpretations of the reported findings difficult.

In brief, the findings suggest but do not prove that amnioinfusion may be useful in preventing MAS where traditional perinatal care is not available. Beyond that, there is no support for its role in treating meconium-stained amniotic fluid to prevent newborn respiratory impairment.

T.H. Kirschbaum, M.D.

Clinical Chorioamnionitis and the Prognosis for Very Low Birth Weight Infants

Alexander JM, Gilstrap LC, Cox SM, et al (Univ of Texas, Dallas)

Obstet Gynecol 91:725–729, 1998 4–8

Background.—Eschenbach recently reported that chorioamnionitis may be primarily an infection of the fetus, rather than of the mother. Other recent reports suggest there may be long-term consequences of such infection, such as cerebral palsy, resulting from maternal mediators of infection that cross the placenta. Preterm infants may be especially vulnerable to the negative effects on the brain caused by chorioamnionitis.

Methods.—An observational cohort analysis was performed in a hospital of all singleton, very low birth weight infants born at 24 weeks' gestation or later. Chorioamnionitis was diagnosed based on maternal fever of 38°C and clinical evidence, such as fetal tachycardia, uterine tenderness, malodorous infant, and no other source of infection. Outcome was analyzed by multiple logistic regression.

Results.—Of 1,397 very low birth weight infants, 95 were born to mothers with chorioamnionitis. After adjusting for preterm ruptured membranes, pregnancy-associated hypertension, cesarean birth, gestational age, and birth weight, it was noted that the rate of neonatal sepsis, respiratory distress syndrome, seizure in the first 24 hours, intraventricular hemorrhage grade 3 or 4, and periventricular leukomalacia was signifi-

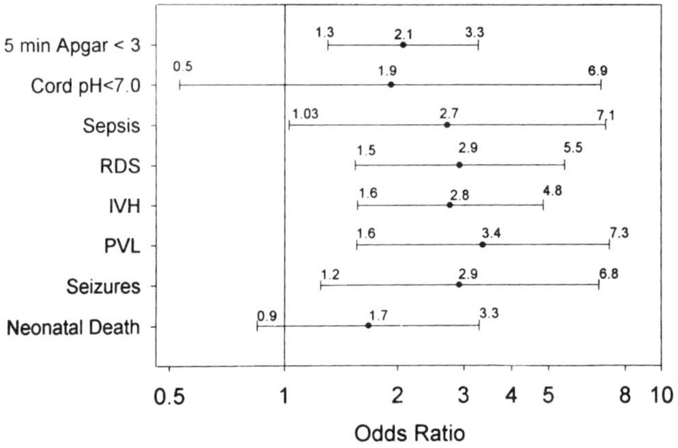

FIGURE 1.—Odds ratio and 95% confidence intervals for neonatal complications associated with intrauterine infection, after adjusting for risk factors. *Abbreviations*: *IVH*, intraventricular hemorrhage (grade 3 or 4); *PVL*, periventricular leukomalacia; *RDS*, respiratory distress syndrome (requiring mechanical ventilation in first 24 hours). (Courtesy of Alexander JM, Gilstrap LC, Cox SM, et al: Clinical chorioamnionitis and the prognosis for very low birth weight infants. *Obstet Gynecol* 91:725–729, 1998. Reprinted with permission of the American College of Obstetricians and Gynecologists.)

cantly higher in infants exposed to chorioamnionitis. Analysis showed an odds ratio of 2.8 for intraventricular hemorrhage grade 3 or 4, periventricular leukomalacia, and seizures in the first 24 hours (Fig 1).

Discussion.—These findings suggest there is a relation between chorioamnionitis and several indices of morbidity in very low birth weight infants. In this study, the preterm infants born to mothers with chorioamnionitis were 2–3 times more likely to have morbidity than infants born to mothers who did not have chorioamnionitis. It appears that the brains of very low birth weight infants are especially susceptible to neurologic damage from chorioamnionitis.

▶ The epidemiologic link between chorioamnionitis and newborn brain injury has grown increasingly strong[1-3] (Abstract 9–11) and has been bolstered by experimental evidence that fetal administration of inflammatory cytokines and endotoxin are capable of inducing fetal brain injury. This 9-year study of infants born past 24 weeks' gestational age with birth weights of less than 1.5 kg provides some direct, controlled evidence very suggestive of a direct relationship between maternal chorioamnionitis and neonatal brain injury. An essential part of the study is the use of multiple logistic regression to correct for the possible confounding effects of gestational age, birth weight, maternal hypertension, premature rupture of membranes, and abdominal birth on fetal brain trauma. As expected, chorioamnionitis was associated with increased risks of preterm delivery and premature rupture of membranes in predominantly older multiparous women. A significantly increased risk of impaired 5-minute Apgar score without increased risk of cord blood acidosis speaks against newborn asphyxial injuries as a cause. Nevertheless, odds ratios for intraventricular hemorrhage, periventricular leukomalacia, and seizures were increased roughly threefold. The high rate of respiratory distress syndrome in these suggests the failure to use corticoids, which would have, diminished respiratory distress, in the newborns years of this nine-year data collection. The risk of neonatal death was not increased in very low birth weight infants born with exposure to chorioamnionitis, suggesting again moderately specific CNS effects of infectious disease. The authors correctly cite the evidence that maternal antibiotics given on indication of preterm labor or premature rupture of membranes fail to influence perinatal mortality rates, and that brain injury without injury to other organ systems capable of resulting in neonatal death is the hazard of chorioamnionitis to very low birth weight infants.

T.H. Kirschbaum, M.D.

References

1. 1987 Year Book of Obstetrics and Gynecology, pp 243–245.
2. 1988 Year Book of Obstetrics and Gynecology, pp 116–118.
3. 1995 Year Book of Obstetrics and Gynecology, pp 135–138.

Maternal Infection and Cerebral Palsy in Infants of Normal Birth Weight

Grether JK, Nelson KB (California Dept of Health Services, Emeryville; Natl Inst of Neurological Disorders and Stroke, Bethesda, Md)

JAMA 278:207–211, 1997 4–9

Background.—Cerebral palsy is a life-limiting disability. There is evidence that exposure to maternal or placental infection may increase the risk of cerebral palsy, and may be associated with brain lesions predictive of cerebral palsy in very low birth weight infants. There are few data on the association between exposure to maternal infection and risk of cerebral palsy in normal birth weight infants, who make up 95% of births and more than 50% of cases of cerebral palsy.

Methods.—In a population-based, case-control study, 46 study children with disabling spastic cerebral palsy who had no prenatal brain lesions were studied, along with 378 control children weighing at least 2,500 g at birth and surviving to age 3 years. Disabling spastic cerebral palsy and signs of neonatal morbidity were the main outcome measures.

Results.—Maternal fever higher than 38°C during labor and a diagnosis of chorioamnionitis were associated with a higher risk of unexplained cerebral palsy. In 2.9% of control children, 22% of children with cerebral palsy, and 37% of children with the spastic quadriplegic subtype of cerebral palsy, one or more indicators of maternal infection were seen. Study and control newborns who had been exposed to maternal infection were more likely to have 5-minute Apgar scores lower than 6 than newborns not exposed to maternal infection. Of children with cerebral palsy, those born to mothers with infection were more likely to be hypotensive, need intubation, have neonatal seizures, and receive a diagnosis of hypoxic-ischemic encephalopathy.

Discussion.—Infants of normal birth weight who had intrauterine exposure to maternal infection had a significantly higher risk of cerebral palsy. Maternal infection was also associated with various signs often attributed to birth asphyxia, such as low Apgar scores, other evidence of hypotension, and need for resuscitation. Perhaps further research will show that the risk of cerebral palsy in term infants can be lowered by treating maternal infection or the inflammatory response to infection.

▶ It has been clear for more than 10 years that maternal chorioamnionitis is a significant risk factor for cerebral palsy (CP) in infants weighing less than 2.5 kg at birth.[1] That observation was derived from the federally sponsored Collaborative Perinatal Project with data collected in the late 1950s to early 1960s. Here, a more recent data source collected by the California Birth Defects Monitoring Program[2] uses 155,636 deliveries during 1983–1985 with infants surviving to 3 years of age to evaluate maternal infection as a risk factor for term infants by weight. A case-control study based on 84 infants with CP derived from singleton pregnancies with adequate records followed. The diagnosis of maternal infection disclosed in chart review was based predominantly on clinical evidence and systematic collection of data pertaining to maternal infection and its treatment was often lacking. It is likely maternal infection was underdiagnosed during this time, both in pregnancies resulting in CP and in normal infants, but it is hard to estimate the significance of that effect. What resulted was strong evidence that maternal fever in labor, chorioamnionitis, and evidence of placental infection were significant risk factors for CP in singlet fetuses weighing more than 2.5 kg at birth who survived to 3 years of age.

In an associated finding, the important issue of confounding variables was explored by stratifying the data for each of a large series of potential confounders (maternal age, race, pay status, hospital care level, etc.) and using stepwise logistic regression to adjust the risk ratios that remained statistically significant. Significant risk ratios prove covariance of maternal infection and cerebral palsy in term size infants. This does not prove infection causes CP nor does it allow accurate measurements of predictability to be made. More infants exhibiting CP were born prematurely than at term and the majority of infants with subsequent CP born to infected women did not have recognizable infection during labor. It is therefore uncertain how this information might have been used to prevent brain injury if the presence of infection had been recognized before birth. It does underline, however, the importance of maternal infection not only in preterm birth and newborn cardiovascular depression, but also in the development of newborn brain injury.

T.H. Kirschbaum, M.D.

References

1. 1987 Year Book of Obstetrics and Gynecology, pp 243–245.
2. 1988 Year Book of Obstetrics and Gynecology, pp 116–118.

The Correlation Between Placental Pathology and Intraventricular Hemorrhage in the Preterm Infant

Hansen A, the Developmental Epidemiology Network Investigators (Children's Hosp, Boston; Michigan State Univ, East Lansing, Mich; Bellevue Research Found, Niskayuna, NJ; et al)

Pediatr Res 43:15–19, 1998 4–10

Objective.—It is hypothesized that whereas morphological correlates of pregnancy-induced hypertension (PIH) are associated with a decreased risk of intraventricular hemorrhage (IVH), morphological correlates of amniotic sac inflammation (ASI) are associated with an increased risk of IVH. Results of a prospective study of 2 clusters of placental morphologic features among very low birth weight infants, associated either with ASI or with PIH/preeclampsia, reveal the relationship between number of features of a cluster and risk of IVH for the infant (lower for PIH and higher for ASI).

Methods.—Placentas of 1,095 very low birth weight infants were examined histologically, neonatal cranial ultrasound examinations were performed, and maternal and neonatal data were subjected to univariate and multivariate analysis. Cluster analysis was used to determine the relationship of characteristics, based on observed versus expected results. Logistic regression was used to evaluate the relationship between each component of the 2 clusters and the risk of IVH. The IVH risk of infants with PIH placentas was compared to that of control infants, and the IVH risk of infants with ASI placentas was compared to that of control infants.

Results.—All PIH component cluster patterns except maternal decidual arteriolar pathology were associated with a decreased risk of IVH, compared with placentas with no PIH component cluster patterns. IVH risk was increased in placentas with ASI components. When histologic features and demographic and clinical factors were taken into account using multivariate analysis, only chorionic or umbilical vasculitis had an elevated odds ratio. In infants with placentas having only components of the PIH cluster, the IVH risk was similar to that of control infants. In infants with placentas having components of the ASI cluster, the IVH risk was significantly higher than for control infants.

Conclusion.—Infants with placentas having at least 1 component of the ASI cluster have up to 3 times the risk of IVH compared with infants having placentas without any components of the ASI cluster.

▶ The logic of this study is clear but subtle. There are fairly good epidemiologic data suggesting a deficit of cases of neonatal IVH in infants born of women with pregnancy-induced hypertension, and a surplus of such infants born of women whose pregnancies are complicated by chorioamnionitis. The authors' hope is that these relationships might have correlated placental pathology that makes prediction of infants destined for IVH possible, and that prophylactic management might be tested on each of such subsets. The problem is circularity in logic. Chorioamnionitis can be defined by its placental pathology and its implications for IVH are known. Nothing more is learned by demonstrating the same covariance of IVH with placental pathology as is seen with the clinical diagnosis of chorioamnionitis. What is interesting here is that no (inverse) relationship with IVH is seen with the clusters of placental pathologic findings identified in women with PIH. The American College of Obstetrician and Gynecologists Committee on Obstetrics was correct in pointing to the lack of productive research in linking placental pathology to obstetric abnormalities (see ACOG Committee Opinion 125- July, 1993).

T.H. Kirschbaum, M.D.

Prenatal Events and the Risk of Cerebral Palsy in Very Low Birth Weight Infants

O'Shea TM, Klinepeter KL, Dillard RG (Wake Forest Univ, Winston-Salem, NC)

Am J Epidemiol 147:362–369, 1998 4–11

Background.—Greater survival of very low birth weight infants in the 1980s and 1990s was associated with an increase in the rate of cerebral palsy in this group. It is estimated that very low birth weight infants make up 25% or more of all new cases of cerebral palsy. Studies have indicated that prenatal factors may be related to the etiology of cerebral palsy in these infants.

Methods.—Associations between prenatal factors and risk of cerebral palsy were analyzed in very low birth weight infants. Associations were analyzed separately for hemiplegia, diplegia, and quadriplegia, and for cerebral palsy with and without antecedent major cranial ultrasound abnormalities. There were 80 study infants; all study and control infants had a birth weight of 500–1,500 g and were born between 1978 and 1989.

Results.—The following factors had the strongest association with a higher risk of cerebral palsy: multiple gestation, chorioamnionitis, maternal antibiotics, antepartum vaginal bleeding, and labor lasting less than 4 hours. A decreased risk of cerebral palsy was seen with preeclampsia and delivery without labor. Except for chorioamnionitis and labor lasting less than 4 hours, there was evidence of confounding for all factors. Diplegia had a stronger association with chorioamnionitis than did hemiplegia or quadriplegia. Cerebral palsy without major cranial ultrasound abnormalities also had a stronger association with chorioamnionitis. The increased risk associated with antepartum vaginal bleeding and the decreased risk associated with pre-eclampsia were stronger for cerebral palsy with major cranial ultrasound abnormalities (Table 4).

Discussion.—Further etiologic studies should address the association between cerebral palsy and chorioamnionitis, while focusing on pathophysiologic mechanisms not involving intracranial hemorrhage. Further studies should also address the causes of rapid labor, which was a risk factor for cerebral palsy in this study. The strength of the associations

TABLE 4.—Associations Between Prenatal Factors and Cerebral Palsy for 45 Singleton Cases of Cerebral Palsy Who Underwent Cranial Ultrasound Examination in Infants Born Between 1982 and 1989 to Mothers Residing in a 17-County Region of Northwest North Carolina*

Factor	Infants with normal ultrasound or uncomplicated SEH/IVH†				Infants with major ultrasound abnormality			
	Unmatched controls		Matched controls		Unmatched controls		Matched controls	
	OR†	95% CI†	OR	95% CI	OR	95% CI	OR	95% CI
Antepartum bleeding	1.3	0.5–3.5	1.1	0.4–3.1	2.3	0.7–7.6	1.9	0.5–6.7
Preeclampsia	0.6	0.1–2.2	0.6	0.1–2.7	0.3	0.1–2.2	0.3	0.1–2.6
Chorioamnionitis	4.1	1.3–12.4	3.2	0.9–10.8	1.6	0.3–7.1	1.2	0.2–6.1
Maternal antibiotics	3.4	1.3–8.9	2.4	0.8–7.8	0.4	0.1–2.9	0.3	0.1–2.3
Delivery without labor	1.1	0.4–3.0	0.8	0.1–3.4	0.6	0.1–2.4	1.5	0.4–4.7
Labor <4 hours	1.4	0.4–4.2	2.5	0.4–12.1	1.6	0.5–5.5	2.2	0.5–9.6
Magnesium sulfate	0.6	0.2–1.6	0.6	0.2–1.7	0.6	0.2–2.1	0.6	0.1–2.2

*Associations are listed for a stratum of cases with normal ultrasound or uncomplicated subependymal/intraventricular hemorrhage (28 cases) and a stratum with major cranial ultrasound abnormality (posthemorrhagic hydrocephalus, persistent ventricular enlargement, or parenchymal echodensity/echolucency [17 cases]).

Abbreviations: CI, confidence interval; *OR*, odds ratio; *SEH/IVH*, subependymal/intraventricular hemorrhage.

(Courtesy of O'Shea TM, Klinepeter KL, Dillard RG: Prenatal events and the risk of cerebral palsy in very low birth weight infants. *Am J Epidemiol* 147:362–369, 1998.)

between prenatal factors and risk of cerebral palsy may depend on the presence or absence of major cranial ultrasound abnormalities.

▶ With time, patterns in the etiologic basis of cerebral palsy (CP) have changed, and a number of new questions have arisen that were not considered in Nelson and Ellenburg's classic analysis of data from the 1950s and 1960s,[1, 2] or from the Northern California study done on births from 1983 to 1985.[3] A major change in the evolving relationships has been an increase in the rates of very low birth weight (VLBW) infants and the increasing fraction of cases of CP derived from this newborn population weighing 0.5–1.5 kg at birth. In this study, the data are from births in 1978–1989 conducted at the Bowman Gray School of Medicine. This cohort study was based on evaluation of children without anomalous development at 1 year of age who had been found to have CP after discharge from the NICU. Typical of the evaluation of the relationship of prenatal events and eventual CP is the confounding effect of gestational age, which varies sharply in significance over a range from 22 to 33 weeks of gestational age. In this study, the importance of gestational age was managed using separate gestational age–matched and unmatched controls, and ultimately by multivariant regression analysis. The analytic strategy was to use a series of univariant analyses for dichotomized (either/or) or nondichotomized continuous variables and then to evaluate them for the possible impact of gestational age. Finally, prenatal factors were stratified against both types of CNS injury and the presence or absence of major ultrasound abnormalities. Of 651 infants surviving infancy at 1 year of age, 80 exhibited CP with a 12% incidence of that event in this VLBW group.

What emerged from the analysis was that chorioamnionitis and labor lasting less than 4 hours were most strongly associated with CP, and antepartum bleeding and maternal antibiotics use were less strongly but significantly associated. Chorioamnionitis and maternal antibiotic use tended to coexist to some extent. Preeclampsia and delivery without labor were associated with a significantly decreased risk of CP in comparison with controls. No beneficial effects of magnesium sulfate administration were seen. Chorioamnionitis tended to be associated with spastic diplegia without ultrasound abnormalities, whereas antepartum bleeding tended to be associated with ultrasound abnormalities in the affected infant. This study highlights the importance of considering fetal cranial ultrasound examinations as independent variables in future research in CP, and reemphasizes the grave significance of chorioamnionitis which, without structural change in the nervous system, is clearly an important potential cause of CP in this gestational age group.

T.H. Kirschbaum, M.D.

References

1. 1987 Year Book of Obstetrics and Gynecology, pp 243–245.
2. 1988 Year Book of Obstetrics and Gynecology, pp 116–118.
3. 1995 Year Book of Obstetrics and Gynecology, pp 135–138.

Elevated Umbilical Cord Plasma Erythropoietin Levels in Prolonged Pregnancies

Jazayeri A, Tsibris JCM, Spellacy WN (Univ of South Florida, Tampa)

Obstet Gynecol 92:61–63, 1998 4–12

Background.—Fetal oxygenation may be compromised in some pregnancies that extend past their expected delivery date. Erythropoietin levels in umbilical cord plasma were measured as an index of fetal oxygenation in normal pregnancies delivered from 37 to 43 weeks' gestation.

Methods.—One hundred twenty-four appropriately grown newborns were studied. All infants were the product of an uncomplicated labor and delivery, and none had evidence of fetal stress or meconium. Infants born at 37–40 weeks' gestation were compared with those born at 41–43 weeks' gestation.

Findings.—The 2 groups did not differ in cord blood gases or Apgar scores at 1 and 5 minutes. Delivery after 41 completed weeks of gestation was associated with significantly greater cord plasma erythropoietin levels. Compared with pregnancies extending to 37–40 weeks, erythropoietin levels were significantly increased in pregnancies extending to 41–43 weeks' gestation (Fig 1).

Conclusions.—Cord plasma erythropoietin concentrations are significantly increased in pregnancies reaching 41 weeks or longer, which indi-

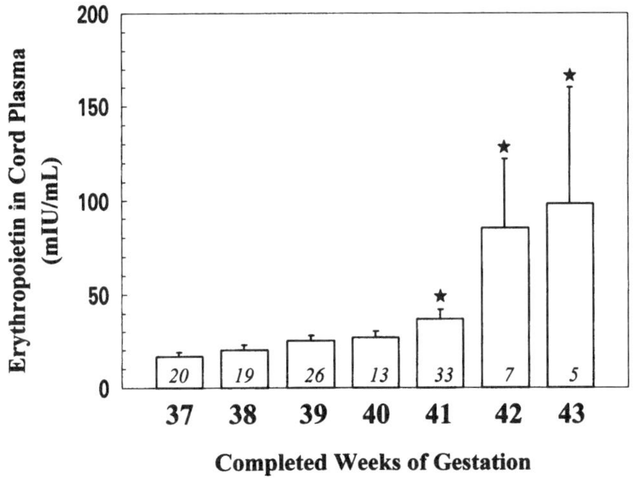

FIGURE 1.—Umbilical cord plasma erythropoietin levels (mean ± SEM) at 37–43 weeks' gestation. Analysis of variance revealed a significant difference between the groups ($P < 0.001$). Post hoc analysis by Dunnett t test using the 37–40 weeks' gestation as the control group and each gestational age after 40 weeks as a separate subgroup revealed significant elevation of fetal erythropoietin in the post-term subgroups ($^*P < 0.02$). *Numbers* inside the *bars* indicate the number of infants tested. (Courtesy of Jazayeri A, Tsibris JCM, Spellacy WN: Elevated umbilical cord plasma erythropoietin levels in prolonged pregnancies. *Obstet Gynecol* 92:61–63, 1998. Reprinted with permission from the American College of Obstetricians and Gynecologists.)

cates altered fetal oxygenation in some. These data support the practice of close fetal surveillance of prolonged pregnancies.

▶ This interesting observation is worth comment because much of the authors' interpretation rests on the assumption that elevated umbilical blood erythropoietin is synonymous with chronic fetal hypoxia. Erythropoietin, interleukin-3, and possibly other cytokines act to stimulate erythropoiesis through inhibition of red blood cell apoptosis, allowing production rates of red blood cells to exceed destruction rates. As other active cytokines are identified, additional mechanisms may come to light. Inhibition of hepatic erythropoiesis and what seems to be compensatory increases in plasma erythropoietin have been identified in fetuses of hypertensive gravidas (Abstract 3–4) and in intrauterine infection in growth-retarded infants who were not post dates. More work needs to be done to clarify the mechanics of erythropoietin production and release before assuming that it is associated with fetal hypoxia or even hypoxemia.

T.H. Kirschbaum, M.D.

Spontaneous Vaginal Delivery: A Risk Factor for Erb's Palsy?

Gherman RB, Ouzounian JG, Miller MA, et al (Univ of Southern California, Los Angeles)

Am J Obstet Gynecol 178:423–427, 1998 4–13

Introduction.—Erb's palsy, which results from injury to the fifth and sixth cervical nerve roots, is often associated with shoulder dystocia. In some cases, however, Erb's palsy occurs without antecedent shoulder dystocia. The records of infants with brachial plexus palsy after vaginal delivery were compared for maternal and fetal characteristics, time course of resolution, and rate of persistent injury at 1 year.

Methods.—During a 2-year period, 126 cases of shoulder dystocia occurred among 9,071 vaginal deliveries (1.4%). There were 40 cases of Erb's palsy, 23 associated with shoulder dystocia and 17 without identifiable shoulder dystocia (defined as the need for ancillary obstetric maneuvers other than gentle downward traction after delivery of the fetal head). Maternal charts, neonatal charts, and orthopedic and physical therapy records of the 2 groups were compared.

Results.—The risk of Erb's palsy was 18.3% and the risk of permanent palsy was 1.6% among infants with shoulder dystocia. Antepartum maternal characteristics were similar in cases of Erb's palsy with and without antecedent shoulder dystocia. Those without shoulder dystocia had an increased incidence of second-stage labor length less than 15 minutes and showed a trend toward smaller birth weight. Cases without shoulder dystocia had a significantly higher rate of palsy persistence at 1 year (41.2%) than cases with shoulder dystocia (8.7%) and took longer to resolve (mean 6.4 vs. 0.7 months).

Conclusion.—Brachial plexus injury has been thought to result from excessive lateral head flexion during delivery, with stretching of the nerve roots causing transient dysfunction. Not all Erb's palsies, however, appear to be related to traction. Erb's palsy with and without shoulder dystocia may be 2 quantitatively different injuries, the latter resulting from in utero forces.

► The incidence of permanent brachial plexus injury after vaginal vertex delivery is small, and its relationship to fetal macrosomia is by no means strong. More than half of the reported incidences of shoulder dystocia occur with fetuses that are not of excessive body weight.[1-2] These authors suggest quite strongly that the relative relationship between Erb's palsy and macrosomia does not have a simple relationship to shoulder dystocia. In the 2-year review of 9,071 deliveries, the incidence of shoulder dystocia was 1.4%, of early Erb's palsy 0.44%, and of permanent upper brachial plexus injury 0.1%. The incidence of permanent injury was higher than most reported experiences, but the reason is a disproportionate incidence of permanent injury among infants born with Erb's palsy but without shoulder dystocia. The risk of permanent injury was 41% among those 17 infants; 42% of all victims of Erb's palsy were born without shoulder dystocia. The comparable figure for permanent injury after shoulder dystocia was 8.7%, a rate comparable to that seen elsewhere. This disproportion in infants without shoulder dystocia has been reported by others.[3] Among infants without shoulder dystocia, mean birth weight at term was 3,561 g. There were high incidences of second stages of less than 15 minutes and of clavicular fractures in that group of infants. The authors point to the probability that a significant number of infants with permanent brachial plexus palsy sustain their injury before the time of delivery. That probability makes it even more likely than earlier realized that birth trauma to the brachial plexus can never be totally eliminated from obstetrical morbidity.

T.H. Kirschbaum, M.D.

References

1. 1987 Year Book of Obstetrics and Gynecology, pp 186–187.
2. 1994 Year Book of Obstetrics and Gynecology, pp 187–188.
3. 1996 Year Book of Obstetrics and Gynecology, pp 188–189.

Fetal and Neonatal Mortality in the Postterm Pregnancy: The Impact of Gestational Age and Fetal Growth Restriction

Divon MY, Haglund B, Nisell H, et al (Albert Einstein College of Medicine, Bronx, NY; Natl Board of Health and Welfare, Stockholm; Karolinska Inst, Stockholm)

Am J Obstet Gynecol 178:726–731, 1998 4–14

Background.—Pregnancies that progress beyond term are at greater risk of perinatal morbidity and mortality. Various studies have addressed this risk based on gestational age as the only contributing factor, although most did not include US (for dating). Another contributing factor may be intrauterine growth restriction (IUGR). Thus, the associations of gestational age and IUGR with fetal and neonatal mortality in the postterm pregnancy was evaluated.

Methods.—Review of the National Swedish Medical Birth Registry identified 480,772 postterm deliveries (40 weeks' gestational age or greater) from 1987 through 1992. Strict inclusion criteria (singleton pregnancy, reliable dating through second semester US, and a maternal age of 15–44 years) reduced the study population to 181,524 newborns. Logistic regression analysis (controlling for the sex of the fetus and maternal age, parity, and smoking history) was used to assess the effect of gestational age at delivery on intrauterine death and on neonatal death (within 28 days of delivery of a live-born infant). Adjusted odds ratios were also calculated for the risk of intrauterine or neonatal death as a function of IUGR (defined as birth weight less than 2 standard deviations below the mean for gestational age). Intrauterine and neonatal death rates at 40 weeks' gestation were used as reference levels.

Findings.—From 41 weeks' gestation on, the risk of intrauterine death rose slightly but significantly compared with reference values (odds ratios at 41, 42, and 43 weeks were 1.5, 1.8, and 2.9, respectively) (Table 2). The risk of neonatal mortality, while although increasing to 1.9 at 43 weeks, was not significantly different from reference values. Intrauterine growth restriction had independent effects on both intrauterine and neonatal deaths at each postterm gestational week (Table 3): Compared with ref-

TABLE 2.—Adjusted Odds Ratios for Perinatal Mortality as a Function of Gestational Age

Gestational age (wk)	*Intrauterine fetal death: Odds ratio and 95% CI*	*Neonatal mortality: Odds ratio and 95% CI*
40	1.0 (ref)	1.0 (ref)
41	1.48 (1.13–1.95)*	1.24 (0.90–1.70)
42	1.77 (1.22–2.56)*	1.44 (0.92–2.24)
≥43	2.90 (1.27–6.61)*	1.89 (0.60–5.99)

*$P < 0.05$ (over reference).

Abbreviation: CI, confidence interval.

(Courtesy of Divon MY, Haglund B, Nisell H, et al: Fetal and neonatal mortality in the postterm pregnancy: The impact of gestational age and fetal growth restriction. *Am J Obstet Gynecol* 178:726–731, 1998.)

TABLE 3.—Adjusted Odds Ratios for Intrauterine Fetal Death and Neonatal Mortality for Infants With and Without Intrauterine Growth Restriction in Relation to Gestational Age

Gestational age	*Intrauterine fetal death: Odds ratio and 95% CI*	*Neonatal mortality: Odds ratio and 95% CI*
40 wk		
Non-IUGR	1.0 (ref)	1.0 (ref)
IUGR	7.17 (4.06–12.66)*	3.45 (1.39–8.55)*
41 wk		
Non-IUGR	1.47 (1.10–1.98)*	1.18 (0.84–1.64)
IUGR	10.03 (5.56–18.07)*	7.19 (3.30–15.69)*
≥42 wk		
Non-IUGR	1.94 (1.33–2.82)*	1.31 (0.82–2.08)
IUGR	7.11 (2.87–17.63)*	9.38 (3.77–23.34)*

*$P < 0.05$ (over reference).
Abbreviation: CI, confidence interval.
(Courtesy of Divon MY, Haglund B, Nisell H, et al: Fetal and neonatal mortality in the postterm pregnancy: The impact of gestational age and fetal growth restriction. *Am J Obstet Gynecol* 178:726–731, 1998.)

erence values, odds ratios for fetal death ranged from 7.1 to 10.0 and odds ratios for neonatal death ranged from 3.5 to 9.4.

Conclusion.—Whereas gestational age in the postterm pregnancy is a significant factor in intrauterine deaths, it is not a significant factor in neonatal mortality. In contrast, IUGR greatly increases the risk for both fetal and neonatal death at each week post term. Methods for identifying the fetus with IUGR prospectively could pave the way for interventions to improve the perinatal outcome of these fetuses.

▶ Because the incidence of perinatal mortality associated with a postdate pregnancy is so small, large data collections are required to provide meaningful estimates of its size. Here, nearly the entire delivery experience reported to the National Swedish Medical Birth Registry for 6 years provides the data. Only 26% of data entries were used for this analysis. The bulk of the exclusions likely represent pregnancies delivered before 40 weeks' gestational age and, therefore, not the recipients of second trimester US to confirm dating, a requirement for entry into the study.

With a 74% exclusion rate, it would be helpful to compare the population excluded for lack of US with the demographic characteristics of those 181,524 women enrolled in the study. The data showed that pregnancy past 40 completed weeks of gestational age is associated with a significantly increased risk of fetal, but not neonatal, mortality, but the differences in mean fetal death rates cited are about 0.5 per 1,000 births per week. Fetal growth restriction risk is defined so as to approximate the lowest 2.5 percentile at stated gestational age and although it is not apparent that growth retardation increases significantly as a function of gestational age past 40 weeks, at each weekly interval, odds ratios for both fetal and neonatal mortality are greater for growth retarded compared with non-growth retarded infants.

Bear in mind that the increased fetal mortality in post dates pregnancy represents a failure of antepartum testing to prevent fetal death by recognizing fetuses in jeopardy. Remember, too, that perinatal mortality post dates is the sum of the intrinsic risk of post datism independent of management plus the possible morbidity and mortality associated with the induction of labor and the use of abdominal birth for failed inductions. Clearly, the process of attempting to deal with post date pregnancy carries with it morbidity of its own. It remains clear that we do not yet know how to manage post date pregnancy to avoid the small risk to the fetus that it may represent.

T.H. Kirschbaum, M.D.

Early Transvaginal Ultrasound Following an Accurately Dated Pregnancy: The Importance of Finding a Yolk Sac or Fetal Heart Motion

Deaton JL, Honoré GM, Huffman CS (Wake Forest Univ, Winston-Salem, NC)

Hum Reprod 12:2820–2823, 1997 4–15

Objective.—Studies using transvaginal ultrasonography (TVU) to distinguish between normal and abnormal pregnancies have been difficult to interpret because they typically date from the last menstrual period. The predictive value of a yolk sac or fetal heart motion during early accurately dated TVU were studied in women with a known date of fertilization or ovulation.

Methods.—Transvaginal ultrasonography was performed in 225 consecutive pregnancies, 5–6 weeks after the known date of ovulation, to follow fetal heart motion, and in 63 pregnancies, 22–32 days after in vitro fertilization (IVF), to study yolk sac formation. Pregnancies were followed up until a live birth or spontaneous abortion occurred.

Results.—Of the 65 yolk sacs in the 63 IVF patients, 61 sacs became ongoing. Of 20 patients without yolk sacs, 16 ultimately underwent a spontaneous abortion. The presence of a yolk sac between 22 and 32 days after fertilization predicted development of fetal heart motion in 94% of patients. There was a significant difference in spontaneous abortion rates between women aged 35 years or younger and those older than 35 (4.5% vs. 18%).

Conclusions.—Early TVU provides information to infertile couples about the quality of the pregnancy as soon as possible. The presence of a yolk sac was significantly predictive of fetal heart motion. Women aged 35 years and older are at increased risk of spontaneous abortion.

▶ Improvements in technology and the use of vaginal ultrasound transducers has improved early fetal visualization to the point where we can now do better in judging viability in the early first trimester than by looking for fetal heart motion. The yolk sac can often be seen at 5–6 weeks after the last menstrual period or 22–29 days postconception. Accurate dating here was obtained by studying women conceiving by in vitro fertilization. If a yolk sac is visualized at 5 weeks' gestational, the odds are 94% that fetal heart motion will subsequently appear. The absence of the yolk sac at that point means the odds are 73% for spontaneous abortion and 27% for subsequent normal pregnancy. The prognosis for continuing pregnancy is affected by maternal age, but all that can be said from these data is that given fetal heart audible in 225 normal pregnancies, the risk of spontaneous abortion is greater for women 35 years of age, averaging about 18% vs. 5% for women 35 years or less. Data of this sort are useful in counseling, especially for infertility patients who are anxious to learn, day by day, the likelihood of normal fetal development.

T.H. Kirschbaum, M.D.

5 Antepartum Fetal Surveillance

Fetal Assessment Based on Fetal Biophysical Profile Scoring: VIII. The Incidence of Cerebral Palsy in Tested and Untested Perinates

Manning FA, Bondaji N, Harman CR, et al (Univ of Manitoba, Winnipeg, Canada; Columbia Presbyterian Med Ctr, New York)

Am J Obstet Gynecol 178:696–706, 1998 5–1

Background.—The authors had 4 goals in undertaking this study: (1) to determine the rate of cerebral palsy in a large population in Manitoba over a 5-year period; (2) to assess whether performing the fetal biophysical profile made a difference in cerebral palsy incidence compared with a group of untested patients; (3) to examine the relationship between cerebral palsy and the last fetal biophysical profile score; and (4) to evaluate clinical characteristics of cerebral palsy in tested and untested patients.

Methods.—Chart review of Manitoba Health Agency data from 1987 through 1991 was used to identify children up to 4 years of age who had cerebral palsy. Data extracted included the antepartum obstetric history, gestational age at delivery, birth weight, age at diagnosis, the presumed timing and cause of the injury that caused the brain damage, and any prenatal biophysical profile scores.

Findings.—Chart review identified 313 children with proven cerebral palsy out of 84,947 live births, for an incidence of 3.68 per 1,000 live births. Of the live births, 26,290 (31%) were referred for fetal biophysical testing; 35 were subsequently identified as having cerebral palsy, for an incidence of 1.33 per 1,000 live births. Of the remaining 58,659 live births that did not undergo fetal testing, 278 cases of cerebral palsy occurred, for an incidence of 4.74 per 1,000 live births. These incidence rates between the tested and untested groups were significantly different. Yearly incidence rates in the tested group did not change over the 5-year period, but rates in the untested population declined linearly and significantly. Among all the tested patients, there was a significant relationship between a last normal fetal biophysical profile score and an increased incidence of cerebral palsy (Fig 2): incidence rates ranged from 0.7 per 1,000 live births for a normal profile score, to 13.1 per 1,000 live births for an equivocal score (6 on a 10-point scale), to 333 per 1,000 live births for a score of 0.

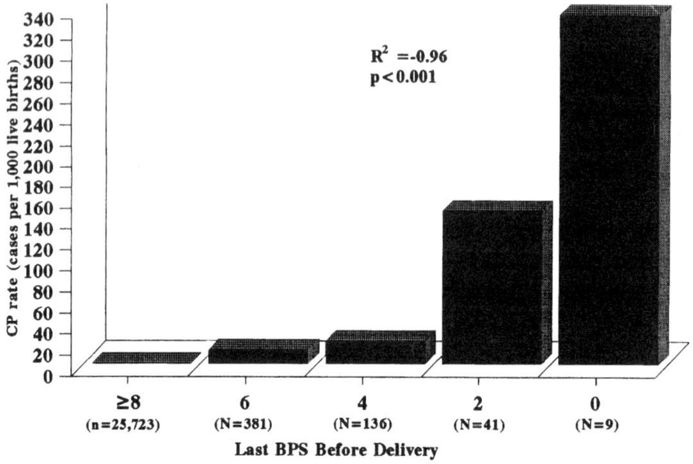

FIGURE 2.—Relationship between last fetal biophysical profile score (*BPS*) and incidence of cerebral palsy (*CP*). An inverse, exponential, and highly significant relationship is observed ($r^2 = -0.965$, P less than 0.001). (Courtesy of Manning FA, Bondaji N, Harman CR, et al: Fetal assessment based on fetal biophysical profile scoring: VIII. The incidence of cerebral palsy in tested and untested perinates. *Am J Obstet Gynecol* 178:696–706, 1998.)

A normal biophysical profile had a negative predictive value of 99.3% and a specificity of 97.98%. Positive predictive values varied with the abnormal test result, ranging from 1.31% for an equivocal score to 33.3% for a score of 0. Lumping all scores of 6 or less together gave a sensitivity of 49%. Neither gestational age, birth weight, assumed timing, nor the cause of the injury were related to the incidence of cerebral palsy.

Conclusion.—In the population as a whole, cerebral palsy incidence rates declined over the 5 years of this study. In the patients who were referred for fetal biophysical profiling, the incidence of cerebral palsy was significantly reduced compared with those who did not undergo testing. Furthermore, the more abnormal the last biophysical profile score, the greater the risk of cerebral palsy. Thus, antenatal testing may play some role in the assessment of infants for cerebral palsy.

► In developing and evaluating the results of the biophysical profile,[1-3] this group of investigators has established the procedure as a potentially useful technique for fetal assessment. In this retrospective cohort study, they compare rates of occurrence of cerebral palsy in women screened and not screened. In 26,288 pregnancies seen for fetal assessment at the University of Manitoba Department of Obstetrics and Gynecology (see table II of original article)—31% of all infants born in Manitoba during the time interval 1987–1991—they define the rate of cerebral palsy as 0.13% in tested pregnancies and 0.47% in untested pregnancies. The latter figure represents the largest rate of occurrence of cerebral palsy in a presumably normal population ever reported. The authors conclude that their data are "the first reported to demonstrate a beneficial effect of antepartum testing in general and fetal biophysical profile scoring in particular." Their attribution of value in prevention through use of the test is valid only if one grants the following implicit assumptions:

1. Tested and untested populations are comparable with respect to known correlates of cerebral palsy and that the incidence of preterm birth, very low birth weight infants, chorioamnionitis, hypertensive disease of pregnancy, birth trauma, third trimester bleeding, socioeconomic status, and access to quality obstetrical care was the same in both groups. No data are available regarding these points.
2. The diagnosis of cerebral palsy was accurate. The authors provide support for consistency in checking that the same diagnosis was made by the neonatologist, the neonatal ICU director, and the provincial registry. However, because the diagnosis was most often not made at the University of Manitoba but by physicians diverse in training, experience, and skill, this assumption seems hazardous.
3. The record review of cases managed elsewhere was sufficiently detailed to attempt a meaningful estimate of the time of fetal brain trauma in the course of labor and delivery. Compare these authors' efforts with those of Blair and Stanley who found that the time of injury could be fixed in only 50% of the cases after extensive record analysis.[4]
4. Obstetric management was the same for normal and abnormal pregnancies throughout the practice in academic communities in Manitoba. Could differences in outcome be attributed to differences in the quality of medical care throughout the province? I leave the answer to the reader.
5. In saying that "the relationship between the last biophysical profile score and cerebral palsy was inverse, reciprocal, exponential, and highly significant," the authors conclusion rests solely with 50 cases, that is, 0.19% of the total with biophysical profiles scores equal to or less than 2. There is no way to rule out the possibility that those fetuses were already brain damaged in utero at the time of their antepartum fetal assessment.

The authors provide some interesting data, but the data cannot be interpreted to mean that use of a biophysical profile was the sole, or even an important, reason for the reported differences cited.

T.H. Kirschbaum, M.D.

References

1. 1987 Year Book of Obstetrics and Gynecology, pp 156–159.
2. 1988 Year Book of Obstetrics and Gynecology, pp 137–138.
3. 1992 Year Book of Obstetrics and Gynecology, pp 132–133.
4. 1995 Year Book of Obstetrics and Gynecology, pp 131–134.

Increased Nuchal Translucency at 10–14 Weeks of Gestation as a Marker for Major Cardiac Defects

Hyett JA, Perdu M, Sharland GK, et al (King's College Hosp, London; Guy's Hosp, London)

Ultrasound Obstet Gynecol 10:242–246, 1997 5–2

Background.—Cardiac defects account for 40% of perinatal deaths and 60% of postneonatal deaths from congenital abnormalities. Sonographic examination of the 4-chamber view of the fetal heart at 16–22 weeks of gestation can identify 26% of major cardiac defects. Increased nuchal translucency thickness at 10–14 weeks of gestation is seen in about 75% of fetuses with chromosomal abnormalities, and a high percentage of these fetuses have congenital heart abnormalities.

Methods.—The prevalence of cardiac defects was determined in 1,427 fetuses who were chromosomally normal, but who had increased nuchal translucency thickness at 10–14 weeks of gestation. Cardiac defects were diagnosed by postmortem examination in cases of termination of pregnancy and intrauterine or neonatal deaths, or by clinical examination and investigation in live infants.

Results.—Of the 1,427 fetuses, there were 1,343 live births, 31 intrauterine or neonatal deaths, and 53 terminations of pregnancy. Cardiac defects were diagnosed in 8 of the 1,343 live births, and 4 of these defects were considered major. Pathological examination of the heart was performed in 17 of the 31 cases of intrauterine or neonatal deaths, and a major cardiac defect was diagnosed in 4. The 53 terminations of pregnancy were divided into 3 groups. In the first group of 9 cases, a major cardiac defect was diagnosed antenatally and confirmed at postmortem examination in all 9. In the second group of 23, termination was performed for other fetal abnormalities. Pathological examination of the heart was performed in 14 cases and major abnormalities were confirmed in 5. In the third group of 21, termination was performed although there was no specific fetal abnormality. Pathological examination of the heart was performed in 6 cases and major abnormalities were confirmed in 2. In the 1,389 live births or postmortem examinations after intrauterine death or termination of pregnancy, there were 24 cases of major cardiac defects (17/1,000). The incidence of defects increased from 5.4/1,000 with nuchal translucency thickness of 2.5–3.4 mm at 10–14 weeks of gestation to 233/100 with nuchal translucency thickness of 5.5 mm or greater.

Discussion.—These findings indicate that fetuses with increased nuchal translucency thickness at 10–14 weeks of gestation have a high incidence of major cardiac defects. This incidence increases as translucency thickness increases. These findings are consistent with the recognized association between cardiac defects and abnormal accumulation of nuchal fluid in the second trimester of pregnancy. Measurement of nuchal translucency thickness at 10–14 weeks of gestation may be a valuable method of detecting cardiac abnormalities as well as chromosomal defects.

► Nuchal translucency in the range of 3–4 mm thickness on fetal ultrasound in the first trimester defines a subset of fetuses at increased risk for aneuploidies, especially trisomies 21, 18, and 13. How effective such an observation is in a prospective sense is debatable.[1] Though estimates vary with the criteria used to define abnormal translucency, sensitivity for the prediction of aneuploidies among unselected patients ranges around 30%, with a 10% false positive rate. However, nuchal translucency may represent either lymphatic collection caused by faulty lymph vascular development adjoining the jugular veins, as in aneuploidy, or cardiac defects which generate high venous filling pressures and surplus lymph. The latter is useful as a screen for congenital cardiac disease, which might increase the present 26% cardiac anomaly detection rate, which is based on fetal ultrasound and the 4-chamber cardiac view at 16–22 weeks.[2] Here 1,427 euploid fetuses with nuchal translucency greater than 2.5 to 3.4 mm in the first trimester are reported, and the findings compared with findings on autopsy, cardiac microdissection, and clinical examination of the heart. With a prevalence of cardiac defects of 1.7% of the total population, the predicted incidence was 2.2%, using a 2.5–3.4 mm cutoff value,[3] and 25% using 5.5 mm. Whether this detection method will prove valuable in a prospective sense remains to be determined. In a small group of 12 of 984 infants with first trimester nuchal translucency greater than 5 mm in thickness, 40% of the infants were normal at birth.[4]

T.H. Kirschbaum, M.D.

References

1. 1996 Year Book of Obstetrics and Gynecology, pp 112–113, 130–131.
2. Tegnandar CE, Eikides SH, Johansen SJ, et al: Prenatal detection of heart defects after routine fetal examination at 18 weeks. *Ultrasound Obstet Gynecol* 5:372, 1995.
3. 1997 Year Book of Obstetrics, Gynecology, and Women's Health, pp 128–130.
4. Fukada CY, Yosumzu T, Takizawa M, et al: The prognosis of fetuses with nuchal translucency. *Acta Obstet Gynecol Scand* 76:913, 1997.

Uncomplicated Baseline Fetal Tachycardia or Bradycardia in Postterm Pregnancies and Perinatal Outcome

Sherer DM, Onyeije CI, Binder D, et al (Albert Einstein College of Medicine, Bronx, NY)

Am J Perinatol 15:335–338, 1998 5–3

Background.—A fetal heart rate (FHR) range of 120–160 beats/min is widely accepted as normal. However, the lower limit of this range may be too stringent, because an uncomplicated baseline FHR of less than 120 beats/min is not uncommon in normal, uncompromised fetuses. Neonatal outcomes in postterm pregnancies in which FHR monitoring demonstrated an uncomplicated FHR above or below the limits of the generally accepted normal range were reported.

Methods and Findings.—Between 1989 and 1995, 1,390 women (6.8% of the general population) were postterm. Thirty-one fetuses (2.2%) had a baseline FHR of 160 beats/min or higher, and 76 fetuses (5.5%) had a baseline FHR of 120 beats/min or lower. Two or 3 control patients were matched for each case of uncomplicated baseline fetal tachycardia or bradycardia. The 2 groups did not differ significantly in the incidence of cesarean delivery, presence of nuchal cord at delivery, meconium-stained amniotic fluid, 5-minute Apgar scores of less than 7, fetal growth restriction, meconium aspiration syndrome, or incidence of neonatal ICU admissions.

Conclusions.—In postterm patients, uncomplicated baseline fetal tachycardia or bradycardia is uncorrelated with an increase in the incidence of adverse perinatal outcomes. Thus these findings support the suggested modification of the FHR normal range.

▶ Despite the failure of 2 large, prospective, randomized studies to prove the benefit of induction of labor in postdate pregnancy,[1] antenatal assessment units continue to evaluate large numbers of postdate women with nonstress and biophysical profile testing. Gradually, the focus of surveillance has changed from those who have completed 42 weeks of gestation to those approaching 41 completed weeks of pregnancy. As the first chapter of *Williams Obstetrics* to be devoted to postterm pregnancy indicates, this change has the effect of increasing the numbers of American pregnancies under fetal surveillance by about 500,000 per year.[2] This gradual change has taken place despite the lack of evidence that such an approach diminishes perinatal morbidity and mortality rates. As a result, given the large number of false-positive results, especially from nonstress testing, the presence of women past 41 weeks' gestational age undergoing labor induction despite unfavorable cervices has become commonplace in labor units. This study gains its importance from its support at least for excluding women with uncomplicated pregnancies and simple tachycardia or bradycardia, the least ominous of all FHR deviations from modal values, from the mistaken perception of need for induction. Using 2 sets of triple controls matched for age and parity for both the 31 women with resting FHRs of greater than 160 beats/min and the 76 with FHRs of less than 120 beats/min, accounting for about 8% of the 1,390 women being evaluated for postdate pregnancies, the authors found no significant differences from controlled incidence rates of indices of neonatal morbidity. Excluding these women from antenatal testing would be a start in reducing the number of pregnant women under surveillance for postdatism in a direction that more closely fits available clinical data.

T.H. Kirschbaum, M.D.

References

1. 1995 Year Book of Obstetrics and Gynecology, pp 74–76.
2. Cunningham EG, MacDonald PC, Gant NE, et al (eds): *Williams Obstetrics*, ed 20. Stamford, Conn, Appleton and Lange, 1997, pp 827–837.

The Effect of Uterine Contractions on Intrapartum Fetal Heart Rate Analyzed by a Computerized System

Zimmer EZ, Paz Y, Copel JA, et al (Rambam Med Ctr, Haifa, Israel; Yale Univ, New Haven, Conn)

Am J Obstet Gynecol 178:436–440, 1998 5–4

Introduction.—The interpretation of electronic fetal heart rate (FHR) tracings often varies between observers. With a computerized monitoring system, FHR indexes can be objectively assessed with the same criteria for all fetuses. A study of 26 healthy women in active labor was designed to evaluate the effect of uterine activity on FHR indexes with a computerized FHR monitoring system.

Methods.—All women had normal singleton pregnancies at term and were studied in the active phase of labor with a cervical dilatation of 4–7

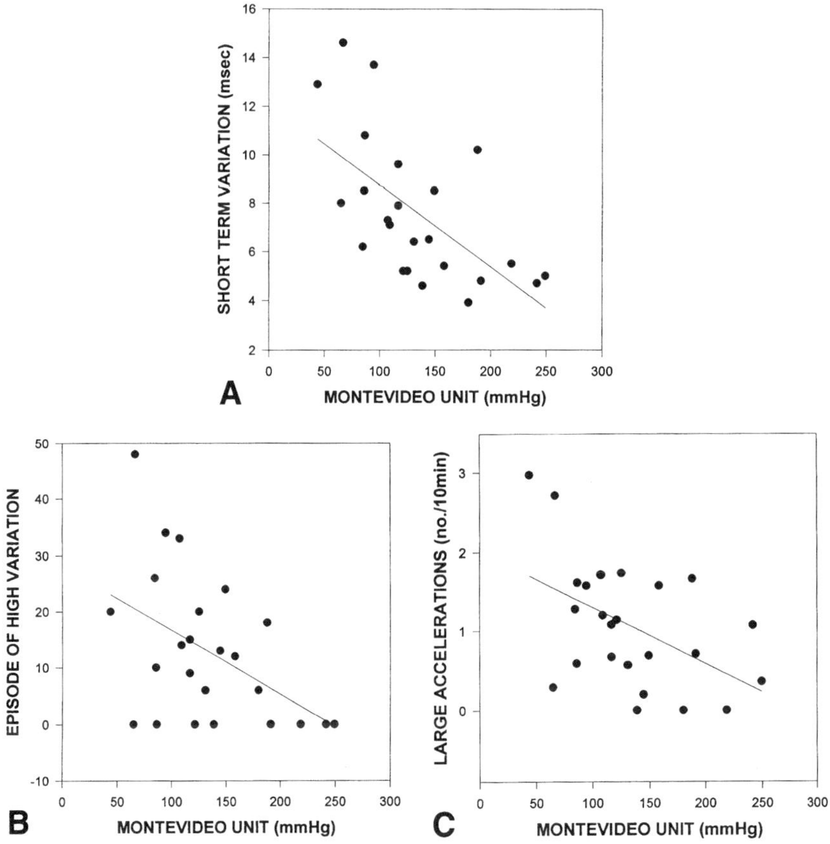

FIGURE 1.—Correlation between MU and short-term variation A, episodes of high variation B, and frequency of FHR accelerations C. *Abbreviation: FHR*, fetal heart rate. (Courtesy of Zimmer EZ, Paz Y, Copel JA, et al: The effect of uterine contractions on intrapartum fetal heart rate analyzed by a computerized system. *Am J Obstet Gynecol* 178:436–440, 1998.)

cm. None received analgesia before or during the study period. Fetal heart rate was analyzed with the Sonicaid System 8000, a computerized system that provides a numeric analysis of the FHR indexes. Quantitative assessment of uterine contractions was performed by measuring 2 parameters: Montevideo units (MU) and Alexandria units (AU). The study continued as long as patients did not request analgesia.

Results.—Duration of the recordings ranged from 28 to 64 minutes (mean 40.2 minutes). The mean MU and AU values were 134 mm Hg and 187 mm Hg × average duration (minutes), respectively. A significant correlation was found between MU and short-term variation (r = -0.62), episodes of high (r = -0.48) and low (r = -0.58) fetal heart rate variation, and frequency of large accelerations (r = -0.49) (Fig 1). Correlations were also significant for AU and short-term variation (r = -0.645), episodes of high FHR variation (r = -0.58), and the frequency of large accelerations (r = -0.49). Correlations were poor between MU and AU and baseline FHR, small accelerations, and frequency of decelerations.

Conclusion.—Variability in active labor FHR was found to be significantly affected by the intensity and duration of contractions. Increases in uterine activity were associated with decreases in FHR variability. Despite changes in FHR indexes, fetal outcome in these low-risk pregnancies was favorable.

▶ The introduction of instrumentation and programming for computer evaluation of fetal heart pulse intervals as a function of baseline and changing fetal heart rates has both objectified electronic fetal heart rate evaluation and brought enhanced sensitivity to the analysis. Here, an inverse relationship between uterine contractile activity in Montevideo units recorded by standard monitoring and beat-to-beat variability emerges in 26 normal term labors. Variability is measured from the baseline fetal heart rate as short-term variation (mean variation of frequencies among 3.75-second time intervals), high variation (the number of instances in which 5–6 consecutive minutes showed pulse intervals greater than 32 msec), and large accelerations (fetal heart rate more than 10 beats per minute greater than baseline for at least 15 seconds). All the data arrays showed that increasing uterine activity decreased fetal heart rate variability, but without adverse fetal effects in low-risk patients. Remember that pattern recognition in visual fetal heart rate analysis is based on a retrospective search for patterns of heart rate change after the delivery of depressed infants. Perhaps the evidence of altered variability here is too small to be discerned by earlier relatively crude attempts at visual pattern recognition. In any event, this observation casts doubt on one of the tenets of fetal heart rate analysis: reduced beat-to-beat variability may not be an accurate reflection of fetal jeopardy at all.

T.H. Kirschbaum, M.D.

Long Term Outcome After Artery Acidaemia at Term Birth: Influence of Gender and Duration of Fetal Heart Rate Abnormalities

Ingemarsson I, Herbst A, Thorngren-Jerneck K (Univ Hosp, Lund, Sweden)

Br J Obstet Gynaecol 104:1123–1127, 1997 5–5

Introduction.—Many labor units regularly analyze acid-base balance at birth. However, many infants with a very low pH (of less than 7·05) will have a normal development because severe fetal hypoxia of short duration that results in a profound cord artery acidaemia can easily be compensated by the newborn once gas exchange is restored. Infant outcome should be correlated with the duration of hypoxia by measuring the occurrence of pathological fetal heart rate patterns in labor. Gender of the infant may also affect the outcome.

Methods.—There were 154 infants with an umbilical artery having a pH of less than 7·05 at term birth. A comparison was made between infants with acidaemia and controls having a pH greater than 7·10 to determine neonatal outcome and the result of developmental screening. A review was conducted of fetal heart rate traces in infants with acidaemia. An analysis was performed of the relationship between outcome and duration of fetal heart rate changes.

Results.—Ten of 154 newborns with acidaemia at birth had encephalopathy. Two of these had cerebral palsy and 2 died. Eight of these 10 infants had a pH of less than 7·00, and 9 of the 10 infants were boys. Pronounced acidaemia with a pH of less than 7·00 was seen more often in male newborns, of which there were 39, than in female newborns, of which there were 22. At follow-up, infants born with acidaemia had speech problems significantly more often than the controls (19/102 vs. 8/98), although few infants had severe impairment. At age 4 years, neonatal encephalopathy and speech problems were significantly associated with duration of abnormal fetal heart rate changes in infants with acidaemia.

Conclusion.—At 4 years of age, neonatal encephalopathy and speech problems were associated with acidaemia at term birth. A more often pronounced acidaemia and a complicated course was seen with boys. Poor outcome was associated with a protracted abnormal fetal heart rate trace.

▶ Though this study of 154 infants born severely acidotic provides important information about the risk of short term and long term central nervous system impairment, it cannot be used to evaluate the role of fetal heart monitoring in prediction or prevention of CNS injury. False-positive rates for electronic fetal heart rate monitoring are not provided and retrospective evaluation of fetal heart tracings which disclosed a 26% incidence of abnormality lasting more than 60 minutes, was not blinded and is therefore subject to unevaluable observer bias. In the 136 cases where the discrimination between metabolic and respiratory acidosis could be made, 96% showed evidence of metabolic acidosis. Short-term outcome included evidence of encephalopathy in 6% (10 cases), perinatal mortality in 1.2%, and cerebral palsy in 1.2% (2 cases). Long-term morbidity in surviving infants followed at least one and a half years was confined to an increased incidence of speech problems compared to normal controls, even in the absence of earlier evidence of encephalopathy. Not reported before, I believe, was an increased preponderance of male gender among infants with either cord blood pH <7.0 or a neonatal neurological complication. This study confirms the absence of a strong relationship between cord blood acidemia and newborn central nervous system injury. The reasons rest with the ability of the fetus and neonate to accommodate to severe hypoxemia of short duration, using respiratory and renal mechanisms together with preferential shunting of cardiac output to favor cerebral blood flow at the expense of peripheral organ perfusion.

T.H. Kirschbaum, M.D.

Home Uterine Activity Monitoring in the Prevention of Very Low Birth Weight

Kempe A, Sachs BP, Ricciotti H, et al (Harvard Med School, Boston; Harvard School of Public Health, Boston; Boston Univ)
Public Health Rep 112:433–439, 1997 5–6

Introduction.—The Genesis Home Uterine Activity Monitor (HUAM), designed to detect early preterm labor in women with previous preterm deliveries, was approved by the United States Food and Drug Administration (FDA) in 1991. Use of HUAM is controversial, however, because indications for its use have expanded, and there is evidence that the monitor does not prevent premature births. The medical records of very low birth weight (VLBW) infants were reviewed to determine which of the mothers would have qualified for HUAM as it is now licensed and in which it could have been used to prolong gestation.

Methods.—Three sets of eligibility criteria for HUAM use were retrospectively applied to 1,440 mothers of VLBW infants born in 5 areas of the United States. Criteria were as follows: (1) a previous preterm birth, the current Food and Drug Administration (FDA) licensing criterion; (2) indications for HUAM commonly cited in published reports; and (3) the presence of any medical or reproductive condition that might predispose to premature delivery. To be included in the study, infants had to weigh between 500 gm and 1,499 gm and to have been born alive. Case records were examined to determine the conditions that precipitated delivery and whether HUAM and tocolytic therapy might have prolonged gestation.

Results.—The percentage of mothers who would have been placed on home monitoring was 18.1% using the FDA criterion, 39.6% using published criteria, and 78.8% using the broadest indication for monitoring. Of the group selected by the FDA criterion, only 24.6% had the potential to benefit from HUAM (based upon conditions precipitating delivery). Monitoring might have benefited 29.3% of those identified with published criteria and 25.8% identified with the broad criteria. The value of HUAM was reduced, however, when the numbers of cases that might have benefited were shown in relation to all pregnancies resulting in VLBW births: 4.4% in the FDA group, 11.6% in the published criteria group, and 20.3% in the broad criteria group.

Conclusion.—To prevent preterm delivery, HUAM must detect early uterine activity and tocolytic therapy used successfully to stop this activity. But the most common precipitating condition for preterm delivery, chorioamnionitis/premature rupture of membranes, would not have been predicted by HUAM. This technology is not likely to reduce current levels of VLBW births.

► A number of studies done with objectivity by investigators without financial interest in HUAM have failed to yield objective evidence of benefit in preventing preterm birth and its attendant costs.[1-3] This retrospective case-control study of women delivering infants in the VLBW range in Massachusetts, Maine, Mississippi, and Colorado attacks a different but related issue, i.e., how many women would be eligible for its use if the device were effective.? There are 2 questions to be answered: how many women meet eligibility criteria and how many have obstetrical complications for which tocolysis is contraindicated? Examples of the latter are chorioamnionitis, placental abruption, and severe hypertensive disease.

Using criteria proposed by the FDA when, in 1991, it approved use of the device, it was found that only 4.4% of women delivering VLBW infants had the potential for benefit. Using the broadest possible criteria proposed by proponents of its use—including some criteria with no definite link to preterm birth—only 20.3% of women could possibly have benefitted. In the minds of many obstetricians, FDA approval of HUAM devices was premature and now, in the face of considerable evidence of failure of benefit by reputable investigators, FDA approval should be withdrawn.

T.H. Kirschbaum, M.D.

References

1. 1993 Year Book of Obstetrics and Gynecology, pp 152–157.
2. 1994 Year Book of Obstetrics and Gynecology, p 165.
3. 1997 Year Book of Obstetrics, Gynecology, and Women's Health, p 152.

Multicenter Study on the Clinical Value of Fetal Pulse Oximetry: II Compared Predictive Values of Pulse Oximetry and Fetal Blood Analysis

Carbonne B, Langer B, Goffinet F, et al (Maternité Port Royal-Baudelocque, Paris; Hôpital Hautepierre, Strasbourg, France; Hôpital Antoine Béclère, Clamart, France; et al)

Am J Obstet Gynecol 177:593–598, 1997 5–7

Introduction.—Few studies have studied the clinical value of pulse oximetry as a tool for fetal monitoring in neonates with suspicious fetal heart

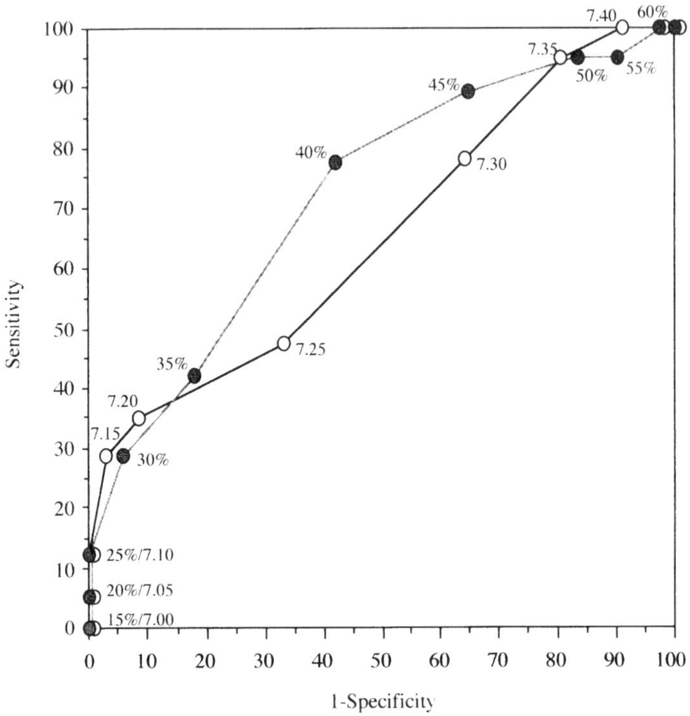

FIGURE 1.—Receiver-operator characteristic curve of values of fetal blood analysis (*open circles*) and fetal oxygen saturation (*solid circles*) in diagnosis of abnormal neonatal outcome expressed as sensitivity (*y axis*) as function of 1–Specificity (*x axis*). Values mentioned on *curve* are thresholds used for each *point*. (Courtesy of Carbonne B, Langer B, Goffinet F, et al: Multicenter study on the clinical value of fetal pulse oximetry: II Compared predictive values of pulse oximetry and fetal blood analysis. *Am J Obstet Gynecol* 177: 593–598, 1997.)

rates. Provided that the neonatal outcome is not compromised, the success of fetal pulse oximetry will depend on its ability to reassure the obstetric team in cases of abnormal fetal heart rate. Information provided by fetal pulse oximetry was compared with information provided by fetal scalp blood analysis to determine their diagnostic value on adverse neonatal outcome.

Methods.—During an abnormal fetal heart rate during labor, fetal oxygen saturation was continuously recorded with a Nellcor N-400 fetal pulse oximeter. The neonatal status was compared with simultaneous readings of fetal oxygen saturation and fetal blood analysis obtained before birth. An abnormal neonatal outcome was defined as when a neonate had a combined variable including 5-minute Apgar score of less than or equal to 7, umbilical arterial pH less than or equal to 7.15, secondary respiratory distress, transfer in a neonatal care unit, or when there was neonatal death. An abnormal neonatal outcome was also defined as when a neonate had an umbilical arterial blood pH less than or equal to 7.15.

Results.—Fetal blood analysis had a similar predictive value as fetal pulse oximetry. There was a 7.20 threshold for fetal scalp pH and 30% for fetal oxygen saturation. Tests were conducted on an arterial umbilical pH less than or equal to 7.15 and for an abnormal neonatal outcome. Both techniques had a similar receiver-operator characteristic curve with a cutoff value of less than or equal to 7.20 for fetal blood pH and less than or equal to 30% for fetal oxygen saturation (Fig 1). At higher thresholds, fetal pulse oximetry became superior.

Conclusion.—The predictive value of fetal blood analysis can be favorably compared to intrapartum fetal pulse oximetry. To assess the potential clinical benefits of this new tool, randomized controlled management trials should be performed.

► The past 10 years have seen a rebirth of interest, principally in Europe, in pulse oximetry as a means of appraising fetal well being during labor. This report represents a trial of feasibility by a French multicenter randomized, prospective trial of pulse oximetry's usefulness in clinical application. The method employs reflected light from a source placed at the side of the fetal head during labor with the intensity of reflected light filtered through two channels, each corresponding to the reflectance maximum of either oxidized or reduced hemoglobin. In an analog system, the relative intensity of light of those 2 wavelengths is used to estimate the percent oxyhemoglobin saturation in the fetal scalp and, depending on the value of saturation deemed appropriate to define abnormality, to predict fetal jeopardy. In order to avoid the inevitably high specificity rates that stem from attempts to predict an uncommon event, 174 records from women felt to have abnormal fetal heart rate tracings were studied. Of these, 134 had oximetry measurements, and 78 received fetal blood analysis (FBA). During the 30 minutes prior to birth in 71 cases, both determinations were performed and could be directly compared. The ability of each technique to predict abnormal cord blood pH (less than or equal to 7.15) and abnormal newborn outcome (impaired 5-minute Apgar, respiratory distress syndrome, NICU admission, or neonatal death) were then compared. Strangely, both FBA and oximetry performed badly in predicting cord blood acidosis with sensitivities of 40% and specificities in the range of 90% to 94%. FBA showed a 60% false-positive rate with oximetry exhibiting a 40% false-positive and 31% false-negative rate. In predicting abnormal fetal outcome, both showed sensitivities in the range of 35% with 50% false-positive rates for FBA and 31% for oximetry. Receiver operating curves revealed the improved predictive capacity of oximetry, but the differences are small, and even using 30% oxyhemoglobin saturation to define abnormality, the false-positive rate for oximetry is 57% and the false-negative rate is 13%. Using a cut-off of 40%, hemoglobin saturation increases sensitivity from 30% to 80% but at the cost of decreasing specificity and raising the false-positive rate to 73%. In brief, pulse oximetry performed roughly as well as FBA in predicting fetal acidosis or abnormal fetal outcome. Regrettably, neither method offers much future promise, nor have either shown evidence of past utility.

T.H. Kirschbaum, M.D.

Antenatal Corticosteroid Therapy and Fetal Behaviour: A Randomised Study of the Effects of Betamethasone and Dexamethasone

Mulder EJH, Derks JB, Visser GHA (Univ Hosp, Utrecht, The Netherlands)

Br J Obstet Gynaecol 104:1239–1247, 1997 5–8

Objective.—Corticosteroid therapy for threatened preterm delivery heightens the development of the fetal lung. Whereas long-term studies have demonstrated no adverse effects on fetal development, recent studies have shown decreased fetal movement and a rise in fetal heart rate variation after dexamethasone administration. The effects on fetal behavior and heart rate of betamethasone or dexamethasone administration were compared in a prospective randomized study.

Methods.—Either betamethasone (group 1, n=30) or dexamethasone (group 2, n=30) was administered to pregnant women between 26 and 33 weeks of gestation because of premature contractions or risk of preterm delivery. Median medication duration was 26 days in group 1 and 32 days in group 2. Observations were not completed in 4 group 1 women and 6 group 2 women. Fetal heart rate and fetal body and breathing movements were monitored. Group measurements were compared statistically.

Results.—Compared with day 0 measurements, day 2 measurements of body and breathing movements were significantly reduced by 48.8% and 84.6% respectively in group 1. Fetal heart rate variation was significantly reduced on days 2 and 3 in group 1 women for both the long-term (18.9% and 13.8%) and the short-term (12.5% and 11.7%). In group 2, day 1 fetal heart rate short-term variation increased significantly by 23.7%. All changes in both groups returned to baseline by day 4.

Conclusion.—Betamethasone has more transient effects on the fetus than dexamethasone. Because only betamethasone has been shown to have a significant effect of reducing neonatal mortality, its use in high-risk pregnancy is justified even though it hampers assessment of the fetal condition.

► The introduction of digital computer analysis to continuous fetal heart rate recording has made fetal heart rate analysis a more objective process, reducing some of the subjectivity which has impaired its effectiveness over the past 4 decades. The methodology has been described here several times.[1-4] It has made possible discernment of fetal heart rate responses of great subtlety and in this article, its use was supplemented by online recording of fetal body and respiratory movements after administration of 12 mg of betamethasone twice over 48 hours to women with threatened preterm labor. What followed was significant reduction of fetal body and respiratory movements for a period of 2½ to 3 days after the beginning drug dosage, and somewhat longer periods of reduced short- and long-term fetal heart rate variability without change in baseline fetal heart rate. Use of dexamethasone results in somewhat different changes, but since betamethasone has a longer period of bioactivity and is more important in affording lung maturity than is dexamethasone, the differences are interesting but of no clinical relevance. The changes are subtle and have eluded subjective fetal heart rate analysis for decades. Their meaning is important only to those who believe fetal heart variability and fetal movement frequency are useful in evaluating fetal well-being in women at risk of preterm delivery, despite the absence of prospective data supporting that contention. Perhaps the authors are revealing part of the basis for the difficulty in demonstrating the usefulness of antepartum testing in this important subset of women threatening to deliver prematurely.

T.H. Kirschbaum, M.D.

References

1. 1989 Year Book of Obstetrics and Gynecology, pp 117–118.
2. 1990 Year Book of Obstetrics and Gynecology, pp 129–131.
3. 1993 Year Book of Obstetrics and Gynecology, pp 144–145.
4. 1994 Year Book of Obstetrics and Gynecology, pp 160–161.

Congenital Heart Defects: Natural Course and In Utero Development

Yagel S, Weissman A, Rotstein Z, et al (Hadassah Med Ctr, Mount Scopus, Jerusalem; Chaim Sheba Med Ctr, Tel Hashomer, Israel; Tel Aviv Univ, Israel)

Circulation 96:550–555, 1997 5–9

Introduction.—With prenatal transvaginal (TV) or transabdominal (TA) US, most fetal congenital heart defects can be diagnosed between the early second trimester and midgestation. However, even with detailed echocardiography, the diagnosis of some cardiac malformations is delayed. There is evidence that progressive cardiac disease can be observed in utero with advancing gestational age. The evolution and in utero development of fetal cardiac anomalies were studied retrospectively.

Methods.—The study included 22,050 pregnant women, divided into 2 groups, depending on their timing and type of US examination. Group A (31%) underwent initial TV US at 13–16 weeks' gestation, followed by TA US at 20–22 weeks'. Group B (69%) underwent initial TA US at 20–22 weeks'. Another examination was performed during the third trimester. The babies were evaluated by certified pediatricians at birth. The findings of patients in whom the diagnosis of fetal cardiac defects was missed during the initial examination but recognized subsequently were reviewed.

Results.—A total of 168 cases of congenital heart defects were diagnosed, 66 in group A and 102 in group B. Of the cases in group A, 64% were recognized at the initial TV US examination, whereas 17% were diagnosed at the subsequent TA US examination. Of the rest, 4% were detected during the third trimester, and 15% were detected after birth. Of the cases in group B, 78% were detected at the initial, midtrimester TA US examination. Another 7% were detected in the third trimester, and 15%

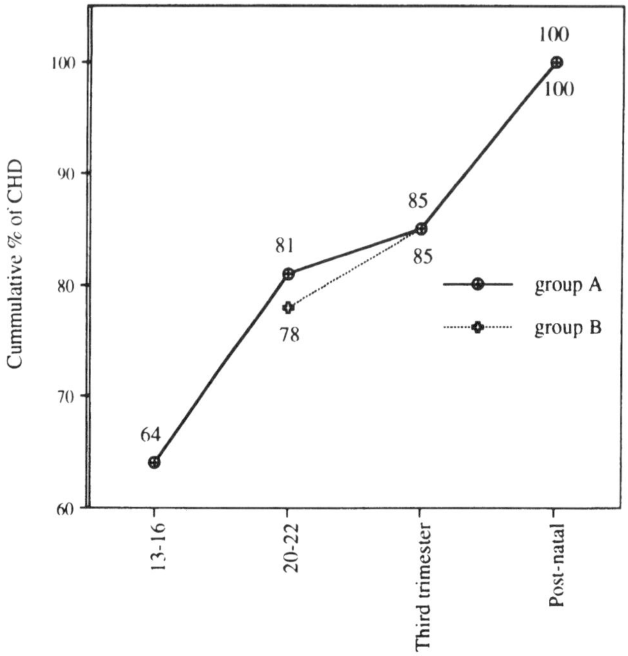

FIGURE 2.—Accumulation of CHD detected by TVS and TAS. (Courtesy of Yagel S, Weissman A, Rotstein Z, et al: Congenital heart defects: Natural course and in utero development. *Circulation* 96:550–555, 1997. Reproduced by permission of *Circulation*. Copyright 1997 American Heart Association.)

were detected postnatally (Fig 2). Overall, 10 cardiac anomalies went unrecognized until the third trimester. These were 2 cases of aortic stenosis, 2 cases of cardiac rhabdomyoma, and 1 case each of subaortic stenosis, tetralogy of Fallot, aortic coarctation, sealed foramen ovale, ventricular septal defects, and hypertrophic cardiomyopathy. Of fetuses with cardiac anomalies, 39% died.

Conclusions.—The appearance of fetal cardiac anomalies can vary during fetal development and evolve in utero. Approximately one fifth of defects may be missed by early second-trimester TV or midgestation TA US examination. If early second-trimester TV US is performed, it should be followed up by a midgestation scan. Currently, late second-trimester or third-trimester scans are indicated only for high-risk patients.

▶ This longitudinal study of 22,050 gravidas who received fetal ultrasonography allows conclusions about the natural course of some cardiac lesions as well as optimal timing for detection by US. About one third of the women had a vaginal US examination between 13 and 16 weeks, and two thirds were examined between 20 and 22 weeks by the abdominal route. A total of 168 congenital lesions identified after birth accounted for a 0.76% incidence, and 85% of these were identified antenatally. It is important that early second trimester vaginal ultrasounds failed to disclose 36% of the lesions and that abdominal US at 20–22 weeks and in the third trimester missed only

15% to 20% of fetal heart abnormalities. The reasons for failure of detection were partly technical but represented the tendency for some cardiac lesions to require sufficient cardiovascular development to make them discernable. Examples of such lesions are stenosis of aortic and pulmonary outflow tracts, aortic coarctation, hypertropic cardiomyopathy, and endocardial fibroelastosis. The most commonly missed lesion, the ventricular septal defect, is often too small to identify in early pregnancy, but it can be readily identified with color flow Doppler imaging later on.

The most important point here is that in terms of optimal detection, a first-trimester vaginal US examination needs to be supplemented with second- or third-trimester abdominal scans to avoid missing a significant number of congenital cardiac lesions.

T.H. Kirschbaum, M.D.

Middle Cerebral Artery Velocimetry: Different Clinical Relevance Depending on Umbilical Velocimetry

Strigini FAL, De Luca G, Lencioni G, et al (Univ of Pisa, Italy)

Obstet Gynecol 90:953–957, 1997 5–10

Objective.—There is no general agreement on the value of cerebral velocimetry for predicting fetal growth restriction. The authors present results of a study evaluating whether Doppler velocimetry recorded from the middle cerebral artery can provide more information than umbilical velocimetry for predicting adverse perinatal outcome in high-risk pregnancies.

Methods.—Umbilical velocimetry and middle cerebral artery pulsatility index were measured in fetuses aged 25 to 41 weeks in 576 high-risk pregnancies. Umbilical artery systolic-diastolic ration was recorded. The contribution of these tests to the ability to predict small for gestational age (SGA) newborns was evaluated by using multiple logistic regression analysis. SGA was defined as birth weight below the 10th centile. Adverse perinatal outcomes were defined as fetal death or death before hospital discharge, 5-minute Apgar score less than or equal to 7, or fetal heart anomalies.

Results.—Both abnormal umbilical and cerebral velocimetry tests were significantly predictive of SGA fetuses and adverse outcome. Interaction between the 2 tests did not improve predictive power of umbilical velocimetry alone ($\kappa = 0.37$ vs. 0.41). Within the group of high-risk pregnancies, fetuses with abnormal umbilical systolic-diastolic rations (relative risk of SGA = 6.1) and with an abnormal cerebral Doppler (relative risk = 1.3) had double the risk of being SGA and having an adverse outcome (relative risk = 2.1).

Conclusion.—Whereas cerebral Doppler velocimetry for high-risk pregnancies adds little information to that already provided by umbilical velocimetry, it does identify those infants with SGA and an abnormal umbilical velocimetry who are likely to have a poor perinatal outcome.

▶ This group of obstetricians assume there is value in routine umbilical artery Doppler-based predictions of fetal growth retardation and wish to evaluate the utility of adding middle cerebral artery Doppler studies in that undertaking. Their data fail to support either Doppler approach. Outcome measures, grouped as adverse perinatal outcome, include abnormal fetal heart rate patterns leading to cesarean section, a criterion which overstates fetal abnormality, since most such newborns are normal at birth. Umbilical artery Doppler fails to detect 63% of growth-retarded infants and bears a 27% false-positive rate. The predictive efficiencies are worse for adverse perinatal outcome. Combining small for gestational age and abnormal perinatal outcome as dependent variables increases sensitivity a bit but at the cost of increasing false-positives to 60% to 64%. The value of adding middle cerebral artery to umbilical artery Doppler analysis cannot be evaluated because the use of fetal heart rate analysis leading to cesarean section is notoriously replete with delivery of normal infants. Umbilical artery velocimetry continues to be a poor means of predicting or detecting fetal growth retardation.[1]

T.H. Kirschbaum, M.D.

Reference

1. 1995 Year Book of Obstetrics and Gynecology, pp 166–167.

A Comparison of Clinical and Ultrasonic Estimation of Fetal Weight

Sherman DJ, Arieli S, Tovbin J, et al (Assaf-Harofeh Med Ctr, Zerifin, Israel)

Obstet Gynecol 91:212–217, 1998 5–11

Objective.—No method of estimating fetal weight has proved to be more accurate than any other. The accuracy of birth weight estimation by routine antepartum sonogram was compared with clinical examination on admission to the labor and delivery ward.

Methods.—Between January 1990 and April 1995, 1,717 women were admitted in early labor within 1 week of an ultrasound for estimated fetal weight (EFW). Clinical EFW was estimated by a senior resident, unaware of the ultrasound EFW, using uterine palpation. Weights were stratified into 3 groups, less than 2,500 g, 2,500–4,000 g, and greater than 4,000 g. Percentage error, absolute percentage error, and proportion of estimates within 10% of actual birth weight were compared for both methods.

Results.—Actual birth weights ranged from 690 to 5,320 g, and 84.6% of deliveries were term. Both methods consistently overestimated actual birth weight in low birth weight infants. In the middle range of birth weights, the ultrasound method underestimated the actual birth weight. In the high birth weight group, both methods underestimated the actual birth weight. The standard deviation of the clinical method was significantly

TABLE 3.—Studies Comparing Clinical and Ultrasonic Estimated Fetal Weight

Reference	No. of patients	Gestational age (wk)	Birth weight (g)	Method of estimation	Mean absolute % error	BW ± 10% (% of estimates)	Findings
Patterson 1985[15]	43/62	>37	3330 ± 445	Clinical	NA	NA	Clin ≤ U/S
				Warsof et al[13]			
				Campbell[15]			
Watson 1988[16]	100	>37	2280–4650	Clinical	8.2%	66%	Clin = U/S
				Shepard et al[5]	7.9%	67%	
Raman et al 1992[17]	50	NA	1800–4500	Clinical	NA	NA	Clin > U/S
				Shepard et al[5]			
				Osaka University[17]			Clin = U/S (BW >4 kg)
				Hadlock et al[22]			
Chauhan et al 1992[20]	106	>37	2440–5225	Clinical	9.0%	66%	Clin = U/S
				Hadlock et al[22]	15.6%	42%	
				Patient	8.7%	70%	
Chauhan et al 1993[19]	200	>37	2440–5225	Clinical	9.1%	65%	Clin > U/S
				Warsof et al[13]	10.7%	56%	
Shamley et al 1994[18]	223	35–42	2028–4678	Clinical	8.4%	66%	Clin ≤ U/S
				Hadlock et al[22]	6.2%	79%	
				Shepard et al[5]	6.1%	77%	Clin > U/S (in labor)
				Rose and McCallum[14]	7.6%	71%	
				Sabbagha et al[6]	7.8%	70%	
Chauhan 1995[21]	602	>37	2302–5225	Clinical	NA	NA	Clin ≥ U/S*
				8 U/S formulas			
Chauhan 1995[21]	67†	>37	NA	Clinical	9.9%	54%	Clin ≥ U/S
				4 U/S formulas	11.4–16.6%	36–51%	
Present study	1717	24–43	690–5320	Clinical	7.9%	72%	Clin ≥ U/S
				3 U/S formulas	8.4%	69%	Clin < U/S (BW <2.5 kg)

*Prediction of macrosomia.
†BW > 4kg.
Abbreviations: BW, birth weight; *NA*, not available; *Clin*, clinical; *U/S*, ultrasound; *Clin>U/S*, clinical estimation significantly more accurate than ultrasonic estimations; *Clin≥U/S*, clinical estimation significantly more accurate or not significantly different from ultrasonic estimations; *Clin=U/S*, accuracy of clinical estimation not significantly different from ultrasonic estimations; *Clin≤U/S*, clinical estimation significantly less accurate or not significantly different from ultrasonic estimations; *Clin<U/S*, clinical estimation significantly less accurate than ultrasonic estimations.
(Courtesy of Sherman DJ, Arieli S, Tovbin J, et al: A comparison of clinical and ultrasonic estimation of fetal weight. *Obstet Gynecol* 91:212–217, 1998. Reprinted with permission from The American College of Obstetricians and Gynecologists.)

smaller than that of the ultrasound method. Accuracy of the ultrasound method compares favorably with results of other studies (Table 3).

Conclusion.—Clinical estimation of birth weight is sufficiently accurate for nearterm or term deliveries. Ultrasound EFW is beneficial for preterm deliveries.

► Though estimates of fetal weight are currently being made through ultrasonic body measurements, and a variety of empirically-defined polynomial expressions of estimated fetal weight as a function of those measurements, it is still not possible to prove that ultrasonic estimates are more highly predictive than clinical estimates based on uterine palpation.[1] This comparative study benefits from the largest number of comparative cases reported to date, but at the cost of data collections from various centers with varying ultrasonic expertise, and of differing formulas from which estimated fetal weights are calculated. The authors' rebuttal is that no single formula or set of formulas has proven superior to others and that the large number of cases tends to minimize variability among centers through regression to the mean. Then too, the mean error of 8% to 8.4% in this case is similar to that reported by groups using a single protocol. Data are evaluated based on absolute and relative differences between estimated fetal weight and birth weight, a process which precludes any comment about the error in diagnoses of macrosomia. Ultrasound proves superior in the 8% of infants weighing less than 2.5 kg at birth, but for all others, clinical estimate is better (in the 81% of infants weighing 2.5 to 4.0 kg) or equally accurate (infants weighing more than 4.0 kg). The authors are correct in pointing out that around the mean birth weight of 3.3 kg, birth weight correlation with gestational age is so good that a reasonable birth weight estimate can be calculated directly from gestational age without examining the patient in any way. In any event, this study highlights our need to continue to teach the art of clinical estimate of fetal weight as an inexpensive and effective means of evaluating the anticipated size of the fetus.

T.H. Kirschbaum, M.D.

Reference

1. 1990 Year Book of Obstetrics and Gynecology, pp 102–103.

Fetal Heart Rate Observations in 300 Term Brain-damaged Infants

Phelam JP, Ahn MO (Pomona Valley Hosp Med Ctr, Calif; Cha Women's Hosp, Seoul, Korea)

J Matern Fetal Invest 8:1–5, 1998 5–12

Background.—A relationship may exist between long-term neurologic impairment in the fetus and a persistent nonreactive fetal heart rate (FHR). These authors retrospectively analyzed FHR patterns through fetal monitoring strips in term infants born with neurologic impairment.

Methods.—Chart review indicated 300 infants who were born with brain damage. All were singleton births at term without traumatic delivery. Fetal monitoring strips were assessed for reactivity every 30 minutes for the first 2 hours of monitoring and for the last 2 hours. Patterns were noted as reactive (FHR acceleration of 15 beats/min for 15 seconds from 1 baseline measurement to the next during a 30-minute period) or nonreactive (no FHR accelerations over 120 minutes).

As described by Hon, monitoring strips were also assessed for the first 2 hours and the last 1 hour for decelerations. Decelerations were noted as variable (typical or atypical), late (repetitive FHR pattern or a deceleration that started at the peak of the uterine contraction, was at its lowest at the offset of the contraction, and had a symmetric waveform), or prolonged (decline from baseline that persisted until delivery). Infants were divided into groups based on whether the FHR at admission was reactive (*N* = 152, or 51%), nonreactive (*N* = 135, or 45%), bradycardic (*N* = 9, or 3%) or unclassifiable (*N* = 4, or 1%).

Findings.—Three patterns were observed in the group with a reactive FHR pattern at admission. In 24 patients (26%), the FHR pattern was persistently reactive; this seemed to indicate that the neurologic injury occurred early in pregancy or during the postnatal period. In 67 patients (44%), a Hon-type FHR pattern emerged, with the abnormal FHR pattern developing over time; this indicated intrapartum asphyxia. The remaining 61 patients (40%) had a sudden FHR deceleration that lasted until delivery; clinical events leading to this pattern included uterine rupture, cord prolapse, maternal arrest, and abruption. Three patterns were also observed in the group with a nonreactive stress pattern at admission. In 97 patients (72%) the baseline FHR continued through to delivery. In 12 patients (9%), an FHR deceleration occurred that lasted until delivery. The remaining 26 patients (29%) experienced progressive deceleration of the FHR until death ("stair steps" pattern) or bradycardia.

Conclusion.—During the intrapartum period, term infants who would be born with brain damage exhibited identifiable FHR patterns. Infants in the nonreactive group had an FHR pattern that did not change from baseline or showed steady and progressive deceleration. These infants should be monitored continuously in the hospital, and additional tests might be needed to determine the status of the fetus. In the reactive group, the 2 main patterns were the Hon pattern of intrapartum asphyxia (which evolves over time) and a sudden prolonged deceleration (which indicates a more immediate clinical event). Recognizing these patterns may help the obstetrician (in concert with the mother) make decisions regarding delivery.

▶ With this publication, the senior author joins Dr. Barry Shifrin in proposing continuous integrated FHR tracings "probably consistent with asphyxia and fetal brain injury" can be identified.[1] In both cases, the investigators' approach was the same. Intrapartum FHR tracings of what proved to be brain damaged infants born at term were studied and common patterns sought. In both cases, the patterns described were somewhat similar: reduced baseline variability; normal or elevated baseline heart rate; a pattern of repeated decelerations; and then progressive reduction in rate, either slowly or abruptly. The patterns "can be easily categorized and identified."

The problems with this sort of analysis have been known for 4 decades. The observations are uncontrolled. Those who use FHR analysis to evaluate fetal well being regularly overdiagnose impairment in fetal function. Loss of beat-to-beat variability often reflects change in fetal sleep and wake state. Without knowing how often a FHR pattern is seen in normal fetuses, nothing can be said about predictability of fetal injury in those in whom it is. In both instances, the authors are interested and experienced expert witnesses in claims against professional liability and litigation. It is disturbing to see how little they value the fundamental tenants of scientific inquiry by failing to carry out controls for their observations.

T.H. Kirschbaum, M.D.

Reference

1. Shields JR, Shifrin BS: Perinatal antecedents of cerebral palsy. *Obstet Gynecol* 71:899, 1988.

6 Fetal Therapy

Antibiotic Therapy for Reduction of Infant Morbidity After Preterm Premature Rupture of the Membranes: A Randomized Controlled Trial

Mercer BM, for the National Institute of Child Health and Human Development Maternal-Fetal Medicine Units Network (Univ of Tennessee, Memphis)

JAMA 278:989–995, 1997 6–1

Introduction.—Many cases of preterm premature rupture of the membranes (PPROM) appear to be caused by intrauterine infection. Because 70% to 80% of women will deliver within 1 week of PPROM, various means of prolonging pregnancy have been sought. A randomized, double-blind, placebo-controlled trial assessed the ability of antibiotic treatment to reduce infant morbidity after PPROM.

Methods.—Study participants were drawn from 11 clinical centers. Eligible women had spontaneous PPROM at 24 weeks to 32 weeks gestation, membrane rupture occurring within 36 hours of randomization, cervical dilatation of 3 cm or less, and 4 or fewer contractions in the hour before randomization. None had recently been treated with antibiotics or corticosteroids. Active treatment was IV ampicillin (a 2-g dose every 6 hours) and erythromycin (a 250-mg dose every 6 hours) for 48 hours, followed by oral amoxicillin (a 250-mg dose every 8 hours) and erythromycin base (a 333-mg dose every 8 hours) for 5 days. Those randomized to placebo received a visually indistinguishable IV and oral regimen. Patients were expectantly managed in the hospital unless fluid leakage stopped and normal amniotic fluid volume returned. Corticosteroid and tocolytic therapy were not allowed after enrollment, but group B streptococcus carriers were identified and treated.

Results.—Three hundred women were randomized to the antibiotic regimen and 314 to placebo. Study outcomes were fetal or infant death, respiratory distress, severe intraventricular hemorrhage, stage 2 or 3 necrotizing enterocolitis, or sepsis within 72 hours of birth. In the group B streptococcus–negative cohort, combined adverse outcomes were significantly lower in the antibiotic group (44.5%) than in the placebo group (54.5%). The incidence of respiratory distress syndrome was 40.8% among infants of mothers who received antibiotics vs. 50.6% among those whose mothers were given placebo. Antibiotic treatment also reduced infant morbidity in the total study population.

Conclusion.—Antibiotic treatment proved effective in reducing infant morbidity after PPROM. Clinical amnionitis was less frequent, pregnancy was prolonged, and there were fewer cases of respiratory distress, necrotizing enterocolitis, and other morbidities.

► Although the use of antibiotic therapy in the prevention of preterm birth has been reviewed several times,[1] this product of the Maternal-Fetal Medicine Units Network sponsored by the National Institute of Child Health and Human Development provides authoritative recommendations based on careful experimental design and analysis. Typically, only one third of eligible study candidates with spontaneous PROM membranes occurring between 24 and 32 weeks' gestation and within 36 hours of randomization without evidence of labor survived the extensive list of exclusion factors designed to reduce confounding variables. It is noteworthy that corticosteroids were not used to allow isolation of the effects of antibiotics. Intravenous ampicillin and erythromycin were given for 2 days, followed by amoxicillin, 0.75 g, and erythromycin, 1 g, every day for 5 days.

Comparing randomized placebo and antibiotic therapy, group B streptococcus (GBS)-negative women had a reduced incidence of newborn respiratory distress syndrome, early onset sepsis and pneumonia, and persistent patent ductus arteriosus. No benefit was discernable among GBS-positive patients, apparently a reflection of inadequate power to identify benefit among low-prevalence negative outcomes. When GBS-positive and GBS-negative women were grouped together, significantly less necrotizing enterocolitis and bronchopulmonary dysplasia were also noted. Prolongation of the latency interval from PROM to delivery in treated vs. placebo women was noted (median value, 6.1 and 2.9 days, respectively). The effect was discernable for as long as 2 weeks after discontinuance of the antibiotic. A decreased incidence of clinical evidence of amnionitis was noted, but no difference in postpartum endometritis nor cesarean section rate was seen.

There were no significant maternal complications of antibiotic use. The conclusion is solidly based: women with spontaneous PROM remote from term should receive antibiotics to decrease fetal morbidity.

T.H. Kirschbaum, M.D.

Reference

1. 1997 Year Book of Obstetrics, Gynecology, and Women's Health, pp 33–37.

Endoscopic Laser Coagulation in the Management of Severe Twin-to-Twin Transfusion Syndrome

Ville Y, Hecher K, Gagnon A, et al (Hôpital Antoine Béclère, Paris; Barmbek Hosp, Hamburg, Germany; King's College, London)

Br J Obstet Gynaecol 105:446–453, 1998 6–2

Introduction.—Outcome is generally quite poor in monochorionic twin pregnancies with severe twin-to-twin transfusion syndrome. Preliminary

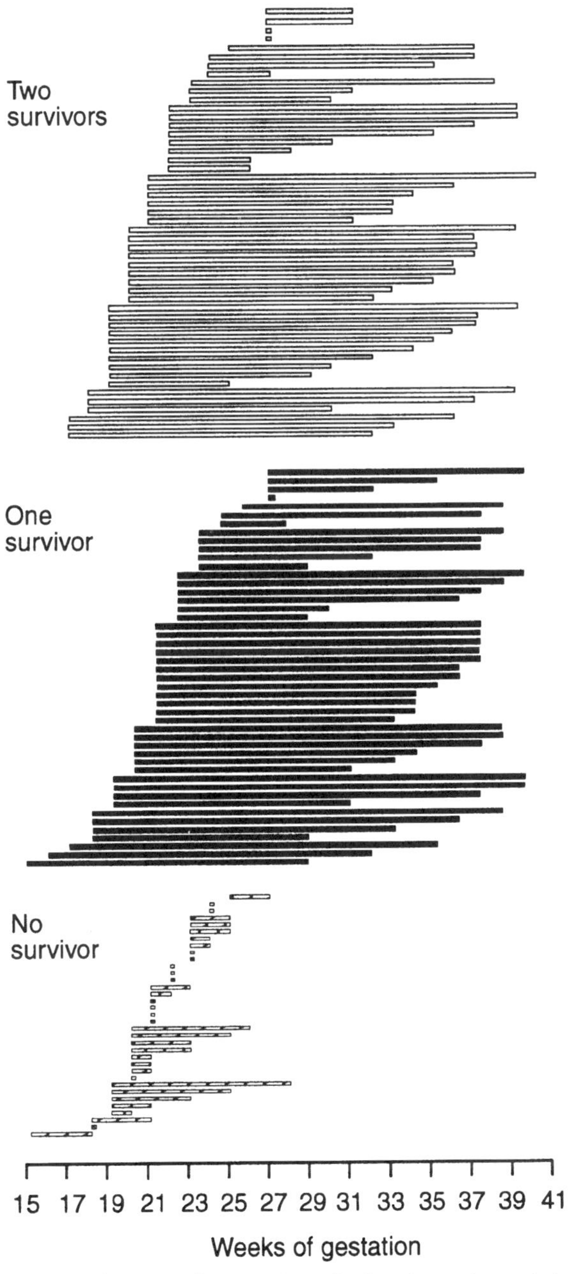

FIGURE 2.—Outcome of endoscopic laser coagulation for the twin-to-twin transfusion syndrome. The *lines* represent the length of time between the procedure and the delivery for each of the 132 pregnancies treated. In 35 pregnancies, the fetuses did not survive; in 50, 1 of the 2 infants survived, and in 47 both infants survived. (Courtesy of Ville Y, Hecher K, Gagnon A, et al: Endoscopic laser coagulation in the management of severe twin-to-twin transfusion syndrome. *Br J Obstet Gynaecol* 105:446–453, 1988. Published by Blackwell Science Ltd.)

data suggest that survival can be improved and the risk of handicap reduced when fetoscopy and laser coagulation are used to interrupt the placental vascular communications between the twins. Results of endoscopic laser coagulation were reported from a multicenter study of 132 pregnancies with severe twin-to-twin transfusion syndrome.

Methods.—Sonoendoscopic laser coagulation was carried out in the second trimester of pregnancy. All cases were confirmed at US to have the characteristic features of twin-to-twin transfusion syndrome, including polyhydramnios surrounding the recipient fetus whose bladder was enlarged and oligohydramnios around the smaller donor fetus whose bladder was collapsed. Laser coagulation was performed after detailed US and umbilical artery Doppler were carried out. The crossing vessels were coagulated, using an output of 30–50 watts for 1–3 seconds.

Results.—Cases were followed for maternal and pregnancy complications, perinatal death, and morbidity. The endoscopic laser was applied at a median gestation of 21 weeks. One woman died 4 weeks after endoscopic surgery, but her death was not attributed to the procedure. There was at least 1 survivor in 97 of the twin pregnancies (73%), and 144 (55%) of the infants survived. Both twins survived in 47 pregnancies (36%) (Fig 2). Twelve infants died in the neonatal period from prematurity-related complications or congenital anomalies. Of 144 survivors followed for 12 to 51 months, 138 are developing normally and 6 are handicapped or may become handicapped.

Conclusion.—Compared with serial amniodrainage, endoscopic surgery for severe twin-to-twin transfusion syndrome achieves at least an equivalent fetal survival rate and a much lower rate of handicap among survivors. A randomized trial of the 2 procedures should be conducted to demonstrate significant difference in survival.

▶ Twin-to-twin transfusion syndrome in monochorionic twin pregnancies results when umbilical vascular shunts between the 2 fetuses do not allow reciprocal return of blood shunted from one to the other. Arterial-to-arterial and venous-to-venous anastomoses seldom cause problems, but the syndrome emerges with arterial-to-venous shunting without sufficient compensatory reverse venous-to-venous shunts to prevent a net flux of umbilical blood flow from one to the other fetus.

Although some of these shunts are visible from within the amniotic cavity between the amnion and the chorionic plate, others lie within the body of cotyledons and are not visualizable on the surface of the chorion, except for possible associated peripheral branches. This remarkable collaborative work of investigators in London, Paris, and Hamburg shows what can be accomplished by Nd–YAG laser coagulation of communicating vessels that lie just under the amnion traversing the diamniotic membrane which separates the twins.

The results are impressive but fall short of an ultimate solution. In 38% of the pregnancies, there was a single surviving infant after laser application; in 35%, both twins survived, whereas both twins were lost in 26%. With laser therapy done at about 21 weeks' gestational age, continuing pregnancies were complicated by spontaneous abortion, recurrent hydramnios, preterm rupture of membranes, and preterm delivery. Sixty-three pregnancies—48% of the total—survived to or past 35 weeks' gestational age, and the evidence of neural handicap at follow-up of 1 year was 4.2%. These talented obstetricians show us that the superficial vessels connecting the fetuses in twin-to-twin transfusion syndrome are important, although not the sole source of uncompensated net blood shunting in this syndrome that is so perilous to fetal well being.

T.H. Kirschbaum, M.D.

Direct Administration of Insulin-like Growth Factor to Fetal Rhesus Monkeys (*Macaca mulatta*)

Tarantal AF, Hunter MK, Gargosky SE (Univ of California, Davis; Oregon Health Sciences Univ, Portland)

Endocrinology 138:3349–3358, 1997 6–3

Introduction.—Intrauterine growth restriction is a major cause of perinatal morbidity and mortality. Some infants with intrauterine growth restriction show catch-up growth after birth, but others have irreversible growth disorders with a high risk of life-long consequences. Insulin-like growth factor-I (IGF-I) is a key modulator of fetal growth. In vivo fetal treatment with IGF-I may be effective in treating fetal growth failure.

Methods.—Insulin-like growth factor-I, 80 µg/kg, was administered with US guidance to healthy rhesus monkey fetuses every other day between gestational days 110–120 and 130–140. Pregnancies were monitored sonographically. Complete blood counts, immunophenotyping, and biochemical analyses were performed in fetal and maternal blood samples. At fetal necropsy or term delivery, blood samples, external measures of the fetus and newborn, and tissue and organ weights were obtained.

Results.—There was no evidence of hypoglycemia in the fetus or dam during the treatment period. Levels of circulating fetal IGF-I increased with treatment, but maternal levels did not. There was no change in serum IGF-II or increase in IGF-binding protein 3 compared to historical control values. Increases were seen in fetal lymphocytes and select red cell parameters. There was also a significant increase in circulating B cells and CD4/CD8 ratios in fetal lymph nodes (Figs 4 and 5). Although there were no changes in body weight, there were increases in thymic, splenic, and kidney weights, and small intestine lengths.

Discussion.—These findings demonstrate the safety of administering IGF-I to fetal rhesus monkeys. Administration of IGF-I caused transient increases in circulating IGF-I, had a significant effect on fetal hematopoietic and lymphoid tissues, and increased select fetal organ weights and measures. It may be possible to treat human fetuses in utero with intrauterine growth restriction with IGF-I.

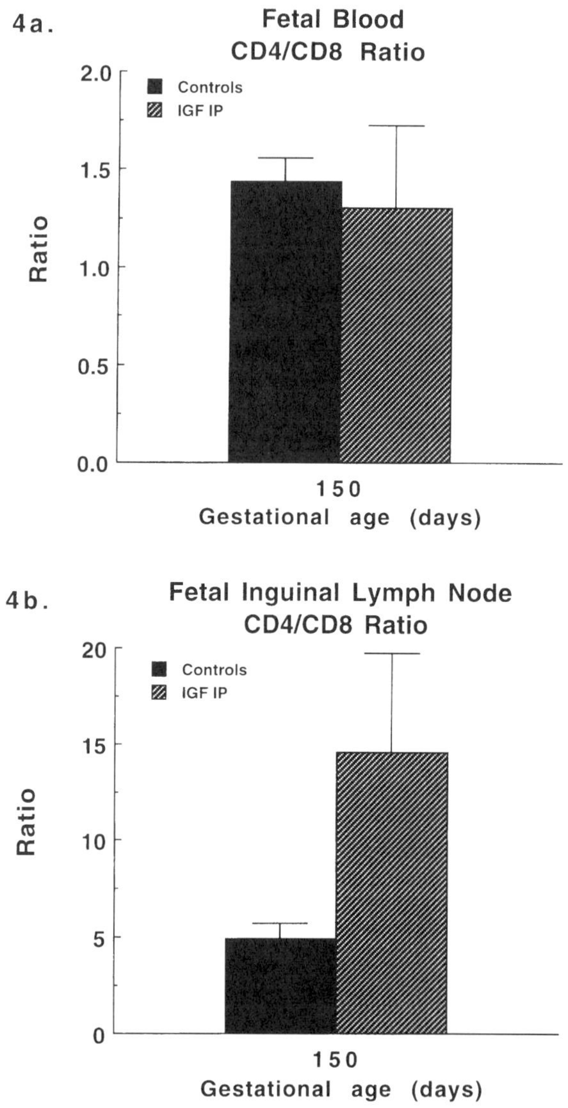

FIGURE 4.—Fetal blood samples collected for immunophenotyping did not indicate any differences in CD4/CD8 ratios for insulin-like growth factor-treated fetuses compared to nontreated controls (**A**, mean ± SEM). Although most fetal tissues (liver, spleen, thymus, and bone marrow) did not show any differences, there was a significant elevation in CD4/CD8 ratios in all fetal lymph nodes evaluated (axillary, inguinal, and mesenteric; inguinal lymph node is shown; **B**, $P < 0.05$). These findings correlated with an increased density of lymphocytes in the cortical region of all lymph nodes assessed histologically. (Courtesy of Tarantal AF, Hunter MK, Gargosky SE: Direct administration of insulin-like growth factor to fetal rhesus monkeys (*Macaca mulatta*). *Endocrinology* 138:3349–3358, 1997. Copyright The Endocrine Society.)

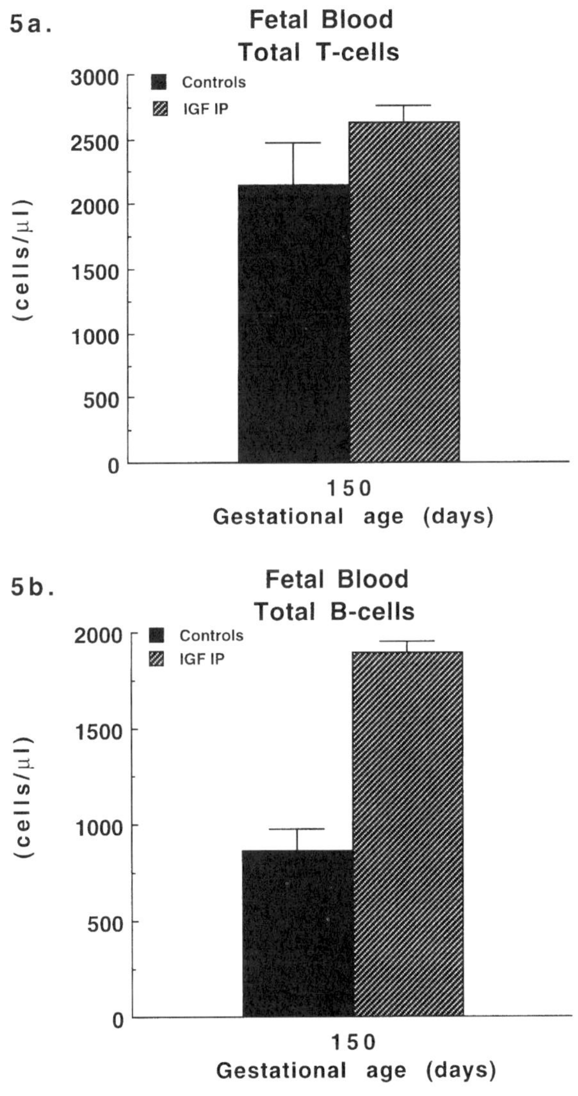

FIGURE 5.—Assessment of fetal blood samples on gestational day 150 showed an increase in total T cells **A**, and a statistically significant rise ($P < 0.05$) in total B cells **B** when comparing historical controls to insulin-like growth factor-I–treated fetuses. (Courtesy of Tarantal AF, Hunter MK, Gargosky SE: Direct administration of insulin-like growth factor to fetal rhesus monkeys (*Macaca mulatta*). *Endocrinology* 138:3349–3358, 1997. Copyright The Endocrine Society.)

▶ Insulin-like growth factors, controlled in part by growth hormone stimulation in adult life, are, after birth, produced by a variety of fetal tissues, differing locally by the amount produced and by the local production of each receptor-binding protein (IGF-BPs). The binding proteins serve as specific inhibitors or facilitators of IGF action—to facilitate glucose and amino acid uptake and inhibit proteinolysis. Despite the apparent complexity of their distribution and regulation, IGF-I and IGF-II have been shown to repair effects of catabolism and malnutrition in a variety of experimental animals and adult human volunteers. Their production rates appear to be in part autoregulated, increasing in activity in times of nutrient need. Insulin-like growth factor-I appears to be more important in growth regulation after embryonic implantation than IGF-II, which appears important in development of the preimplantation embryo.[1] Gene knock-out experiments for IGF receptor peptide results in severe growth retardation and often fetal death. This work is part of an important series of requisites needed to justify antenatal human use of IGF-I in intrauterine growth restriction (IUGR) resulting from deficient nutrient access, but it says something important about normal fetal growth regulation as well.

Insulin-like growth factor-I was given fetal rhesus monkeys intraperitoneally in 2 series with 6 injections each over a period of 10 days. No changes in growth of the biparietal diameter or femur length in the normal fetuses were seen in comparison to normal controls. After each series of IGF-I administrations, lymphocytosis and erythrocytosis as well as increases in platelet and reticulocyte counts were seen, but subsided after 10 days. This raises the possibility that increases in fetal blood erythropoetin activity in the IUGR fetus may derive from increased IGF-I production, not as some believe from chronic hypoxemia. The noted increase in fetal lymphocyte B cells may be part of the dominance of humoral and relative inhibition of cellular immunity noted in normal pregnancy. Finally, hypoglycemia was not noted in either the mother or the fetus. There was no evidence of fetal to maternal transfer of IGF-I nor changes in fetal IGF-BP3, its major regulatory binding protein. Clearly, fetal administration is safe and the next step is to prove the capacity of IGF-I to repair IUGR resulting from impaired nutrient transfer. The growing evidence for potential human use makes it important to develop precise measurements of impaired fetal nutrition to define the subset of human fetuses for which IGF-I therapy may well be important.

T.H. Kirschbaum, M.D.

Reference

1. 1998 Year Book of Obstetrics, Gynecology, and Women's Health, pp 34, 46, 61.

Fetal Renal Biopsies in Obstructive Uropathy: Feasibility and Clinical Correlations—Preliminary Results

Bunduki V, Saldanha LB, Sadek L, et al (Univ of São Paulo, Brazil)

Prenat Diagn 18:101–109, 1998 6–4

Background.—Determining the outcome of fetal obstructive uropathy is difficult. Ultrasonography, fetal urine electrolytes, and β-2–microglobulin have been found to be useful. When renal function is unclear, a US-guided fetal kidney biopsy may be performed to probe for histologic features of

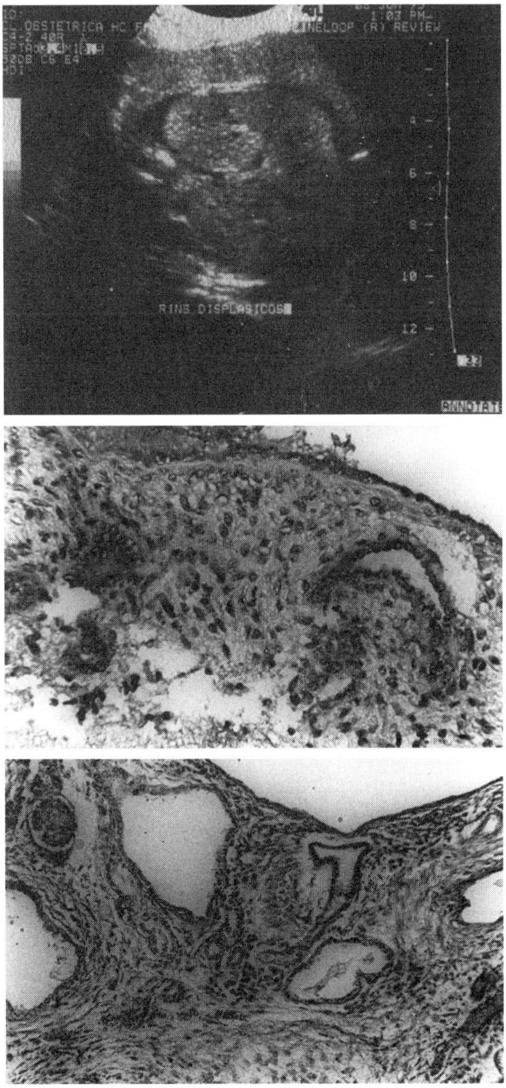

FIGURE 1.—A, ultrasound scan of large dysplastic kidneys at 29 weeks; B, histology of renal biopsy; and C, necropsy. Biopsy and necropsy revealed a highly disorganized parenchyma, with cysts and fibroconnective proliferation. (Courtesy of Bunduki V, Saldanha LB, Sadek L, et al: Fetal renal biopsies in obstructive uropathy: Feasibility and clinical correlations—preliminary results. *Prenat Diagn* 18:101–109, copyright 1998. Reprinted by permission of John Wiley & Sons, Ltd.)

renal dysplasia. Results of a preliminary study of the feasibility and possible risks of this approach were reported.

Methods and Findings.—Eleven severely malformed fetuses underwent biopsy after fetal death. Three had associated renal abnormalities. Renal material was successfully obtained in 63.6% of the fetuses, with no maternal complications. Ten biopsies and urine collections were then performed in fetuses with bilateral obstructive uropathy, with a 50% success rate and no complications. Eighty percent of the fetuses had normal renal histologic findings. In 1 fetus with normal electrolytes, renal dysplasia was demonstrated and was subsequently well correlated with outcome (Fig 1).

Conclusion.—Fetal kidney biopsy for obstructive uropathy is a feasible procedure. Additional research is needed to determine its clinical relevance and risks.

► As the title accurately describes it, this is a feasibility study, but it is also a preliminary attempt to evaluate the accuracy of the diagnosis of renal dysplasia made by fetal US and an extension of 3 initial cases of fetal renal biopsy reported by others.[1] The authors first practiced the procedures on a group of 11 nonliving anomalous fetuses, at an average of 26.5 weeks' gestational age, awaiting induction. Their success rate was 63%, and renal dysplasia was confirmed in 2 of 3 cases. Biopsies done in 10 living fetuses with US evidence suggestive of dysplasia proved possible in 50%; of the 5 biopsies performed, the ultrasound pattern was confirmed in 4.

Urine samples were aspirated from the renal pelvis before biopsy was conducted. In 2 cases, the biopsy results changed management. One case involved US evidence of renal dysplasia with normal urine and normal kidney biopsy results. In the second case, a biopsy diagnosis of severe dysplasia confirmed the US picture despite false negative urinalysis results. The US diagnosis of dysplasia was based on demonstration of thin, hyperechoic cortical parenchyma with cysts and no corticomedullary sonic differentiation. There were no maternal complications among the 21 women whose fetuses were submitted to biopsy and no evident fetal complications. Although additional feasibility and safety data would be desirable, this may be a useful approach in evaluating fetal obstructive uropathy when US data and chemical data appear to differ.

T.H. Kirschbaum, M.D.

Reference

1. Greco P, Loverro G, Caruso G, et al: The diagnostic potential of fetal renal biopsy. *Prenat Diagn* 13:551–556, 1993.

In Utero Lysis of Amniotic Bands

Quintero RA, Morales WJ, Phillips J, et al (St Joseph's Women's Hosp, Tampa, Fla)

Ultrasound Obstet Gynecol 10:316–320, 1997 6–5

Objective.—Amniotic band syndrome is a relatively rare occurrence that can result in amputations, constrictions, and other deformities of the fetus. Release of the constriction has restored the anatomy and functionality of the limb in sheep but the procedure has not been performed in

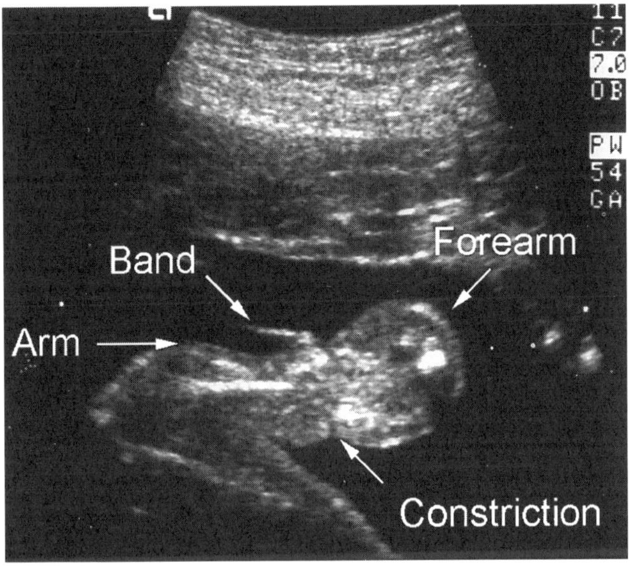

FIGURE 1.—Ultrasound image of amniotic band attached to lower third of left arm. Marked edema of the forearm was present. (Courtesy of Quintero RA, Morales WJ, Phillips J, et al: *In utero* lysis of amniotic bands. *Ultrasound Obstet Gynecol* 10:316–320, 1997.)

humans. Two cases are presented in which a constricting band around a limb was released through minimally invasive surgery.

Case 1.—A 21-week fetus with amniotic bands attached to the face and left arm had a markedly edematous left forearm on ultrasonography (Fig 1). Diagnostic fetoscopy, performed using a 2.7-mm 5 degree endoscope at 22 weeks under general anesthesia, revealed a bilateral cleft lip. When a second trocar was inserted to allow the use of scissors under endoscopic guidance, uterine bleeding occurred, and the second port was removed. The band was cut with scissors under ultrasound guidance, using the remaining port. Microphthalmia or anophthalmia, detected at 32 weeks, was not present at 22 weeks. When electively delivered at 39 weeks, the baby had a bilateral cleft lip, a type 4 Tessier craniofacial cleft, right microphthalmia, and radial paresis and mild hypoplasia of the left hand.

Case 2.—A 23-week fetus, with a thick band constricting the left ankle, had marked edema of the foot and ankle. Because a 2.7-mm 5 degree endoscope did not reveal toes, it was replaced by a 70 degree, endoscope that revealed toes. When a second port was inserted, uterine bleeding required removal, and a 2.4-mm 0 degree operating endoscope with a 400-γ contact yttrium aluminum garnet laser fiber was used to release approximately 85% of the band. Risk of injury to the ankle did not allow complete release. Foot edema decreased and arterial blood flow to the distal foot improved. When spontaneously delivered at 34.5 weeks, the baby had successful repair of the amniotic band with Z-plasties. Full use of the foot is anticipated.

Conclusion.—This is the first antenatal experience with surgical treatment of amniotic bands *in utero* using minimally invasive surgery.

▶ This report of 2 cases of successful lysis of amniotic bands by amnioscopy demonstrates that the technique is possible, though not easy. In both cases, bands constricted fetal extremities with marked distal edema and with blood flow through the stricture site (though minimal in 1 case) based on Doppler velocity shift. In both cases, lysis of the adhesive band resulted in prompt relief of edema and normalization of extremity positioning. Both extremities were normal at birth, exempting minor residual skin changes at the constriction site. However, the procedures were complicated. In both cases, attempts to use a second trochar failed because of uterine bleeding. In the first case, unrecognized anomalies, together with anophthalmia related to an unrecognized additional band, were seen at birth. In a second case, an yttrium aluminum garnet laser was cautiously used, because of failure of fetal positioning adequate for scissor application to the band. With fetoscopy done at 22 to 23 weeks gestational age, it is not surprising that both pregnancies delivered prematurely. A companion article describes serial ultrasound observations with a banded extremity that subsequently showed distal edema, disappearance of a Doppler signal, and spontaneous limb amputation. It is useful to know that, in principal, it is possible to avoid amputation through fetal surgery, however complicated it might be.[1]

T.H. Kirschbaum, M.D.

Reference

1. Tadmor OP, Kreisberg GA, Achiron R, et al: Limb amputation in amniotic band syndrome. *Ultrasound Obstet Gynecol* 10:312, 1997.

7 Labor, Operative Obstetrics, and Anesthesia

Randomized Study of Non-closure of Peritoneum in Lower Segment Cesarean Section

Grundsell HS, Rizk DEE, Kumar RM (United Arab Emirates Univ, Al-Ain)

Acta Obstet Gynecol Scand 77:110–115, 1998 7–1

Objective.—Several studies have demonstrated that nonclosure of the peritoneum after cesarean section does not increase postoperative morbidity and reduces operative time. Most of these studies were small and short-term. The long-term and short-term postoperative effects of closure of the visceral and parietal peritoneum were compared in a prospective, randomized study with nonclosure of both layers at lower segment cesarean section (LSCS) performed through a lower midline or a low transverse abdominal incision.

TABLE 2.—Operative and Postoperative Outcome in Study Patients

	Closure of the peritoneum (n=182)	Non-closure of the peritoneum (n=179)	Significance
Operating time (minutes)	41.3±6.9*	33.4±6.2	p<0.01
Febrile morbidity	35 (19.2)†	14 (7.8)	p<0.001
Endomyometritis	9 (4.9)	9 (5.0)	NS
Wound infection	7 (3.2)	4 (2.2)	p<0.05
Urinary tract infection	9 (4.9)	9 (5.0)	NS
Fever of unknown origin	7 (3.8)	3 (1.7)	p<0.05
Wound dehiscence (6 weeks postoperatively)	1 (0.05)	1 (0.06)	NS
Opening of bowels (days)	1.8±0.7	1.1±0.5	NS
Admission days	6.4±1.0	5.3±1.0	p<0.01
Ileus	1	0	NS

*Mean ± SD.
†Values in parentheses are percentage of the total number in each group. n = 182 in the closure group and n = 179 in the nonclosure group.
Abbreviation: NS, not significant.
(Courtesy of Grundsell HS, Rizk DEE, Kumar RM: Randomized study of non-closure of peritoneum in lower segment cesarian section. *Acta Obstet Gynecol Scand* 77:110–115. Copyright 1998, Munksgaard International Publishers Ltd., Copenhagen, Denmark.)

Methods.—Between November 1991 and July 1994, 361 women delivered by LSCS were randomly assigned to closure (n = 182) or nonclosure (n = 179) of both visceral and parietal peritoneum. Patients were followed up after discharge at 6 weeks, 6 months, and 1 year by blinded obstetricians and nursing staff.

Results.—Operating time, febrile morbidity incidence, wound infection incidence, and admission days were significantly lower in the nonclosure group than in the closure group (Table 2). Incidence of urinary tract infection and ileus, postoperative wound dehiscence, and time of first bowel movement were similar in both groups. The potential cost saving per patient with nonclosure vs. closure was $330.

Conclusions.—Nonclosure of the peritoneum after cesarean section resulted in fewer complications, less operating time, and a savings of $330 per patient.

▶ When Munro Kerr introduced the lower uterine segment incision for cesarean section, he suggested that closure of both visceral and parietal peritoneum might safely be deleted, and evidence is now quite strong that he was correct in that contention. This prospective randomized study of 361 women, 201 of them receiving primary cesarean section prior to the onset of labor, showed no increased incidence of wound dehiscence, bladder infection, or ileus as a result of nonclosure of visceral and parietal peritoneum. Indeed, the incidence of febrile morbidity and wound infection was less, and hospitalization days were fewer in the nonclosure group for reasons that are not clear. There was a small surplus of women with primary cesarean sections in the closure group in which febrile morbidity might be expected to occur more often as a result of labor preceding the operative procedure. This article includes references to 2 smaller and 1 larger prospective trials showing the same findings. It is an important strength that follow-up was conducted for 2–5 years in this group, failing to show any long-term sequelae as a result of adhesions and related changes. The possibilities are that preperitoneal fat inclusion in the peritoneal closure may impede healing, and that the risk of vesico-uterine scarring is increased by visceral and parietal closure. The peritoneum is replaced de novo from its underlying connective tissue layer rather from the cut mesothelial margins. It is intriguing that open subperitoneal connective tissue surfaces may actually speed removal from the peritoneal cavity of bacteria and potential media through uncomplicated stromal contact. Those who continue peritoneal closure in the lower cervical transverse cesarean section have little evidence to support their position beyond tradition.

T.H. Kirschbaum, M.D.

Nulliparous Active Labor, Epidural Analgesia, and Cesarean Delivery for Dystocia

Bofill JA, Vincent RD, Ross EL, et al (Wright State Univ, Dayton, Ohio; Univ of Alabama, Birmingham; Univ of Mississippi, Jackson)

Am J Obstet Gynecol 177:1465–1470, 1997 7–2

Background.—The effect of epidural analgesia on the rate of cesarean delivery performed for dystocia is debated. The effect of epidural analgesia on the rate of cesarean delivery for dystocia was studied prospectively in actively laboring nulliparous women.

Methods.—One hundred women were randomly assigned to receive epidural analgesia or narcotics. The presence of active labor was verified by uterine contractions, cervical dilatation of 4 cm, effacement of 80%, and fetopelvic engagement. The protocol for labor management was strict. Using a visual analogue scale, patients assessed their level of pain at randomization and at hourly intervals.

Findings.—The cesarean delivery rates in the 2 groups did not differ significantly, being 8% in the epidural group and 6% in the narcotic group. Also, there were no significant differences in the lengths of first or second stages of labor or in any other time factor. Operative vaginal delivery was done more commonly in the women given epidural analgesia. At randomization, pain scores were equivalent but differed greatly at each hour thereafter (Fig 1).

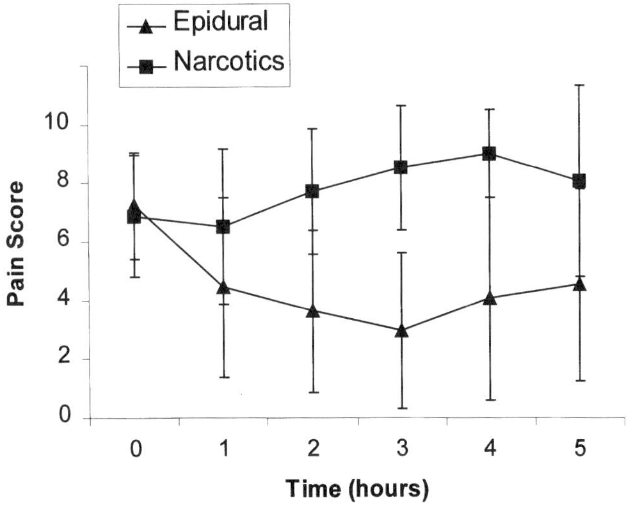

FIGURE 1.—Pain scores are recorded on the *y* axis, whereas time (in hours) is recorded on the *x* axis. Pain scores for the epidural group are shown as *triangles*. Pain scores for the narcotics group are shown as *squares*. *Error bars* denote 1 SD. At randomization, there is no significant difference in pain scores ($P = 0.26$). Differences in pain scores at hours 1–4 are significant ($P < 0.001$). Difference in pain scores at 5 hours is also significant ($P = 0.01$). Data were analyzed with analysis of variance. (Courtesy of Bofill JA, Vincent RD, Ross EL, et al: Nulliparous active labor, epidural analgesia, and cesarean delivery for dystocia. *Am J Obstet Gynecol* 177:1465–1470, 1997.)

Conclusions.—These data showed no increase in dystocia-related cesarean delivery with epidural analgesia. Strict criteria for the diagnosis of labor and a rigid protocol for labor management were used.

▶ This most recent prospective randomized trial designed to test the relationship between epidural anesthesia and the risk for cesarean section for dystocia is well designed but has 2 defects, one of them important. The authors included only nulliparous women who showed at least 4 cm of cervical dilatation and an engaged presenting part in the study. They used rigorous uniform labor management protocols, which resulted in an 80% incidence of oxytocin supplementation, and avoided motor blockade in the 49 women randomized to bupivacaine epidural anesthesia. Women undergoing induction of labor or attempts at cervical ripening and those with multiple pregnancies or complicated pregnancies were excluded. Twenty-three percent of women randomized to narcotic use subsequently received epidural anesthesia, but this was aptly managed by the "intent to treat" rule in data analysis. Power spectrum analysis, assuming rates of cesarean section of 10% for epidural users and 5% for women receiving only narcotics, indicated 318 gravidas were sufficient to detect a 10% difference in the rate of cesarean section for dystocia. The trial was discontinued with only 100 patients enrolled, primarily because of defections and crossovers from the nonepidural group. Cesarean section rates were 10.2% for epidural anesthesia, reduced to 8.2% by excluding 1 cesarean section done for abnormal fetal heart rate, vs. 5.9% for the nonepidural users. Patient satisfaction clearly favored epidural use.

The authors' work emphasizes the problems in investigating this issue satisfactorily. No significant difference in cesarean section for dystocia was noted but who knows what might have emerged if, as suggested by power analysis, 3 times more patients had been enrolled in this study.

T.H. Kirschbaum, M.D.

Neonatal Morbidity After Elective Repeat Cesarean Section and Trial of Labor

Hook B, Kiwi R, Amini SB, et al (Case Western Reserve Univ, Cleveland, Ohio)

Pediatrics 100:348–353, 1997 7–3

Introduction.—Because elective repeat cesarean section (ERCS) is associated with both maternal and fetal morbidity, a trial of labor (TOL) after a previous cesarean section has been recommended. Women who delivered after a previous cesarean section were studied to determine neonatal outcome after ERCS vs. TOL.

Methods.—During the period from April 1992 through March 1993, 1007 women with a previous cesarean section delivered singleton infants at a gestation of 37 weeks or longer at 3 hospitals in Cleveland. A repeat cesarean section was planned by 508 women and a TOL by 499; 342

attempting a TOL delivered vaginally (69%) and 157 required a repeat cesarean section (31%). A cohort of 989 mother/infant pairs served as a "routine vaginal delivery" group. Excluded from analysis were 18 infants with major congenital malformations—8 delivered by ERCS, 3 vaginally after a TOL, and 7 after routine vaginal delivery.

Results.—The pregnancy complication rate of the 3 groups was low and similar, except that gestational diabetes was significantly higher in the ERCS group. The mean obstetric gestational age was significantly lower for infants delivered by ERCS compared with the TOL and routine vaginal delivery groups. Transient tachypnea was increased in ERCS (6%) vs. TOL (3%) groups. The adjusted odds ratio of development of any respiratory problem after ERCS (compared with routine vaginal deliveries) was 2.3. Respiratory distress syndrome developed in 2 infants delivered by ERCS; both suspected and proven sepsis occurred significantly more often in infants delivered by TOL. Neonatal outcomes after successful TOL were similar to those of routine vaginal births, but delivery by cesarean section after a failed TOL was associated with increased neonatal morbidity—including respiratory illness and sepsis—and a longer hospital stay.

Conclusion.—Term infants delivered by ERCS remain at increased risk for respiratory problems compared with infants undergoing routine vaginal delivery. Vaginal delivery after a successful TOL yielded neonatal outcomes similar to those of routine vaginal delivery, but cesarean section after a failed TOL was associated with increased neonatal and maternal morbidity.

► In this collection of 1,007 women who had undergone prior cesarean section in 3 Cleveland hospitals from 1992 to 1993, the rates for acceptance of a TOL was about 50%; for success in the TOL the rate was 62%. Both incidence rates are lower than those reported by other facilities where vaginal birth after cesarean (VBAC) programs resulted in a reduction of cesarean section rates for such women of about two thirds, instead of the one third reported in this series.

However, the strength of this article rests with the observations regarding the neonates that make clear the trade-offs inherent in a VBAC program. Elective repeat cesarean section is associated with significantly increased risk of transient tachypnea of the newborn and of respiratory distress syndrome. The pulmonary problems are, however, infrequent, mild, and not reflected in increased mortality rates. On the other hand, proven and suspected sepsis and newborn laboratory work designed to help with the diagnosis were more frequent in the TOL group, although, again, not expressed in infant mortality.

The general incidence of probable sepsis was greatest in the TOL group, less in the ERCS group, and least of all in the control group. A trial of labor was associated with an incidence of uterine rupture/dehiscence of 1.2%, but as there were no hysterectomies and disruptions were unsuspected, these episodes are likely best characterized as dehiscenses. In this less-than-maximal effort at VBAC, there was not much difference in newborn outcome, and the value of VBAC continues to rest with the avoidance of maternal operative risks, anesthesia, postoperative discomfort, length of hospital stay, and costs.

T.H. Kirschbaum, M.D.

The Case for Trial of Labor in the Patient With a Prior Low-segment Vertical Cesarean Incision

Martin JN Jr, Perry KG Jr, Roberts WE, et al (Univ of Mississippi, Jackson)

Am J Obstet Gynecol 177:144–148, 1997 7–4

Background.—The use of primary and repeat cesarean delivery has increased enormously in the last 20 years. Although the National Institutes of Health Consensus Conference in 1980 recommended that women with otherwise uncomplicated pregnancies and a previous low-segment transverse cesarean incision should be encouraged to undergo a trial of labor, the management of patients with a previous low-segment vertical cesarean incision remains controversial. Outcomes of pregnancy in patients with this incision were analyzed.

Methods.—A review was conducted of 10 studies from the American obstetric literature with information about pregnancy outcome in patients with a previous low-segment vertical cesarean incision. All abstracts presented annually since 1981 to the Society of Perinatal Obstetricians were also reviewed.

Results.—Analysis was performed of subsequent pregnancy outcome in 382 patients with a previous low-segment vertical cesarean incision. Complete patient population information was available for 372 patients. Among these 372 patients, safe vaginal delivery occurred in 306 patients (Table 1). Four uterine ruptures were reported; only 1 occurred after a single previous unextended low-segment vertical cesarean incision, 2 occurred elsewhere on the lateral or posterior aspect of the uterus in later pregnancies, and 1 occurred at the juncture of previous low vertical and transverse cesarean incisions. There were no reports of perinatal mortality or permanent perinatal morbidity in these pregnancies.

Discussion.—Among women with otherwise uncomplicated pregnancies, those with a single previous nonextended low-segment vertical cesarean incision should be considered to have a previous low-segment scar and be candidates for trial of labor in a current singleton pregnancy. Such patients should receive the same care, counseling, and caution as patients with a previous low-segment transverse incision.

► The relative hazards and success rates for trial of labor (TOL) after previous low-segment transverse and fundal cesarean sections are quite well known, but the implications of a vertical low-segment incision are uncertain. These authors have performed a service in collecting accounts of attempts at vaginal birth after cesarean section (VBAC) in 382 such women from the obstetric literature of the years 1983–1986. Part of their motivation appears to stem from local Mississippi custom that has favored the low-

TABLE 1.—Cumulative Published United States Experience With Trial of Labor After Low-segment Vertical Cesarean Delivery

Year	*Site*	*No. of patients*	*No. of successful trials of labor*	*Success (%)*	*No. of uterine dehiscences*	*No. of uterine ruptures*
1983	Jackson, Miss.	12	6	50	0	0
1984	Los Angeles, Calif.	4	NA	NA	0	0
1987	Memphis, Tenn.	64	57	89	2	0
1988	Houston, Tex.	2	2	100	0	0
1988	Houston, Tex.	5	NA	NA	0	0
1989	Norfolk, Va.	36	25	69	0	0
1992	Jackson, Miss.	7	6	86	0	0
1995	Jackson, Miss.	174	144	83	3	2
1996	Jacksonville, Fla.	77	66	86	0	1
1996	Fort Worth, Tex.	1	NA	NA	0	1
TOTAL		382	306	82*	5	4

*Based on 306 of 372 trials in series with available denominators to permit this calculation.
Abbreviation: NA, not available.
(Courtesy of Martin JN Jr, Perry KG Jr, Roberts WE, et al: The case for trial of labor in the patient with a prior low-segment vertical cesarean incision. *Am J Obstet Gynecol* 177:144–148, 1997.)

segment vertical cesarean incision in the past. Although the success rates are comparable to experience with VBAC in general, the incidence of rupture of 1% and of dehiscence, that is, bloodless wound separations, of 1.3% is slightly larger than rates reported with experience of TOL with known previous lower segment transverse incisions.[1] Individual rates from the 3 largest reported experiences in Mississippi, Florida, and Tennessee reveal virtually the same and somewhat smaller mean values as the aggregate incidence figures for successful VBAC with transverse lower segment scars. Clearly, some vertical low-segment incisions done during labor do not enter the uterine fundus and it is hazardous to make comparisons between disparate numbers of gravidas, but the data here suggest the risks might be slightly increased with TOL with a vertical scar, but not prohibitively so.

T.H. Kirschbaum, M.D.

Reference

1. Famer RM, Kirschbaum TH, Potter D, et al: Uterine rupture during trial of labor after previous cesarean section. *Am J Obst Gynecol* 165:996–1001, 1991.

Perinatal Mortality and Route of Delivery in Term Breech Presentations

Lindqvist A, Nordén-Lindeberg S, Hanson U (Örebro Med Ctr Hosp, Sweden)

Br J Obstet Gynaecol 104:1288–1291, 1997 7–5

Objective.—Risk of mortality in fetuses older than 34 weeks was compared for vaginal vs. caesarean section delivery for breech births.

Methods.—A register-based nationwide study conducted in Sweden from 1991 to 1992 examined 246,344 deliveries of which 6,542 were breech. Gestational age, intrapartum and early neonatal death, stillbirths, low Apgar score (less than 7 at 5 minutes), and mode of delivery were recorded.

Results.—Of the 6,542 breech deliveries, 2,349 (35.9%) were vaginal, 1,761 (26.9%) were elective caesarean section, and 2,358 (35.9%) were emergency caesarean section. The mortality rate was 60 (0.92%). When 36 term infants who died, 18 stillbirths, and 2 vaginal deliveries resulting in death were excluded, the rate of intrapartum and early neonatal death among infants born vaginally was 2 per 2,248 (0.09%) and among infants born by caesarian section it was 2 per 4,029 (0.05%). The relative risk of 1.81 for vaginal deliveries was not significant. The incidence of low Apgar scores was 69 (3.1%) for vaginal births, 21 (0.93%) for elective caesarean section births, and 28 (1.7%) for emergency caesarean section births. The relative risk of low Apgar scores was significantly higher in the vaginal delivery group compared with the elective caesarean section group (3.28) and with the emergency caesarean section group (1.85).

Conclusion.—There was no increased risk of mortality in breech births for vaginal delivery compared with caesarean section. Whether the lower Apgar scores in breech vaginal deliveries have long-term consequences needs to be investigated further.

► This retrospective cohort study of Swedish singlet pregnancies in at least the 35th week of gestation examines the result of 642 breech births, 35.9% delivered vaginally compared with 62.8% delivered abdominally. Cases with lethal anomaly and antepartum fetal deaths were excluded, as were 2 fetal deaths in which delivery took place outside the hospital. Intrapartum and early neonatal death during the first 7 days of life occurred in 0.09% of the vaginal and 0.05% of abdominal births; there was no significant difference between these rates. The results differ from a recent Danish study similar in general organization.[1] Mortality rates in the Danish study were generally higher (0.26%), and relatively fewer vaginal deliveries were carried out (20.8% of the total). The problem remains that retrospective results reflect both the inherent irreducible hazard of breech presentation and the skill and experience of the operators. The data suggest that continued familiarity with the management of vaginal breech delivery of a sizeable number of women presenting in labor near term results in low perinatal death rates, indistinguishable from the results of abdominal delivery. Although this study may not convince those who feel vaginal breech delivery is unsafe, it at least demonstrates that retaining experience in vaginal breech deliveries can be done safely and at the benefit of reduced cesarean section rates.

T.H. Kirschbaum, M.D.

Reference

1. 1997 Year Book of Obstetrics, Gynecology, and Women's Health, pp 189–190.

Obstetric Anesthesia Work Force Survey, 1981 Versus 1992

Hawkins JL, Gibbs CP, Orleans M, et al (Univ of Colorado, Denver)

Anesthesiology 87:135–143, 1997 7–6

Introduction.—A national survey of obstetric anesthesia conducted in 1981 found a need for improvement in the availability of obstetric anesthesia personnel. A follow-up survey to update the 1981 information was performed in 1992 with the collaboration of the American Society of Anesthesiologists and the American College of Obstetricians and Gynecologists.

Methods.—The original survey instrument was expanded to include newer issues. Questionnaires were sent to 2,265 hospitals, with 3 strata distinguished on the basis of the hospitals' reported number of annual deliveries: 1,500 or more births, 500 to 1,499 births, and fewer than 500 births. Two copies of the survey were sent to each hospital, 1 for the chief of obstetrics and 1 for the chief of anesthesiology.

Results.—Data from the American Hospital Association revealed an overall reduction in the number of hospitals providing obstetric care from 1981 (4,163) to 1992 (3,545). The percentage of hospitals with 1,500 or more deliveries per year increased significantly from 14% to 23%. Surveys were returned from 740 hospitals (902 surveys), for a response rate of

TABLE 4.—Types of Analgesia Provided for Patients in Labor and Anesthesia Provided for Patients Undergoing Cesarean Section

	Stratum I (≥1,500 births)		Stratum II (500–1,499 births)		Stratum III (<500 births)	
	1981	1992	1981	1992	1981	1992
Labor						
None (%)	27	11	33	14	45	33
Parenteral (%)	52	48	53	60	37	48
Paracervical (%)	5	2	5	4	6	7
Spinal (%)	0	4	0	4	0	4
Epidural (%)	22	51	13	33	9	17
Cesarean section						
Epidural (%)	29	54	16	45	12	29
Spinal (%)	33	35	35	40	37	49
General (%)	35	12	45	15	46	22

(Courtesy of Hawkins JL, Gibbs CP, Orleans M, et al: Obstetric anesthesia work force survey, 1981 versus 1992. *Anesthesiology* 87:135–143, 1997.)

33%. Responses came from an approximately equal number of anesthesiology (49%) and obstetric (51%) departments. More women received some type of analgesia during labor in 1992, and the use of epidural analgesia increased 100% (Table 4). Regional anesthesia was unavailable in 20% of the smallest hospitals. The use of general anesthesia was considerably reduced; 78% to 85% of patients undergoing cesarean section had regional anesthesia. Obstetricians provided 30% of epidural analgesia for labor in 1981, but only 2% in 1992. Nurse anesthetists provided anesthesia for cesarean section without the medical direction of an anesthesiologist in only 4% of the largest hospitals but in 59% of the smallest hospitals (Table 5). Anesthesia personnel provided neonatal resuscitation in 23% of cesarean deliveries in 1981, but in only 10% in 1992.

TABLE 5.—Personnel Providing Epidural Analgesia for Labor and Anesthesia for Cesarean Section

	Stratum I (≥1,500 births)		Stratum II (500–1,499 births)		Stratum III (<500 births)	
	1981	1992	1981	1992	1981	1992
Labor						
Anesthesiologist* (%)	70	95	61	79	35	42
Independent CRNA† (%)	4	4	8	16	10	55
Obstetrician (%)	26	0	31	5	46	3
Cesarean section						
Anesthesiologist* (%)	90	96	81	88	51	41
Independent CRNA† (%)	7	4	15	12	36	59
Obstetrician (%)	3	0	4	0	9	0

*Personally performed or medically directed resident or certified registered nurse anesthetist.
†Not medically directed by an anesthesiologist.
Abbreviation: CRNA, certified registered nurse anesthetist.
(Courtesy of Hawkins JL, Gibbs CP, Orleans M, et al: Obstetric anesthesia work force survey, 1981 versus 1992. *Anesthesiology* 87:135–143, 1997. Copyright American Society of Anesthesiologists, Inc. used with permission of Lippincott-Raven Publishers.)

Discussion.—The 1992 survey indicates that regional anesthesia and analgesia are more available for obstetric patients than in 1981. There is a decline in the use of general anesthesia for cesarean section. Obstetricians are less likely to provide epidural analgesia and anesthesia personnel are less involved in newborn resuscitations. The smallest hospitals are often unable to provide regional anesthesia and have only nurse anesthetists available for cesarean section anesthesia.

► This is a repeat of the Obstetric Anesthesia National Survey, conducted a decade ago,[1] which revealed widespread deficiencies in anesthetic availability. This survey of 902 respondent facilities represents 61% of American births in 1992 and shows improvements and changes in practice patterns. Data are stratified by numbers of births, training of those responsible for anesthesia, hospital type, and services for labor analgesia and anesthesia for abdominal birth.

There is need for caution in interpreting comparative percentages because obstetric units with less than 500 births per year (stratum III) accounted for 45% of respondents but only 9% of deliveries. Larger units with more than 1,500 deliveries annually (stratum I) accounted for 23% of respondents but delivered 64% of the newborns.

Only in stratum III units was labor analgesia not given to a sizeable fraction of parturients, roughly one third. The use of epidural procedures doubled at all levels, both for labor analgesia and cesarean section anesthesia. Use of parenteral analgesia also increased in strata II and III. Spinal opioid techniques were reported in 4% of the deliveries.

Obstetricians as purveyors of epidural techniques have virtually disappeared, as anesthesiologists account for 72% and certified registered nurse anesthetists for 24% of reported procedures. In stratum III facilities, independently functioning certified registered nurse anesthetists account for 60% of labor and cesarean section procedures, especially in the central portion of the country. However, problems of access persist in stratum III hospitals, where regional anesthesia is not available for labor in 20% or for abdominal birth in 2%, and where the number of available staff anesthesiologists has remained unchanged since 1980, despite increases in their numbers nationally.

T.H. Kirschbaum, M.D.

Reference

1. 1988 Year Book of Obstetrics and Gynecology, pp 164–165.

Pethidine

Cesarean Delivery: A Randomized Trial of Epidural Versus Patient-controlled Meperidine Analgesia During Labor

Sharma SK, Sidawi JE, Ramin SM, et al (Univ of Texas, Dallas)
Anesthesiology 87:487–494, 1997 7–7

Introduction.—A number of studies have concluded that the use of epidural analgesia for pain relief during labor increases the incidence of cesarean deliveries. Because few controlled studies have examined this issue, a randomized trial was designed to compare the rate of cesarean deliveries using epidural analgesia and patient-controlled IV analgesia (PCIA) during labor.

Methods.—Women eligible for the study had a singleton cephalic gestation and were in spontaneous active labor at full term. They were randomized to epidural analgesia or meperidine PCIA but were told that they could switch to an alternative type of analgesia if needed for pain relief. Standard labor management was used in both groups and oxytocin was administered according to a written protocol. Epidural analgesia was maintained in 358 women with a continuous infusion of 0.125% bupivacaine with 2 μg/mL of fentanyl. The 357 women randomized to PCIA could receive 10 to 15 mg of meperidine every 10 minutes as needed. The 2 groups were similar in demographic characteristics.

Results.—The study protocols were followed by 243 women (68%) in the epidural group and 259 (73%) in the PCIA group. Only 5 women who received PCIA according to the protocol crossed over to epidural analgesia to obtain better pain relief. Using intention-to-treat analysis based on the original randomization, the rate of cesarean deliveries was 4% in the epidural group and 5% in the PCIA group. The type of analgesia used appeared to have no deleterious effect on neonatal Apgar scores or acid-base condition. Administration of epidural analgesia prolonged the first stage of labor and increased the use of oxytocin and low forceps delivery. Epidural analgesia provided superior pain relief; 24 hours after delivery, 90% of women who received epidural analgesia vs. 65% who received PCIA rated their satisfaction as good to excellent.

Discussion.—Although epidural analgesia affected the duration of labor and the use of low forceps, the incidence of cesarean deliveries was not increased relative to meperidine PCIA in this group of healthy women at full term in spontaneous labor. Epidural analgesia is a superior method of pain relief, but PCIA is quite effective and less expensive.

► The first round in what has become a skirmish between obstetricians and anesthesiologists over this issue was the work by J.A. Thorp, et al. indicating that the rate of cesarean section for dystocia was 5–6 times greater among women who received epidural analgesia than among those who did not.[1] This was, however, a retrospective, nonrandomized case-controlled study. In a similarly retrospective case-controlled study[2] a byproduct of the clinical trial of active management of labor in Boston,[3] women who requested and received epidural analgesia had more intrapartum temperature elevation and longer labors than those who did not. However, the possibility that patients correctly discerned painful and/or slow labor as a basis for their request for epidural anesthesia cannot be ruled out and that alone could have accounted for the observation.

This is the second of 2 prospective, randomized trials involving epidural analgesia from the University of Texas at Dallas. The first[4] has been criticized because 35% of women randomized to epidural analgesia did not receive it and 24% randomized to IV meperidine received another mode of pain management. In the study abstracted here, the alternative to epidural analgesia was patient-controlled analgesia using meperidine coupled with an initial dose of promethazine. This alternative was chosen to make the lack of epidural analgesia more acceptable to women in labor. Of 358 women randomized to epidural analgesia, 115 delivered too rapidly to receive it and 37, having initially accepted that technique, declined it during labor. Similarly for the PCIA Group, 97 women either delivered too quickly or refused analgesia, whereas only 5 received epidural medication. The sum of patients who failed to receive prescribed management was about half as many as in the earlier Dallas study. Based on patients chosen for intent to treat, primigravid status, or successful compliance with group protocols, no differences in cesarean section rates were noted between the epidural and control groups. Women receiving epidural medication had lower pain scores and more often received oxytocin, and sedation was more common than in the PCIA group.

However, it is well to remember the population under study here. The patients at Parkland Memorial were largely indigent and overwhelmingly nonwhite. They were admitted with cervices dilated 3 to 5 cm and given oxytocin unless the spontaneous rate of cervical dilatation was at least 1 cm per hour. The cesarean section rates for all patients in the study ranged from 1% to 5%, and the general applicability of these results can, therefore, be questioned. Perhaps the best course for obstetricians still troubled by this controversy is to read Dr. David Chestnut's masterful editorial in the same issue of this journal.

T.H. Kirschbaum, M.D.

References

1. 1993 Year Book of Obstetrics and Gynecology, pp 182–183.
2. 1998 Year Book of Obstetrics, Gynecology, and Women's Health, pp 41–42.
3. 1997 Year Book of Obstetrics, Gynecology, and Women's Health, pp 184–185.
4. 1997 Year Book of Obstetrics, Gynecology, and Women's Health, pp 186–187.

Laparoscopy During Pregnancy: A Study of Five Fetal Outcome Parameters With Use of the Swedish Health Registry

Reedy MB, Källén B, Kuehl TJ (Texas A&M Univ, Temple; Univ of Lund, Sweden)

Am J Obstet Gynecol 177:673–679, 1997 7–8

Introduction.—Many laparoscopy procedures have been performed successfully during pregnancy, such as cholecystectomy, appendectomy, ovarian torsion, and management of adnexal masses. There has been no evaluation of the safety of laparoscopy in pregnancy. Sweden's national health registry was reviewed during a 20-year period to compare the fetal outcomes of laparotomy vs. laparoscopy performed during pregnancy.

Methods.—There were 2,181 laparoscopies and 1,522 laparotomies of singleton pregnancies with nonobstetric operations between the 4th and 20th weeks of gestation in a 20-year period. The study was limited from the 4th to 20th weeks because too few were performed after this time (Fig 1). The 2 groups had no differences in demographic variables. Comparisons were made between pregnancies with operations and pregnancies without operations for gestational duration, growth restriction, weight, infant survival, and fetal malformations.

Results.—For infants in the laparoscopy and laparotomy groups, there was an increased risk to weigh less than 2,500 gm (Fig 2), to be delivered before 37 weeks and to have an increased incidence of growth restriction

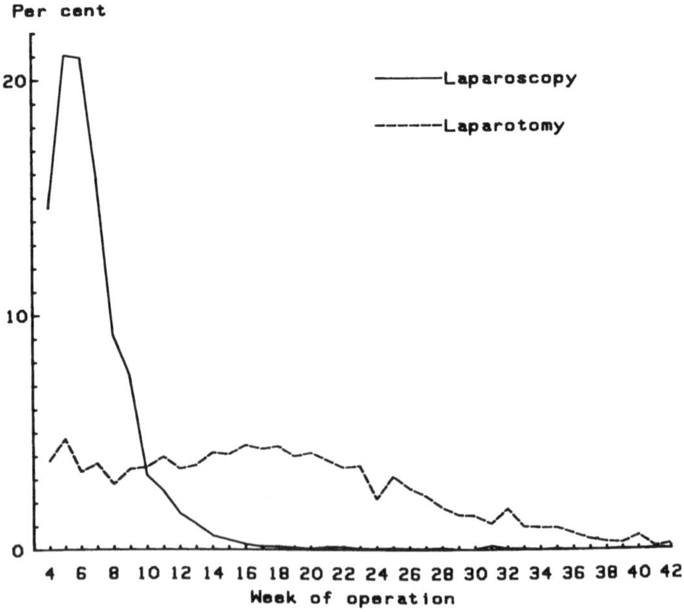

FIGURE 1.—Distribution of operations in pregnancy by week of gestation. (Courtesy of Reedy MB, Kallen B, Küehl TH: Laparoscopy during pregnancy: A study of five fetal outcome parameters with use of the Swedish Health Registry. *Am J Obstet Gynecol* 177:673–679, 1997.)

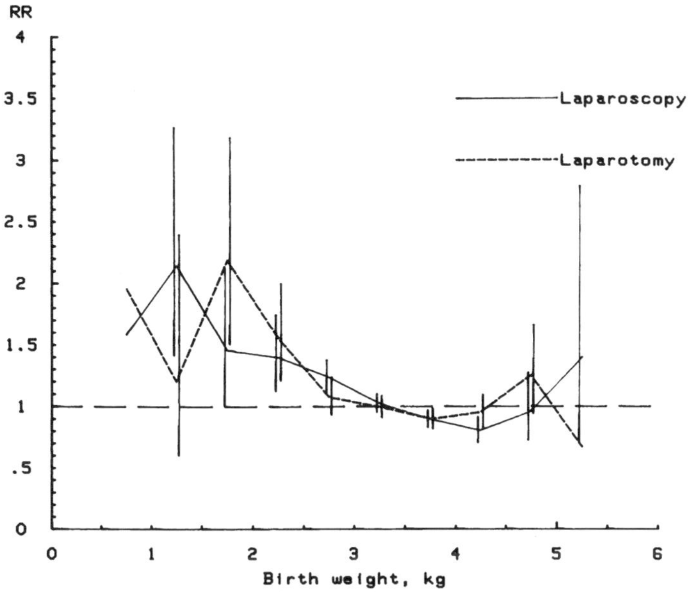

FIGURE 2.—Comparison of birth weight in laparoscopy and laparotomy cohorts with total population. *RR*, Risk ratio. (Courtesy of Reedy MB, Kallen B, Küéhl TH: Laparoscopy during pregnancy: A Study of five fetal outcome parameters with use of the Swedish health registry. *Am J Obstet Gynecol* 177:673–679, 1997.)

when compared with the total population. In cumulative infant survival up to 1 year, there was no difference between laparoscopy and laparotomy. Between these 2 groups and the total population, there was also no difference in the rate of fetal malformations. The laparoscopy group had 9 deaths and the laparotomy group had 6 deaths. When restricted to singleton deliveries with operations performed between the 4th and 20th weeks, there appears to be no difference in cumulative infant deaths between laparoscopy, laparotomy, and the total population.

Conclusion.—For patients having laparoscopy vs. laparotomy in singleton pregnancies between 4 and 20 weeks of gestation, there is no difference in 5 fetal outcome variables.

► This analysis of the Swedish National Health Registry evaluates the relative risk of laparoscopy vs. laparotomy for nonobstetrical procedures done during pregnancy, but it provides information regarding the general impact of surgery on the integrity of pregnancy as well. Distribution by gestational age differs strikingly between the 2 groups, with most of 2,233 laparoscopies being done by the 10th week of pregnancy. Two thousand four hundred and ninety-one laparotomies were identified from records of 2,015,000 deliveries done between 1973 and 1995. As in a prior report from this group no data are available to evaluate abortion incidence following surgical procedures, and anesthesia type has not been recorded by the Registry since 1983. The general approach was to calculate risk ratios from both laparoscopic and laporatomy groups against general population norms, and to stratify results in terms of birth weight, maternal and gestational age, growth retardation, malformations, and infant survival by maternal age, parity, and the year of surgery. No differences in outcome measures could be discerned between laparoscopy and laparotomy, except for a statistically significant but clinically irrelevant difference in mean birth weight. As before, both procedures were associated with an increased risk of premature birth and delivery, and of infant growth retardation. Whether these differences arose from the surgical procedure, the underlying disease process which nessitated surgery, or anesthesia cannot be evaluated. The results validate the safety of laparoscopy in the first trimester pregnancy, with reservations only for the risk of spontaneous abortion, which could not be evaluated from this data.

T.H. Kirschbaum, M.D.

Reference

1. 1991 YEAR BOOK OF OBSTETRICS AND GYNECOLOGY, pp 137–138.

Obstetric Embolotherapy: Effect on Menses and Pregnancy

Stancato-Pasik A, Mitty HA, Richard HM III, et al (Mount Sinai Med Ctr, New York)

Radiology 204:791–793, 1997 7–9

Objective.—Although transcatheter embolization as a safe and effective technique for management of pelvic hemorrhage is more likely to preserve the uterus, its long-term effects on a woman's menstrual cycle and reproductive capacity have not been well studied. The long-term effects of uterine embolotherapy with gelatin sponge pledgets on menses and fertility were determined.

Methods.—Between June 1990 and December 1995, uterine embolotherapy using gelatin sponge pledgets was performed on 17 women, aged 20–44 years, with severe, pregnancy-related bleeding. In 7 women, the procedure was performed on an emergency basis. In 10 the risk of bleeding was recognized ahead of time. In 4 of these 10 women, the fetus did not survive. Five of 17 women had a hysterectomy and were excluded from follow-up. Twelve patients or their doctors were contacted during a follow-up period of 1 to 6 years to determine if and when menses returned, if they had tried to conceive, if they had conceived, whether they were using birth control and if so, what type, and if menses were normal when they started to use contraceptives.

Results.—All but 1 of 12 women reported that normal menses returned 3–8 months after uterine embolotherapy or cessation of breast feeding. Eight women were practicing contraception. The 3 women who had attempted to conceive were successful. One patient whose menses had not returned is receiving medroxyprogesterone for bleeding secondary to a uterine arteriovenous malformation.

Conclusion.—Although this study is small, it showed that all but 1 pregnant patient had normal menses resume within 3–8 months after embolotherapy and that those patients who wished to conceive were able to do so.

▶ As transcatheter embolization of the posterior segment of hypogastric arteries has proved effective and acutely safe in controlling intraoperative pelvic hemorrhage uncontrolled by other methods, long-term safety has loomed as a secondary concern. Since gelatin sponge pledgets usually resorb after about 2 weeks, it seems unlikely that they would result in chronic reproductive dysfunction. It is useful, however, to see this group of 12 women treated by embolectomy, who did not require subsequent hysterectomy, provide some reassurance. All but 1 patient returned to normal menstrual function in the absence of breast feeding in 6 to 8 weeks after the procedure. The exception was a patient pharmacologically rendered amenorrheic in order to control bleeding from a uterine arteriovenous malformation. Of 3 women who sought subsequent pregnancy, all successfully conceived. The authors list 7 case reports with similar findings. Their experience provides reassurance for women who have received embolization about prospects for future fertility.

T.H. Kirschbaum, M.D.

8 Genetics and Teratology

Identification of Fetal DNA and Cells in Skin Lesions From Women With Systemic Sclerosis

Artlett CM, Smith JB, Jimenez SA (Thomas Jefferson Univ, Philadelphia)

N Engl J Med 338:1186–1191, 1998 8–1

Objective.—Systemic sclerosis is a connective tissue disease affecting 8 times as many women as men. The highest incidence occurs in the 45- to 55-year age group and has features similar to those of graft-vs.-host disease. Because fetal stem cells are transferred to the mother during pregnancy, it has been suggested that microchimerism established by fetal cells with appropriate activation may produce a chronic graft-versus-host disease. The male-specific Y-chromosome sequence DYZ1—a marker for fetal cells in affected tissues from women with systemic sclerosis—was identified using the polymerase chain reaction (PCR).

Methods.—DNA was extracted from the peripheral blood cells of 69 women with systemic sclerosis, from 25 normal women, and from biopsy specimens of active skin lesions of 19 women (16 previously pregnant) with systemic sclerosis. Y-chromosome–positive cells were identified using PCR, and the 148–base pair product was sequenced. Peripheral blood cells and paraffin-embedded skin-biopsy specimens were tested by fluorescence in situ hybridization.

Results.—The Y-chromosome sequence was identified in peripheral blood cells of 32 women with systemic sclerosis and in 1 normal woman. Y-chromosome–specific DNA was found in skin lesions of 11 women with active lesions but in none of the 68 women with osteoarthritis or their relatives. Results of PCR showed a male pattern. CD3 T cells or CD14 and CD45 cells from women who had male children had Y-chromosome sequences. No Y-chromosome sequences were found in women depleted of CD14 and CD45 cells or of CD3 cells, in normal women, or in a woman who had never been pregnant. Nucleated cells containing Y chromosomes were found in skin biopsy specimens of all 7 women with systemic sclerosis but not in specimens from normal women. All but 2 of the women with systemic sclerosis had carried male children. Of the 8 women with systemic sclerosis and negative PCR skin biopsy specimen results, 3 had never been pregnant, 2 had had daughters, and 3 were dead.

Conclusion.—Fetal graft-vs.-host disease may cause systemic sclerosis in some women who have born male children.

▶ Efforts to identify and collect fetal cells from the blood of pregnant women—initially aimed at enabling fetal diagnosis without invading the uterine cavity—have, in this study, come to play a potentially important role in what appears to be autoimmune disease for which the stage was set by fetal-to-maternal transfers 2–3 decades before diagnosis. Fetal-to-maternal cell transfer is quite common in pregnancy, with 99.3% of maternal blood samples containing fetal cells at a concentration, on average, of 1.2 cells per mL of maternal blood (Abstract 2–21). Such fetal cells may survive for decades in the maternal host.[1] Although maternal-to-fetal cell transfer during pregnancy occurs, it is less common and, apparently, less numerous. It has been estimated by some that maternal cells may comprise as much as 4% of cord blood leukocytes at the time of delivery, and they, too, may persist in infants for years.[2]

These authors provide a 10-year cohort study of women attending the Scleroderma Center of Jefferson University Hospital. Three sets of observations were employed, all using fluorescence in situ hybridization for cell detection.[3] First, peripheral blood from 69 women with scleroderma was compared with that of controls after sorting out cells bearing clonal designators for T lymphocytes (CD3), mononuclear cells (CD14), and leukocytes (CD45), using colloidal magnetic tags to monoclonal antibodies. Fluorescence probes were constructed to cDNA to a known 148–base pair segment of the Y chromosome, and 46% of females with scleroderma showed evidence of male DNA material, presumably transferred from a male fetus. A comparable incidence figure for normal control women was 4%. Fluorescence in situ hybridization demonstrated circulating male cells in 3 women with scleroderma, and none were found in controls.

Finally, in 7 women with systemic sclerosis whose skin lesions were biopsied, all had male fetal DNA segments in tissue sections, with none found in normal females. In what has come to be known as microchimerism, immunocompetent fetal cells transferred across the placenta take up chronic residence in gravidas, resulting in a maternal antibody response which is not autoimmunity, as the sensitizing antigens are not maternal but fetal epitopes presenting as graft-versus-host disease. As is common with graft-versus-host disease, the skin, lungs, and esophagus bear the bulk of the injury; in this case, systemic sclerosis or scleroderma is the ultimate result.

Much remains to be done to identify this role of fetal-to-maternal cell transfer during pregnancy in the generation of what appears to be autoimmunity occurring as it does primarily in women in the fourth to sixth decade of life. What generates such diseases in the few true nulliparas and men in whom scleroderma develops remains to be explained.

T.H. Kirschbaum, M.D.

References

1. 1997 Year Book of Obstetrics, Gynecology and Women's Health, pp 202–203.
2. Tyndall A, Gratwoh HA: Microchimerism, friend or foe. *Nat Med* 4:386–388, 1988.
3. 1994 Year Book of Obstetrics, Gynecology and Women's Health, pp 215–217.

PCR Quantitation of Fetal Cells in Maternal Blood in Normal and Aneuploid Pregnancies

Bianchi DW, Williams JM, Sullivan LM, et al (Tufts Univ, Boston; The Prenatal Diagnostic and Imaging Ctr, Sacramento, Calif; et al)

Am J Hum Genet 61:822–829, 1997 8–2

Purpose.—Fetal-maternal erythrocyte transfusion, which leads to maternal alloimunization and fetal anemia, has long been recognized. However, it has only recently been realized that fetal cells in maternal blood can be useful for noninvasive prenatal cytogenetic diagnosis. A polymerase chain reaction (PCR) technique of quantifying male fetal cell DNA equivalents was used to determine the number of fetal cells circulating in maternal whole blood, and whether the fetal karyotype influences this number.

Methods.—Peripheral blood specimens from 199 pregnant women carrying chromosomally normal fetuses and 31 with male aneuploid fetuses were analyzed. A Y-chromosome–specific sequence was amplified by PCR

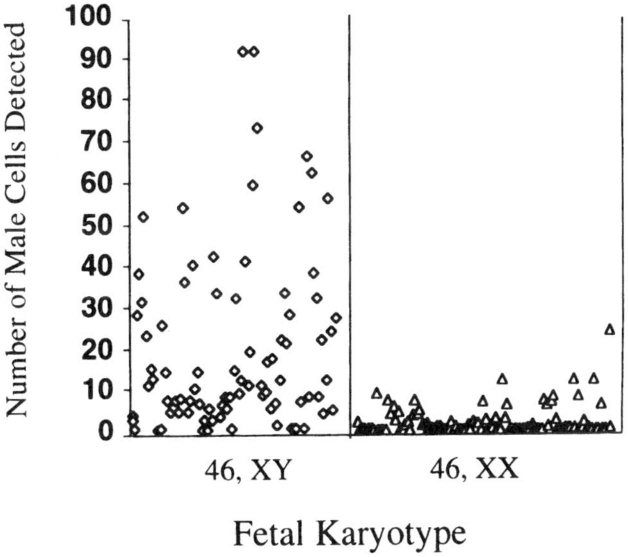

FIGURE 3.—Dot plots demonstrating number of male fetal cell DNA equivalents detected in 16-mL maternal samples from women carrying fetuses with normal karyotypes. The range of the number of male fetal cell DNA equivalents detected is shown for 46,XY (left) and 46,XX fetuses. (Courtesy of Bianchi DW, Williams JM, Sullivan LM, et al: PCR quantitation of fetal cells in maternal blood in normal and aneuploid pregnancies. *Am J Hum Genet* 61:822–829, 1997. Published by The University of Chicago Press.)

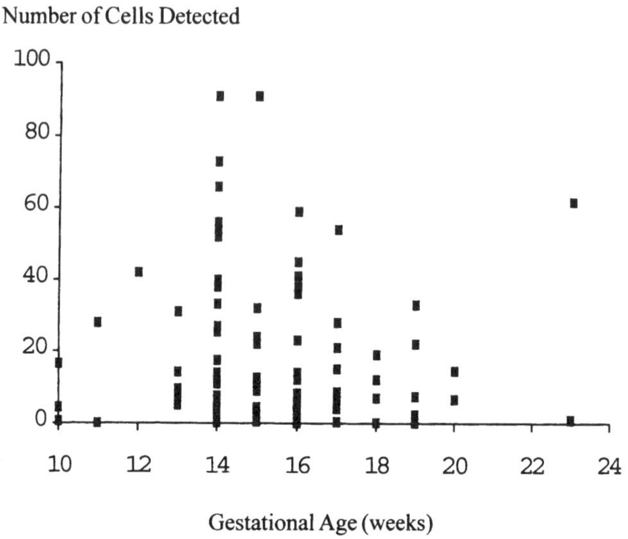

FIGURE 4.—Number of male cell DNA equivalents detected, as a function of gestational age. Data are shown for 46,XY fetuses only. (Courtesy of Bianchi DW, Williams JM, Sullivan LM, et al: PCR quantitation of fetal cells in maternal blood in normal and aneuploid pregnancies. *Am J Hum Genet* 61:822–829, 1997. Published by The University of Chicago Press.)

for quantification of the male fetal cell DNA equivalents. This number was compared with a PCR product amplified from known, simultaneously run concentrations of male DNA. The findings were analyzed to determine whether the fetal cell number in maternal blood was influenced mainly by fetal karyotype, which has a biological effect on the fetoplacental unit, or by the laboratory method of cell separation.

Findings.—In a 16-mL blood specimen, the mean number of male fetal cell DNA equivalents was 19 in samples from women with 46,XY fetuses vs. 2 in women with a 46,XX fetus (Fig 3). The number of male cells detected was not significantly related to the gestational age at the time of sampling (Fig 4). The differences in number of cells detected was highly significant when the fetus was male versus female. The number of fetal cells detected in maternal blood was greater when the fetus was aneuploid. For mothers with fetuses of karyocyte 47,XY,+21, the mean number of male fetal cell DNA equivalents was 110, significantly higher than in 46,XY fetuses.

Conclusions.—Fetal karyotype has a substantial effect on fetal-maternal transfusion of nucleated cells. For fetuses with trisomy 21, the number of fetal cells is elevated six-fold, suggesting the possibility of noninvasive cytogenetic diagnosis of this abnormal karyotype. Other fetal cytogenetic abnormalities are also associated with increased fetal-maternal transfusion, including Klinefelter's syndrome and 47,XXY+inv-(dup)15. Surprisingly, some women with normal female fetuses have low numbers of circulating male fetal cells.

▶ This collection of 230 maternal venous samples obtained from women undergoing genetic amniocentesis represents the largest collection of material employed in the effort to quantitate fetal nucleated cell availability in maternal blood to date, and benefits by the careful work of a pioneer in this undertaking. The benefit of access to fetal cells without invading the placenta for fetal genetic diagnosis is clear to everyone. The primary goal here is to obtain firm estimates of the concentration of fetal cells and to resolve the relatively wide range of concentration by other workers.[1, 2]

After hemolysis, isolation and purification of DNA samples, PCR was performed using primers specific to the long arm of the Y chromosome, thereby employing the search for male genetic material in pregnant women as a means of identifying fetal cells. The method was calibrated using 6 different ratios of known male and female nucleated cells. The results demonstrated a mean of 1.2 fetal cells/mL of maternal blood with a wide range (0 to 5.7 cells/mL), with maximal concentration in the second trimester. Using a 16-mL maternal sample, fetal cells could be found in 99.3% of cases. In addition, as noted earlier in about one fourth of cases, male cells could be detected in the presence of a female fetus. As before, this evidence suggests retention of cells from a prior pregnancy consisting of a male fetus, of the possibility of a "lost male twin," transfusion from a male donor, or the "grandmother hypothesis." A principal finding is the presence of roughly 4 times more fetal cells per maternal blood volume in pregnancies bearing fetuses with trisomies 13, 18, 21, and Kleinfelter's syndrome. This finding both explains the high density of fetal cells noted by investigators studying aneuploid pregnancies and points to facility in using fetal cell isolates to diagnose aneuploid pregnancies. The basis for the larger number of fetal and maternal cell transfers is intriguing and invites further study.

T.H. Kirschbaum, M.D.

References

1. 1990 Year Book of Obstetrics and Gynecology, pp 178–180.
2. 1993 Year Book of Obstetrics and Gynecology, pp 199–201.
3. 1997 Year Book of Obstetrics, Gynecology, and Women's Health, pp 202–203.

Quantitative Analysis of Fetal DNA in Maternal Plasma and Serum: Implications for Noninvasive Prenatal Diagnosis

Lo YMD, Tein MSC, Lau TK, et al (Chinese Univ, Shatin, Hong Kong; John Radcliffe Hosp, Oxford, England)

Am J Hum Genet 62:768–775, 1998 8–3

Background.—Maternal plasma and serum DNA may be a useful source of material for the noninvasive prenatal diagnosis of certain genetic disorders. A real-time quantitative TaqMan polymerase chain reaction assay was developed for measuring the copy numbers of fetal DNA molecules in maternal plasma and serum.

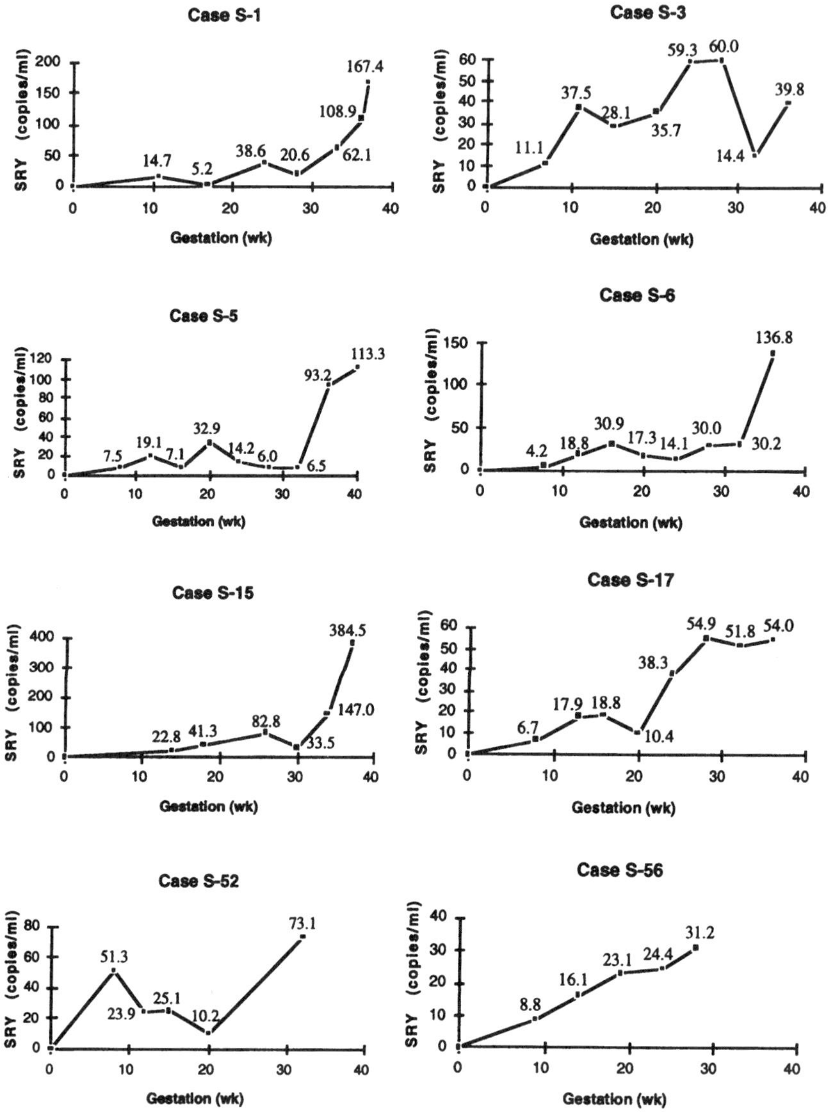

(Continued)

Methods and Findings.—Samples for analysis were collected from women at different points in pregnancy. Fetal DNA was found in high concentrations in maternal plasma, reaching means of 25.4 and 292.2 genome equivalents/mL in early and late pregnancy, respectively. These levels correspond to 3.4% and 6.2%, respectively, of the total plasma DNA. Follow-up of women conceiving by in vitro fertilization demonstrated that fetal DNA is detectable in maternal serum as early as week 7, the concentrations increasing as pregnancy progresses (Fig 2).

FIGURE 2 (cont.)

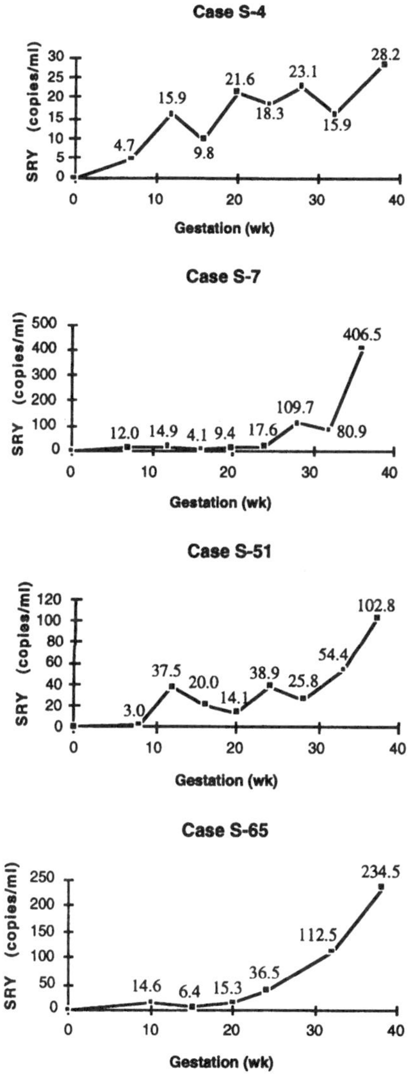

FIGURE 2.—Sequential study of 12 women, bearing male fetuses, who conceived by in vitro fertilization. Each case is denoted by a unique recruitment case number. The *X-axis* denotes the gestational ages at which serum samples were obtained. A gestational age of 0 denotes the preconception sample. The *Y-axis* denotes the concentration of fetal SRY in maternal serum, expressed in copies per milliliter. The scale has been optimized for the concentration range for each case. (Courtesy of Lo YMD, Tein MSC, Lau TK, et al: Quantitative analysis of fetal DNA in maternal plasma and serum: Implications for noninvasive prenatal diagnosis. *Am J Hum Genet* 62:768–775, 1998, published by The University of Chicago Press.)

Conclusion.—This newly developed assay allows continuous optical monitoring of the progress of an amplification reaction, yielding accurate target quantitation over a wide concentration range. By using this assay, fetal DNA can be readily identified in maternal plasma and serum, which may be a valuable source of material for noninvasive prenatal diagnosis.

▶ Stimulated by the ability to identify large quantities of tumor DNA in blood samples from cancer patients, these investigators have demonstrated the ability to detect fetal DNA in maternal plasma and serum.[1] This is a further application of molecular genetic techniques beyond identifying fetal cells circulating in maternal blood as reported by Bianci et al. (Abstract 8–2), which appears to increase available fetal DNA for diagnostic evaluation.

Here the authors provide quantitative data and demonstrate the ability to detect fetal DNA sequences extracted from maternal plasma and serum. The method involves simultaneous polymerase chain reactions (PCRs) with 2 sets of primers. The first is directed at amplification of a DNA sequence housed in the Y chromosome (SRY) and the second, an adaptation of the Taq polymerase method designed for cyclic base sequencing, using a dual-labeled fluorescent probe. The TagMan probe contains a fluorescent dye linked by intervening nucleotide sequences to a second dye which quenches it. During each PCR cycle, a polymerase that acts between primers chosen to allow separation of the quenching flour and the availability of the fluorescent marker at 518 MU, allows expression of the quantity of copied DNA. Using standard DNA amplification plots for the SRY gene, the authors prove sensitivity to the DNA from a single gene copy, albeit only after 30 PCR cycles. A parallel calibrating curve is run with each sample from which the identity of 6.6 pg of DNA to 1 cell copy, was derived to allow expression of results in terms of cell copy number.

The authors demonstrate increasing quantities of fetal DNA with gestation; it is about 12 times more abundant in late than in early gestation. In early pregnancy, fetal DNA averages 25.4 gene copies per mL of plasma and 28.7 copies per mL of serum. In late pregnancy, corresponding values are 292.2 copies per mL of plasma and 342.1 copies per mL of serum. These concentrations are roughly 20–24 times greater than the equivalent yield of fetal cells obtained from maternal blood in the same intervals of pregnancy. In all of 20 cases, fetal sex was accurately predicted from the analysis of the SRY gene products.

As described, this methodology is faster, more sensitive, and less likely contaminated by maternal DNA than any process reported to date for this purpose. This contribution may well open the door wider to noninvasive fetal DNA analysis.

T.H. Kirschbaum, M.D.

Reference

1. Lo YMD, Corbetta N, Chamberlain PF, et al: Presence of fetal DNA in maternal plasma and serum. *Lancet* 350:485–487, 1997.

Maternal Uniparental Disomy of Chromosome 2 and Confined Placental Mosaicism for Trisomy 2 in a Fetus With Intrauterine Growth Restriction, Hypospadias, and Oligohydramnios

Hansen WF, Bernard LE, Langlois S, et al (Univ of North Carolina, Chapel Hill; British Columbia's Children's Hosp, Vancouver, Canada)

Prenat Diagn 17:443–450, 1997 8–4

Background.—In confined placental mosaicism (CPM), a cell line is present in the placenta that has different chromosomes from the cell line found in the fetus. This situation can result either from a diploid zygote through mitotic error (in which case the fetus inherits a homologue from each parent [biparental disomy]), or from a trisomic zygote through mitotic loss of the trisomic chromosome (in which case the fetus can inherit both homologues from a single parent [uniparental disomy]). Confined placental mosaicism is associated with a poor pregnancy outcome, intrauterine growth restriction (IUGR), and stillbirth, and fetal uniparental disomy (UPD) can contribute to a poor outcome. These authors report a case of UPD for chromosome 2 in which only the placenta had the trisomy 2 line and the nonmosaic fetus had maternal UPD.

> *Case Report.*—Woman, 23 (G2P1) was seen at 24 weeks of pregnancy because of IUGR and oligohydramnios. No cause of these abnormalities was apparent, and a placental biopsy was performed. The biopsy specimen showed chromosomal mosaicism with trisomy 2. Amniocentesis was not helpful in karyotyping because of the lack of amniotic fluid, but the parents were counseled regarding the poor prognosis. An elective cesarean section was performed at 36 weeks' gestation, and the infant was live born with a birth weight of 510 g. The fetal-placental weight ratio at birth was 2:1 (normal at term is 6:1). The infant died of severe pulmonary hypoplasia within 2 hours of birth. At autopsy, brain gyral development, kidneys, and ureters were normal, but there was a hypospadia with chordee. Chromosomes from the placenta and fetus underwent DNA analysis with chromosome 2 microsatellite markers.

Findings.—Placental biopsy samples at 24 weeks' gestation and at term showed high levels of trisomy 2, particularly in the trophoblast and the stroma. However, fetal tissues did not have trisomy 2, and cell lineages were consistently diploid. Furthermore, fetal tissues had no paternal alleles, but there were 2 heterozygous chromosome 2 alleles from the mother (i.e., maternal UPD). Placental tissues contained 2 maternal alleles and 1 paternal allele. The most likely cause of the trisomic zygote was an error in maternal meiosis phase I.

Conclusion.—In this case, fetal UPD for chromosome 2 occurred but there was no evidence of trisomy 2 mosaicism in the fetus. The occurrence of trisomy 2 in the placenta seems likely to account for the placental insufficiency; in fact, all 3 reported cases of UPD for trisomy 2 have involved IUGR and oligohydramnios. How CPM and/or UPD for trisomy 2 causes IUGR and oligohydramnios has yet to be determined, but current data support 2 possible mechanisms. First, the high levels of trisomy 2 in the placenta may be directly responsible for placental dysfunction. Alternatively, imprinted genes on chromosome 2 may be responsible for fetal, placental, and postnatal growth beyond what we already know to be the case.

▶ This well-investigated case of maternal UPD nicely illustrates what is emerging as a likely sequence in the evolution of this genetic abnormality. The initial disturbance is abnormal meiosis in an early embryo, resulting in trisomic chromosome 2 in which two heploid chromosome sets are derived from 1 parent (here, the mother), and 1 set from the father.

Because triploid fetuses with triploid placentaes are seldomly reported, it is likely that this is a lethal combination and results in abortion or early fetal death. Occasionally in the course of further development of the trisomic embryo, trisomic rescue takes place with the expulsion of 1 haploid chromosome set (in this case, including the extra chromosome 2). With 2 maternal and 1 paternal chromosome in 2 out of 3 random selections of paired chromosomes, a normal maternal-paternal fetal set will emerge, but in 1 of 3 cases, the ultimate rescued diploid line will be composed of 2 sets from the same parent (in this case, from the mother); hence, the origin of UPD. The result is the original trisomy—in this case, of chromosome number 2 present in the placenta with UPD of chromosome 2 in the fetus.

Although the role of CPM in which the trisomic state arises from a mitotic error after differentiation of placental from fetal cells has occurred in embryogenesis, it is debated as a cause of IUGR. Certainly UPD is associated with growth retardation fairly commonly.[1] The later in the course of placental development the mitotic error occurs, the smaller the clonal fraction of placental tissue containing the mitotic error and the less the functional significance. Although CPM is a common event and occurs in about 2% of pregnancies, its association with profound growth retardation raises the likelihood of high-order fetal mosaicism or UPD and requires a genetic search using fetal and parental cell lines.

T.H. Kirschbaum, M.D.

Reference

1. 1998 Year Book of Obstetrics, Gynecology, and Women's Health, pp 2–3 and 6.

Prospective Prenatal Investigations on Potential Uniparental Disomy in Cases of Confined Placental Trisomy

Opstal DV, van den Berg C, Deelen WH, et al (Erasmus Univ, Rotterdam, The Netherlands)

Prenat Diagn 18:35–44, 1998 8–5

Objective.—Uniparental disomy (UPD) refers to the presence of a chromosome pair derived from a single parent in a diploid offspring. Initially reported cases of UPD associated with confined placental mosaicism (CPM) demonstrated a high level of mosaicism or full trisomy in the chorionic villi. However, these findings could not demonstrate whether fetal UPD was also present in the more common low levels of mosaicism. The incidence of UPD associated with CPM was prospectively evaluated in a series of chorionic villus (CV) samples.

Methods.—The 4-year study included 3,958 consecutive CV samples. From these were identified 29 cases of trisomy CPM. In 23 of these, the level of mosaicism in the CV was studied extensively with interphase in situ hybridization. Cultured amniotic fluid cells were used to study the parental origin of the particular chromosome pair. Uncultured amniotic fluid cells were studied to rule out the presence of generalized mosaicism.

Results.—Of the 23 cases studied, 22 had had normal biparental chromosome contributions. The remaining case showed maternal heterodisomy for chromosome 16. Pregnancy complications occurred in 7 of the 23 cases, but were not caused by UPD.

Conclusions.—A very low incidence of UPD was found among a series of CPM cases. The trisomic cell line in CV most often originates from somatic duplication, consistent with the low level of mosaicism found in most of these cases. Intrauterine growth retardation, intrauterine death, and other obstetric complications are not related to UPD.

► UPD involves the transmission of both pairs of a chromosome pair from 1 parent. Interest in the finding followed demonstration of a 1% to 2% incidence of trisomy confined to placental cells on chorionic villus biopsy in which amniocentesis and fetal cell karyotype have demonstrated that in most cases, the associated fetus was genetically normal. In such cases, placental trisomy appears to arise from post zygotic nondisjunction in somatic placental cells. In many cases of UPD, the mechanism appears to be trisomic rescue in which trisomy in embryonic meiosis results in expulsion of 1 surplus chromosome, leaving a pair of chromosomes derived from the same parent. The appearance of the fetus (its phenotype) is usually not altered unless UPD allows expression of a recessive trait not manifest in either parent but homozygous in the inherited chromosomal pair, or through the result of imprinting. Imprinting results in a difference in gene expression based on the origin of the gene pair from one or another parent. An example stems from UPD in chromosome 15, which yields Prader-Willi syndrome if the origin is maternal chromosomes, or Angleman syndrome if they are paternal. As information has accumulated, there is increasing reason to feel that UPD is an infrequent event, seldom associated with antenatal pregnancy abnormalities.

In contrast to earlier cohort studies, this is a prospective analysis of 3,958 chorion villus biopsies obtained largely for advanced paternal age and the risk of inheritance of a deleterious recessive trait. The incidence of CPM was 1.7% and of an associated trisomy, 0.7%. In 3 of those 29 fetal trisomics, the aneuploidy was not mosaic but general throughout the fatal body in 1 case resulting in fetal death. Flourescent in situ hybridization to flourescent-tagged chromosomal markers proved to be an effective means of estimating the extent of fetal mosaicism and was far faster than karyotypic analysis. In this 4-year experience with 23 cases of CPM that could be investigated by DNA fingerprinting, UPD was present in only 1 case. In none of the 7 women with confined placental trisomy and pregnancy abnormalities such as intrauterine growth retardation and preterm birth was the aneuploidy etiologic. Fetal trisomy occurs most often in association with chromosomes 16 and 22, and occasionally chromosome 9. A trisomy arises from meiotic error in such cases, and the incidence of mosaic abnormalities in the fetuses is large as a result. Most trisomic fetuses associated with CPM have sustained somatic disjunctional errors and have lower-order mosaicisms expressing the relatively small clones of trisomic cells, and rarely exhibit a phenotypic abnormality.

T.H. Kirschbaum, M.D.

Increased Nuchal Translucency as a Marker for Fetal Chromosomal Defects

Taipale P, Hiilesmaa V, Salonen R, et al (Jorvi Hosp, Helsinki; Univ Central Hosp, Helsinki)

N Engl J Med 337:1654–1658, 1997 8–6

Introduction.—An established practice in many countries is to perform maternal serum screening for fetal trisomy 21 (Down's syndrome) at 15–16 weeks of gestation. The average maternal serum concentrations of chorionic gonadotropin are higher than normal, and those of alpha-fetoprotein and estriol are lower than normal, in the presence of fetal trisomy 21. Increased nuchal translucence can be detected on US and is caused by the subcutaneous accumulation of fluid in the neck of a fetus. Because of advanced age or positive serum screening tests for trisomy 21, most ultrasound studies have been performed on mothers at elevated risk for fetal trisomy. There are little data on the usefulness of increased nuchal translucency as a primary screening method for fetal chromosomal abnormalities. In a population of pregnant adolescents and women, the frequency of increased fetal nuchal translucency was defined.

Methods.—In 10,010 unselected adolescents and women younger than 40 years of age with live singleton fetuses at 10–15.9 weeks of gestation, transvaginal ultrasonography was performed (Figure 1, B). An area of translucency at least 3 mm in width was the definition of increased fetal

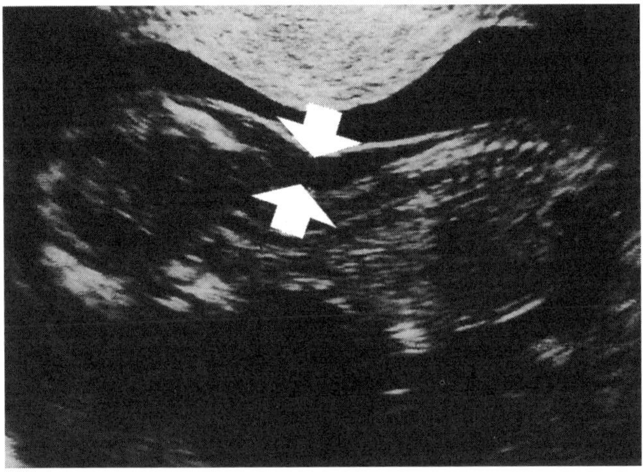

FIGURE 1,B.—Sagittal Transvaginal Ultrasonographic Images. Panel B shows a zone of nuchal translucency of 6 mm (arrows) in a 14-week fetus with trisomy 21. (Reprinted by permission of *The New England Journal of Medicine* from Taipale P, Hiilesmaa V, Salonen R, et al: Increased nuchal translucency as a marker for fetal chromosomal defects. *N Engl J Med* 337:1654–1658, copyright 1997, Massachusetts Medical Society. All rights reserved.)

nuchal translucency. Septated, fluid-filled sacs in the nuchal region were the definition of cystic hygromas. Fetal karyotyping was offered to mothers whose fetuses had these characteristics. Hospital records, national birth, and malformation registries were analyzed to obtain information on pregnancies, deliveries, and neonates.

Results.—In 76 fetuses (0.8%), nuchal translucency or cystic hygroma was seen. Of those who had nuchal translucency, 18 (24%) had an abnormal karyotype. There was a 62% sensitivity for trisomies 21, 18, and 13 combined in 13 of 21 fetuses. There was a 54% sensitivity for trisomy 21 alone in 7 of 13 fetuses.

Conclusion.—For fetal aneuploidy, the use of transvaginal ultrasonography to detect increased nuchal translucency and cystic hygroma is a sensitive test. Transvaginal ultrasonography decreases the need for chorionic-villus sampling or amniocentesis and can be done earlier in pregnancy than serum screening. Other currently-used methods should be compared with transvaginal ultrasonography to identify the most cost-effective combinations for detecting fetal aneuploidy.

► There is no question that nuchal translucency observed on ultrasound between 10 and 15 weeks of pregnancy is associated with an increased risk of trisomy 21 and other aneuploidies. This group from Helsinki University is exploring the possible use of routine ultrasound screening at that gestational age for case detection. The current standard for case detection in a low-risk population, using biochemical screening, leads to recognition of 65%-80% of cases, with a false-positive rate of about 5%. Here, a low rate of prevalence of nuchal translucency (0.8%), and sensitivity of 54% for Down syndrome and 69% for all aneuploidies, makes the proposition tempting. In a population of 10,000 screened gravidas, there would be 61 false positives among those predicted to have aneuploid fetuses. But the results reported by other investigators do not appear equally favorable. The definition of the thickness of maximum translucency deemed normal varies among reported groups, and unsuccessful ultrasound evaluation at this gestational age has been reported in as many as 25% of cases. The incidence of aneuploidy among fetuses with nuchal translucencies varies widely among reporting groups, as does the base incidence of nuchal translucency. Physicians need more uniform reported experience before deciding on incorporation of routine assessment of nuchal translucency as part of the standard of obstetrical care.

T.H. Kirschbaum, M.D.

Human Leukocyte Antigen Matching and Fetal Loss: Results of a 10 Year Prospective Study

Ober C, Hyslop T, Elias S, et al (Univ of Chicago; Thomas Jefferson Univ, Philadelphia; Baylor College of Medicine, Houston; et al)

Hum Reprod 13:33–38, 1998 8–7

Objective.—Maternal-fetal HLA compatibility may result in increased risk of spontaneous abortion. The role of HLA compatibility in pregnancy was evaluated in a 10-year prospective study of the Hutterites, a communal population of European ancestry living in South Dakota, characterized by a limited number of HLA haplotypes and a high fertility rate.

Methods.—Information was collected on 251 pregnancies in 111 women aged 20–42 years. Genetic typing was performed, and couples were classified according to whether they shared no alleles or 1 or more alleles at specified loci. All spontaneous abortions and tubal pregnancies that occurred at less than 20 weeks' gestation were recorded. Fetal HLA genotypes were determined and characterized as homozygous for the shared haplotype, heterozygous and identical to the mother, or heterozygous and different from the mother.

Results.—There were 38 (15.6%) fetal losses, at an average of 9.5 weeks, in 27 women, 26 of whom had at least 1 prior live birth and 21 of whom had at least 2 prior live births. Of 68 haplotypes present in the Hutterite population, 37 were found in the women who had fetal loss. The relative frequencies of these 37 haplotypes were the same as the relative frequencies of these same haplotypes in the Hutterite population. Fetal loss rates were highest among couples with matching alleles at all 16 loci (odds ratio, 4.39). Matching alleles at loci HLA-B, HLA-C, or at the complement component C4 were significant predictors of fetal loss. When the 30 couples with matching alleles at all 16 loci were excluded, loss rates associated with HLA-B were no longer significant. Matching class I, class II, and class III regions were also significantly associated with fetal loss. There was a 13.6% deficiency of living children heterozygous and identical to the mother among couples matching for HLA-B, and a 21% deficiency of living children heterozygous and identical to the mother among couples matching for the haplotype.

Conclusions.—Couples sharing the HLA-B antigens and/or the 16–locus HLA haplotype are at increased risk of fetal loss.

▶ Genetic homogeneity among parent animals prejudices against reproductive efficiency. The same conclusion has come from the analysis of some, but not all, retrospective cohort studies in the human, enrolling women with a past history of recurrent abortion. This human study is unique in its prospective design and its study population—111 Hutterite women residing in relatively closed communities in South Dakota. Hutterites are of highly inbred European origin with high fertility rates and a high incidence of genetic homogeneity. Over 10 years, 251 pregnancies occurred in this population, all with known HLA sex cell composition (haplotype) with respect to HLA class I and II alleles, as well as some other genetic histocompatability loci. The first identified HLA complex (HLA-A) was characterized by 16 of its gene loci in this analysis. Of the resulting 251 pregnancies occurring over 10 years, there was an overall fetal loss rate of 15.6% (38 spontaneous abortions and/or ectopic pregnancies). Most strongly predictive of reproductive failure was maternal-paternal sharing of all 16 gene states (alleles) in the HLA-A-haplotype and somewhat less strong evidence for the importance of HLA-B maternal incompatibility. Because of Hutterite inbreeding, only 16 haplotypes were associated with fetal death, and it is important that the incidence of this haplotype was the same in those with normal as in abnormal pregnancies. This makes the chance of one or more lethal factors within the haplotype unlikely. Ultimately, the goal is to identify one or more gene loci that will account for the increased fetal jeopardy in these patients, and only then will genetic screening become useful in repeated reproductive failure. Until then, we can only be certain that some instances of pregnancy wastage occur on the basis of genetic factors beyond the extent of our current knowledge.

T.H. Kirschbaum, M.D.

α-Fetoprotein, Free β-Human Chorionic Gonadotropin, and Dimeric Inhibin A Produce the Best Results in a Three-Analyte, Multiple-Marker Screening Test for Fetal Down Syndrome

Wenstrom KD, Owen J, Chu DC, et al (Univ of Alabama, Birmingham)

Am J Obstet Gynecol 177:987–991, 1997 8–8

Objective.—There are 6 second-trimester maternal markers of Down syndrome. The best 3-analyte combination for detecting Down syndrome was determined.

Methods.—Serum α-fetoprotein (AFP), unconjugated estriol, intact human chorionic gonadotropin (hCG), free β-human chorionic gonadotropin (β-hCG), CA 125, and dimeric inhibin A levels were analyzed in stored sera from 33 Down syndrome pregnancies. Median values for free β-hCG, 125, and dimeric inhibin A kits were determined, using stored sera from 45 to 50 euploid pregnancies at each week between 14 and 20 weeks' gestation. The screen-positive rates and Down syndrome detection rates at several risk cutoff points were retrospectively determined and compared for each 3-analyte combination.

Results.—The average maternal age was 35.6 in the euploid patients and 36.3 in the Down syndrome population. Free β-hCG and intact hCG were highly correlated. Dimeric inhibin A was correlated with free β-hCG and intact hCG. The best 3-analyte combination was serum AFP, free β-hCG, and dimeric inhibin A, detecting 97% of all Down syndrome fetuses, with a false-positive rate of 16% at a cutoff value of 1:300.

Conclusion.—The best 3-analyte combination for detecting Down syndrome was serum AFP, free β-hCG, and dimeric inhibin A. These results should be confirmed by large prospective studies in women of a variety of ages.

► The dynamics of serum dimeric inhibin A in normal pregnancy, its increase in concentration in Down syndrome, its usefulness in detecting Down syndrome and its possible relationship to hCG production have been discussed here earlier.[1] This group explores the use of dimeric inhibin A in conjunction with other biochemical markers of Down syndrome, and in particular the value of substituting it for unconjugated estriol in conjunction with α-fetoprotein and free β-hCG. Determinations were done on samples obtained from 313 women with euploid fetuses at regular intervals from 14–20 weeks' gestational age. Stored samples from 33 women with Down syndrome infants were then analyzed and various combinations of 6 laboratory determinations were analyzed for their predictive value, correcting for variability in pair-wise intercorrelations previously calculated. Replacing unconjugated estriol with inhibin A assays resulted in improved detection rates and reduced false-positive rates at each of 3 cutoff values. Using AFP, free β-hCG, and dimeric inhibin, a detection rate of 90%, with a false-positive rate of 11%, emerges—a clear improvement over existing approaches. These results must now be verified through a prospective study.

T.H. Kirschbaum, M.D.

Reference

1. 1997 Year Book of Obstetrics, Gynecology, and Women's Health, pp 166–170.

Congenital Malformations in Offspring of Women With Hyperglycemia First Detected During Pregnancy

Schaefer UM, Songster G, Xiang A, et al (Univ of Southern California, Los Angeles; Humboldt Univ, Berlin)

Am J Obstet Gynecol 177:1165–1171, 1997 8–9

Objective.—Women with type I or II diabetes are at risk for having an infant with congenital anomalies. There is also probably a significant, although not quantified, risk that women with gestational hyperglycemia could deliver an infant with congenital anomalies. The incidence of major and minor congenital anomalies in infants of women with gestational hyperglycemia, and the clinical parameters that can be used to quantify the risk in individual patients, were identified.

Methods.—Between January 1987 and July 1995, records of 3,743 women with pregnancies complicated by gestational diabetes, who delivered at more than 20 weeks' gestation, were reviewed for the presence of congenital malformations in their infants. Genetic anomalies were excluded. One-hour screening glucose concentration, fasting serum glucose

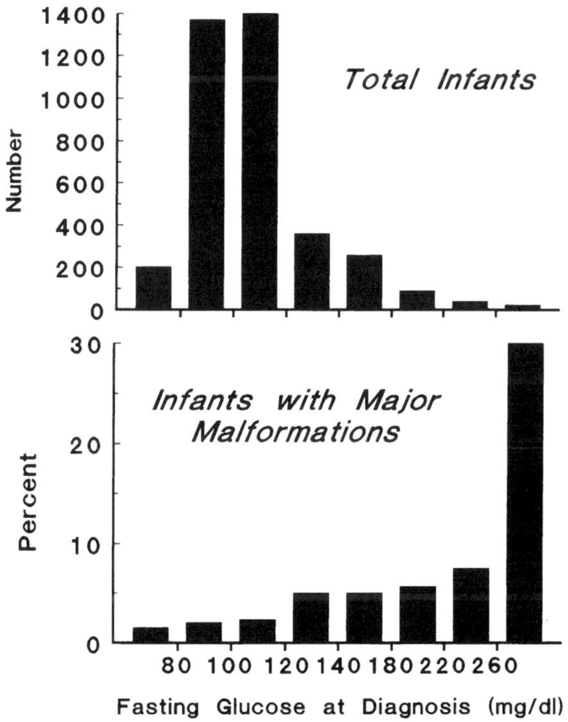

FIGURE 1.—Rates of major congenital anomalies in women with hyperglycemia detected during pregnancy. Cohort was divided into 8 subgroups according to fasting serum glucose level at initial diagnosis of hyperglycemia. **Top panel**, number of infants with major anomalies. (Courtesy of Schaefer UM, Songster G, Xiang A, et al: Congenital malformations in offspring of women with hyperglycemia first detected during pregnancy. *Am J Obstet Gynecol* 177:1165–1171, 1997).

level at the time of diagnosis of gestational diabetes mellitus, hourly postchallenge serum glucose concentrations from the diagnostic oral glucose tolerance test, highest fasting glucose concentration, and hemoglobin A_{1c} were examined for ability to predict risk for anomalies.

Results.—There were 199 infants with 1 or more congenital anomalies, 108 major and 91 minor. The most common major anomalies affected the cardiovascular, musculoskeletal, and central nervous systems. The most common minor abnormalities were dermatologic and craniofacial. Fasting glucose concentrations were the best predictors of risk for major anomalies, according to multivariate regression analysis. Highest fasting glucose concentration was the only independent risk factor for risk of malformations (odds ratio, 1.13) in the regression model. When women were stratified by initial fasting glucose concentrations, those with levels higher than 260 mg/dl had a 30.4% rate of major malformation, those with levels between 121 and 260 mg/dl a 5.2% rate, and those with levels lower than 120 mg/dl a 2.1% rate (Fig 1).

Conclusion.—Maternal fasting glucose concentration was a predictor of major infant malformations. Patients with fasting glucose concentrations greater than 120 mg/dl had double the risk of having an infant with major malformations.

▶ In women with established diabetes mellitus, it is clear that early-pregnancy hyperglycemia and elevated glycosylated hemoglobin values are reliable predictors of anomalous development in the cardiovascular system, central nervous system, and axial skeleton. That's not to say that non-genetically-determined anomalies can be prevented by prepregnancy therapy, perhaps because the teratogenic influence appears to take place during the first 6 weeks post conception, before motivation and resources can be effectively mustered. If the teratogen is simple hyperglycemia, the relationship to anomaly should be the same for gestational diabetics with early diagnosis as it is for type I and type II established diabetics. The problem rests with finding estimates of glycemic control prior to the establishment of the diagnosis of gestational diabetes, often made only at the start of the third trimester. Here the incidence of anomaly in 3,544 patients with gestational diabetes was stratified by fasting serum glucose level at the time of diagnosis, and the results are at least compatible with and supportive of hyperglycemia as a cause. In women with a fasting serum glucose level greater than 260 mg/dL, the 30% anomaly rate compares with the rate in women with pre-existing diabetes during pregnancy. Even in the range of 120 mg/dL to 140 mg/dl as the screening detection value of serum glucose, the risk of major anomaly was twice the control value. Glycosylated hemoglobin values were available in only 40% of these women, but the mean value, even so, was significantly higher than in controls. Aside from these theoretical considerations, there is little hope of effective prevention in such pregnancies, since that would mean routine glycemic testing at a threshold value of less than 120 mg/dL of serum glucose, but these authors strengthen the evidence for hyperglycemia as the basis for abnormal fetal development in the dominant organ systems involved.

T.H. Kirschbaum, M.D.

Contribution of Parental Blood Pressures to Association Between Low Birth Weight and Adult High Blood Pressure: Cross Sectional Study

Walker BR, McConnachie A, Noon JP, et al (Univ of Edinburgh, Scotland; Univ of Glasgow, Scotland)

BMJ 316:834–837, 1998 8–10

Introduction.—Recent epidemiologic studies in several countries report a relationship between low birth weight and increased blood pressure later in life. Because both birth weight and blood pressure are influenced by hereditary factors, the assessment of parental background is important. A cross-sectional study was designed to examine the potential contribution of parental blood pressure to the relation between low birth weight and subsequent hypertension.

Methods.—The study cohort was drawn from 603 families who received medical care at a primary care center in Edinburgh, Scotland. Blood pressure had been measured in adults in 1979 and in their young adult offspring in 1986. In 1994, all 603 mothers were asked to report the birth weight of their offspring; case records and replies from 398 mothers provided information for 545 offspring. Analyses were performed on data from 452 offspring, 1 selected at random from each family.

Results.—Blood pressure in young adult offspring was higher in men than in women and showed a positive correlation with current body weight. There was also an association between higher maternal or paternal systolic blood pressure and higher systolic blood pressure in their children and between higher maternal systolic blood pressure and lower birth weight in offspring. When parental blood pressures were not considered, a 1-kg decrease in birth weight was associated with a 2.24-mm Hg increase in systolic blood pressure of offspring. With correction for parental blood pressure, a 1-kg decrease in birth weight was associated with only a 1.71-mm Hg increase in systolic blood pressure.

Conclusion.—Findings suggest that low birth weight is one of the features of the inherited contribution to hypertension. Mothers with elevated blood pressure in later life have babies with lower birth weight, and these offspring also have higher blood pressures as they grow older.

▶ This study adds important information to a currently popular clinical research effort exploring the hypothesis constructed by David Barker to the point that low birth weight predisposes the infant to adult hypertension, dyslipidemia, coronary disease, diabetes, and diabetic complications.[1] Data collected from 504 products of 398 pregnancies delivered in 1986 in Edinburgh, part of a Medical Research Council study of hypertension, were employed. When midwife-registered birth weights were compared with mother's recall, the range of probable error in the latter proved to be plus or minus 1 pound, a major error implicit in earlier cohort studies done by recall of birth weight after several years. Paternal blood pressures recorded at the time of pregnancy were also studied, and the data were analyzed appropriate to the group's interest in the epidemiology of hypertension.[2] Like others, these authors found that birth weight was influenced by gender and maternal age as well as by current body weight. In addition, both maternal and paternal blood pressure was found to be directly correlated with offspring blood pressure to an extent which suggested that 24% of the incidence of offspring hypertension was associated with hereditary factors. Reduced infant birth weight was associated with maternal but not paternal blood pressure elevation.

Barker et al have proposed that low birth weight and hypertension in later life stem primarily from inadequate fetal nutrition or placental dysfunction which, in turn, programs the infant to pathology later in life. An equally valid hypothesis suggested here is that maternal hypertension results in small infants who simultaneously inherit the genetic tendency to hypertension present in the mother and possibly the father. This genetic predisposition with or without environmental factors results in later life pathology in the infants who are small for gestational age. An analogous argument may be made for insulin resistance as a confounding variable affecting newborn weight while simultaneously predisposing the offspring to abnormal lipid and carbohydrate metabolism in later life. Both alternative explanations need to be explored before the Barker hypothesis can be taken seriously.

T.H. Kirschbaum, M.D.

References

1. 1998 Year Book of Obstetrics, Gynecology, and Women's Health, pp 39–41.
2. Watt GCM, Fox CJW, Holten DW, et al: Prediction of high blood pressure in young people. *J Hypertension* 9:55, 1991.

Hyperhomocysteinaemia and Protein S Deficiency in Complicated Pregnancies

de Vries JIP, Dekker GA, Huijgens PC, et al (Free Univ Hosp, Amsterdam)
Br J Obstet Gynaecol 104:1248–1254, 1997 8–11

Objective.—Studies have found that maternal hyperhomocysteinemia and/or thrombophilic disorders are risk factors for placental abruption, intrauterine fetal death, and small for gestational age infants, but only 1 study described the presence of hypertension. The occurrence of metabolic and/or hemostatic abnormalities was evaluated in carefully selected pregnancies complicated by placental abruption, intrauterine fetal death, and small for gestational age infants in women without hypertension before and during pregnancy.

Methods.—Between January 1994 and December 1995, 62 women were admitted to the hospital with placental abruption (PA) (n = 31),

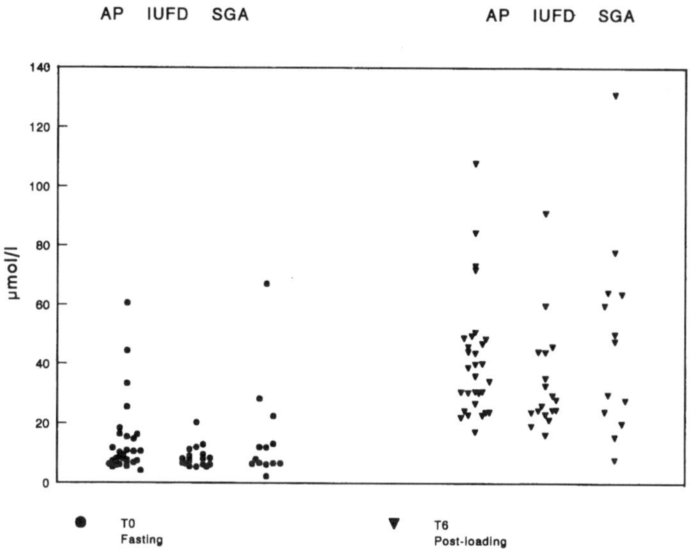

FIGURE 1.—Fasting and post-load total homocysteine levels in patients with placental abruption (PA, n=31), (IUFD, n=18), and (SGA, n=13). *Abbreviations: PA*, placental abruption; *IUFD*, intrauterine fetal death; *SGA*, small for gestational age. (Courtesy of de Vries JIP, Dekker GA, Huijgens PC, et al: Hyperhomocysteinaemia and protein S deficiency in complicated pregnancies. *Br J Obstet Gynaecol* 104:1248–1254, 1997 Blackwell Science Ltd.).

intrauterine fetal death (IUFD) (n = 18), or small for gestational age (SGA) infants (n = 13). Serum total homocysteine, protein S, protein C, antithrombin III, activated protein C resistance, factor V Leiden mutation, Lupus anticoagulant, and immunoglobulin (Ig) and Ig anticardiolipin antibodies were assessed at least 10 weeks after delivery. A methionine loading test was performed 2–4 weeks later. Women with hyperhomocysteinemia were given daily oral doses of pyridoxine (250 mg) and folic acid (5 mg).

Results.—At least 1 abnormality was found in 20 (65%) women in the PA group, 10 (56%) women in the IUFD group, and 11 (85%) women in the SGA group (Fig 1). Hyperhomocysteinemia was present in 15 (24%) of women, protein S deficiency in 16 (26%), protein C deficiency in 4 (6%), activated protein C resistance in 3 of 33 (9%), factor V Leiden mutation in 2 of 33 (6%), lupus anticoagulant in 1 (2%), anticardiolipin Ig 6 in 7 (11%), and anticardiolipin IgM in 1 (2%). After 6 weeks of vitamin-supplement therapy, fasting homocysteine levels had been reduced by 68% and post-load values had decreased by 65%.

Conclusion.—Women with PA, IUFD, or SGA should be evaluated for metabolic and/or hemostatic abnormalities even in the absence of thromboembolic disorders.

► Hyperhomocysteinaemia has been implicated as the possible cause of endothelial injury in pregnancy-induced hypertension (Abstract 3–9) and this cohort study explores the possible relationship between mild hyperhomocysteinaemia and placental abruption, fetal death, and intrauterine growth retardation in normotensive gravidas. Mild hyperhomocysteinaemia is marked by elevated plasma values less than 200 micro moles per liter after a provocative dose of methionine (0.1 gram per kilo). The upper limit of normal plasma concentration is in some dispute and has recently been altered as a result of an international conference on homocystine metabolism in 1995. In this report of the study of 62 puerperas, half have suffered a placental abruption and the remainder delivered a growth-retarded infant or sustained a fetal death. Provocative methionine testing was done 1 to 2 months after delivery, together with a series of related blood assays designed to demonstrate hypercoagulant tendencies. Some abnormality was noted in 41 women or two thirds of the study population. Most common was protein S deficiency in 26%, evidence of mild hyperhomocysteinaemia in 24%, and anticardiolipin antibody in 16%. The incidence of protein C deficiency and the Factor V Leiden mutation was not increased compared to controls. Six weeks of therapy with folic acid and pyridoxine in 9 women reduced post methionine load values of homocystine in several. This is part of an extended effort to explain pregnancy wastage not related to anatomic or developmental abnormalities or to the birth process. Perhaps there are patterns of metabolic abnormalities, genetically or environmentally conditioned or both. It is a worthwhile job and suggestive data such as this should stir continued efforts to clarify what at present are uncertain relationships.

T.H. Kirschbaum, M.D.

Randomised Trial to Assess Safety and Fetal Outcome of Early and Midtrimester Amniocentesis

Wilson RD, and the Canadian Early and Mid-trimester Amniocentesis Trial (CEMAT) Group (Univ of British Columbia, Vancouver)
Lancet 351:242–247, 1998 8–12

Background.—Midtrimester amniocentesis at 15–16 weeks of gestation is commonly used to diagnose chromosomal anomalies. However, an earlier, first-trimester amniocentesis at 11–12 weeks of gestation would be preferable for optimizing management of the pregnancy. The safety and fetal outcomes of amniocenteses performed either early or midtrimester were compared in a multicenter study.

Methods.—Women were randomly assigned to undergo early amniocentesis (n = 2,183), or midtrimester amniocentesis (n = 2,185). All patients were contacted at 20–22 weeks gestation and at 3–5 weeks after the infant's birth to determine the pregnancy outcome.

Findings.—The 2 groups did not differ significantly in the number of cases of premature rupture of membranes after 22 weeks, preterm delivery, or intrauterine or neonatal death at or after 20 weeks. However, the group undergoing early amniocentesis had a significantly increased total pregnancy loss rate (7.64%) compared with the group undergoing midtrimester amniocentesis (5.92%). Furthermore, amniotic fluid leakage was significantly more common in the early amniocentesis group (3.5%) than in the group tested midtrimester (1.7%). Congenital anomalies at birth occurred in both groups, but talipes equinovarus was significantly more common in the early amniocentesis group (29 cases) than in the midtrimester group (2 cases). Even within the early amniocentesis group, talipes equinovarus was significantly more common when the procedure was done at 11 weeks rather than at 12 weeks.

Conclusions.—Amniocentesis at 11–12 weeks gestation was associated with significantly increased risks for pregnancy loss, amniotic fluid leakage, and talipes equinovarus.

► Certainly genetic amniocentesis performed in the first rather than the second trimester of pregnancy is preferable in the event that the results constitute an indication for induced abortion. An interest in first-trimester maternal serum biochemical screening for Down syndrome recently reported has the same motivation. (Abstract 4–1) Although studies of the relative merits of first- and second-trimester amniocentesis have been reported[1] this Canadian collaborative study involving 12 centers and almost 4,400 women prospectively randomized between first- and second-trimester amniocenteses is by far the largest and most authoritative such work. Patients were divided into 2 study groups, one at 10–12 completed weeks of gestation and the other at 15–17 completed weeks. After the procedure, phone contact was made at 20–22 weeks of gestation and 3–5 weeks after the EDC. Eighty to ninety percent of patients underwent amniocentesis at the time designated at randomization.

First-trimester amniocentesis resulted in a larger total pregnancy loss (7.6 % vs. 5.9%), a larger number of failed diagnostic attempts (1.7% vs. 0.2%), and a higher incidence of fetal euploid anomalies (3.9% vs. 2.4%) than did second-trimester procedures. The surplus anomaly rate resulted almost entirely from an increased risk of talipes equinovarus in the first-trimester cohort (1.3% vs 0.1%). The occurrence of talipes appeared to center about amniocenteses done at 12 weeks gestational age. This finding appears to reflect the longer increased risk of amniotic fluid leak from 12–22 weeks in the first-trimester group than in the midtrimester group. This hypothesis is supported by the 15% incidence risk of talipes with amniotic fluid leak vs. the 1% incidence in second-trimester amniocentesis without leaks. Although the postamniocentesis spontaneous pregnancy loss rate was greater in the first-trimester group (2.6% vs. 0.8%), comparisons are difficult because the first-trimester group had a longer postamniocentesis interval at risk than did the second-trimester group. No differences in rates of perinatal death, neonatal death, preterm delivery, or premature rupture of membranes after 22 weeks were seen between the groups. Besides providing clarification of the causes of some cases of talipes equinovarus, this study provides the clearest view to date of the complication rates of early diagnostic amniocentesis. The advantages of early diagnostic amniocentesis must be weighed against the increased rate of complications.

T.H. Kirschbaum, M.D.

Reference

1. 1992 Year Book of Obstetrics And Gynecology, pp 95–96.

Pregnancy Outcome Following Maternal Use of the New Selective Serotonin Reuptake Inhibitors: A Prospective Controlled Multicenter Study

Kulin NA, Pastuszak A, Sage SR, et al (Univ of Toronto; Teratogen Information Service, Tampa, Fla; Pennsylvania Hosp, Philadelphia; et al)

JAMA 279:609–610, 1998 8–13

Background.—Selective serotonin reuptake inhibitors, introduced about 10 years ago, are now used for depression by millions of individuals around the world. Fetal safety is a major concern because more than 50% of all pregnancies are unplanned, and an estimated 8% to 20% of all women have depression. Studies of pregnancy outcome after maternal exposure to fluoxetine have reported no evidence of major malformations or behavioral teratology, although women exposed to fluoxetine throughout their pregnancy did have more perinatal complications and minor malformations. New selective serotonin reuptake inhibitors have been introduced in the last few years. There is no data on their reproductive safety in humans.

Methods.—Nine teratology information service centers in the United States and Canada participated in a study of fetal safety and risk of fluvoxamine, paroxetine, and sertraline. The rate of major congenital malformations was determined in women who were counseled during pregnancy and followed up after exposure to fluvoxamine, paroxetine, or sertraline. The rate of major congenital malformations was also determined in a group of control subjects who were counseled after exposure to nonteratogenic agents.

Results.—There were 267 women who took fluvoxamine, paroxetine, or sertraline for depression in the first trimester of pregnancy; 267 control subjects were also analyzed. Exposure to the selective serotonin reuptake inhibitors was not associated with a higher risk of major malformations or a higher rate of miscarriage, stillbirth, or prematurity. The mean birth weight and gestational age were similar in both the study and control groups.

Discussion.—These findings indicate that fluvoxamine, paroxetine, and sertraline do not increase the risk of major congenital malformations in pregnant women when used at recommended doses. On all measured pregnancy outcomes, these results were well within the results reported for the general population.

▶ Originally introduced in the form of fluoxetine (Prozac), this class of agents acts to increase CNS serotonin activity by inhibiting its reuptake after release by serotonergic neurones in the brain stem, thalamus, and hypothalamus. The impact of these drugs is to decrease depressive ideation and symptoms. Their use has proliferated enormously and a number of products with similar actions have been marketed over the past few years. Exposure of a pregnant woman to these agents before or, during labor, or both, has become commonplace, and questions regarding their safety have increased in number in parallel. Evidence that the drug is not harmful to the developing fetus can never be totally conclusive, but security in its use rests in the number of well-conducted studies that have sought, but failed, to find any deleterious effects.

A study of the infants of 80 women using these agents has failed to find evidence of intellectual, language developmental or behavioral abnormality as an associated finding.[1] This report of 267 women contacting 1 of 9 teratology information centers in the United States and Canada and interviewed at contact and 6–9 months after giving birth comes from the Division of Clinical Pharmacology and Toxicology at Toronto's Hospital for Sick Children. The cohort study using controls matched for parity, age, spontaneous abortions, and alcohol use (but not for gravidity, abortion procedures, or tobacco use), found no surplus of major malformations, fetal deaths, reduced birthweight or gestational age at birth, or spontaneous abortions among antidepressant users. It can be fairly said that, after a reasonable search, no teratologic effects from this class of agents has yet been found.

T.H. Kirschbaum, M.D.

Reference

1. 1998 Year Book of Obstetrics, Gynecology, and Women's Health, pp 215–216.

Isolated Single Umbilical Artery Anomaly and the Risk for Congenital Malformations: A Meta-analysis

Thummala MR, Raju TNK, Langenberg P, et al (Univ of Illinois, Chicago; Univ of Maryland, Baltimore)

J Pediatr Surg 33:580–585, 1998 8–14

Background.—Single umbilical artery occurs in many chromosomal abnormalities and congenital malformations, but it can also occur as an isolated anomaly. It is unclear how much diagnostic intervention and follow-up study we need in infants with single umbilical artery as an isolated anomaly.

Methods.—A meta-analysis was conducted of 37 studies of single umbilical artery that were published between 1952 and 1995. The studies were divided into 2 groups. In group 1, the diagnosis of single umbilical artery was made using specimens from early abortuses, fetal deaths, or autopsies. In group 2, the diagnosis was made using placental and umbilical cord specimens from live-born infants, or using the umbilicus soon after birth.

Results.—The incidence of single umbilical artery was 2.13% in group 1 and 0.55% in group 2. The incidence of congenital malformation associated with single umbilical artery was 66.3% in group 1 and 27.0% in group 2. These differences were considered significant. In group 2, further urologic examinations were performed in 7 of 26 studies in a total of 204 infants with single umbilical artery as an anomaly. Of these 204 infants, 33 had a renal anomaly, but 18 of the 33 were minor or self-limiting. In a cost-benefit analysis, it was determined that 14 cases of isolated single umbilical artery anomaly needed to be investigated to detect 1 major renal malformation. The value of early detection was unclear because most of these malformations would have been revealed in a good pediatric examination.

Discussion.—In the case of isolated single umbilical artery anomaly in an infant who is otherwise healthy, a small increase in risk of renal malformation exists. This risk is similar to the risk of another anomaly in the presence of 1 anomaly. In infants with isolated single umbilical artery anomaly, most renal malformations are minor and self-limiting. Major malformations are of the type that would be diagnosed during a good examination with a thorough evaluation of the urogenital system. These findings do not support extensive urologic radiographic studies in asymptomatic infants with isolated single umbilical artery anomaly, unless there are additional risk factors for renal malformation.

► The authors use meta-analysis to estimate the occurrence rate of single umbilical artery (SUA) at birth and the frequency of associated urinary tract anomaly. As always, the problem with meta-analysis is with the assumption that all aggregated studies are fundamentally the same. Here, differences in experimental design, the nature of controls, variation between reported cohorts, the nature of newborn workups, and differences between trivial and consequential anomalies all represent challenges. Most useful are 26 reports of examinations of live-born infants, 16 reports using pathological confirmation of the SUA diagnosis and 7 using urologic workups, in 204 cases of isolated SUA with no overt evidence of anomaly. The mean incidence of associated developmental urinary anomaly was 11.3%. But the range of incidence (9% to 50%) among various reports attests to differences in cohort composition and to problems with comparisons. Among the 204 cases in which urologic evaluation was done, the incidence of major occult urinary tract anomaly was 7.4%. Cost-benefit analysis based on such small populations is hazardous, but the authors' conclusion seems appropriate. In the absence of evident anomaly, urologic workup should not be routinely done on infants with SUA, should be done but only if the newborn exhibits abnormal findings, or if problems in subsequent development appear. It is interesting that SUA occurs twice as often in white as in black patients, on the basis of 2 studies.

T.H. Kirschbaum, M.D.

9 The Newborn

The Effect of Antenatal Phenobarbital Therapy on Neonatal Intracranial Hemorrhage in Preterm Infants

Shankaran S, Papile L-A, Wright LL, et al (Wayne State Univ, Detroit; Univ of New Mexico, Albuquerque; Natl Inst of Child Health and Human Development, Bethesda, Md; et al)

N Engl J Med 337:466–471, 1997 9–1

Background.—Prevention of cerebral, intraventricular, and periventricular hemorrhage in preterm infants may be attempted by the use of drugs such as indomethacin or phenobarbital. Although such interventions may reduce the likelihood and severity of intracranial hemorrhage, nearly 50% of hemorrhages occur before postnatal intervention can be attempted. Previous studies have suggested that administration of phenobarbital during the antenatal period may decrease intracranial hemorrhage frequency and severity in infants. The effectiveness of antenatal phenobarbital administration in the prevention of intracranial hemorrhage and early death in preterm infants was further evaluated in this study.

Methods.—Six hundred ten women between 24 and 33 weeks pregnant and expected to deliver within the subsequent 24 hours were included in the study. Phenobarbital, at 10 mg/kg body weight, was infused intravenously over 20–40 minutes in 309 women, and a saline placebo was administered to the remaining 301 women. Women who failed to deliver within 24 hours were given 100 mg of phenobarbital or placebo orally, once daily, until delivery or maintenance of the pregnancy beyond 33 weeks. The clinical outcome of each infant was monitored until the 120th day of hospitalization, discharge from the neonatal ICU, or death. Infants were monitored for intracranial hemorrhages by intracranial ultrasonography.

Results.—Three hundred forty four infants were born to the 309 women in the phenobarbital group, and 324 infants to the 301 women in the placebo group. Intracranial hemorrhage or death in the 72 hours following birth occurred in 24% of infants in the phenobarbital group (relative risk of 1.1) and 23% of those in the placebo group. Of infants born before a gestational age of 34 weeks, the incidence of intracranial hemorrhage was 23% in both the phenobarbital and placebo groups, for a relative risk of 1.0 for the phenobarbital group. No difference in hemorrhage severity between the two groups was noted.

Conclusions.—There is apparently no protective effect of antenatally administered phenobarbital on intracranial hemorrhage in preterm infants. The use of phenobarbital in the antenatal period as prophylaxis for neonatal intracranial hemorrhage is not supported based on the results of this trial.

► In 1992, the publication entitled *Effective Care of the Newborn* provided results of a meta-analysis that indicated the potential value of maternal phenobarbital prior to delivery in preventing neonatal intracranial hemorrhage (ICH). The rationale was, at least in part, that sedative effect in the newborn might reduce the large variations of premature newborn blood pressure, particularly as they struggle against cyclic endotracheal ventilation. Despite 3 subsequently generally supportive publications, this prospective randomized controlled study conducted under the auspices of the National Institute of Child Health and Human Development Neonatal Research Network failed to show any benefit from 10 mg per kilo maternal weight of phenobarbital administered more than 2 hours before birth in 610 gravidas. Study entry was confined to 24–33 weeks' gestational age and there was a high incidence of preterm birth, with all but 7% of women delivering before 35 weeks' gestation. This generated a large population of newborns at risk for ICH. Newborn evaluation was made at the time of discharge from the NICU and at 12–22 months of age thereafter. At neither interval were significant differences in outcomes seen between phenobarbital treated and control infants. Perhaps the recommendation for phenobarbital was valid in an earlier decade before advances in neonatal care began to reduce the incidence of ICH. There is no evidence here that the drug is useful in this regard.

T.H. Kirschbaum, M.D.

Reference

1. Sinclair JC, Bracken MB (eds). *Effective Care of the Newborn.* London, 1992, p. 562.

Outcome of Infants Born at 24–26 Weeks' Gestation: I. Survival and Cost

Kilpatrick SJ, Schlueter MA, Piecuch R, et al (Cardiovascular Research Inst, San Francisco; Univ of California, San Francisco)
Obstet Gynecol 90:803–808, 1997 9–2

Introduction.—In even very preterm infants, including those born before 28 weeks' gestation, antenatal steroids and exogenous surfactant treatment improve morbidity and mortality. For fetuses born at 24–26 weeks' gestation where antepartum steroids and exogenous surfactant were routinely used, morbidity and mortality were determined. The hospital cost to care for these infants was also determined.

TABLE 1.—Prenatal Characteristics

	24 Weeks (n = 42)	25 Weeks (n = 42)	26 Weeks (n = 54)	P
Maternal age (y)	26 ± 6	29 ± 6	26 ± 7	.058
Nulliparity	26 (62%)	13 (31%)	25 (46%)	.017
Race*				.267
White	15 (41%)	18 (50%)	26 (52%)	
Black	11 (30%)	2 (6%)	8 (16%)	
Latina	7 (19%)	11 (31%)	13 (26%)	
Asian	3 (8%)	4 (11%)	3 (6%)	
Other	1 (3%)	1 (3%)	0	
Betamethasone	28 (67%)	37 (88%)	49 (91%)	.004
Multiple gestation	6 (14%)	12 (29%)	7 (13%)	.106
Indication for delivery				
Preterm labor	20 (48%)	16 (38%)	18 (33%)	.35
PROM	19 (45%)	18 (43%)	25 (46%)	.94
Medically indicated	3 (7%)	8 (19%)	11 (20%)	.172

SD = standard deviation; PROM = premature rupture of membranes.
Data are presented as mean ± standard deviation or n (%).
*Percentages are adjusted for missing data.
(Courtesy of Kilpatrick SJ, Schlueter MA, Piecuch R, et al: Outcome of Infants Born at 24–26 Weeks' Gestation: I. Survival and Cost. *Obstet Gynecol* 90:803–808, 1997. Reprinted with permission from The American College of Obstetricians and Gynecologists.)

Methods.—For pregnancies delivered at 24 to 26 weeks during 5-year period, survival, short-term outcome, and initial hospital charges were compared in this retrospective study by using the corresponding institutional cost-charge ratio, hospital costs for each year were calculated. There were 42 infants born at 24 weeks, 42 born at 25 weeks and 54 born at 26 weeks. There were 41% to 52% white babies and 6% to 30% black babies (Table 1).

TABLE 4.—Neonatal Morbidity of Surviving Infants

	24 Weeks (n = 18)	25 Weeks (n = 31)	26 Weeks (n = 45)	P
Retinopathy of prematurity ≥ stage III	6 (33%)	4 (13%)	2 (4%)	.008
Chronic lung disease	6 (33%)	5 (16%)	3 (7%)	.026
Necrotizing enterocolitis	2 (11%)	1 (3%)	4 (9%)	.52
Intracranial hemorrhage ≥ grade 3	2 (11%)	5 (16%)	2 (4%)	.23
Periventricular leukomalacia without intracranial hemorrhage	0	2 (6%)	2 (4%)	.56
Positive culture*	14.8	17.3	13.0	
Hospital days†	120 ± 39 (48–220)	86 ± 27 (28–132)	80 ± 33 (18–179)	<.001
Days mechanical ventilation‡	76 ± 25 (41–133)	58 ± 19 (21–90)	45 ± 19 (4–81)	<.001

Data are presented as mean ± standard deviation (range) or n (%).
*Positive culture included positive blood, cerebral spinal fluid, and urine cultures reported as number of episodes of infection per 1,000 hospital days.
†Significantly different between 24 and 25 weeks and between 24 and 26 weeks but no significant difference between 25 and 26 weeks by Scheffe post hoc test.
‡Significantly different between all gestational ages by Scheffe post hoc test.
(Courtesy of Kilpatrick SJ, Schlueter MA, Piecuch R, et al: Outcome of Infants Born at 24–26 Weeks' Gestation: I. Survival and Cost. *Obstet Gynecol* 90:803–808, 1997. Reprinted with permission from The American College of Obstetricians and Gynecologists.)

TABLE 5.—Cost for Surviving Infants

	24 Weeks	25 Weeks	26 Weeks	Total
Total infants*	32†	37‡	54	123
Total cost (millions)	$5.3	$5.6	$7.5	$18.4
Surviving infants	18	31	45	94
Total hospital days for surviving infants	2167	2652	3610	8429
Total cost for surviving infants (millions)	$4.4	$5.4	$7.1	$16.9
Cost per day for surviving infants	$2028	$2042	$1975	$2010
Cost per survivor	$294,749	$181,062	$166,215	$195,724

*Excludes stillborn and nonresuscitated infants.
†No cost data available for 2 infants.
‡No cost data available for 3 infants.
(Courtesy of Kilpatrick SJ, Schlueter MA, Piecuch R, et al: Outcome of Infants Born at 24–26 Weeks' Gestation: I. Survival and Cost. *Obstet Gynecol* 90:803–808, 1997. Reprinted with permission from The American College of Obstetricians and Gynecologists.)

Results.—After excluding infants with severe anomalies, 138 infants were included in the study. The survival rate was 43% at 24 weeks, 74% at 25 weeks and 83% at 26 weeks. Antenatal steroids were given to the majority of women and exogenous surfactant was given to the majority of surviving neonates. From 24 to 26 weeks, there was a significant decrease in severe retinopathy of prematurity and chronic lung disease (Table 4). At 24 weeks, the likelihood of having a surviving infant without severe retinopathy or chronic lung disease was 35%. At 26 weeks, this increased to 78%. For the 29 nonsurvivors, hospital costs were $1.46 million. For the 94 surviving infants, hospital costs were $16.9 million. At each gestational age, the cost per day was similar. To produce a survivor at 24 weeks, the cost was $294,649; at 25 weeks, it was $181,062; and at 26 weeks, it was $166,215 (Table 5).

Conclusion.—Despite treatment with antenatal steroids and exogenous surfactant, survival at 24 weeks was only 43%. For infants born at 24 weeks, the cost per survivor was higher than the cost for those born after 1 more week in utero. There was a marked improvement in outcome between 24 and 26 weeks. There are large economic differences in the small differences in gestational age. Pregnancy should be prolonged, and treatment options including nonintervention should be available to parents of 24-week gestation if prolongation is unsuccessful.

▶ Survival data for very low birth weight infants vary considerably with time and with the availability and employment of steroids and surfactant administration from 1 center to another. This retrospective cohort study of infants born from 24–26 weeks' gestational age at UCSF between 1990 and 1994 reflects current nearly optimal neonatal care with 100% of 138 newborns receiving surfactant and 84% exposed to antenatal corticosteroids. Data analysis is well done, and fetal deaths and infants not resuscitated are included in outcome data, making it particularly useful for counseling. In only 40% of cases was spontaneous labor the cause of immature birth. The rest followed spontaneous premature membrane rupture or delivery opted for obstetrical complications. Total survival for infants completing 24 weeks' gestation was 43%, an order of magnitude less than survival at 25 and 26 completed weeks. In addition, 24-week survivors showed a 33% incidence of severe retinopathy and chronic lung disease. With each subsequent week of fetal life, the incidence of those 2 dominant complications halved and survival increased dramatically. Cost estimates from hospital records adjusted by Medicare cost to charge ratios are not easy to interpret. Though costs per survivor are large for 24 week infants, that figure is dependent on the fetal death rate and the length of life among the 38% who succumbed in the hospital. Cost per day per survivor, roughly the same for all 3 groups, reflects the shortened cost interval for neonatal and fetal deaths and the shortened hospitalization interval for 26-week pregnancies. One conclusion seems clear. In the interest of intact survival, completion of the 25th gestational week in utero is very important. Every perinatal unit should have data of this sort available to inform women with spontaneous premature rupture of membranes or severe complications sufficient to motivate premature delivery of the implications. This fine unit provides a basis for comparing quality of perinatal care among other units as well.

T.H. Kirschbaum, M.D.

Outcome of Infants Born at 24–26 Weeks' Gestation: II. Neurodevelopmental Outcome

Piecuch RE, Leonard CH, Cooper BA, et al (Univ of California, San Francisco; California School of Professional Psychology, Alameda)

Obstet Gynecol 90:809–814, 1997 9–3

Introduction.—Before the routine use of exogenous surfactant, infants born between 23–25 weeks' gestation had a 32% to 67% rate of handicap that was defined as cerebral palsy, blindness, deafness, and low Bayley Mental Development Index scores. In very premature infants, medical risk factors and social risk factors have been associated with poor outcome.

TABLE 2.—Neurologic and Cognitive Outcome

	24 Weeks	25 Weeks	26 Weeks
No. of infants followed	18	30	38
Neurologically normal	12 (67%)	22 (73%)	34 (89%)
Neurologically suspicious	4 (22%)	2 (7%)	0
Cerebral palsy	2 (11%)	6 (20%)	4 (11%)
Normal cognitive development	5 (28%)	14 (47%)	27 (71%)
Borderline cognitive development	6 (33%)	7 (23%)	7 (18%)
Deficient cognitive development	7 (39%)	9 (30%)	4 (11%)

Data are presented as *n* (%).

Kruskal-Wallis $\chi 2 = 10.6542$, $P = 0.005$ for cognitive outcome and gestational age.

(Courtesy of Piecuch RE, Leonard CH, Cooper BA, et al: Outcome of infants born at 24–26 weeks' gestation: II: Neurodevelopmental outcome. *Obstet Gynecol* 90:809–814, 1997.)

TABLE 3.—Neurologic and/or Cognitive Deficits

	24 Weeks	25 Weeks	26 Weeks
No. of infants	18	30	38
No deficit	5 (28%)	14 (47%)	24 (63%)
One deficit	7 (39%)	7 (23%)	13 (34%)
Two or more deficits	6 (33%)	9 (30%)	1 (3%)

Data are presented as *n* (%).
Kruskal-Wallis $\chi 2 = 9.5813$, $P = 0.008$
(Courtesy of Piecuch RE, Leonard CH, Cooper BA, et al: Outcome of infants born at 24–26 weeks' gestation: II: Neurodevelopmental outcome. *Obstet Gynecol* 90:809–814, 1997. Reprinted with permission from The American College of Obstetricians and Gynecologists.)

Infants born at extremely low gestational age were followed up to evaluate their outcome and to determine whether gestational age is related to outcome.

Methods.—After pregnancies of 24–26 weeks' gestation in a 5-year period, there were 138 nonanomalous infants born. There were 94 infants that survived to discharge and 86 that were followed up in a nursery for outcome. An analysis was conducted of any association between neurodevelopmental outcome, gestational age, and risk factors and outcome. At follow-up, the mean age was 32 months.

Results.—In the 3 groups, the frequency of cerebral palsy did not differ, with 11% at 24 weeks, 20% at 25 weeks, and 11% at 26 weeks (Table 2). Gestational age at birth was significantly associated with the incidence of normal cognitive outcome with 28% normal at 24 weeks, 47% normal at 25 weeks, and 61% normal at 26 weeks (Table 3). The medical risk factor of intracranial hemorrhage grade 3 or 4 or periventricular leukomalacia was associated with poor neurologic outcome. Medical and social risk factors were associated with poor cognitive outcome. Regardless of the relationships of any other risk factors to cognitive outcome, lower gestational age was associated with poor cognitive outcome.

Conclusion.—The high percentage of infants born at 24–25 weeks' gestation with cognitive deficits is of concern, although the incidence of cerebral palsy was low in these 3 groups.

► This companion to the previous report provides an account of neurodevelopmental studies done on 86 infants born between 24–26 weeks' gestation who survived to be discharged from the NICU. The follow-up evaluations were done for at least the first year of life at 3 month intervals, and they provide some new associative interpretations regarding short- and long-term outcomes. The incidence of neurologic abnormalities increased with gestational age, but the increase did not reach levels of statistical validity. Probably the reason for this increase was that neurologic impairment depended so heavily on the occurrence of intracranial hemorrhage and periventricular leukomalacia, both of which were more likely related to NICU events than to birth trauma. There was, however, a significant inverse relationship between gestational age and evidence of cognitive impairment and of multiple neurologic and/or cognitive defects. This was true even when multiple regression was used to control for covariants such as social risk, substance abuse, chronic newborn lung disease, and intracranial hemorrhage. Much of what has been learned about perinatal brain injury has been based on the occurrence of cerebral palsy, and this is a first convincing attempt to deal with the occurrence of what have been termed "soft" neurologic deficits in prematures related to perinatal events. In summary, the probability that an infant surviving after 24 completed weeks' gestation will have normal or borderline cognitive function is 26%. At 25 weeks it is 52%, and at 26 completed weeks it is 74%. Combining this derived data with the chances for survival, the preceding yields probabilities of survival with intact cognitive development of 11% at 24 weeks, 39% at 25 weeks, and 61% at 26 weeks. It is important that this information be shared with women undergoing medically indicated delivery during this gestational interval.

T.H. Kirschbaum, M.D.

The Addition of Indomethacin to Betamimetics for Tocolysis: Any Benefit for the Neonate?

Van Overmeire B, Slootmaekers V, De Loor J, et al (Univ Hosp of Antwerp, Belgium)

Eur J Obstet Gynecol Reprod Biol 77:41–45, 1998 9–4

Introduction.—Indomethacin is used as a tocolytic agent, either initially or as a secondary agent when betamimetics fail to inhibit preterm uterine contractions. In this setting, indomethacin inhibits prostaglandin synthesis, but complications may also occur. A retrospective study compared outcome in 2 groups of low-birth-weight infants: those whose mothers received both betamimetics and indomethacin (study group) and those whose mothers were treated with betamimetics alone (control group).

Methods.—The gestational age of all 76 infants was less than 33 weeks. The 2 treatment groups were closely matched for gestational age and birth weight and had similar rates of preterm premature rupture of membranes and prenatal corticosteroid treatment. When IV betamimetics failed to arrest uterine contractions, indomethacin was given according to the obstetrician's discretion. Most patients received 2 doses of 12 mg betamethasone 24 hours apart. Indomethacin was administered intrarectally (50 mg 3 times daily).

Results.—The groups receiving betamethasone alone and betamethasone plus indomethacin were similar in neonatal characteristics. The incidence of respiratory distress syndrome (RDS) was significantly increased, however, in the study group (97%) vs. the control group (45%). Treatment with both agents was also associated with an increased need for surfactant administration (68% vs. 26%), more ventilation days and more days on supplemental oxygen, and an increased incidence of bronchopulmonary dysplasia (BPD, 47% vs. 24%) (Table 2). Three independent risk factors were identified for RDS (indomethacin treatment, gestational age, and

TABLE 2.—Respiratory Evolution of Neonates*

	Control group (n=38	Study group n=38	P
RDS	17 (45)	37 (97)	≅001
Surfactant use	10 (26)	26 (68)	<0.001
Surfactant doses	17	59	<0.01
Ventilation days	363	589	0.01
Oxygen days	604	1015	0.1
BPD	9 (24)	18 (47)	0.03
Pneumothorax	1 (3)	2 (5)	0.50

*Results in numbers (%) or totals.

Abbreviations: RDS, respiratory distress syndrome; *BPD*, bronchopulmonary dysplasia.

(Courtesy of Van Overmeire B, Slootmaekers V, De Loor J, et al: The addition of indomethacin to betamimetics for tocolysis: Any benefit for the neonate? *Eur J Obstet Gynecol Reprod Biol* 77:41–45, 1998.)

Apgar score at 5 minutes) and 2 for BPD (gestational age and antenatal indomethacin treatment). The 2 groups were similar in occurrence of pneumothorax and incidence of death, necrotizing enterocolitis, sepsis, and intraventricular hemorrhage grades II to IV.

Conclusion.—The addition of indomethacin to betamethasone did not significantly prolong gestation in women with premature uterine contractions. Indomethacin was associated with an increased incidence of RDS, surfactant use, and BPD.

► The effects of indomethacin given after betamethasone with premature rupture of membranes to infants at less than 32 weeks of gestation include an impressive array of side effects—intraventricular hemorrhage, necrotizing enterocolitis, and premature closure of the ductus arteriosus.[1] The agent freely crosses the placenta, it has a long half-life, and often the resultant fetal oliguria appears to help guarantee prolonged fetal exposure to the drug will follow maternal dosage. Here the question is, given 76 pregnancies of less than 33 weeks' gestation treated unsuccessfully with Ritodrine, what is the positive effect of adding indomethacin as a secondary agent? Although the control group, which did not receive the prostocycline synthetase inhibitor, was well matched for premature membrane rupture incidence (approximately 50%), there was a surplus of women receiving betamethasone in the study group (84% vs. 68%), which should have, if anything, resulted in somewhat less likelihood of respiratory distress syndrome in the indomethacin-treated group. The incidence of respiratory distress syndrome is not significantly different between treated and untreated groups, primarily because of small sample sizes. The same problem deprives the greater death rate among study participants receiving indomethacin of statistical significance (16% vs. 5%). The important conclusion here stems from multivariate analyis and the increased incidence of newborn respiratory problems—respiratory distress syndrome, need for ventilation support, and bronchopulmonary dysplasia. Indomethacin use in prematurity appears significantly related to both respiratory distress syndrome and bronchopulmonary dysplasia, independent of confounding variables in the infant. Prostaglandin species play such an important nearly ubiquitous role in fetal physiology that it seems dangerous to administer an agent that inhibits their formation as a tocolytic, ignoring the implications of that step to fetal organ systems. Even as a tocolytic, it didn't prove of value here.

T.H. Kirschbaum, M.D.

Reference

1. 1995 Year Book of Obstetrics, and Gynecology, pp 246–248.

Neonatal Effects and Serum Cortisol Levels After Multiple Courses of Maternal Corticosteroids

Terrone DA, Smith LG Jr, Wolf EJ, et al (Saint Barnabas Med Ctr, Livingston, NJ)

Obstet Gynecol 90:819–823, 1997 9–5

Introduction.—It is now common practice to administer parenteral corticosteroids to mothers at risk for preterm birth. In newborns whose mothers were treated with antenatal corticosteroids, neonatal survival had improved and frequency of respiratory distress syndrome and intraventricular hemorrhage had decreased. After a period of treatment for 7 days, the benefits of therapy seem to dissipate, thus some protocols suggest repeating corticosteroids doses each week until delivery or 34 weeks' gestation, although this practice remains controversial. This prospective observational study was conducted to determine whether multiple doses of antenatal corticosteroids resulted in cumulative suppression of day 1 and day 3 neonatal serum cortisol levels or neonatal Cushing syndrome.

Methods.—The study included 79 mother-infant pairs delivered between 24 and 36 weeks'gestation. They were divided into 3 groups according to the number of courses of betamethasone received—those receiving no courses, one course, or 2 or more courses. On days 1 and 3 of life, physical examinations were performed and serum glucose, electrolyte, and cortisol levels were measured.

Results.—The mean number of courses for those receiving multiple courses of betamethasone was 5.3 ± 0.4 and a mean total dose of 125 ± 10.7 mg. Cushing syndrome was not seen in any of the neonates. In those receiving no courses, day 1 cortisol level was 12.6 ± 2.4; for those receiving 1 course, the level was 5.3 ± 3.2; and for those receiving 2 or more courses, the level was 4.4 ± 1.8 µg/dL. When corrected for multiple variables, the differences were not significant. There were no significant differences among the 3 groups in day 3 cortisol levels. Day 1 cortisol levels were not lower than normal in any of the neonates in the group receiving no courses of betamethasone. Day 1 levels were lower than normal in 22% of those receiving one course and were 11% for those receiving two or more courses. Serum cortisol levels were also lower than normal on day 3 for 15% of those receiving 1 course and for 10% of those receiving 2 or more courses. A low cortisol level was not seen for any who had no courses.

Conclusion.—There is no suppressive effect with repeated dosing because it was found that serum cortisol levels were independent of the number of courses or total dose of corticosteroids given or, in a subpopulation, were associated with increasing levels with increasing doses.

▶ Since the 1994 recommendation by the National Institutes of Health Consensus Development Conference that the effects of repeated maternal betamethasone administration on the newborn warranted study, a number of studies such as this, often comprised of small numbers of cases, have appeared and some publications from the 1980s have gained renewed interest. It is reasonably clear, however, that fetuses are partially protected from glucocorticoid administration by placental 11 beta hydroxysteroid dehydrogenase activity which converts 11 hydroxysteroids to their relatively inert keto forms. Thirty-two of the 79 newborns in this study were from the first of multiple pregnancies. The endpoint is newborn blood cortisol concentrations, half obtained on day 1 and half on day 3 of life. Aggregated data comparing untreated controls with infants receiving one course (18 infants) and two or more courses (43 infants) showed lower newborn cortisol mean values in infants of treated mothers. However, when multivariate regression was employed to eliminate the possible effects of race, fetal number, gestational age and birth weight, severity of respiratory distress syndrome (RDS), serum glucose, and electrolyte concentrations, no significant differences suggestive of fetal adrenal suppression could be demonstrated. It is likely the lack of control of age at sampling and the relationship of first to multiple siblings cloud the issue in this case. However, others have demonstrated reduced serum cortisol concentration in such infants[1] as well as impaired adrenal response to neonatal ACTH administration.[2] As in this case, the value of steroid administration in reducing the incidence of RDS remains unchallenged. Despite occasional claims of minor growth retardation in such infants, no deleterious effects in clinical performance have been demonstrated in infants exposed to multiple maternal dosage to this point.

T.H. Kirschbaum, M.D.

References

1. Teramo K, Hallman M, Raivio KO. Maternal glucocorticoid in unplanned premature labor. Controlled study on the effects of betamethasone phosphate on the phospholipids of gastric aspirate and on the adrenal cortical function of the newborn infant. *Pediatr Res* 1980; 14:326–329.
2. Evans MI, Chrousos GP, Mann DW. Pharmacologic suppression of the fetal adrenal gland in utero. *JAMA* 1985; 253:1015–1020.

Disproportionate Consumption of Ventilator Resources by Very Preterm Survivors Persists in the 1990s

Amir I, Doyle LW, Davis P, et al (Royal Women's Hosp, Carlton Victoria, Australia)

Am J Perinatol 15:187–190, 1998 9–6

Background.—Using data from 1977 to 1985, these authors found that as the gestational age of newborns decreased, their duration of hospitalization and use of nursery resources (particularly assisted ventilation) increased. In this report, they expand upon their previous studies, by including current data (up to 1995) on the use of ventilator and nursery resources by preterm infants (before 31 weeks' gestational age).

Methods.—All liveborn infants between 23 and 30 weeks (inclusive) of gestation born between 1977 and 1995 at a tertiary perinatal center were included, except for those with lethal congenital abnormalities and those who were transferred to another level III nursery. Infants were stratified according to their era of birth: 1977–1985 (N = 1,108), when systematic ventilation came into use; 1986–1990 (N = 835), before the use of exogenous surfactant; and 1991–1995 (N = 858), during the era of exogenous surfactant. The duration of an infant's use of assisted ventilation of any sort was recorded as patient-days of assisted ventilation (partial days were counted as whole days), and the patient-days off ventilation but before discharge were also recorded.

Findings.—Over the study period, the survival rate to hospital discharge for these very preterm infants increased significantly (odds ratio, 2.11) for each week of increase in gestational age. Furthermore, the survival rate increased significantly with time (Table 2). In fact, in the first 2 time periods, no infants born before 24 weeks' gestational age survived, whereas in the third era, 7 of 37 of these premature infants (18.9%) did so. Along with increased survival came significantly more patient-days of assisted ventilation as the eras progressed (mean, 7.4 ± 12.9, 11.5 ± 17.7,

TABLE 2.—Survival Rates to Hospital Discharge by Gestational Age for Each Era

Era—years of birth		*Gestational Age (Weeks)*								
		23	*24*	*25*	*26*	*27*	*28*	*29*	*30*	*23–30*
1977–1985	Livebirths (n)	32	68	67	129	112	180	145	274	1007
	Survivors (n)	0	2	10	60	77	148	123	254	674
	(%) survived	0	2.9	14.9	46.5	68.8	82.2	84.8	92.7	66.9
1986–1990	Livebirths (n)	32	32	53	80	100	104	154	181	736
	Survivors (n)	0	0	21	56	78	84	142	179	560
	(%) survived	0	0	39.6	70.0	78.0	80.8	92.2	98.9	76.1
1991–1995	Livebirths (n)	37	45	76	82	77	121	133	181	752
	Survivors (n)	7	22	52	72	69	116	128	177	643
	(%) survived	18.9	48.9	68.4	87.7	89.6	95.9	96.2	97.8	85.5

Note: Figures exclude infants with lethal abnormalities and those transferred to other level III nurseries.

(Reprinted with permission from the *American Journal of Perinatology* courtesy of Amir I, Doyle LW, Davis P, et al. Disproportionate consumption of ventilator resources by very preterm survivors persists in the 1990s. *Am J Perinatol* 15:187–190, 1998. Thieme Medical Publishers, Inc.)

TABLE 4.—Consumption of Nursery Resources by Gestational Age for Survivors Between Eras

Era—years of birth	*Gestational Age (Weeks)* 23	24	25	26	27	28	29	30	23–30
				Mean days of assisted ventilation					
1977–1985	na	43.0	38.9	24.1	11.0	7.3	4.3	2.5	7.4
1986–1990	na	na	43.1	37.1	19.4	9.2	5.0	2.4	11.5
1991–1995	77.4	62.3	52.0	36.7	23.7	12.5	7.3	3.3	18.5
				Mean days in hospital with no assisted ventilation					
1977–1985	na	81.0	88.4	80.0	76.2	70.4	64.9	54.0	65.0
1986–1990	na	na	70.3	62.1	64.4	59.2	45.9	33.8	49.1
1991–1995	61.4	63.0	53.2	52.5	46.6	45.0	39.3	32.4	42.9

Abbreviation: na, not applicable.

(Reprinted with permission from the *American Journal of Perinatology* courtesy of Amir I, Doyle LW, Davis P, et al. Disproportionate consumption of ventilator resources by very preterm survivors persists in the 1990s. *Am J Perinatol* 15:187–190, 1998. Thieme Medical Publishers, Inc.)

and 18.5 ± 23.0 days, respectively). Conversely, patient-days in the nursery not requiring ventilation dropped significantly (65.0 ± 24.3, 49.1 ± 29.4, and 42.9 ± 24.4 days, respectively). In infants of 23 to 27 weeks' gestational age, each week of decrease in gestational age was associated with an extra 12.9, 13.4, and 13.5 days of assisted ventilation across the eras. In infants of 28 to 30 weeks' gestational age, each week of decrease in gestational age was associated with only an extra 2.3, 3.3, and 4.6 days of assisted ventilation across the eras (Table 4). The differences in ventilation use were significant between the first 2 eras, but ventilator use in the third era did not differ significantly from that in the second time frame. Whereas in 1977–1985 only 12.2% of survivors were discharged to level I or II nurseries, in 1986–1990, 47.9% were, and in 1991–1995 slightly over half (50.4%) were.

Conclusion.—Despite advances in perinatal care, the duration of assisted ventilation in very premature infants has not changed significantly. However, at each gestational age, more infants are now surviving. The decrease in patient-days off the ventilator over the eras reflects changes in transfer practices from level III to level II or I nurseries. For these infants, each week of gestational age spent in utero before 27 weeks avoids about 2 weeks of assisted ventilation.

▶ This comparative review of neonatal ICU utilization measured by infant ventilator days for infants born before 31 weeks' gestational age over 5- to 9-year intervals during the past 2 decades is designed to illuminate patterns in neonatal care for very low birth weight infants, but it has an additional singular message for obstetricians. The 2,495 births were evenly divided among the 3 time intervals studied. Especially for infants born at less then 28 weeks' gestational age, survivorship increased exponentially among those most immature of newborns. At 24 weeks' gestational age, there were virtually no survivors until 1991 to 1995 when 48.9% of 45 infants are listed as survivors.

Net respiratory support increased over time as smaller infants progressively survived to discharge, or at least to live longer than in earlier decades. Time off respirator support decreased progressively as nursery facilities were more rapidly cleared of newborns no longer in need of respiratory support, making room for sicker infants. But for obstetricians, the message is the same as from earlier reports from this Melbourne unit. The information now extends backward as far as 23 weeks' gestational age. Each week of in utero residence maintained from 23 to 27 weeks' gestation saves, on average, about 2 weeks of ventilator support in the neonatal ICU.

T.H. Kirschbaum, M.D.

Transmission of Cytomegalovirus to Preterm Infants Through Breast Milk

Vochem M, Hamprecht K, Jahn G, et al (Univ of Tuebingen, Germany)
Pediatr Infect Dis J 17:53–58, 1998 9–7

Objective.—There is evidence that mothers with cytomegalovirus (CMV) infection can transmit the virus to their infants through breast milk. The risk of serious or fatal complications from this transmission is particularly high for premature infants. The incidence of virolactia in mothers of preterm infants, the rate of CMV transmission, and the onset of infection in small, premature infants were determined.

Methods.—Screening for CMV infection and excretion was performed prospectively in 67 premature infants at day 7 after birth and at 3 to 6 months. Immunoglobulin G and immunoglobulin M antibodies to CMV were measured in breast milk, urine samples, ear swabs, and throat washes of 56 mothers using enzyme-linked immunosorbent assay. DNA for CMV was performed, and fibroblast monolayers were cultured. The study lasted 12 months.

Results.—Of the 29 women with CMV immunoglobulin G antibodies, 27 breast-fed their infants. Of 27 seronegative women, 24 breast-fed their infants. None of the seronegative breast-feeding women shed CMV into breast milk. CMV DNA was found in breast milk of 25 of 27 seropositive breast-feeding mothers, and CMV was isolated from 23 (85%). In 2 seropositive breast-feeding women, CMV was not isolated. Viral excretion into breast milk was detected within the first 4 weeks postpartum in 21 of 23 women with positive CMV isolates, and in the remaining 2 women in the sixth and eighth weeks. Seventeen (59%) of 29 exposed infants acquired CMV infection. CMV was detected in 12 infants after 8 weeks and in 5 very low birth weight infants before 2 months, acute CMV in 4 of them.

Conclusion.—A significant percentage of mothers with CMV infection shed the virus in breast milk. Very low birth weight infants are at highest risk for early, acute infection.

► This study, originally performed to look for special susceptibility of preterm infants to postnatal maternal-fetal infection, demonstrated an increased risk in immature infants for the acquisition of early and symptomatic CMV infection. The implication of the 1% to 1.5% incidence of maternal infection in term infants is well known.[1] The risks of fetal transmission are higher in women lacking maternal antibody, although the antibody fails to be completely protective. Of those women who acquire primary CMV infection, the risk of fetal transmission is 40% and 10% to 15% of those infants (4% to 6% of infants born after primary maternal infection) have clinically apparent infection at birth, with late sequelae common in clinically infected newborns and present in 10% of asymptomatic infected newborns. In this study of 56 preterm births, the prevalence of CMV antibody positivity was 52%, and among seropositive women, breast milk was positive for virus by culture in 85% and by PCR in 93%. Presence of virus reached a maximum incidence at 2–3 weeks of newborn age, during which time viral replication in breast tissue, though not in salivary nor renal tissue, took place. Fetal transmission occurred in 92% of women with virolactia, producing an overall transmission rate of 59% in CMV-exposed infants. In view of these very high rates of transmission and their implications for newborn care, the authors recommend inactivating virus in the expressed milk of seropositive women by either Pasteurization or freezing. Their recommendations seem well founded.

T.H. Kirschbaum, M.D.

Reference

1. 1987 YEAR BOOK OF OBSTETRICS AND GYNECOLOGY, pp 80–85.

Prognostic Value of ^{1}H-MRS in Perinatal CNS Insults

Shu SK, Ashwal S, Holshouser BA, et al (Loma Linda Univ, Calif)

Pediatr Neurol 17:309–318, 1997 9–8

Objective.—Predicting outcome for neonates with severe CNS insults is difficult. Proton magnetic resonance spectroscopy (^{1}H-MRS) has been used to detect neuronal markers after severe perinatal asphyxia. The value of (^{1}H-MRS) for assessing the long-term prognosis for neonates with a wide variety of perinatal CNS insults was determined.

Methods.—Proton magnetic resonance spectroscopy (1.5T, 8 cm^3 vol, stimulated spin echo acquisition mode sequence, TE = 20 ms, TR = 3,000 ms) of occipital gray matter and parietal white matter was performed in 37 term neonates with severe perinatal encephalopathy. Peak area metabolite ratios (*N*-acetyl aspartate/creatine [NAA/Cr], NAA/Cho [choline], Cho/Cr) for spectra obtained at the end of the study and repeated later were calculated, and the 2 measurements were averaged. Lactate analysis was also performed. Acute CNS injuries stemmed from asphyxia in 18 neonates, sepsis in 4, meningitis in 4, metabolic disorders in 5, stroke in 4, and trauma in 2. Patient outcome was evaluated at 6 to 12 months with the Pediatric Cerebral Performance Scale.

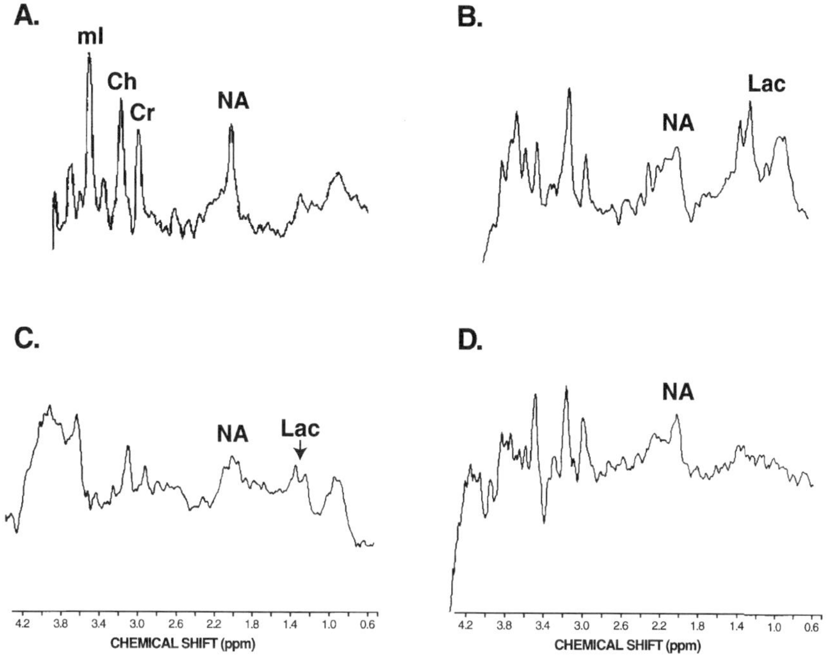

FIGURE 1.—A, occipital spectra from a control term neonate, showing the typical relatively low *N*-acetyl aspartate (*NAA*) and creatine (*Cre*) and high choline (*Cho*) peaks as compared with that seen in children more than 18 months of age. In addition, the myoinositol peak (*m*I) is prominent in neonates. **B**, occipital spectra from a term infant with severe traumatic brain injury. The MRI showed multiple hemorrhagic infarcts and proton magnetic resonance spectroscopy (^{1}H-MRS) demonstrated a marked reduction in NAA and Cr and a prominent lactate (*Lac*) doublet. The infant is severely disabled. **C**, occipital spectra in a term infant with meconium aspiration syndrome and severe hypoxic-ischemic encephalopathy (HIE) shows a Lac peak and virtually complete absence of NAA. The patient is severely disabled. **D**, occipital spectra from a term infant with cardiac arrest and severe HIE whose ^{1}H-MRS showed only a mild reduction in NAA without lactate and whose outcome was normal. (Reprinted by permission of the publisher from Shu SK, Ashwal S, Holshouser BA, et al: Prognostic value of ^{1}H-MRS in perinatal CNS insults. *Pediatr Neurol* 17:309–318, copyright 1997 by Elsevier Science Inc.)

Results.—The ^{1}H-MRS was performed at a median of 6 days after insult. Patients were followed for an average of 15 months. NAA, Cr, and Cho levels were lower in normal infants than in infants with acute CNS injuries (Fig 1). The mean occipital NAA/Cho was significantly lower and the mean occipital and parietal Cho/Cr were significantly higher in the 16 patients with poor outcome (severe disability, persistent vegetative state, death) than in the 21 patients with good/moderate outcome (good, mild, or moderate disability). Patients with a good/moderate outcome had metabolite ratios 2 standard deviations from the mean. The absence of lactate was significantly associated with a good/moderate outcome. The addition of metabolite ratio information significantly enhanced the correlation between these prognostic factors and outcome, using clinical and neurodiagnostic evaluations.

Conclusion.—The ^{1}H-MRS improves prediction of neurologic outcome in term neonates with a variety of CNS insults.

▶ In 1952, F. Block and E.M. Purcell received Nobel awards for their description of magnetic nuclear resonance. The method exposes tissues to a strong magnetic field and radio frequency electromagnetic waves with a frequency chosen to be resonant with atoms of special interest. In theory, any atom with an odd atomic number sufficient to render it a magnetic dipole can be studied. Interruption of the radio frequency wave field allows the magnetic dipolar atoms of interest to rotate in a magnetic field, generating a current capable of detection and analysis.[1]

A common atom of interest is ^{31}P, which is useful in studying cell energetics expressed in activities of adenosine triphosphate and phosphocreatine. These authors use radio frequencies resonant with protons (^{1}H), a relatively difficult task because of the ubiquity of protons and the strong signals obtained from water molecules, both of which diminish resolution. However, the Loma Linda investigators are able to define signals reflecting markers of neuronal metabolic activity (NAA), cell energy availability as phosphocreatine (Cr), lactate indicating levels of anaerobic glycolysis (Lac), and intracellular choline compounds released during cytolysis (Cho). Studying 37 term infants with suspected neonatal brain injury from a variety of sources, it was possible to demonstrate that decreased NAA and Cr with increased Lac and Cho correlated roughly with the severity and permanence of brain injury. Because of the inability to standardize tissue levels, ratios of relative concentrations had to be used for the inferences they made.

The use of physical methods noninvasively to explore the cellular biology of the brain in vivo is an extraordinarily useful approach and is destined to see wider use. The results, using ^{1}H-MRS, help to confirm the validity of data already available from ^{31}P MRS and support future biomedical development and use of this approach.

T.H. Kirschbaum, M.D.

Reference

1. 1990 Year Book of Pediatrics, pp 206–207.

Changes in Oxygenation and Pulmonary Haemodynamics in Preterm Infants Treated With Inhaled Nitric Oxide

Subhedar NV, Shaw NJ (Univ of Liverpool, England; Liverpool Women's Hosp, England)

Arch Dis Child 77:F191–F197, 1997 9–9

Background.—Interest in the neonatal use of inhaled nitric oxide (NO) in the treatment of hypoxemic respiratory failure has been increasing in recent years. To date, controlled studies confirming the short- and/or long-term benefits of NO have included only term infants with persistent pulmonary hypertension of the newborn (PPHN). Changes in oxygenation, respiratory support, and pulmonary hemodynamics in high-risk preterm infants treated with inhaled NO were investigated.

Methods.—By random assignment, 20 infants received inhaled NO and 22 did not, the latter serving as a control group. Inhaled NO treatment was given for 72 hours. Doses ranged from 5–20 ppm, with a median of 5 ppm.

Findings.—Median oxygenation index (OI) declined by 17% in the treated infants within 30 minutes. This drop in OI differed significantly from the response in control subjects until 96 hours. Treated infants had a rapid response, with a median 0.04 increase in accelerated time to right ventricular ejection time ratio (AT:RVET) within 30 minutes. This change was significantly different from that in control subjects until 4 hours. Median systolic pulmonary artery pressure decreased by 6.1 mm Hg in treated infants within 1 hour. Changes in OI were significantly correlated with changes in pulmonary blood flow but not with changes in AT:RVET.

Conclusions.—Inhaled NO treatment rapidly improves oxygenation and reduces pulmonary artery pressure in preterm infants. However, these effects are transient. Long-term outcomes are unaffected.

► Nitric oxide serves as a potent dilator of the pulmonary vasculature in normal pregnancy and its near instant inactivation by hemoglobin allows the effect to be confined to the pulmonary parenchyma, avoiding systemic hypotension and other extrapulmonary affects. After an initial series of encouraging case reports concerning its use in infants with respiratory distress syndrome, this is a first randomized prospective trial in a series of 42 very low birth weight infants with randomized entry into the study, all of them with evidence of chronic lung disease at 96 hours of life. The relatively small number of cases and the tendency for untreated newborns in retrospect to have less severe lung dysfunction than those treated with NO complicates data evaluation.

Using NO at an initial 20 ppm concentration and weaning it to 5 ppm over 72 hours resulted in improved arterial oxygenation and decreased pulmonary artery pressure, both effects noted 30 minutes after NO administration. The effects, however, showed wide individual differences and variable duration. There was indirect evidence of a small increase in pulmonary blood flow rates. In about one third of the 20 infants treated, no or minimal effects were noted. In another third, the effects lasted no longer than 24 hours. No overall effects on birth rate, gestational age at birth, persistent patent ductus arteriosus, or pulmonary hemorrhage were noted. All infants received 2 doses of surfactant as part of their care. Presumably, NO acts by inducing pulmonary vasodilatation, increasing the efficiency of lung tissue showing unequal perfusion diffusion and shunting of pulmonary blood through lung segments deprived of adequate circulation. General vasodilatation per se may be expected to be beneficial only if the relative volume of unaerated lung tissue decreases and shunting decreases; presumably the latter was not prominent during this study. The authors' work suggests NO effects some transient basis for improvement, but its long-term effectiveness rests with multiple factors having little directly to do with pulmonary circulatory events.

T.H. Kirschbaum, M.D.

Correlation of Neonatal Nucleated Red Blood Cell Counts in Preterm Infants With Histologic Chorioamnionitis

Leikin E, Garry D, Visintainer P, et al (New York Med College, Valhalla)
Am J Obstet Gynecol 177:27–30, 1997 9–10

Background.—Recent studies suggest that an elevated nucleated red blood cell (RBC) count in umbilical cord blood may indicate chronic intrauterine hypoxia. Recently, elevated nucleated RBC counts were associated with clinical and histologic chorioamnionitis in preterm infants after preterm premature rupture of membranes and preterm labor. It was suggested that a higher nucleated RBC count may be a response to inflammation, not fetal tissue hypoxia. No evaluation was done of the effect of gestational age and birth weight percentile, which are both inversely related to nucleated RBC counts. Nucleated RBC counts in response to clinical and histologic chorioamnionitis were evaluated while controlling for gestational age and birth weight percentile.

Methods.—There were 359 preterm infants delivered after preterm labor or preterm premature rupture of membranes. Nucleated RBC counts were obtained. Patients were divided according to clinical and histologic chorioamnionitis. Nucleated RBC counts were compared. Regression analysis was performed while controlling for gestational age and birth weight percentile.

Results.—There was a significant correlation between measures of infection status and higher nucleated red blood cell counts. Regression analysis showed that histologic chorioamnionitis was significant, but clinical chorioamnionitis was not.

Discussion.—These findings show that histologic chorioamnionitis elicits an erythropoietic response in the fetus. It is unclear whether fetal erythropoiesis is a direct response to inflammation or the result of a rise in erythropoietin. After controlling for gestational age and birth weight percentile, the relationship of nucleated RBC count to clinical chorioamnionitis could not be confirmed.

► This study attempts to comment on the hypothesis that chorioamnionitis is associated with increased cord blood normoblast counts through a mechanism other than fetal hypoxemia. Although it is not clear that such a mechanism exists, this is a search for correlative information, which might support a search for an etiologic link between infection and erythropoiesis. Unfortunately, the results are difficult to evaluate and not very helpful. The authors chose to define normoblast counts per hundred white blood cells rather than per hundred red blood cells or per unit blood volume. The resulting problem rests with the tendency for the reference denominator to vary with infection. Newborn leukocytosis could tend to reduce and leukopenia increase the apparent nucleated red blood cell (NRBC) density, though the NRBC density might remain unchanged in absolute numbers. The observed incidence of histologic chorioamnionitis 2½ times greater than the incidence of clinical chorioamnionitis in the 330–360 women studied, and the failure to do cultures, raise the real possibility that meconium staining of amniotic fluid, associated possibly with fetal hypoxemia, may have caused the 50% incidence of leukocytic infiltration of membranes noted in the group of low-birth weight newborns. Perhaps this is the reason histologic but not clinical chorioamnionitis remained a significant correlate of NRBC on multiple regression. Inclusion of discontinuous variables (mortality, histologic amnionitis) requires use of logistic multiple regression. Because the variance ratio (R^2) for the multiple regression equation accounts for only 10% of the observed variance in NRBC counts, it is hard to know how to interpret the significance of the regression coefficients. In brief, the results here do little to support the hypothesis of erythropoiesis resulting from chorioamnionitis, particularly because newborn hypoxemia is an unmeasured and uncontrolled covariant.

T.H. Kirschbaum, M.D.

Comparison of Ring Block, Dorsal Penile Nerve Block, and Topical Anesthesia for Neonatal Circumcision: A Randomized Controlled Trial

Lander J, Brady-Fryer B, Metcalfe JB, et al (Univ of Alberta, Edmonton, Canada)

JAMA 278:2157–2162, 1997 9–11

Background.—Because of beliefs about the safety and efficacy of current anesthetics, many newborns are circumcised without the benefit of anesthesia. Ring block, dorsal penile nerve block, a topical eutectic mixture of local anesthetics (EMLA), and topical placebo were compared during neonatal circumcision.

Methods.—Fifty-two healthy, full-term boys aged 1–3 days were enrolled in the randomized, controlled trial. The main outcome measures were heart rate, cry, and methemoglobin level.

Findings.—Untreated newborns showed homogeneous responses consisting of sustained increases in heart rate and high-pitched cry during and after circumcision. Two boys in this group became ill after the procedure, experiencing choking and apnea. Crying and heart rates were significantly reduced in the 3 active treatment groups during and after circumcision. The ring block was equally effective throughout all stages of the circumcision. The dorsal penile nerve block and EMLA were ineffective during foreskin separation and incision. Methemoglobin levels were greatest in the boys given EMLA, though none of the infants needed treatment.

Conclusions.—An anesthetic should be administered to infants before circumcision is performed. In this series, the ring block was the most effective anesthetic for neonatal circumcision, and EMLA was the least effective.

▶ The evaluation of pain in newborns is complicated by their limited behavioral repertoires and by the absence of language skills. Argument that a newborn doesn't experience or remember pain with circumcision is meaningless because pain is a personal experiential event that is communicable to others only behaviorally. The authors handle this issue by observing that infants who did not receive an anesthetic "suffered great distress during and following the circumcision." Most would agree, but this largely subjective observation, bolstered by measurements of newborn tachycardia and time spent crying, suffices to deal with the first hypothesis, which was that newborns treated with the placebo would experience more pain. The other aims were to decide whether a topical anesthetic causes less pain response than an infiltration technique (it does) and whether distress in placebo-treated infants is greater than that caused by anesthetic infiltration. Here there are problems, partly because the experiment was truncated at the point where only 11 infants received placebo compared with 26 who had infiltration with lidocaine and 15 who had topical anesthesia, "because of obvious differences in behavior." Also data during the period of drug infiltration had to be compared with data derived from the 11 placebo recipients during circumcision, events separated by time spent in restraint. The principal conclusion here is that the procedure of lidocaine infiltration is safe in terms of operative complications and that methemoglobinemia was largely confined to the topical anesthetic group. If you share the authors' conclusion that local anesthesia is warranted for this procedure, and I do, the study suggests that either ring infiltration or dorsal penile infiltration of 0.8 mL of 1% lidocaine without epinephrine is a safe option.

T.H. Kirschbaum, M.D.

Blood Flow Distribution in the Normal Human Preterm Brain

Børch K, Greisen G (Copenhagen Univ)

Pediatr Res 43:28–33, 1998 9–12

Objective.—One of the main causes of brain damage in neonates is disturbance in cerebral blood flow (CBF). Most studies that have measured regional CBF (rCBF) had no estimates of normal rCBF available for comparison purposes. The relative flow to gray and white matter regions of the neonatal brain was compared with results from animal and other human studies.

Methods.—RCBF flow was measured in 12 normotensive and normoxic preterm infants (6 girls), mean gestational age 27.7 weeks, during and between episodes of hypotension and hypoxemia. Measurements were performed using a fast-rotating 4-head multidetector system, specially

TABLE 4.—rCBF of Neonates Compared to rCBF of Dog, Lamb, and Piglet

	Specimen and methodology			
Region	Dog, microspheres 4-iodo-[^{14}C]antipyrine (n = 70)	Piglet, microspheres (n = 14)	Lamb, microspheres (n = 24)	Infant, ^{99m}Tc-HMPAO SPECT (n = 12)
Subcortical white matter	0.33 (0.30, 0.37)	0.44 (0.31, 0.57)	0.72 (0.56, 0.90)	0.23 (0.19, 0.26)
Lateral cortex		0.94 (0.71, 1.16)		
Frontal	1.07 (0.81, 1.32)		0.64 (0.55, 1.06)	0.47 (0.41, 0.53)
Fronto-temporal	0.98 (0.92, 1.05)		0.68 (0.48, 0.88)	0.43 (0.38, 0.5)
Occipitotemporal	1.28 (1.13, 1.42)		0.94 (0.71, 1.17)	0.44 (0.38, 0.5)
Occipital	0.97 (0.87, 1.07)		0.98 (0.73, 1.22)	0.43 (0.37, 0.49)
Cerebellum	1.13 (0.97, 1.28)	0.89 (0.67, 1.11)	1.17 (0.89, 1.45)	0.97 (0.66, 1.28)
References	27, 28, 33, 34, 37–40	36	35	The present study

Values are given as fraction of flow to the basal ganglia.
Abbreviation: RCBF, regional cerebral blood flow.
(Courtesy of Børch K, Greisen G: Blood flow distribution in the normal human preterm brain. *Pediatr Res* 43:28–33, 1998.)

designed for neonatal studies, within 1–2 hours after injection of ^{99m}Tc-labeled hexamethylpropylenamine oxime (4 MBq/kg). All neonates had a normal ultrasonographic examination.

Results.—The rCBF of the subcortical white matter was 0.53 of the global CBF. After correction for scattered radiation, the flow was reduced to 0.39. The flow to the basal ganglia was 2.33 times the global CBF. Although the cortical flow was underestimated, using a correction for the partial-volume effect provided an estimate of the cortical flow of 5 times the global CBF. The flow to the mesial cortex was 1.30 times the global CBF, significantly higher than the flow to the lateral cortex. After correcting for the partial-volume effect, cortical flow was 3.6 times the global CBF. The flow to the motor cortex was significantly higher than the flow to other areas of the lateral cortex, and the flow to the mesial cortex was significantly higher in the frontal lobes than in the occipital lobes. Flows to the cerebellum and basal ganglia were of the same magnitude, but cerebellar flows show significantly more variation. Studies of newborn mammals show a significantly higher ratio of basal ganglia flow to white matter flow than studies of newborn humans do, possibly indicating a reduced flow to white matter, in humans compared to animals (Table 4).

Conclusion.—Blood flow to the white matter of preterm human neonates is very low, perhaps predisposing this area of the brain to hypotension.

▶ Noninvasive analysis of the brains of preterm newborns continues to show surprising results. An estimate of cerebral oxidative metabolism using PET, based on ^{15}0 labeled water, shows intervals of virtually zero oxygen consumption in the brains of preterm infants who subsequently grew to become normal neonates.[1] This study measures regional cerebral blood flow using Technicium (^{99}TE) labeled tracer to record relative regional blood flow rates and a xenon clearance technique to record total or global cerebral blood flow. Multiplying 133 xenon-based value by each regional fractational flow value yields a series of estimates of regional absolute blood flow. Distribution patterns of ^{99}TE tracer are generated from 8 coronal slices of the newborn head from a rotating array of sensors. Blood flow in subcortical white matter, the site of germinal matrix hemorrhage was extremely low, representing only 23% of blood flow to the cerebellum and basal ganglia and about 50% of blood flow to the cortex. The differences are most striking in view of the tendency to underestimate cortex blood flow, because of small sampling volume, and to overestimate white matter flow, because of low tracer density. In this group of 12 newborns, averaging 915 g at 27.7 weeks gestational age, the very low white matter blood flow rates are congruent with the low rates of oxidative metabolism shown by PET in preterm infants especially at the most likely sites of neonatal parenchymal hemorrhage. These studies clarify the physiologic basis for neonatal intraventricular hemorrhage after periods of hypotension or hypoxemia which preceded these studies by 1 to 7 days.

T.H. Kirschbaum, M.D.

Reference

1. 1998 Year Book of Obstetrics, Gynecology, and Women's Health, pp 243–245.

GYNECOLOGY

10 Gynecologic Urology

Open Compared With Laparoscopic Approach to Burch Colposuspension: A Cost Analysis

Kohli N, Jacobs PA, Sze EHM, et al (Univ of Cincinnati, Ohio)

Obstet Gynecol 90:411–415, 1997 10–1

Background.—The most effective surgical treatment for female genuine stress urinary incontinence has not been established definitively. Because the cost-effectiveness of surgical procedures is being increasingly scrutinized, the cost of the open approach to Burch colposuspension was compared with that of the laparoscopic approach in women with genuine stress urinary incontinence.

Methods.—All patients undergoing open or laparoscopic Burch colposuspension by 1 surgeon in a 2-year period were identified by a retrospective chart review. Twenty-one had had the open procedure, and 17, the laparoscopic procedure.

Findings.—The operative times associated with the laparoscopic and open procedures were 110 and 66 minutes, respectively, a significant difference. In addition, the laparoscopic procedure had greater operating room charges ($3,479 vs. $2,138). Estimated blood loss and change in postoperative hematocrit in the 2 groups did not differ. There were no major intraoperative complications. Mean length of hospital stay was 1.3 and 2.1 days for the laparoscopic and open groups, respectively. However, the total hospital charges were still significantly higher for those undergoing the laparoscopic procedure than for those undergoing the open procedure ($4,960 vs. $4,079).

Conclusions.—Although patients undergoing laparoscopic Burch colposuspension had a shorter length of hospitalization than those undergoing open colposuspension, the former procedure was significantly more costly than the latter. This was because of the expense associated with increased operative time and the use of laparoscopic equipment.

Prospective Comparison of Laparoscopic and Traditional Colposuspensions in the Treatment of Genuine Stress Incontinence

Su T-H, Wang K-G, Hsu C-Y, et al (Taipei Med College, Taiwan; Li-Shin Hosp, Chungli, Taiwan)

Acta Obstet Gynecol Scand 76:576–582, 1997 10–2

Background.—The use of minimally invasive procedures, such as laparoscopic colposuspension, has become a trend in the treatment of genuine stress incontinence (GSI). The results of laparoscopic and traditional colposuspensions for GSI were compared.

Methods.—Ninety-two patients with GSI proved urodynamically were included in the study. Half were assigned randomly to laparoscopic colposuspension, and half to traditional procedures. In all patients, studies were repeated at least 3 months postoperatively.

Findings.—In both groups, the bladder neck position was increased significantly after surgery at rest or during straining. However, it was higher in the traditional group during straining. Preoperative and postoperative urodynamics in both groups showed significantly increased minimal urethral resistance and improved pressure transmission ratios at the proximal urethra. The patients undergoing laparoscopy had less blood loss. After laparoscopy, the duration of bladder drainage was shorter and unaffected by subsequent laparotomy. Operative times were almost the same in the 2 groups. The success rates of the laparoscopic and traditional procedures were 80.4% and 95.6%, respectively. The respective complication rates were 10.8% and 17.4%.

Conclusions.—Anatomical and functional assessments attest to the efficacy of laparoscopic colposuspension in the treatment of GSI. However, the success rate associated with this procedure is still lower than that of the traditional procedure.

► The question of whether "minimally invasive" is "maximally effective" in reconstructive pelvic surgery is not solved. There are very few comparative studies on this subject and no prospective randomized comparative works. This well-designed study by Su et al. is an important step in the right direction.

Kohli et al. (Abstract 10–1) show that laparoscopic surgery for stress incontinence does not save money. Su et al. indicate that, although effective, laparoscopic bladder neck suspension is not as effective as an "open" operation. An 80% cure rate is a very good result for stress incontinence, but a 95% cure rate with the "open Burch" on similar patients is better. When comparing laparoscopic with open operations, laparoscopic procedures have the advantage if they are safe and cost-effective and offer a shorter hospital stay and faster return to work or regular activities while having similar results to the open operation. Su et al. demonstrate that the "laparoscopic Burch" is doable and safe.

Is it more cost-effective than open Burch? While offering a shorter hospital stay, there is no cost saving in the laparoscopic compared with open bladder suspension (Kohli et al.). Is a faster return to work an advantage after bladder suspension? Probably not. We encourage patients not to lift heavy objects and to avoid strenuous exercise after bladder neck suspension, even if they feel they can do so. Are the end results comparable? Su et al. found the open operation (95% cure) to be superior to the laparoscopic approach (80% cure).

If more prospective comparative studies will support these results, then one should keep in mind that the laparoscopic Burch is doable, safe, and good, but the open Burch still has a higher cure rate.

A. Bergman, M.D.

Multichannel Urodynamic Evaluation of Laparoscopic Burch Colposuspension for Genuine Stress Incontinence

Ross JW (Ctr for Reproductive Medicine and Laparoscopic Surgery, Salinas, Calif)

Obstet Gynecol 91:55–59, 1998 10–3

Background.—Though several investigators have reported experiences with laparoscopic bladder suspension, some did not follow the Tanagho modification, lacked multichannel urodynamics, and did not include long-term data. In the current study, the 2-year outcomes of multichannel urodynamics with the laparoscopic Burch colposuspension using the Tanagho modification were reported.

Methods.—Forty-eight consecutive patients with genuine stress incontinence were included in the prospective study. All were followed up for 30–41 weeks after laparoscopic Burch colposuspension. All had had a routine urogynecologic assessment, including multichannel urodynamics before and after surgery.

Findings.—The cure rate was 98% at 6 weeks, 93% at 1 year, and 89% at 2 years. Urethral hypermobility was decreased significantly, and urethral pressure transmission ratios were increased significantly. Eighty-one percent of the patients voided spontaneously within 24 hours. No clinically significant pelvic organ prolapse was noted at 2 years.

Conclusions.—The 2-year cure rate and multichannel urodynamic findings associated with laparoscopic Burch repair are comparable to those associated with laparotomy. The early results of prophylactic apical vault suspension suggest that the incidence of prolapse after routine retropubic urethropexies may be decreased.

► Laparoscopic bladder neck suspension may be a reasonable choice for some women with stress incontinence (i.e., for women without significant pelvic relaxation). It may be even more attractive for women with stress incontinence whose physicians plan laparoscopic operation for other pelvic pathology. This series suggests that laparoscopic bladder neck suspension is effective. An 89% cure rate of stress incontinence is equivalent to any other good operation.

When performing abdominal hysterectomy and bladder neck suspension, closure of the Douglas pouch is recommended, to prevent future prolapse and enterocele formation. Dr. Ross performed uterosacral plication to prevent vault prolapse; this approach should be kept in mind by surgeons performing laparoscopic bladder neck suspensions.

A. Bergman, M.D.

Feasibility of Outpatient Percutaneous Bladder Neck Suspension Under Local Anesthesia

Haab F, Leach GE (Tenon Hosp, Paris; Univ of California, Los Angeles)
Urology 50:585–587, 1997 10–4

Background.—Percutaneous bladder neck suspension (BNS) is a relatively noninvasive procedure that can be performed on an outpatient basis with local anesthesia. The feasibility of outpatient percutaneous BNS with local anesthesia in the treatment of stress urinary incontinence (SUI) in women was investigated.

Methods.—Forty women with SUI underwent the procedure since October 1994. Mean patient age was 59.6 years. Outpatient percutaneous BNS was performed with "Z" suture anchoring of the anterior vaginal wall and pubocervical fascia.

Findings.—Ninety-eight percent of the procedures were performed successfully using local anesthesia. One patient required conversion to general anesthesia because of knee pain in the lithotomy position. No major complications occurred. On a scale of 0 (no pain) to 5 (severe pain), perioperative pain was rated as a mean of 1. Pain medications were needed for a mean of 2.4 days after surgery. The mean duration of recovery was

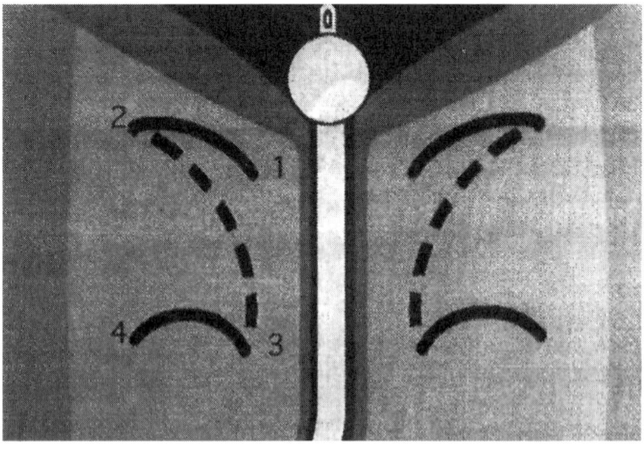

FIGURE 1.—Suspension suture: configuration of the vaginal anchoring; the four sequential vaginal wall perforation sites are shown. (Courtesy of Haab F, Leach GE: Feasibility of outpatient percutaneous bladder neck suspension under local anesthesia. *Urology* 50:585–587. Copyright 1997, by Elsevier Science, Inc. Reprinted by permission.)

2.2 weeks. Ninety-two percent of the patients were continent postoperatively. There was no recurrence of urethral hypermobility (Fig 1).

Conclusions.—Outpatient percutaneous BNS with local anesthesia is feasible in patients with SUI. No significant morbidity occurred in the current series. The long-term efficacy of this procedure has yet to be demonstrated.

▶ Needle suspension operations for SUI did not have the same long-term effect as abdominal retropubic procedures. One of the possible explanations is that needle suspensions attached "soft tissue" to "soft tissue," whereas the abdominal Burch anchored strong fascia to a bony ligament. The current modification of the needle suspension seems to get closer, by concept, to the abdominal urethropexy by anchoring the periurethral tissue to a bony structure.

When analyzing failures of the needle suspension technique, mainly recurrences of bladder base hypermobility, a question was raised regarding which suture failed in suspending the bladder base. Was it the abdominal suture or the vaginal one? The current technique offers good anchoring of the "abdominal suture." The strength of the "vaginal suture" anchor and the possibility of it pulling through the tissue still exist.

Needle suspensions were designed to simplify bladder suspension operation. In spite of early enthusiasm and reported good results, they were modified and improved again and again, indicating some problems with the technique. Whether the current modification is the ultimate one remains to be seen, although first results, like the current report, are encouraging.

A. Bergman, M.D.

A Method for Intraoperative Adjustment of Sling Tension: Prevention of Outlet Obstruction During Vaginal Wall Sling bladder

Rovner ES, Ginsberg DA, Raz S (Univ of California, Los Angeles)

Urology 50:273–276, 1997 10–5

Background.—Slings are being used increasingly to treat all types of stress urinary incontinence (SUI) in women. The intraoperative adjustment of the tension on the suspending sutures of the sling is of concern, because too much tension can result in bladder outlet obstruction, whereas too little tension may not coapt the urethra effectively. A simple, effective technique for adjusting intraoperative tension on the suspending sutures of a vaginal wall sling placed for SUI treatment was described.

Methods.—Data on the first 160 patients undergoing a vaginal wall sling that used the new technique were analyzed. A cystoscope sheath was placed in the urethra and inclined to 20 to 30 degrees relative to horizontal. The suspension sutures were then directly tied down onto the rectus fascia without indenting it. The sheath could be rotated easily in the vertical plane in the urethral lumen, to maintain elastic mobility as the sutures were tied (Fig 2).

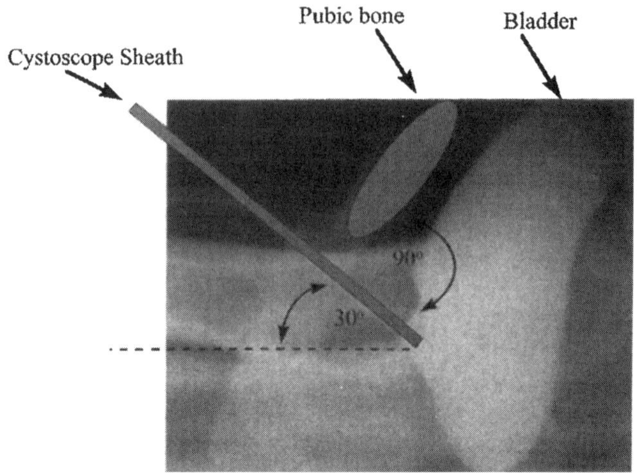

FIGURE 2.—Postoperative lateral cystogram demonstrating the ideal relationship between the cystoscope sheath, pubic bone, bladder neck, and the horizontal plane as the sutures are tied. (Reprinted by permission of the publisher from A method for intraoperative adjustment of sling tension: Prevention of outlet obstruction during vaginal wall sling. Rovner ES, Ginsberg DA, Raz S, *Urology* 50:273–276, Copyright 1997 by Elsevier Science, Inc.)

Outcomes.—None of the patients had unexpected permanent urinary retention. Less than 7% continued to have urgency incontinence postoperatively, and 6.8% had recurrent SUI during follow-up.

Conclusions.—Properly adjusting suture tension during a sling procedure for SUI is essential to prevent urethral obstruction. The method described in this article is simple, reproducible, and very effective.

▶ More and more pelvic surgeons are choosing sling operation as their primary choice for SUI procedure. It has several advantages. Sling is effective in correcting SUI of low urethral pressure and of the intrinsic sphincter deficiency type, as well as the "regular" stress incontinence and bladder base hypermobility. Sling's disadvantages are that many times it trades incontinence with retention and inability to void. Voiding difficulties after sling are quite common, as well as pulling of sutures through the urethra.

The current technique, by Dr. Rovner et al., seems to reduce the risk of postoperative retention and pulling of sutures through the urethra, by minimizing pressure on sutures. In a large series, this group reports no significant problem of urinary retention. The technique is simple and should be kept in mind by pelvic surgeons performing sling operations for stress incontinence.

A. Bergman, M.D.

Treatment Results Using Pubovaginal Slings in Patients With Large Cystoceles and Stress Incontinence

Cross CA, Cespedes RD, McGuire EJ (Univ of Texas, Houston; Wilford Hall Med Ctr, Lackland Air Force Base, Tex)

J Urol 158:431–434, 1997 10–6

Background.—Anterior vaginal wall prolapse is a serious problem. Large defects—grade III or IV cystoceles—are especially difficult to treat. The efficacy of a pubovaginal sling performed concurrently with a formal cystocele repair in women with grade III to IV cystoceles was determined.

Methods.—Forty-two women with diagnoses of grade III to IV cystoceles based on physical assessment and videourodynamics were included. Twenty-two percent had intrinsic sphincter deficiency diagnosed by an abdominal leak point pressure of less than 60 cm H_2O. Fifty-seven percent had type II stress incontinence with urethral hypermobility and an abdominal leak point pressure of more than 90 cm H_2O. A pubovaginal sling and anterior colporrhaphy were done along with other indicated vaginal procedures.

Findings.—Thirty-six patients were available for postoperative pelvic examinations at 3-month intervals. Mean follow-up was 20.4 months, with a range of 12–39 months. At follow-up, only 3 patients had symptomatic grade III cystoceles, and 2 had enteroceles. Two patients needed collagen injections. Another 2 underwent a repeated pubovaginal sling.

Conclusions.—A pubovaginal sling and anterior colporrhaphy are effective in the treatment of incontinence and the reduction of the cystocele in patients with large cystoceles and stress urinary incontinence. The fascial sling also appears to provide additional support to the bladder base, which improves the durability of the anterior colporrhaphy.

► Women with significant pelvic relaxation (large cystocele) and stress urinary incontinence are a surgical challenge in pelvic reconstruction. Treatment of stress incontinence only, i.e., retropubic procedures and needle suspension, does not reduce a large cystocele. Anterior colporrhaphy for reduction of a cystocele is not effective in curing stress incontinence. A combined approach of reducing the cystocele and suspending the bladder neck should be undertaken. Cross et al. report on their results with patients having stress incontinence and large cystoceles. The cure rate of 89% is a very good outcome for these patients. Sling procedures have their problems, mainly postoperative voiding difficulty and urinary retentions. In this study, 30% of patients required a catheter for more than a week, and 2 patients required self-catheterization for 3 months.

Another option for patients with large cystoceles and stress incontinence is vaginal colporrhaphy combined with retropubic bladder neck suspension (Burch type), although that approach was not studied in this series.

A. Bergman, M.D.

The Results of Laparoscopic Adhesiolysis for Intractable Urinary Frequency

Chen G-D, Lin L-Y, Gardner JD (Chung Shan Med and Dental College, Taichung, Taiwan, Republic of China; Harvard Univ, Boston)

J Urol 158:1714–1716, 1997 10–7

Background.—Laparoscopic adhesiolysis performed to treat chronic lower abdominal pain from pelvic adhesions appears to incidentally and concomitantly resolve urinary frequency problems. To date, no one has reported that pelvic adhesions may cause urinary symptoms. Whether pelvic adhesions may cause urinary dysfunction was prospectively studied.

Methods.—Ten women, aged 29–49, underwent laparoscopic adhesiolysis for diagnosis and treatment. All had previous pelvic surgery, after which urinary frequency problems developed. Conservative therapy had failed in these patients. Before and after the current procedure, urinary signs and symptoms were recorded, a urinary diary was kept, and cystometry was performed.

Findings.—Varying degrees of pelvic adhesions were observed, primarily around the bladder. After surgery, urinary frequency and urgency were improved in 9 patients. At follow-up, improvement was noted in urinary diary and cystometry parameters.

Conclusions.—Adhesions involving the bladder wall may restrict bladder distention. Laparoscopic adhesiolysis is useful for diagnosing and treating affected patients

► This well-designed prospective study suggests that postoperative pelvic adhesions can cause bladder dysfunctions. This is an interesting and new concept that has not been previously studied. The bladder is considered an extraperitoneal organ, and, as such, peritoneal adhesions are not supposed to affect it. Chen et al. suggest that they do. Lysis of adhesions affected not only perception of bladder irritation, such as urgency frequency, but also affected objective urodynamic parameters.

Whatever the mechanism of lysis of adhesions is in alleviating symptoms of bladder irritation, the results cannot be disputed.

Laparoscopy should be considered whenever severe bladder irritation symptoms occur after abdominal-pelvic operation and when conservative treatment fails.

A. Bergman, M.D.

Results of the Anti-Incontinence Operations and Kegel Exercises in Patients With Type II Anatomic Stress Incontinence

Yalcin OT, Hassa H, Ozalp S, et al (Osmangazi Univ, Eskisehir, Turkey)

Acta Obstet Gynecol Scand 77:341–346, 1998 10–8

Background.—Surgical anti-incontinence methods designed to elevate the bladder neck and proximal urethra and fixate them to the intrapelvic region are considered the treatment of choice for type II anatomical stress incontinence. However, conservative therapy has also been proposed for this type of incontinence. The outcomes of Kegel exercises were compared with those of anti-incontinence operations in patients with type II anatomical stress incontinence.

Methods.—Ninety-eight patients with pure type II anatomical stress incontinence were studied. Twenty-seven patients were treated by modified Pereyra procedures, 24 by Burch procedures, and 47 by Kegel exercises. Outcomes were determined by patient questionnaire, 24-hour urinary diary, 1-hour pad tests, and stress tests.

Findings.—At a mean follow-up of 13.7 months, anti-incontinence operations yielded complete cure in 90.2% of the women based on objective criteria and in 94.1% based on subjective criteria. At a mean follow-up of 12.8 months, these rates were 8.5% and 14.9%, respectively, among women treated with Kegel exercises. Among those whose compliance with Kegel exercises was good, these rates were 13.8% and 20.7%, respectively. Women with poor compliance had objective and subjective cure rates of 0% and 5.6%, respectively.

Conclusion.—In these women with type II anatomical stress incontinence, anti-incontinence operations were more effective than Kegel exercises. Further research is recommended to determine the value of regular, intensive Kegel exercise in a greater number of patients followed up in the long term.

▶ With pelvic muscle exercise programs becoming popular and the recommendation of the American Urologic Association that they be tried before resorting to surgery, the practicing physician may get the impression that the exercise is as good as, or almost as good as, operations for stress incontinence. Many studies report "cured and improved" results (usually reported as 1 group) in more than 60% of patients with stress incontinence. Yalcin et al. put results in a different perspective. When comparing only cures, surgical procedures for primary noncomplicated stress incontinence were in the 90% range, whereas the Kegel exercises were much less effective in "curing" stress incontinence.

Should Kegel exercise not be offered to patients with uncomplicated stress incontinence because they are less effective than operative procedures? The exercise definitely has a role in treating stress incontinence and should be tried before operation. If improvement is satisfactory, then Kegel exercise can be quite effective. It is simpler and does not carry the risks of operative procedures. However, when discussing treatment options with patients, the physician should make it clear that "simpler," "easier," and "safer" conservative treatment is not as effective as the surgical option.

A. Bergman, M.D.

Effect of Pelvic Muscle Exercise on Transient Incontinence During Pregnancy and After Birth

Sampselle CM, Miller JM, Mims BL, et al (Univ of Michigan, Ann Arbor; Kent State Univ, Ohio)

Obstet Gynecol 91:406–412, 1998 10–9

Background.—Vaginal birth has a major effect on the development of urinary incontinence, although pregnancy with cesarean birth may also be a risk factor. In nonpregnant, incontinent women, pelvic muscle exercise has been shown to increase muscle strength and decrease urine loss. There is little information about the effect of pelvic muscle exercise on urinary incontinence in women of childbearing age.

Methods.—In a prospective, randomized trial, 72 pregnant women were assigned to a treatment group that received instruction in pelvic muscle exercise or to a control group that received routine care with no instruction in pelvic muscle exercise. The women completed a questionnaire concerning symptoms of urinary incontinence, and pelvic muscle strength was measured with an instrumented gynecologic speculum. Data were obtained at 20 weeks and 35 weeks of gestation and at 6 weeks, 6 months, and 12 months after birth.

Results.—Data are reported for 46 women who had either vaginal or cesarean delivery and for a subsample of 37 women who had vaginal delivery. Longitudinal data are reported for women who provided complete data throughout the study. Women in the treatment group had decreased symptoms of urinary incontinence; significant effects of treatment were seen at 35 weeks of gestation and at 6 weeks and 6 months after delivery. A significant interaction between time and treatment for urinary incontinence was shown by a repeated-measures analysis of variance. Initial pelvic muscle strength had a significant effect on pelvic muscle strength during pregnancy and after birth; pelvic muscle strength at 20 weeks of gestation was a significant predictor of strength at 12 months after delivery. Women in the treatment group had greater pelvic muscle strength at 6 weeks and 6 months after delivery than women in the control group, but this difference was not statistically significant.

Discussion.—On the basis of these findings, the authors recommend that women receive instruction in pelvic muscle exercise before and after giving birth. Because of the importance of baseline pelvic muscle strength, it is also recommended that pelvic muscle strength be evaluated in women who are planning a first pregnancy and that those with muscle weakness be encouraged to practice pelvic muscle exercise.

► Kegel exercise was introduced by Arnold Kegel in the 1940s as a postpartum pelvic muscle training program to preserve sexual functions. After proving its efficacy, Dr. Kegel learned that these exercises are helpful for stress-incontinent women with weak pelvic floor support. We have made almost a full circle back to pregnancy, using pelvic muscle training as a "prophylactic" way to prevent future problems, rather than as a program to treat current stress incontinence.

Dr. Sampselle et al., in a well-designed prospective study, proved that a pelvic muscle training program in pregnancy reduces urinary incontinence during late pregnancy and after delivery. Does the effect of pelvic muscle exercise continue in later years and prevent stress incontinence? This study cannot answer that question, although common sense indicates that if the exercise continues, incidence and severity of stress incontinence might be reduced. Should physicians recommend "prophylactic" Kegel exercise to their patients? If we keep in mind that pelvic muscle training exercise is good not only in supporting the bladder but also in supporting the whole pelvic floor integrity, then this may be an idea to keep in mind. This study's results are clearly a recommendation in this direction.

A. Bergman, M.D.

Contribution of the Posterior Compartment to the Urinary Continence Mechanism

Zivkovic F, Tamussino K, Haas J (Univ of Graz, Austria)

Obstet Gynecol 91:229–233, 1998 10–10

Background.—Histologic studies have shown that the smooth muscle, collagen, and elastin fibers of the vaginal wall and paraurethral tissues interdigitate with the muscle fibers of the medial portion of the levator ani around the proximal urethra. In healthy women, urodynamic studies of urethral pressure and power generation during coughing indicate that, in addition to the midurethral closure mechanism, there is a dynamic active closure mechanism at the bladder neck. In women with genuine stress incontinence, power generation is substantially decreased at the bladder neck and midurethra during coughing. DeLancy's "hammock hypothesis" attributes urethral closure during stress to the urethra being pressed against a posterior, hammock-like supportive layer consisting of the endopelvis fascia and anterior vaginal wall.

Methods.—The contribution of the posterior compartment to the urinary continence mechanism was tested in 32 continent women. Urethral pressure profilometry was performed with and without a weighted posterior speculum to displace the posterior vaginal wall and levator ani muscles away from the bladder neck and urethra. The mean patient age was 45.2 years and the median parity was 2.

Results.—In all 32 subjects, insertion of the weighted speculum caused a decrease in pressure transmission ratios in the proximal quarter of the urethra, and in urethral closure pressures under stress in the proximal 2 urethral quarters. Before insertion of the speculum, 20 women had positive urethral closure pressures in the proximal urethra under stress. In these 20 women, insertion of the speculum decreased pressure transmission ratios to the proximal urethral quarter and decreased urethral closure pressures under stress in the proximal 2 urethral quarters. Before insertion of the speculum, 12 women had negative urethral closure pressures in the proximal urethra under stress. In these 12 women, insertion of the speculum did not change profilometry values.

Discussion.—In 12 of these 32 women, there was evidence of bladder neck incompetence in the form of negative urethral closure pressure under stress in the proximal urethra. These findings suggest that the posterior vaginal wall and levator ani muscles contribute to the closure mechanism of the proximal urethra in continent women.

► One of the questions in anti-incontinence operations is "how does it work?" In the early 1960s, Enhorning[1] popularized the theory of abdominal pressure transmission to the urethra by bringing the proximal urethra into the intra-abdominal pressure sphere. In this theory, the bladder and proximal urethra should be above the pelvic diaphragm, i.e., in the same abdominal pressure sphere, so that increase of abdominal pressure during Valsalva's maneuver that is transmitted to the bladder is equally transmitted to the urethra and continence maintained. In women with pelvic relaxation and stress incontinence, the prolapsed urethra is not in the abdominal pressure sphere and operation to restore continence "pulls" the proximal urethra to its "abdominal" position.

In the late 1980s, Dr. Beck et al.[2] hypothesized that continence during Valsalva's maneuver is maintained by a kinking effect. By this theory, the proximal urethra is fixed to a high retropubic position while the bladder base maintains some mobility. During stress, the bladder moves down while the urethra does not, and the kinking in the urethra prevents loss of urine. Surgery for stress incontinence is thus aimed at fixing the proximal urethra in a high retropubic position to enable the kinking effect during stress.

Recently, DeLancy[3] hypothesized that continence during stress is maintained by a "hammock" effect. By this theory, the proximal urethra is supported posteriorly by the fascia of the anterior vaginal wall. Abdominal pressure transmitted anteriorly during stress pushes the urethra against the vaginal wall and closes it. Pelvic relaxation results in mobility of the vaginal wall, which cannot support the urethra during stress. The anti-incontinence operation works by supporting the posterior urethral wall by creating a sling beneath the urethra, restoring the "hammock effect."

The work by Zivkovic et al. is in line with the theory of the "hammock effect." In this study, posterior support to the urethra was interrupted in 32 continent women, resulting in incontinence in most of them. Insertion of a heavy speculum in the posterior vaginal wall, pulling down all the vaginal wall, reduced abdominal pressure transmission to the urethra in 20 of 32 continent women. These results indicate that the vaginal wall support of the urethra is important in the continence mechanism, and that includes the posterior wall of the vagina.

The message to the pelvic surgeon is that the vaginal wall support to the urethra plays a role in continence mechanisms. Therefore, any relaxation of the posterior vaginal wall should be addressed and corrected during the anti-incontinence operation.

A. Bergman, M.D.

References

1. Enhorning GE: Simultaneous recording of intravesical and intraurethral pressure: A study of urethral closure in normal and stress incontinent women. *Acta Clin Scand* 176:1, 1961.
2. Beck RP, McCormick S, Nordstrom L: Intraurethral intravesical cough pressure spike difference in 267 patients surgically cured of genuine stress incontinence of urine. *Obstet Gynecol* 72:302–306, 1988.
3. DeLancy JOL: Structural support of the urethra as it relates to stress urinary incontinence: The hammock hypothesis. *Am J Obstet Gynecol* 170:1713–1723, 1994.

A Population Based, Randomized, Controlled Trial of Conservative Treatment for Urinary Incontinence in Women

Holtedahl K, Verelst M, Schiefloe A (Univ of Tromsø, Norway; Univ Hosp, Tromsø, Norway; Central Hosp, Bodø, Norway)

Acta Obstet Gynecol Scand 77:671–677, 1998 10–11

Background.—Urinary incontinence continues to be an unrecognized, inadequately treated problem in a high proportion of women. A population-based, randomized, controlled study of conservative therapy was reported.

Methods.—Ninety women, aged 50–74, with urinary incontinence were recruited for the general practice study. The treatment group received local estrogen, physiotherapy, and electrostimulation with close follow-up. The control group had delayed treatment.

Findings.—Active treatment decreased the severity and impact of leakage. Nearly one third of the patients did not complete all micturition testing, but, among those who did, the mean number of wet episodes per 24 hours declined with treatment, as did the mean number of micturitions in urge and mixed incontinence. Fifty-six percent of the women were cured or improved after 1 year.

Conclusions.—Older women with urinary incontinence can experience substantial improvement through conservative treatment in a general practice. This study emphasizes the need for individualized treatment and very active patient involvement.

► The current recommendation of the American Urologic Association for treatment of urinary incontinence in women is to try conservative treatment first and to exercise the surgical option for nonresponders. Whether legally that will become "the standard of practice" (ie, offering conservative treatment before surgery) is a question still to be answered. However, nonsurgical modalities should be offered and discussed with patients before surgery. Conservative treatments are less effective than surgical ones. Most patients still report "reduction in wet episodes" rather than "cure." Still, if patients feel better and are happy with their results, then treatment can be considered successful.

The present study points in this direction. Three treatment modalities—local estrogen, physiotherapy, and electrostimulation—were studied in a large population base, and more than half of the patients were pleased with the results. Keeping these numbers in mind, the American Urologic Association's recommendation of conservative treatment first, with operation reserved for noncompliance or unsuccessful treatments, makes sense.

A. Bergman, M.D.

Antecedent History as a Predictor of Surgical Cure of Urgency Symptoms in Mixed Incontinence

Scotti RJ, Angell G, Flora R, et al (Albert Einstein College of Medicine, Bronx, NY; Mount Sinai Hosp, Hartford, Conn)

Obstet Gynecol 91:51–54, 1998 10–12

Introduction.—Mixed incontinence, the copresence of genuine stress incontinence and detrusor instability, may occur in up to 50% of patients seen for urinary incontinence. The hypothesis that patients with mixed incontinence were less likely to be cured of detrusor instability by procedures designed to cure genuine stress incontinence if urgency preceded their symptom of stress was examined. Conversely, a cure was more likely if urge incontinence postdated stress incontinence.

Methods.—Forty-six women with mixed incontinence underwent Burch colposuspension. Patients who could not remember which symptom appeared first and those whose symptoms appeared within 3 months of each other were excluded. The women underwent clinical examination, had a detailed history taken, and had preoperative and postoperative multichannel urodynamic and other functional studies. Cure rates were calculated for the antecedent stress and antecedent urge groups.

Results.—Stress incontinence preceded urgency in 28 patients, whereas urgency occurred first in 18. In the antecedent stress group, 78.6% of patients were cured of urge incontinence and 21.4% had persistent urge incontinence. Urge incontinence was cured in only 22.2% of the antecedent urge group; the remaining 77.8% had persistent urge incontinence. Cure rates of stress incontinence were similar in the antecedent stress group (92.9%) and the antecedent urge group (88.9%). Previous surgery for incontinence had no effect on cure rates.

Conclusion.—Patients with stress incontinence who later experience urge incontinence are 2.5 times more likely to be cured of urge incontinence by Burch colposuspension than those in whom urge incontinence appeared first. Aggressive treatment of detrusor instability may not be necessary for patients with antecedent stress incontinence because of the high postoperative cure rates of their symptoms.

▶ Mixed incontinence, ie., stress and urge incontinence, is associated with a high failure rate of the anti-incontinence operation. The traditional teaching of "treat detrusor instability first and operate only on those who respond"

if urge preceded stress inco.

may leave many of these women with mixed incontinence wet, if they do not respond to medical treatment of detrusor instability. On the other hand, some women with mixed incontinence do respond well, and have a stable bladder after anti-incontinence operations. Can this group of patients be identified preoperatively? Scotti et al. suggest they can.

When urge incontinence preceded stress incontinence, the cure rate for urge incontinence by bladder neck suspension was 78.6%. When stress incontinence symptoms preceded urge incontinence, most women still had urge incontinence after operation (cure for urge incontinence of only 22.2%).

Pelvic surgeons should keep these data in mind, and try to avoid an operation on women with mixed incontinence if urge symptoms preceded stress, and detrusor instability cannot be controlled medically.

A. Bergman, M.D.

Complications of Periurethral Collagen Injection for Stress Urinary Incontinence

Stothers L, Goldenberg SL, Leone EF (Univ of British Columbia, Vancouver, Canada)

J Urol 159:806–807, 1998 10–13

Background.—Previous authors have advocated periurethral collagen injection as a safe, effective method for treating stress urinary incontinence. The complications associated with this treatment were investigated.

Methods.—Three hundred thirty-seven women with at least a 1-year history, physical findings, and urodynamic abnormalities consistent with stress urinary incontinence were included in the prospective cohort study. All required pads or protective clothing. Cystocele was either absent or grade 1.

Findings.—The most common and serious complication was de novo urinary urgency with incontinence, occurring in 12.6% of the patients. In many of these women, the symptoms were irreversible. Hematuria occurred in 5% of the women, and urinary retention in 1.9%. These effects were short-lived and resolved spontaneously. Three patients (0.9%) had delayed reaction at the skin test site; this was associated with arthralgias in 2.

Conclusion.—In this series, the overall incidence of complication risk in any individual was 20%. These findings contradict previous reports that periurethral collagen injection is free of complications.

► Periurethral collagen injections for stress urinary incontinence are considered a simple, risk-free, outpatient or office procedure. Efficacy in selected groups of patients (mainly those with stress incontinence and intrinsic sphincter deficiency) is good and one of the most appealing points of the procedure is that it has been said to be complication free. Stothers et al., in this large series of 337 patients, report that the procedure is not risk free. The authors report a 20% complication rate. Although some of the complications were transient, others, such as de novo urgency and urge incontinence, were persistent. De novo detrusor instability occurred in 12.9% of patients, and in 21%, there was no response to medical treatment.

These numbers are similar to those of reported detrusor instability after bladder suspension operations for stress incontinence. One of the main reasons for failed anti-incontinence operations is detrusor instability and urge incontinence, either previously present or de novo. It seems, from this study, that periurethral collagen injections carry a similar risk. Potential complications, including persistent urgency and urge incontinence, should be discussed with patients before decisions regarding surgical procedures are made.

A. Bergman, M.D.

Delayed Hypersensitivity and Systemic Arthralgia Following Transurethral Collagen Injection for Stress Urinary Incontinence

Stothers L, Goldenberg SL (Univ of British Columbia, Vancouver, Canada)

J Urol 159:1507–1509, 1998 10–14

Background.—Periurethral collagen injection is generally thought to be safe and effective in the treatment of stress urinary incontinence. Three cases of delayed hypersensitivity reactions to bovine collagen injection were described.

Methods and Findings.—These cases were encountered during a prospective cohort study of the efficacy and safety of transurethral collagen injection for stress urinary incontinence. Three hundred thirty-seven women were enrolled in the study. All had a history, physical findings, and urodynamic abnormalities indicative of stress urinary incontinence. All needed pads or protective clothing, and none had cystocele above grade 1. Previously, all study subjects had had negative skin test results. The incidence of delayed reaction at the skin test site was 0.9%. In 2 patients, this adverse reaction was associated with arthralgias.

Conclusion.—Glutaraldehyde cross-linked collagen injection may not be as innocuous as previously believed. Patients should be informed of the unknown long-term outcome of this complication. Clinicians should consider double skin testing before initiating collagen treatment for stress urinary incontinence.

▶ This is the second report in this YEAR BOOK regarding problems with periurethral collagen injection. This series from Canada reports on 3 cases (out of more than 300) of delayed sensitivity to collagen in women who had negative skin test results. Two of the 3 women had systemic manifestations as well. This form of treatment is considered safe and risk free. The 2 reports indicate that there are risks involved in periurethral collagen injection, and both patient and physician should be aware of that fact.

A. Bergman, M.D.

Collagen for Female Genuine Stress Incontinence After a Minimum 2-Year Follow-up

Swami S, Batista JE, Abrams P (Bristol Urological Inst, England)

Br J Urol 80:757–761, 1997 10–15

Background.—Glutaraldehyde cross-linked collagen is now approved for the treatment of genuine stress incontinence (GSI) in the United Kingdom. The medium-term outcome of this agent was investigated.

Methods.—One hundred eleven women, aged 33–90 years, with GSI were treated with paraurethral collagen injections between 1990 and 1995. The patients were followed up prospectively for at least 2 years, with a mean of 3.3 years.

Findings.—At the last follow-up, 25% of the patients were dry, and another 40% were improved. Some urodynamic values were changed significantly, but no factors predicted success. Previous surgery for stress incontinence did not affect outcomes.

Conclusion.—Parauretheral collagen injection is safe and relatively simple and yields acceptable outcomes in the medium term. It may be offered as a primary or secondary treatment to women with GSI who are unable or unwilling to have surgery. No factors of prognostic significance could be identified.

▶ Experience with paraurethral collagen injections in the United Kingdom is longer than it is in this country, and the present series, starting at 1990, adds to our knowledge of long-term effects of this treatment. Paraurethral collagen injection is an attractive alternative to surgery for GSI. Collagen injection can be an office procedure, often requiring only local anesthesia, with no postoperative catheterization or restriction of activity. Simple it is, but is it effective as surgery?

Dr. Swami et al. report a 25% cure and a 40% improvement rate after at least 2 years of treatment. A 65% "cure-improved" rate is quite a good outcome. However, most women required more than 1 treatment. Nonresponders were offered up to 3 treatments, so failures and partial improvement were considered after multiple treatments. Moreover, the success rate (not necessarily after 1 treatment) at 6 months was 85% and later fell to 65%, indicating that good results did not hold up well over time.

The current recommendation for paraurethral collagen injection is for GSI secondary to intrinsic sphincter deficiency and not GSI secondary to bladder-base hypermobility (an anatomical defect). Dr. Swami et al. did not exclude women with GSI and hypermobility from their series.

When reporting results of surgical procedures, "cure" is reported as "dry." By these criteria, a 25% cure rate by collagen injection achieved by multiple treatments is not equivalent to surgery. Still, 65% of women pleased with their outcome by a procedure that is relatively simple is quite a good outcome. Paraurethral collagen injection is a reasonable alternative for women with GSI who cannot or wish not to have an operation for their problem. Paraurethral collagen injection is a primary therapy for women with GSI secondary to intrinsic sphincter deficiency and no bladder-base hypermobility.

A. Bergman, M.D.

The Incidence of Low-Pressure Urethra as a Function of Prolapse-reducing Technique in Patients With Massive Pelvic Organ Prolapse (Maximum Descent at all Vaginal Sites)

Veronikis DK, Nichols DH, Wakamatsu MM (Harvard Med School)
Am J Obstet Gynecol 177:1305–1314, 1997 10–16

Background.—Although the use of various devices for reduction of massive prolapse may reveal urinary incontinence during urodynamic assessment, these devices may conceal the diagnosis of a low-pressure urethra, which can contribute to the failure of standard urethropexy procedures. A standard artifact-free method for reducing massive prolapse during urodynamic testing that would best create the postoperative anatomical relationships preoperatively was developed and compared with other reduction methods.

Methods and Findings.—Thirty consecutive continent patients with grade 4 prolapse at all vaginal sites were included in the preoperative, prospective, repeated-measures, urodynamic study. The maximal urethral closure pressure associated with 4 different techniques was documented. All patients underwent surgery and were followed up clinically for at least 1 year. Twenty patients with grade 0 prolapse composed a control group. The use of the Scopette reduction method to reduce the prolapse linearly during multichannel urodynamics revealed a 56% incidence of low-pressure urethra and an 83% incidence of overall genuine stress urinary incontinence in patients with massive pelvic organ prolapse but without clinical urinary incontinence.

Conclusions.—A linear reduction of the prolapse apparently reveals a low-pressure urethra as the cause of stress incontinence in more than half of the patients. Intrinsic sphincter deficiency should be suspected in patients with massive prolapse. Urethral pressure measurements can be used to reliably assess urethral function in patients with massive prolapse.

► One of the frustrating results for a pelvic surgeon is the appearance of stress incontinence in a previously continent woman after operation to correct pelvic relaxation. It is even more frustrating to face stress incontinence in a previously continent patient after the operation for pelvic relaxation included some form of bladder neck suspension. Veronikis et al. found that the occurrence of "occult" stress incontinence in continent women with massive prolapse was 83%. More important was the finding that ⅔ of continent women with "occult" stress incontinence and massive pelvic relaxation had stress incontinence of the "low urethral pressure type." These women might not have responded well to bladder neck suspension, but would probably benefit from bladder neck obstruction, in the form of a sling operation.

Another important finding of Veronikis et al. is that not all forms of prolapse reduction to detect occult stress incontinence work the same. The Gelhorn pessary, in this study, was less effective in detecting urethral sphincter weakness, than use of the Scopette.

A. Bergman, M.D.

Accuracy of Survey Questions for Geriatric Urinary Incontinence

Kirschner-Hermanns R, Scherr PA, Branch LG, et al Harvard Med School; Ctrs for Disease Control and Prevention, Atlanta, Ga; Duke Univ, Durham, NC; et al)

J Urol 159:1903–1908, 1998 10–17

Background.—Symptoms of bladder dysfunction correlate well with the underlying type of incontinence, especially in the elderly. However, this close correlation occurs only when the clinical assessment is detailed and performed by investigators with expertise in urodynamic testing. In epidemiologic studies, symptoms are typically elicited by short questionnaires completed by the study subjects. The accuracy of a typical questionnaire used in a large epidemiologic study was tested by comparing questionnaire findings with the results of multichannel video urodynamic testing.

Methods and Findings.—A questionnaire was administered to 132 patients, aged 65 years or older, before urodynamic assessment. Eighty percent of the patients were women. All were ambulatory, and none was severely demented. Overall, no analytic strategy could correctly classify more than 67% of patients. None could accurately classify even a single type of incontinence, including stress incontinence.

Conclusion.—Short questionnaires commonly used in epidemiologic studies do not correlate well with the results of urodynamic testing in incontinent elderly persons. Thus, previous reports of the prevalence of incontinence types should be re-examined.

► This is a nice prospective study regarding the accuracy of patients' symptoms in evaluating urinary incontinence. Detrusor instability may simulate stress incontinence symptoms, mainly if bladder contractions are induced by cough. In these cases, patients will tell us they lose urine with cough or sneeze, and the pathology is still detrusor instability. Detrusor instability is the No. 1 reason for failed anti-incontinence operation. In this prospective study using urodynamic evaluation, Kirschner-Hermanns et al. find that questionnaires correlate poorly with video urodynamic testing in incontinent older adults. Should video urodynamics be used routinely to evaluate incontinence? Definitely not. However, relying mainly on history, without any form of cystometric or urodynamic testing, may result in inaccurate diagnoses and unnecessary treatments.

A. Bergman, M.D.

A Medium Term Analysis of the Subjective Efficacy of Treatment for Women With Detrusor Instability and Low Bladder Compliance

Kelleher CJ, Cardozo LD, Khullar V, et al (Kings College, London)

Br J Obstet Gynaecol 104:988–993, 1997 10–18

Background.—Detrusor instability (DI) commonly causes urinary frequency, nocturia, urgency, and urge incontinence. The medium-term subjective outcomes of treatment among women with DI and low bladder compliance were investigated.

Methods.—A total of 1,105 women referred for assessment of urinary symptoms at a urogynecology center were enrolled in a prospective study of long-term outcomes and quality of life. Three hundred forty-eight women had a videourodynamic diagnosis of DI or low bladder compliance. Most of the women subsequently returned to their referring consultant for treatment. This group was contacted at least 6 months after their urodynamic assessment and asked to complete a questionnaire regarding treatment, its efficacy and adverse effects, and residual urinary symptoms.

Findings.—The response rate was 73.6%. Only 5.5% of these women reported cure of their urinary symptoms. Ninety percent had been treated with anticholinergic agents. Only 18.2% continued this treatment for more than 6 months. Residual urinary symptoms were common after diagnosis and treatment (Table 1).

Conclusion.—The medium-term outcomes of DI treatment and compliance are disappointing. Problems with compliance may be caused by low treatment efficacy, adverse effects, or inadequate follow-up after diagnosis and treatment initiation.

▶ Detrusor instability is a difficult problem to treat because, in most cases, its etiology is unknown. Treating an idiopathic condition is always frustrating, and the low cure rate is not surprising. The authors were honest in reporting "cure" and "improvement" rates separately and in using clear criteria for these definitions. In this large series, cure was achieved in only 5.5% of women with DI. Even if "cure" and "improvement" are combined into 1 group (as in most reports), almost half of the women in this series still reported disappointing results. An improvement rate that is similar to the

TABLE 1.—The Subjective Treatment Outcome of Women With Detrusor Instability and Low Compliance

	Cured	Improved	Same	Worse
DI	11 (5·7)	96 (49·7)	75 (38·9)	11 (5·7)
LC	3 (4·8)	27 (42·9)	29 (46·0)	4 (6·3)
TOTAL	14 (5·5)	123 (48·0)	104 (40·6)	15 (5·9)

Note: Figures in parentheses are percentages.

Abbreviations: DI, detrusor instability; *LC,* low compliance.

(Courtesy of Kelleher CJ, Cardozo LD, Khullar V, et al: A medium term analysis of the subjective efficacy of treatment for women with detrusor instability and low bladder compliance. *Br J Obstet Gynaecol* 104:988–993, 1997. Published by Blackwell Science Ltd.)

"placebo effect" in a medication with troublesome side effects indicates that the current treatments are far from satisfactory. It is clear that current treatment modalities do not provide an adequate answer for women with urinary incontinence caused by detrusor instability.

A. Bergman, M.D.

Detrusitol 2 mg bid.

Tolterodine, a New Antimuscarinic Agent: As Effective but Better Tolerated Than Oxybutynin in Patients With an Overactive Bladder

Abrams P, Freeman R, Anderström C, et al (Southmead Hosp, Bristol, England; Derriford Hosp, Plymouth, England; Universitetssjukhuset, Lund, Sweden)

Br J Urol 81:801–810, 1998 10–19

Background.—The overactive bladder, characterized by increased frequency of micturition, urgency, and urge incontinence, is believed to affect 10% or more of the population. Treatment usually consists of antimuscarinic drugs. The efficacy of tolterodine, a new antimuscarinic agent specifically developed for the treatment of overactive bladder, was compared with that of oxybutynin, currently the most commonly used agent.

Methods.—Two hundred ninety-three patients with urodynamically confirmed bladder overactivity, increased frequency of micturition, and urgency or urge incontinence were enrolled in a randomized, double-blind, placebo-controlled, parallel-group, multinational phase III study. Patients were given tolterodine (2 mg twice a day), oxybutynin (5 mg 3 times daily), or placebo. The protocol allowed dose reduction, to prevent withdrawal, to 1 or 2.5 mg, respectively.

Findings.—After 12 weeks of therapy, the mean frequency of micturition declined by 21% in the tolterodine group, 19.5% in the oxybutynin group, and 10.5% in the placebo group. Among those with urge incontinence at entry into the study, the mean number of incontinent episodes declined by 47%, 71%, and 19%, respectively. Tolterodine and oxybutynin were similarly effective in ameliorating these 2 symptoms. Mean volume voided per micturition rose by 27% in the tolterodine group and by 31% in the oxybutynin group, compared with 7% in the placebo group. The most common adverse effect was dry mouth, which occurred more often and with greater intensity in oxybutynin recipients than among tolterodine or placebo recipients. More oxybutynin recipients withdrew because of adverse events, and a greater proportion needed dose reductions because of adverse events.

Conclusions.—Tolterodine, 2 mg twice a day, is as effective as oxybutynin in the treatment of bladder overactivity and is better tolerated. Its superior tolerability allows more patients to continue effective treatment.

▶ Urinary urgency, frequency, and urge incontinence constitute a frustrating condition affecting more than 10% of the population. It is frustrating because, even after establishment of an accurate diagnosis, treatment is empirical and results are less than optimal. Since in the majority of cases the cause is unknown, treatment is nonspecific and long. Because treatment may last many months, annoying side effects are the major reason for stopping treatment, even when it is helpful.

Most of the medications for detrusor instability are anticholinergics, derivatives of atropine. The most common side effect is dryness of the mouth; in fact, this is the main reason to stop treatment.

This prospective randomized study compared a new antimuscarinic medication, tolterodine, to the most commonly used Ditropan, in women with detrusor instability. The new medication had the same efficacy as Ditropan, but with much fewer side effects. This offers a clear advantage, since many women might have benefited from the good effects of Ditropan but stopped taking it because of intolerable dryness of the mouth.

Tolterodine is not a "new" major solution for women with detrusor instability, but it may make treatment more tolerable. These results should be kept in mind by physicians treating women with lower urinary tract disorders.

A. Bergman, M.D.

The Relationship of Body Mass Index to Intra-abdominal Pressure as Measured by Multichannel Cystometry

Noblett KL, Jensen JK, Ostergard DR (Long Beach Mem Med Ctr, Calif)
Int Urogynecol J 8:323–326, 1997 10–20

Background.—Obesity is thought to be a factor in the pathophysiology of genuine stress urinary incontinence (GSI). In theory, obesity may increase intra-abdominal pressure, exposing the pelvic support structures and organs to a chronic state of stress and pelvic floor muscle fatigue. The relationship between body mass index (BMI) and intra-abdominal pressure was investigated.

Methods.—Data were obtained from the records of 136 patients undergoing urodynamic assessment between January 1995 and March 1996. Patient age ranged from 30 to 91. Intra-abdominal pressure was measured by multichannel cystometry.

Findings.—The mean BMI was 27.7 kg/m^2, and mean intra-abdominal pressure was 27.5 cm H_2O. Intra-abdominal pressure was strongly associated with BMI. Intravesical pressure was also strongly correlated with BMI. Forty-eight percent of the patients subsequently received a diagnosis of GSI; 25.7%, GSI and low-pressure urethra; and 13.2%, detrusor instability. Severe prolapse was the diagnosis in the remaining 13.2%.

Conclusion.—Intra-abdominal pressure was significantly correlated with BMI in this series. Obesity may stress the pelvic floor because of chronically increased pressure, thus explaining the mechanism for the role of obesity in the development and recurrence of GSI.

Effect of Preoperative Voiding Mechanism on Success Rate of Autologous Rectus Fascia Suburethral Sling Procedure

Iglesia CB, Shott S, Fenner DE, et al (Rush-Presbyterian-St Luke's Med Ctr, Chicago)

Obstet Gynecol 91:577–581, 1998 10–21

Background.—The suburethral sling procedure is an established treatment for genuine stress incontinence (GSI). Standard urethropexy procedures may be associated with an increased risk of failure in patients with low-leak-point–pressure and low-closure–pressure urethras. The efficacy and adverse effects of the rectus fascia suburethral sling were determined, together with the association of preoperative urodynamic or clinical variables with objective outcomes.

Methods.—The records of 50 patients undergoing the suburethral sling procedure with rectus fascia at 1 center between 1994 and 1996 were reviewed. All had GSI with intrinsic sphincteric deficiency or urethral hypomobility. In all patients, multichannel urodynamics were recorded before surgery. At 3 months postoperatively, urodynamic testing was done in 48 patients.

Findings.—Subjective cure of GSI was achieved in 94% of the patients by 3 months. Objective cure was documented in 73%. Patients with preoperative voiding caused by the Valsalva maneuver had an increased risk of objective failure. Fifty-four percent of the 13 patients in the Valsalva group and 17% of the 35 patients in the non-Valsalva group had objective failure at 3 months. The duration of postoperative catheterization tended to be longer in patients in the Valsalva group than in those in the non-Valsalva group.

Conclusion.—The rectus fascia suburethral sling procedure appears to be effective in carefully selected patients with GSI. Patients with preoperative voiding caused by the Valsalva maneuver have a higher failure rate than those without this cause of voiding.

▶ Sling operation is most effective for women with severe sphincteric weakness such as the sphincter deficiency or low urethral pressure type of stress incontinence. One of the possible complications of the sling procedure is postoperative voiding difficulties and urinary retention. Voiding difficulties result in patients having to use Valsalva maneuvers and increase intra-abdominal pressure. Obesity, as shown in this article by Iglesia et al., produces the same result, i.e., increased abdominal pressure.

Chronic increased abdominal pressure puts a lot of pressure on the bladder, which is in the abdominal pressure sphere, thus weakening its support and resulting in GSI or increased risk of failure after bladder neck suspension operations. It is not surprising that women with preoperative voiding difficulties because of the Valsalva maneuver had a higher sling operation failure rate, as shown by Iglesia et al.

Pelvic surgeons should be aware that any condition resulting in chronic high abdominal pressure, such as obesity or voiding with the Valsalva Manuever, may result in a higher failure rate of bladder neck suspension operations, as shown in these 2 articles (Abstracts 10–20 and 10–21).

A. Bergman, M.D.

Clinical Predictors of Urinary Incontinence in Women

Cundiff GW, Harris RL, Coates KW, et al (Duke Univ, Durham, NC)

Am J Obstet Gynecol 177:262–267, 1997 10–22

Background.—Urodynamic testing is not readily available to all physicians treating women with urinary incontinence. Many physicians must rely on historical and clinical information to determine who needs urodynamic testing. The value of symptoms as predictors of the final urodynamic diagnosis in women with urinary incontinence was determined.

Methods.—Data on 535 consecutive women with final diagnoses of genuine stress incontinence and/or detrusor instability were analyzed. The patients' evaluations included a standardized history, examination, urinary diary, quantitation test, and urodynamics.

Findings.—Half of the women had symptoms of both stress and urge incontinence, whereas only 21% had both genuine stress incontinence and detrusor instability. Fewer than half of the women with diagnosed genuine stress incontinence or detrusor instability had symptoms of, respectively, stress incontinence only or urge incontinence only.

Conclusions.—Symptoms alone identify fewer than half of patients with pure genuine stress incontinence or detrusor instability. Including historical and clinical parameters does not improve the sensitivity of these symptoms.

► The question of whether every patient with urinary incontinence needs a full urodynamic evaluation is very relevant to many clinicians who may not have access to urodynamic equipment. Is a history and a physical evaluation accurate enough so one can establish treatment plans based solely on such findings? Cundiff et al. studied 535 women with urinary incontinence and concluded that pure symptoms of stress incontinence or detrusor instability did not correlate, many times, with the final urodynamic diagnosis.

Should we carry it to the extreme and consider the history in urinary incontinence unreliable and thus unimportant in establishing a diagnosis and building treatment plans? The data of Cundiff et al. do not support it. More than 85% of women who gave symptoms of pure stress incontinence indeed had it by urodynamic testing. Many women who complained about urgency and frequency were found to have stress incontinence, making symptoms not very specific; yet, still most women who complained about stress urinary incontinence (SUI) had it. Are symptoms of SUI sensitive enough to establish a diagnosis and make treatment plans? It depends on what the treatment plans are. If they involve performing surgery, then close to 15% of women with symptoms of pure SUI would have had unnecessary surgery. This is clearly unacceptable. If the plan involves a short trial of nonsurgical treatment, then the answer is perhaps yes. A documented history of pure SUI may be reliable enough to justify a short plan of conservative treatment, but not reliable enough to plan surgery. For symptoms of detrusor instability, sensitivity and specificity were too low to rely on.

Does every woman with SUI need full urodynamic evaluation before planning surgical treatment? This study does not answer this question. It indicates that some form of urodynamic evaluation is needed. Simple cystometry to rule out detrusor instability may be good enough, but the answer to this question is not found in this study.

A. Bergman, M.D.

Transvaginal Gray-scale Imaging of Ureteral Jets in the Evaluation of Ureteral Patency

Harataz-Rubinstein N, Murphy KE, Monteagudo A, et al (Columbia-Presbyterian Med Ctr, NY)

Ultrasound Obstet Gynecol 10:342–345, 1997 10–23

Introduction.—Operative ureteral injuries are a serious complication of pelvic surgery, and most are sustained during gynecologic surgery rather than during general surgery or urologic procedures. The absence of immediate postoperative symptoms does not exclude ureteral damage. Postoperative tests to assess damage are costly, often unpleasant, and may be risky. Fifty women without a history of urinary complaints were recruited for a study of the efficacy of transvaginal gray-scale imaging for the evaluation of ureteral jets to confirm ureteral patency.

Methods.—The women had attended a US unit for various benign gynecologic conditions. The presence or absence of the right and left ureteral jets, as well as the time to detection of the first jet with gray-scale and color Doppler, were recorded for all study participants. Also reported was total scanning time. Sensitivity and positive predictive value of gray-scale imaging for the detection of ureteral jets were calculated, and the technique was compared to color Doppler as the "gold standard."

Results.—Study participants had a mean age of 40.7 years; 76% were Hispanic, 16% were black, and 8% were white. There were no procedure-related complications. On gray-scale US, the ureteral jet appeared as a hyperechoic flame-shaped stream in a lateromedial and anteroposterior direction. Ureters were identified bilaterally in all women using color Doppler sonography and in 28 using gray-scale US. Gray-scale imaging had a sensitivity of 68% and a positive predictive value of 100%. Median time to detection of the first jet was 47 seconds on the right side and 53 seconds on the left side, not a significant difference. The median scanning time was 176 seconds.

Conclusion.—Color Doppler is an expensive diagnostic modality that may not always be available. A useful and reliable alternative for the detection of ureteral jets in the bladder is transvaginal gray-scale imaging. This test is safe, inexpensive, and convenient, and has a positive predictive value of 100%. Transvaginal gray-scale imaging should prove useful when ureteral patency is in question after pelvic surgery.

▶ One of the complications of pelvic and anti-incontinence operations is ureteral injury or blockage. The consequences of not diagnosing this complication on time may be devastating. Cystoscopy to evaluate ureteral patency can be done in the operating room or after operation, when IV pyelography is another option. The problem with cystoscopy is that it requires special equipment and a trained physician to perform the test. Intravenous pyelography is an x-ray procedure that cannot be done in the operating room.

Dr. Harataz-Rubinstein et al. offer another attractive alternative, i.e., vaginal probe US. Sonography is widely available, not invasive, and can be done on the operative table with no problems.

The authors suggest that bilateral ureteral jets can be seen through pelvic sonography. This is a reassuring finding for ureteral patency and rules out ureteral injury. The current series reports a sensitivity of 68% and a positive predictive value of 100%. This is quite good for a simple, inexpensive "screening test."

The clinical message for the pelvic surgeon suspecting ureteral injury is that vaginal sonography can be done to detect ureteral patency. If ureteral jet is identified, the surgeon can be reassured that injury to the ureter did not occur. If ureteral jet cannot be seen sonographically, then the more specific tests of cystoscopy or IV pyelography should be done.

A. Bergman, M.D.

Stress Urinary Incontinence: Laparoscopically Assisted Transvaginal Needle Suspension

Pelosi MA III, Pelosi MA (Pelosi Women's Med Ctr, Bayonne, NJ; New Margaret Womens Health Inst, Secaucus, NJ)

J Reprod Med 42:319–324, 1997 10–24

Background.—Traditional methods of transvaginal needle suspension for stress urinary incontinence have some disadvantages. For example, needle placement relies on digital palpation, surgically induced trauma cannot be reliably detected, and objective cure rates are lower than those of retropubic colposuspension methods. A simplified technique of laparoscopically assisted transvaginal needle urethropexy that eliminates these disadvantages as well as the need for time-consuming laparoscopic suturing was described.

Methods.—Nineteen patients with stress urinary incontinence treated by laparoscopically assisted transvaginal needle suspension were reviewed retrospectively. All patients were assessed at least 1 year after surgery.

Findings.—The procedure was completed successfully in all patients. None of the patients needed conversion to laparotomy. No instances of intraoperative morbidity were attributed to prevesical dissection. The mean operating time was 25 minutes. Average blood loss was 50 mL. None of the patients had infection or bleeding postoperatively. At the

1-year follow-up, all patients were subjectively cured of incontinence, although 2 had transient urinary retention and 1 had transient detrusor instability in the first 3 months after surgery.

Conclusions.—Laparoscopically assisted transvaginal needle suspension allows accurate, visually guided placement of suspension sutures. It may also induce extraperitoneal scarring similar to retropubic colposuspension. These features may enable long-term cure rates that are comparable to those of retropubic colposuspension without the need for endoscopic suturing.

► Needle suspension for stress urinary incontinence was first introduced by Pereyra et al.[1] (and later modified by Stamey, Raz, and Gittes) as a way to simplify bladder neck suspensions. Abdominal retropubic procedures for stress incontinence were introduced by Marshall, Marchetti, and Krantz[2] and later modified by Burch, as ways to permanently anchor the bladder neck to a bony structure for long-term cure of incontinence. Laparoscopic operations were popularized in latter years as a way to simplify and replace abdominal operations. In an era when many abdominal procedures were performed laparoscopically, the surgeon should be careful in patient selection for these procedures. Laparoscopic surgery has an advantage when replacing abdominal operations. It is not designed to replace vaginal operations.

Transvaginal needle suspension is a relatively simple vaginal operation, and laparoscopic guidance of a vaginal operation does not simplify it. Dissection of the retropubic space of Retzius can be done safely and effectively from a vaginal incision. Laparoscopy does not simplify it. Surgical procedures that can be done effectively and safely by vaginal approach do not need laparoscopic assistance.

A. Bergman, M.D.

References

1. Pereyra AJ, Lebherz TB, Growdon WA, et al: Pubourethral supports in perspective: Modified Pereyra procedure for urinary incontinence. *Obstet Gynecol* 59:643–648, 1982.
2. Marshall VI, Marchetti AA, Krantz KE: The correction of stress incontinence by simple vesicourethral suspension. *Surg Gynecol Obstet* 88:509–518, 1949.

11 Infection

Herpes Simplex Virus Type 2 in the United States, 1976 to 1994

Fleming DT, McQuillan GM, Johnson RE, et al (Ctrs for Disease Control and Prevention, Atlanta, Ga; Emory Univ, Atlanta, Ga)

N Engl J Med 337:1105–1111, 1997 11–1

Introduction.—Herpes simplex virus type 2 (HSV-2) infections typically affect the genital area and are usually transmitted sexually. In newborns, the infection may cause severe systemic disease and death. It is difficult to assess the extent of HSV-2 infection in the United States because most of those affected are unaware of the disease and few states require cases to be reported. Serologic methods were used to study the epidemiology of HSV-2 and examine changes in HSV-2 seroprevalence during a 13-year period.

Methods.—A nationally representative serologic survey of HSV-2 was done as part of the third National Health and Nutrition Examination Survey (NHANES III), conducted from 1988 to 1994. This survey included information on behavioral risk factors for HSV-2 infection and the effects of an increased public awareness of genital herpes and other sexually transmitted diseases. Findings of NHANES III were compared with those of NHANES II, conducted between 1976 and 1980. An immunodot assay specific for glycoprotein gG-2 of HSV-2 was used to assess HSV-2 antibody.

Results.—From 1988 to 1994 among study participants 12 years or older, the seroprevalence of HSV-2 was 21.9%, corresponding to 45 million infected individuals in the noninstitutionalized civilian U.S. population. The female-to-male prevalence ratio was 1.4, and the black-to-white prevalence ratio was 2.6. Less than 10% of seropositive individuals reported a history of genital herpes infection. Independent predictors of seropositivity in multivariate analysis were female sex, black race, Mexican-American ethnic background, older age, less education, poverty, cocaine use, and a greater lifetime number of sexual partners. The age-adjusted seroprevalence of HSV-2 rose 30% as compared with the period from 1976 to 1980. The increases in HSV-2 seroprevalence that occurred between NHANES II and NHANES III were found mainly in the younger age groups (Fig 2). Among white teenagers, the seroprevalence quintupled; whites in their 20s had double the seroprevalence compared with the earlier period.

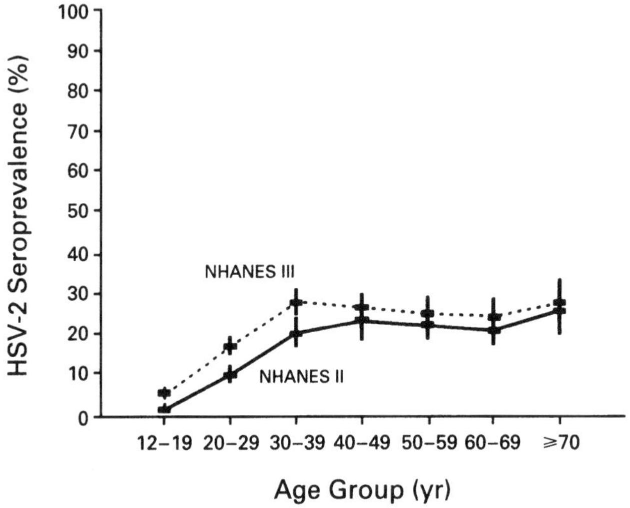

FIGURE 2.—Herpes simplex virus type 2 (*HSV-2*) seroprevalence according to age in the National Health and Nutrition Examination Survey (*NHANES*) II (1976–1980) and NHANES III (1988–1994). *Bars* indicate 95% confidence intervals. (Courtesy of Fleming DT, McQuillan GM, Johnson RE, et al: Herpes simplex virus type 2 in the United States, 1976 to 1994. *N Engl J Med* 337:1105–1111. Copyright 1997, Massachusetts Medical Society. Reprinted by permission of *The New England Journal of Medicine*. All rights reserved.)

Conclusions.—The seroprevalence of HSV-2 in the United States increased by 30% during the period covered by NHANES III as compared with the period covered by NHANES II, and the greatest relative increases were among young whites. Findings emphasize the ongoing need to prevent HSV-2 and other sexually transmitted infections, especially because transmission of HIV may be facilitated by the presence of genital ulcers.

► Although the incidence of clinically recognizable genital herpes infection is only 2.6% of U.S. adults, serologic evidence of infection with this virus was present in 1 of 4 adult females in the United States between 1988 and 1994. Because genital herpes infection occurs on the skin of the perineal area, use of the male condom will not always prevent transmission of this organism. Herpes infection can cause vaginal itching or discharge without the presence of the typical ulcerating lesions. Viral cultures should be performed when the symptoms of vaginitis do not respond to the usual therapies, to determine whether the cause of the infection is HSV-2.

D.R. Mishell, Jr., M.D.

Mortality Related to Sexually Transmitted Diseases in US Women, 1973 Through 1992

Ebrahim SH, Peterman TA, Zaidi AA, et al (Ctrs for Disease Control and Prevention, Atlanta, Ga)

Am J Public Health 87:938–944, 1997 11–2

Background.—In the United States, more than 12 million people are infected with a sexually transmitted disease every year. A method for evaluating sexually transmitted disease-related deaths using the International Classification of Diseases codes for specific sexually transmitted diseases and disease or syndromes caused by sexually transmitted diseases was developed, and deaths from sexually transmitted diseases in women in the United States from 1973–1992 were estimated.

Methods.—Three methods were used to determine the total number of deaths: (1) the actual number of deaths from diseases that are always transmitted sexually, (2) the best estimates of deaths from diseases that are not always sexually transmitted, and (3) reported deaths of women with sexually transmitted HIV. United States national mortality data, AIDS surveillance data, and current literature were used to calculate the total number of deaths from sexually transmitted diseases.

Results.—Approximately 150,600 women aged 15 years or older died of a sexually transmitted disease from 1973 through 1992. From 1973–1984, the number of deaths per year from all sexually transmitted diseases decreased by 24%, from 8,713–6,610. From 1984–1992, however, this number increased by 31% (Fig 1).

The major causes and proportion of deaths from individual sexually transmitted diseases changed during the study period. In 1973, cervical carcinoma, hepatitis B and C virus infection, and syphilis were the leading

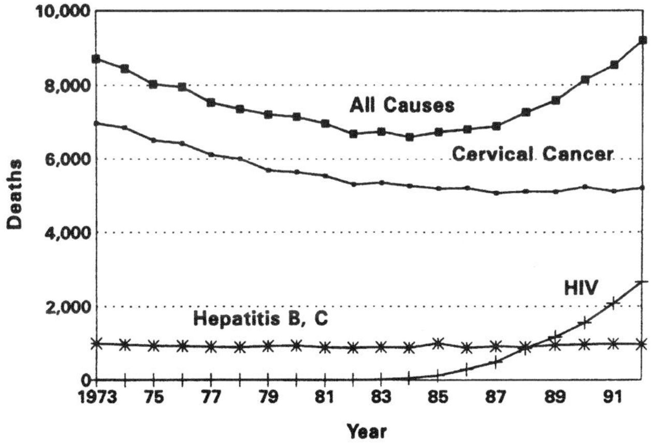

FIGURE 1.—Sexually transmitted disease-related deaths among U.S. women: deaths from all sexually transmitted disease-related causes and deaths attributed to cervical cancer, sexually transmitted HIV, hepatitis B virus, and hepatitis C virus, 1973–1992. (Courtesy of Ebrahim SH, Peterman TA, Zaidi AA, et al: Mortality related to sexually transmitted diseases in US women, 1973 through 1992. *Am J Public Health* 87:938–944, 1997. Copyright American Public Health Association.)

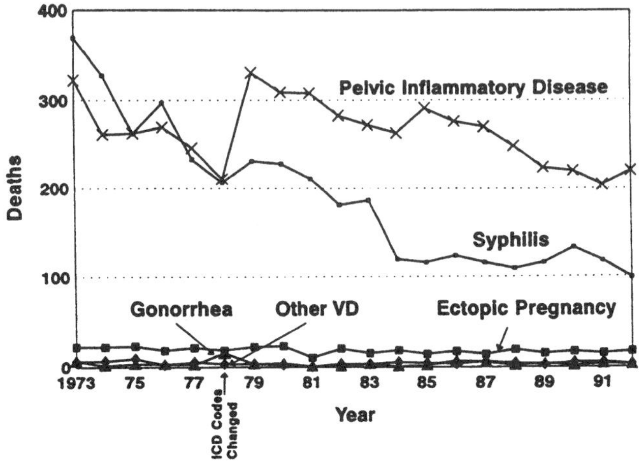

FIGURE 2.—Deaths among U.S. women attributed to sexually transmitted pelvic inflammatory disease, syphilis, ectopic pregnancy, gonorrhea, and other venereal diseases, 1973–1992. *Abbreviation: ICD,* International Classification of Diseases. (Courtesy of Ebrahim SH, Peterman TA, Zaidi AA, et al: Mortality related to sexually transmitted diseases in US women, 1973 through 1992. *Am J Public Health* 87:938–944, 1997. Copyright American Public Health Association.)

causes. Cervical cancer was the main cause of death from sexually transmitted disease throughout the study period. In 1989, there were more deaths related to HIV infection than from hepatitis B and C virus infection. From 1977 to 1986, pelvic inflammatory disease was the third leading cause of death from sexually transmitted diseases, replacing syphilis. From 1989 to 1992, infection from hepatitis B and C virus infection was the third leading cause of sexually transmitted disease-related death. In 1992, cervical carcinoma, HIV infection, and hepatitis B and C virus infection were the 3 leading causes of sexually transmitted disease-related death. Throughout the 20-year study period, death from cervical cancer decreased by 25%, death from syphilis decreased by 73%, and death from sexually transmitted pelvic inflammatory disease decreased by 31% (Fig 2). The most notable change was in heterosexually transmitted HIV-associated death. The first reports of HIV-related deaths were in 1984; by 1992, they had increased to 29% of all sexually transmitted disease-related deaths.

Discussion.—This assessment is the most comprehensive report to date of the risk of mortality associated with sexually transmitted diseases. This estimate includes all currently recognized sexually transmitted diseases and their outcomes based on vital statistics data and the best available estimates on transmission patterns. The report emphasizes various components of sexually transmitted disease-related mortality that have otherwise been neglected. The major causes of sexually transmitted disease-related death, viral sexually transmitted diseases and their outcomes, are generally not recognized as being transmitted sexually. Most deaths from sexually transmitted diseases might be prevented by changing sexual behavior and use of condoms.

▶ It is generally known that sexual transmission of the HIV virus can cause mortality because of the development of AIDS in women and that the number of female deaths resulting from AIDS has been steadily increasing in the past decade in the United States. Sexual transmission of the human papillomavirus is the major cause of development of cervical cancer. In addition, about 25% of hepatitis B virus infections and 10% of hepatitis C virus infections in adults are believed to be sexually transmitted.

Deaths from the sequelae of infection from these types of sexually transmitted viruses accounted for more than 90% of sexually transmitted disease-related deaths in women in the United States after 1990. Women should be advised that sexual contact with possibly infected partners without correct and consistent use of condoms cannot only cause infertility resulting from tubal occlusion and ectopic pregnancy but also death as a result of sexual transmission of viruses. Nearly 10,000 deaths occur among women annually in the United States that are attributable to the sequelae of sexual transmission of various organisms. Sexually transmitted disease-related mortality is one of the 10 leading causes of death in women of all ages in this country.

D.R. Mishell, Jr., M.D.

Vaginal Douching and Adverse Health Effects: A Meta-analysis

Zhang J, Thomas AG, Leybovich E (Mount Sinai School of Medicine, New York; New York Univ)

Am J Public Health 87:1207–1211, 1997 11–3

Background.—Vaginal douching continues to be a common practice, although the benefits and risks have not been clearly defined. Because such a large number of women douche regularly, even a small risk will have an important impact on public health. The current literature describing adverse health effects of vaginal douching was reviewed in a meta-analysis.

Methods and Findings.—Reports published between 1965 and 1995 were considered. All articles analyzed were case-control studies. One third of white women and two thirds of black women of reproductive age reported regular douching. Vaginal douching increased the overall risk of pelvic inflammatory disease by 73% and the risk of ectopic pregnancy by 76%. Frequent douching was highly correlated with pelvic inflammatory disease and modestly associated with cervical cancer.

Conclusions.—The current literature suggests that frequent douching increases the risk of pelvic inflammatory disease, ectopic pregnancy, and possibly cervical cancer. Further research, especially prospective cohort studies, is needed. In the meantime, women should be told that douching is unnecessary and potentially harmful.

▶ It was most interesting to learn how commonly vaginal douching is performed in the United States. A national survey reported that two thirds of black women and one third of white women in the United States douche regularly and that half of the women douche at least once a week. This analysis showed that douching nearly doubled the risk of pelvic inflammatory disease as well as ectopic pregnancy and may be a risk factor for cervical cancer. Women should be counseled about the health risks of frequent vaginal douching.

D.R. Mishell, Jr., M.D.

Antecedent Antimicrobial Use Increases the Risk of Uncomplicated Cystitis in Young Women

Smith HS, Hughes JP, Hooton TM, et al (Univ of Washington, Seattle; Group Health Cooperative of Puget Sound, Seattle)
Clin Infect Dis 25:63–68, 1997 11–4

Objective.—Animal studies have shown that the use of certain antimicrobials can alter the normal vaginal flora. Whether antimicrobial use can predispose women to urinary tract infections (UTIs) is not known. Data were analyzed from 2 cohorts of premenopausal women who were followed up prospectively for 6 months to determine risk factors for UTI.

Methods.—Between 1989 and 1993, a university cohort of 326 young women were examined at enrollment, at weekly intervals for a month, and at monthly intervals for the remaining 5 months, and a cohort of 425 women enrolled in an HMO were seen at enrollment and every 2 months.

Results.—During follow-up, it was found that 20% of the university cohort and 14% of the HMO cohort had a UTI. Approximately one third of participants took antimicrobials for at least 1 day, and antimicrobials were used on 2.5% to 2.9% of total follow-up days. Antimicrobial use during the previous 3, 7, or 14 days did not alter the risk of UTI, whereas antimicrobial use during the previous 15–28 days significantly increased the risk of UTI by a factor of 4. Women using antimicrobials during days 15–28 but not during the prior week were 5.83 times as likely at the HMO and 2.57 times as likely at the university to have UTI than women who did not use antimicrobials. Women who took antimicrobials during the prior week and during days 15–28 had no increased risk of UTI compared with women who took no antimicrobials. The increased risk of UTI was present for all antimicrobials evaluated. The relative risk of UTI for women at the HMO who had taken antimicrobials for UTI during days 15–28 was 6.40, whereas the relative risk of UTI was 3.82 for women at the HMO who took antimicrobials for another reason. Relative risks for university women were similar but lower, with wider confidence intervals.

Conclusions.—The higher risk for HMO women who used antimicrobials for treatment of a condition other than UTI is consistent with the idea that antimicrobial use alters the vaginal flora, thereby predisposing to vaginal colonization with uropathogens.

► The results of this prospective study indicate that use of antimicrobial agents for any reason increases the risk of uncomplicated cystitis developing in young women 2–4 weeks after discontinuation of antimicrobial use. It is likely that the antimicrobials alter the urogenital flora so that colonization with bacteria that can cause cystitis occurs. If a young woman has cystitis 2–4 weeks after discontinuing antimicrobial use, the clinician can inform her about a possible causal relation.

D.R. Mishell, Jr., M.D.

Dermovate

Clobetasol Dipropionate 0.05% Versus Testosterone Propionate 2% Topical Application for Severe Vulvar Lichen Sclerosus

Bornstein J, Heifetz S, Kellner Y, et al (Carmel Med Ctr, Haifa, Israel)
Am J Obstet Gynecol 178:80–84, 1998 11–5

Objective.—The various topical and systemic drugs that have been used to treat lichen sclerosus have not produced satisfactory results. Testosterone propionate 2% has been the treatment of choice because of concern that corticosteroids will exacerbate the atrophy already seen. The corticosteroid clobetasol does not cause atrophy. Topical treatment with testosterone propionate 2% was compared with that of clobetasol 0.05% for lichen sclerosus, for both short- and long-term applications.

Methods.—Between 1988 and 1993, 20 women treated with testosterone propionate 2% and 20 treated with clobetasol 0.05% for lichen sclerosus were followed up for at least 1 year. Patients were evaluated at 3 months and 1 year, and responses and degree of atrophy were recorded.

Results.—Patients were postmenopausal women with an average age of 64 years. At 3 months, subjective outcomes were similar, whereas gynecologic examination indicated that the clobetasol group was significantly more improved than the testosterone group. At 12 months, 90% of the clobetasol group and 10% of the testosterone group had a response (Table 3). Significantly more testosterone patients than clobetasol patients discontinued treatment because of lack of response. Six patients in the testosterone group and 1 patient in the clobetasol group had side effects.

TABLE 3.—Treatment Outcome at 12-Month Follow-up

	Complete response		*Incomplete response*		*No response*		*Total*
	No.	%	No.	%	No.	%	No.
Subjective (symptoms)*							
Clobetasol	10	50	8	40	2	10	20
Testosterone	5	25	3	15	12	60	20
Objective (signs)†							
Clobetasol	10	50	8	40	2	10	20
Testosterone	5	25	3	15	12	60	20

*$P \leq 0.02$.
†$P \leq 0.02$.
(Courtesy of Bornstein J, Heifetz S, Kellner Y, et al: Clobetasol dipropionate 0.05% versus testosterone propionate 2% topical application for severe vulvar lichen sclerosus. *Am J Obstet Gynecol* 178:80–84, 1998.)

Significantly more women in the clobetasol group than in the testosterone group were satisfied with their treatment (18 vs. 7).

Conclusions.—Clobetasol is significantly more effective than testosterone for the treatment of lichen sclerosus and results in fewer side effects.

► For many years, the standard treatment of lichen sclerosus of the vulva has been the local application of 2% testosterone propionate cream. The most common symptom of this disorder is pruritus. However, testosterone cream only relieves these symptoms in a minority of women. Although this study was not a randomized clinical trial, the groups treated with testosterone and the potent corticosteroid clobetasol were similar. The historical control group treated with testosterone had less subjective and objective improvement of the lichen sclerosus than did the women treated with clobetasol. The results of this and other series suggest that the preferred therapy for lichen sclerosus should now be a high-potency cortisol ointment like clobetasol instead of testosterone propionate.

D.R. Mishell, Jr., M.D.

Randomized Trial of Trovafloxacin and Ofloxacin for Single-dose Therapy of Gonorrhea

Jones RB, and the Trovafloxacin Gonorrhea Study Group (Indiana Univ, Indianapolis)

Am J Med 104:28–32, 1998 11–6

Background.—A single dose of a broad-spectrum cephalosporin or a quinolone antibiotic has been recommended for the treatment of uncomplicated gonococcal infections. Presumptive treatment with a regimen effective against *Chlamydia trachomatis* is also recommended for patients treated for gonorrhea. The efficacies of single-dose trovafloxacin, 100 mg, and ofloxacin, 400 mg, were compared in patients with uncomplicated gonorrhea.

Methods.—Six hundred twenty-five women and men with uncomplicated gonococcal urethritis or cervicitis were enrolled in the multicenter, double-blind study. The patients were randomly assigned to trovafloxacin or ofloxacin to be taken under direct supervision.

Findings.—Trovafloxacin treatment was bacteriologically and clinically comparable to ofloxacin. *Neisseria gonorrhoeae* was eradicated in 99% of evaluable trovafloxacin recipients and in 98% of evaluable ofloxacin recipients. Both treatments were tolerated well. The most common adverse effect was vaginitis, occurring in 4% and 7% of the trovafloxacin and ofloxacin groups, respectively (Table 2).

Conclusion.—In this large, randomized trial, single-dose oral therapy with trovafloxacin, 100 mg, was as bacteriologically and clinically effective as single-dose ofloxacin, 400 mg, in women and men with uncomplicated gonorrhea. These agents were effective against urogenital infections as well as infections at sites that were more difficult to treat.

TABLE 2.—Eradication Rate by Source in Evaluable Patients

Gender	Source	Trovafloxacin 100 mg	Ofloxacin 400 mg
Males (%)	Urethra	103/104 (99)	111/111
	Pharynx	5/5	4/4
Females (%)	Cervix	93/94 (99)	112/116 (96)
	Urethra	2/2	0/0
	Rectum	27/27	18/18
	Pharynx	9/9	8/8

(Reprinted by permission of the publisher from Jones RB, and the Trovafloxacin Gonorrhea Study Group. Randomized trial of trovafloxacin and ofloxacin for single-dose therapy of gonorrhea. *Am J Med* 104:28–32, copyright 1998 by Excerpta Medica, Inc.)

▶ The advantage of using quinolones instead of cephalosporins for treating gonococcal infection is that quinolones can be given orally and are less expensive. The results of this large trial indicate that use of a single 100-mg dose of a new quinolone antibiotic, trovafloxacin, is very effective for the eradication of both urogenital gonococcal infection and infection with this organism at other sites. Advantages of trovafloxacin include its effectiveness in eradicating strains of gonorrhea that are resistant to cephalosporin and oflaxacin as well as its effectiveness in the treatment of *Chlamydia trachomatis*, which frequently accompanies gonococcal infection.

D.R. Mishell, Jr., M.D.

Metronidazole Prophylaxis to Prevent Infections After Total Abdominal Hysterectomy

Henriksson L, Colling-Saltin A-S, Frick G, et al (Dept of Gynecology and Obstetrics, Malmö, Sweden; Dept of Gynecology and Obstetrics, Helsingborg, Sweden; Dept of Gynecology and Obstetrics, Karlskrona, Sweden; et al)

Acta Obstet Gynecol Scand 77:116–119, 1998 11–7

Background.—The risk of infection after abdominal hysterectomy is high. The efficacy of IV metronidazole infusion given as the only drug

TABLE 3.—Postoperative Infection; Placebo/Metronidazole; Infected Cases

	Primary analysis	Secondary analysis	*p*-value
Evaluated patients	141/150	124/134	
Number of infected patients	17/9	16/8	0.035/0.028
Percent of	12.1/6.0	12.9/6.0	
Lower pelvis infections	9/5	8/4	
Abdominal wall infection	8/4	8/4	

(Courtesy of Henriksson L, Colling-Saltin A-S, Frick G, et al: Metronidazole prophylaxis to prevent infections after total abdominal hysterectomy. *Acta Obstet Gynecol Scand* 77:116–119, copyright 1998, Munksgaard International Publishers Ltd., Copenhagen, Denmark.)

during and after total abdominal hysterectomies in preventing postoperative infection was studied.

Methods.—Three hundred sixteen women were included in the randomized, double-blind trial. One hundred thirty-four patients received metronidazole, 500 mg, in an IV infusion immediately before abdominal total hysterectomy and again 8 hours later. One hundred twenty-four patients received placebo.

Findings.—Compared with the treatment group, the placebo group had a significantly higher rate of wound infection, longer postoperative hospitalization, and a greater sedimentation rate on postoperative day 6. Postoperative temperatures did not differ significantly between the groups. Six percent of the patients given metronidazole and 12% given placebo had postoperative wound infections. Overall, 8% had urinary tract infections as diagnosed by urine culture (Table 3).

Conclusion.—Intravenous infusion of metronidazole before and after total hysterectomy is recommended for preventing postoperative wound infections. This agent can reduce both the frequency of wound infection and the length of stay after surgery.

▶ Prophylactic antibiotics are usually given in association with vaginal hysterectomy, but their routine use during abdominal hysterectomy has not been consistently found to be effective. The results of this large study suggest that IV infusion of 500 mg of metronidazole before and after abdominal hysterectomy is cost effective and should be used as a routine measure.

D.R. Mishell, Jr., M.D.

12 Endocrinology

The Endocrinology of Aging

Lamberts SWJ, van den Beld AW, van der Lely A-J (Erasmus Univ, Rotterdam, The Netherlands)

Science 278:419–424, 1997 12–1

Objective.—The average life span is 75–78 and will probably increase during the coming decades. Whereas most elderly individuals will die of disease or dementia, the healthy elderly will become disabled as a result of loss of muscle strength that leads to frailty. Frailty can be reduced or prevented by exercise. Changes in the endocrine system may be responsible for changes in body composition leading to frailty. The effect of hormone replacement therapy on body composition, atherosclerosis, cancer formation, and cognitive function was analyzed.

Endocrinology of Aging.—Aging of the thyroid and pancreas leads to the most significant changes, with 40% of individuals aged 65–74 and 50% aged over 80 years having impaired glucose tolerance or diabetes mellitus. The low plasma thyroxine and high thyrotropic concentrations that exist in 5% to 10% of elderly women results from autoimmunity. Whether the elderly would benefit from serum triiodothyronine is not known. Changes in hormone systems lead to menopause in women and andropause in men and adrenopause and somatopause for both sexes. Possibly, medical intervention in these processes could delay or prevent the aging process.

Menopause and Andropause.—Long-term hormone replacement in women relieves the symptoms of menopause but does not appear to increase life span. Hormone replacement therapy does delay atherosclerosis, bone loss, and the onset of Alzheimer's disease but results in an increase in the incidence of breast cancer. Testosterone therapy in men increases muscle mass and strength, but long-term studies have not been conducted.

Adrenopause.—The effect of increasing sex steroid levels on the aging process has been little studied, particularly with regard to the development of ovarian, prostate, and other cancers.

Somatopause.—Healthy 70-year-old men, given long-acting derivatives of hypothalamic peptide growth hormone twice daily, have higher levels of growth hormone and insulin-like growth factor 1 than 35-year-old men, indicating that somatopause is the result of a slowdown in the hypothalamus/pituitary system. Oral growth hormone–releasing peptide derivatives, if as active as subcutaneously administered growth hormone, might be used to reverse somatopause, prevent frailty, and reverse catabolism.

Conclusion.—The goal of increasing life expectancy should be to increase the health and functional capacity of the elderly by developing intervention programs that delay or prevent the aging process.

▶ This excellent review of the endocrinologic alterations that occur in elderly women and men should be read by all gynecologists, as they are becoming the primary health care providers for a large number of elderly women. By providing postmenopausal women with estrogen replacement, the quantity of life is increased by reducing the incidence of coronary heart disease, the major cause of death in women. The quality of life is also improved by estrogen replacement as women are more likely to remain in a self-care environment because of the reduced risk of the occurrence of hip fractures, Alzheimer's disease, and urinary incontinence.

D.R. Mishell, Jr., M.D.

Late Endocrine Effects of Ovarian Electrocautery in Women With Polycystic Ovary Syndrome

Gjønnæss H (Aker Univ Hosp, Oslo, Norway)

Fertil Steril 69:697–701, 1998 12–2

Introduction.—Pregnancy rates near 80% have been found since the original description of ovarian electrocautery in women with polycystic ovary syndrome, and successful ovulation is up to 96%, with resultant decreases in serum concentrations of androgens and luteinizing hormones. The duration of the endocrine changes produced by ovarian electrocautery in women with polycystic ovary syndrome was examined. It was also determined whether late endocrine changes were dependent on body weight.

Methods.—Through the laparoscope, ovarian electrocautery was performed on 165 infertile women with polycystic ovary syndrome. Before the operation and at defined intervals thereafter, blood was sampled. Sampling was performed 1 week before the menstrual period after the establishment of regular cycles. Fifteen women were observed before and at defined intervals after ovarian electrocautery, for up to 20 years. Determinations were made of serum concentrations of hypophyseal and ovarian hormones, including sex hormone-binding globulin.

Results.—A significant decrease in androgens and gonadotropins was seen after ovarian electrocautery, and there was a clear shift from anovulation to ovulatory cycles. There was also an increase in sex hormone-binding globulin. These effects continued for many years. Two thirds of the women were still ovulating after 18–20 years. In normal-weight women, the ovulation rate did not differ significantly from that in overweight women, and the rates were almost identical after 10–20 years.

Conclusion.—Ovarian function, including androgen production, was normalized with ovarian electrocautery for polycystic ovary syndrome. The results seemed to be stable for 18–20 years. Ovarian electrocautery did not appear to increase the risk of early menopause.

▶ The normal changes associated with polycystic ovarian syndrome (PCOS), particularly increased androgenicity, are risk factors for the overall health of women with untreated PCOS. It will be useful to determine whether the beneficial and long-lasting hormonal changes associated with ovarian electrocautery reduce the risk for women with PCOS developing diabetes mellitus, hypertension, or myocardial infarction. These beneficial hormone changes are an additional reason for performing partial ovarian destruction, instead of gonadotropin therapy, for anovulatory women with PCOS who fail to ovulate with clomiphene citrate.

D.R. Mishell, Jr., M.D.

Factors Affecting the Outcome of Laparoscopic Ovarian Drilling for Polycystic Ovarian Syndrome in Women With Anovulatory Infertility

Li TC, Saravelos H, Chow MS, et al (Jessop Hosp for Women, Sheffield, England; Queen Elizabeth Hosp, Lowloon, Hong Kong)

Br J Obstet Gynaecol 105:338–344, 1998 12–3

Objective.—Women with polycystic ovarian syndrome frequently have anovulatory fertility. Treatments to induce ovulation result in a wide variation in pregnancy rates. Results of a retrospective analysis of a consecutive series of women with polycystic ovarian syndrome and either oligomenorrhea or anovulatory infertility, treated with laparoscopic ovarian drilling between January 1991 and December 1995 in a teaching hospital, are presented.

Methods.—The analysis excluded women with blocked tubes or associated male infertility factors. Multiple ovarian drilling and simultaneous application of either argon laser or monopolar diathermy were performed on 111 women, aged 20–39. Outcome measures were ovulation and pregnancy rates.

Results.—The mean number of punctures per ovary was 23.2 by laser and 6.3 by diathermy. The cumulative conception rate at 1 year was 54%. Of the 7 women who had miscarriages, 4 conceived again, making the "take-home" baby rate 56%. The conception rate within 12 months of surgery was 50.1%. Women who conceived tended to be infertile for 3 years or less, younger, treated with diathermy, and to have preluteinizing hormone levels greater than 10 IU/L. Although mild-to-moderate male factors and nonobstructive tuboperitoneal factors did not appear to affect treatment results, women with severe male factors or obstructive tubal disease should seek in vitro fertilization. The spontaneous ovulation rate of 67% was increased by 20%, using clomiphene citrate after surgery.

Conclusion.—Laparoscopic ovarian drilling is an effective treatment for anovulatory infertility resulting from polycystic ovarian syndrome. If treatment with clomiphene fails, laparoscopic drilling is suggested over regular gonadotropic therapy as a more cost-effective procedure.

▶ The initial therapy to induce ovulation in women with polycystic ovarian syndrome (PCOS) is clomiphene citrate. A substantial percentage of women with PCOS fail to ovulate following clomiphene citrate therapy. Induction of ovulation with gonadotropins in women with PCOS who fail to ovulate with clomiphene results in a pregnancy rate of about 20% per treatment cycle but careful monitoring is necessary to prevent the ovarian hyperstimulation syndrome. In addition, compared with clomiphene, with gonadotropins the rate of multiple gestation and spontaneous abortion is increased if pregnancy does occur. Because multiple cycles of gonadotropin therapy are usually necessary to achieve a viable pregnancy, it may be preferable to perform ovarian diathermy and thus induce continuous ovulatory cycles and a 50% incidence of pregnancy during the first year after the procedure. If spontaneous ovulation does not occur after ovarian diathermy, repeated use of clomiphene citrate is more likely to induce ovulation after the procedure than before it was performed.

D.R. Mishell, Jr., M.D.

Effects of Metformin on Spontaneous and Clomiphene-induced Ovulation in the Polycystic Ovary Syndrome

Nestler JE, Jakubowicz DJ, Evans WS, et al (Virginia Commonwealth Univ, Richmond; Hosp de Clinicas Caracas, Venezuela; Univ of Virginia, Charlottesville; et al)

N Engl J Med 338:1876–1880, 1998 12–4

Objective.—Polycystic ovary syndrome is a major cause of infertility. Although clomiphene citrate is the drug of choice for inducing ovulation in women with this syndrome, obese women frequently require multiple treatments, possibly because of the increased hyperinsulinemia that goes along with increasing obesity. Reducing hyperinsulinemia with metformin's effect on the ovulatory response in obese women with polycystic ovary syndrome was examined.

Methods.—Glucose tolerance tests were performed in 61 obese women with polycystic ovary syndrome, before and after administration of either 500 mg of metformin (n = 35) or placebo (n = 26) 3 times daily for 35 days. The 21 women in the metformin group and the 25 women in the placebo group who did not ovulate were also given 50 mg of clomiphene daily for 5 days. Serum progesterone was measured on days 14, 28, 35, 44, and 53. Ovulation was presumed to have occurred if progesterone levels were greater than 8 ng/mL.

Results.—Whereas the average area under the serum insulin curve remained unchanged in the placebo group during the glucose tolerance test, the area decreased significantly in the metformin group (6,598 vs. 3,764 μU/mL/min). The waist-to-hip ratio decreased slightly but significantly in the metformin group, but not in the placebo group, during testing. Nineteen of 21 women in the metformin group and 2 of 25 in the placebo group ovulated after treatment with clomiphene (mean peak serum progesterone level, 23.8 ng/mL.

Conclusion.—Metformin significantly increased the ovulatory response to clomiphene in obese women with polycystic ovary syndrome.

▶ Many anovulatory women with polycystic ovarian syndrome (PCOS) fail to ovulate with the use of clomiphene citrate and require gonadotropin therapy or partial ovarian destruction to induce ovulation. Many women with PCOS also have insulin resistance with hyperinsulinemia. The results of this well-performed randomized clinical trial indicate that when metformin is given to obese women with PCOS and without diabetes mellitus, insulin levels decrease and the ovulatory response to clomiphene citrate increases markedly.

For women with PCOS who fail to ovulate with clomiphene citrate alone, administering metformin for a few weeks prior to and then concurrently with clomiphene citrate is certainly easier than giving gonadotropins, and appears to be very effective for ovulation induction. Because monitoring is not required, the treatment can be performed by all clinicians with infertility training.

D.R. Mishell, Jr., M.D.

Menstrual Cyclicity After Metformin Therapy in Polycystic Ovary Syndrome

Velázquez E, Acosta A, Mendoza SG (Univ of The Andes, Mérida, Venezuela)
Obstet Gynecol 90:392–395, 1997 12–5

Background.—Metformin, a biguanide agent that improves insulin action at the cellular level without affecting insulin secretion, has been found to reduce hyperinsulinemia and hyperandrogenemia in women with polycystic ovary syndrome (PCOS) while facilitating normal menses and pregnancy. The effects of a 6-month course of metformin treatment on menstrual cycle regularity in oligomenorrheic women with PCOS were investigated.

Methods.—Forty oligomenorrheic women with PCOS were enrolled in the prospective clinical study. All were asked to complete at least 6 months of metformin therapy. Twenty-two finished the trial. Parameters were measured before and after 8 weeks of treatment. Menstrual cyclicity and serum progesterone concentrations at the midluteal phase were evaluated at treatment week 30.

Findings.—Menstrual cyclicity was restored in 95.7% of the women. Nineteen percent became pregnant in the sixth or seventh month of treatment, and all were delivered of healthy infants. Thirteen of 15 women whose menses were regular had a serum progesterone concentration within the ovulatory range. After 8 weeks of treatment, fasting and the integrated insulin response to glucose lead declined, accompanied by a significant decrease in the serum luteinizing hormone level, free testosterone level, and luteinizing hormone/follicle-stimulating hormone ratio. There was also a small, significant decrease in body mass index after 8 weeks of therapy.

Conclusions.—In women with PCOS, a 6-month course of metformin therapy may improve menstrual cyclicity and fertility. Insulin-sensitizing agents offer a rational approach to the treatment of the metabolic and endocrine abnormalities in this population.

▶ The results of this study indicate that metformin, given by itself for 6 months to anovulatory women with PCOS, can result in the development of spontaneous ovulatory cycles. Metformin reduces serum insulin levels in these women with insulin resistance and also appears to reduce serum androgen levels. Studies of long-term use of metformin in women with PCOS should be undertaken to determine the drug's effect on the metabolic and endocrine changes associated with PCOS.

D.R. Mishell, Jr., M.D.

Successful Induction of Ovulation in Normogonadotrophic Clomiphene Resistant Anovulatory Women by Combined Naltrexone and Clomiphene Citrate Treatment

'nalorex'

Roozenburg BJ, van Dessel HJHM, Evers JLH, et al (St Elisabeth Hosp, Tilburg, The Netherlands; Academic Hosp Maastricht, The Netherlands)
Hum Reprod 12:1720–1722, 1997 12–6

Background.—Most women with anovulatory subfertility are normogonadotropic with normal levels of follicle-stimulating hormone, but sometimes elevated levels of luteinizing hormone. The preferred treatment is use of antiestrogens, such as clomiphene citrate. About 30% of normogonadotropic anovulatory women are clomiphene citrate-resistant. Naltrexone is an opioid receptor blocker that has been used in patients with anovulation and cycle abnormalities. The occurrence of ovulation after oral naltrexone alone or naltrexone combined with the antiestrogen clomiphene citrate was studied in women with subfertility due to normogonadotropic anovulation who were clomiphene citrate-resistant.

Methods.—There were 22 infertile women (Table 1), 11 with amenorrhea and 11 with oligomenorrhea. All subjects were normogonadotropic and had received clomiphene citrate up to 150 mg for 5 days with no signs of ovulation. Oral naltrexone, 25 mg twice a day, was begun on the first day of a menstrual cycle. If there was no response to naltrexone alone, clomiphene citrate, 100 mg for 5 days, was added to the naltrexone regimen.

TABLE 1.—Patient Characteristics and Median (and Range) Baseline Plasma Concentrations in 22 Normogonadotropic Anovulatory Clomiphene Citrate-Resistant Women

Age (years)	29	(24–35)
Duration of subfertility (years)	2.4	(0.7–10.7)
Luteinizing hormone (IU/l)	9	(1–28)
Follicle stimulating hormone (IU/l)	5	(2–11)
Oestradiol (pmol/l)	219	(88–422)
Testosterone (nmol/l)	1.9	(0.6–5.5)

(Reprinted by permission of Oxford University Press, from Roozenburg BJ, van Dessel HJHM, Evers JLH, et al: Successful induction of ovulation in normagonadotrophic clomiphene resistant anovulatory women by combined naltrexone and clomiphene citrate treatment. *Hum Reprod* 12:1720–1722, 1997. Copyright European Society for Human Reproduction and Embryology, by permission of Oxford University Press.)

Results.—Ovulation occurred in 19 of the 22 subjects; ovulation occurred with naltrexone alone in 4 women and with clomiphene citrate and naltrexone in 18 women. Twelve women conceived during this treatment period: 3 in their first cycle, 4 in their second cycle, 2 in their third cycle, and 2 in their fourth cycle. All women had singleton pregnancies. The median frequency of menstrual periods was 0.5 per year before treatment and 11.5 per year after treatment. Three subjects did not respond to the combined treatment.

Discussion.—This is the first report of successful ovulation induced by an opioid receptor blocking agent and anti-estrogen in normogonadotropic anovulatory women who were clomiphene citrate-resistant. This treatment avoided ovarian hyperstimulation syndrome and multiple pregnancies. The use of naltrexone is a safe, effective, simple, and inexpensive alternative to gonadotropin ovulation induction in women with cycle disturbances who are clomiphene-resistant.

▶ As many as one third of anovulatory women fail to ovulate when treated with progressively increasing doses of clomiphene citrate. Most of these women have polycystic ovarian syndrome. Treatment of these clomiphene citrate-resistant ovulatory women withh human menopausal gonadotropin is expensive, requires daily sonographic monitoring, and frequently produces multiple pregnancies with a high rate of spontaneous abortion.

This initial study in which the opioid receptor blocker, naltrexone, was given to a small group of women who failed to ovulate with 150 mg of clomiphene citrate for 5 days found that use of naltrexone alone or combined with clomiphene citrate resulted in a high rate of ovulation and singleton pregnancies. Further studies are needed to confirm these findings; however, the initial results appear to indicate that naltrexone may be an effective safe alternative to human menopausal gonadotropin therapy for women who fail to ovulate with clomiphene citrate alone.

D.R. Mishell, Jr., M.D.

Mirena IUD

Randomised Comparative Trial of Levonorgestrel Intrauterine System and Norethisterone for Treatment of Idiopathic Menorrhagia

Irvine GA, Campbell-Brown MB, Lumsden MA, et al (Univ of Glasgow, Scotland; Glasgow Royal Infirmary NHS Trust, Scotland)

Br J Obstet Gynaecol 105:592–598, 1998 12–7

Background.—The most common treatment for menorrhagia in the United Kingdom is norethisterone. However, this treatment has been shown to be ineffective at currently recommended dosages. The efficacy and acceptability of the levonorgestrel intrauterine system were compared with those of norethisterone in the treatment of idiopathic menorrhagia.

Methods.—Forty-four women with heavy regular periods and a menstrual blood loss of more than 80 mL were included in the randomized comparative parallel group study. In one half of the women, a levonorgestrel intrauterine system was inserted within the first 7 days of menses; the other half received norethisterone, 5 mg 3 times a day, from day 5 to day 26 of the cycle for 3 cycles.

Findings.—Expressed as a percentage of the control at 3 months, menstrual blood loss was reduced 94% by the levonorgestrel intrauterine system and 87% by oral norethisterone. After 3 cycles of therapy, 76% of those treated with the levonorgestrel intrauterine system wished to continue their treatment, compared with only 22% of those given noresthisterone.

Conclusions.—In this study, both the levonorgestrel intrauterine system and oral norethisterone effectively reduced menstrual blood loss to within normal limits in women with idiopathic menorrhagia. However, patient satisfaction with the levonorgestrel intrauterine system was greater than with norethisterone, and a higher proportion wished to continue treatment. Thus, the levonorgestrel intrauterine system is a valuable alternative to the currently available medical treatment for menorrhagia.

► It is difficult to treat women with excessive menstrual blood loss, regular cycles, and no lesions in the endometrial cavity: a symptom complex called ovulatory dysfunctional bleeding. Because medical therapy of this entity has several side effects and may be ineffective, hysterectomy or endometrial ablation is frequently performed. This study shows that reduction of menstrual blood loss achieved with the insertion of an intrauterine device (IUD) releasing a progestin locally is as effective as that achieved with ingestion of 5 mg of norethindrone 3 times a day from day 5 to 26 of the cycle. The IUD was better tolerated by the women than the oral steroids. Although this type of IUD is currently unavailable in the United States, an IUD releasing progesterone is marketed and can also be used in the treatment of ovulatory dysfunctional bleeding.

D.R. Mishell, Jr., M.D.

Uterine Thermal Balloon Therapy for the Treatment of Menorrhagia: The First 300 Patients From a Multi-centre Study

Amso NN, for the International Collaborative Uterine Thermal Balloon Working Group (Queen Elizabeth Hosp, Gateshead, England; Stanford Univ, Calif; Belfast City Hosp, UK; et al)

Br J Obstet Gynaecol 105:517–523, 1998 12–8

Introduction.—Menorrhagia is traditionally managed by medical therapy with its associated side effects. Dilatation and curettage is a temporary treatment and has limited efficacy. Hysteroscopic treatment is difficult to perform and is associated with serious complications. Uterine balloon therapy is a potentially safer and easier technique for endometrial ablation than hysteroscopy. The safety and efficacy of thermal balloon therapy was assessed in 296 women with menorrhagia.

Methods.—Women with severe menorrhagia from 15 centers in Canada and Europe who failed medical therapy and were suitable candidates for either endometrial ablation or hysterectomy underwent 321 procedures of balloon endometrial ablation. Women with pathology distorting the uterine cavity, atypical endometrial hyperplasia, suspected genital tract infection or malignancy, uterine cavity depths over 12 cm, previous endometrial ablation, or a desire to preserve fertility were excluded. Patients underwent either general anesthesia (61%) or local anesthesia with or without sedation (39%). The balloon was filled with a variable volume of 5% dextrose water at a mean temperature of 87°C for 8 minutes. All patients were discharged within 24 hours and were evaluated at 3, 6, and 12 months postprocedure.

Results.—A comparison of preprocedure and postprocedure pad counts revealed a significant reduction in pad counts after balloon endometrial ablation. Treatment significantly decreased pain severity. Increasing age, higher balloon pressure, smaller uterine cavity, and lesser degree of preprocedure menorrhagia were correlated with significantly better outcome. Further surgery was required in 28 patients (10%) to treat unresolved symptoms; 15 had hysterectomies and 13 had endometrial ablations. There were no intraoperative complications. One patient was treated for postoperative cystitis, 6 were treated for febrile morbidity presumably caused by low-grade endometritis, and 2 were treated for hematometra. The overall minor complication rate was 3%.

Conclusions.—The efficacy of thermal balloon endometrial ablation was 88% to 91%. The procedure was well tolerated in women who underwent general anesthesia or local anesthesia with or without sedation. Twelve of the 28 women who requested further surgery had an average decrease of 54% in menstrual flow. The ease of use of thermal balloon endometrial ablation could possibly become an office procedure, thus decreasing cost and increasing patient and physician convenience.

▶ Menorrhagia without the presence of uterine lesions that fails to respond to medical therapy is the reason why many hysterectomies are performed in the United States. Endometrial ablation with the use of hysteroscopically placed instruments that destroy the endometrium with electrocautery are used by some individuals to treat menorrhagia in uteri without lesions. However, the technique of endometrial ablation with cautery is not as simple to learn or perform as is the use of thermal balloon therapy. Thermal balloon therapy thus provides a more easily performed technique than endometrial ablation to treat menorrhagia in women with normal uteri who do not respond to medical therapy. Thermal balloon therapy can be performed as an outpatient procedure, and is much safer and less expensive than performing a hysterectomy. Also, the time away from work after the procedure is markedly less. Clinicians should consider learning how to use this new modality to treat menorrhagia.

D.R. Mishell, Jr., M.D.

Thermal Balloon and Rollerball Ablation to Treat Menorrhagia: A Multicenter Comparison

Meyer WR, Walsh BW, Grainger DA, et al (Univ of North Carolina at Chapel Hill; Brigham and Women's Hosp, Chestnut Hill, Mass; Wesley Med Ctr, Wichita, Kan; et al)

Obstet Gynecol 92:98–103, 1998 12–9

Background.—Menorrhagia continues to be the reason for more than one third of the hysterectomies performed in the United States. The clinical efficacy of ablation therapy has been documented. In the current study, the clinical effectiveness and safety of a thermal uterine balloon system were compared with those of hysteroscopic rollerball ablation in the treatment of dysfunctional uterine bleeding.

Methods.—Two hundred fifty-five premenopausal women were enrolled in the randomized, multicenter study. Menstrual diary scores and quality-of-life questionnaires were obtained before and after the procedure. Twelve-month follow-up data were available on 239 women.

Findings.—Both procedures significantly decreased menstrual blood flow at 12 months, with no clinically significant difference between the 2. Multiple results from the quality-of-life questionnaires were also comparable, including the percentage of patients highly satisfied with outcomes. More than 60% of the patients in both groups had a 90% reduction in diary scores. Procedural time was decreased significantly in the uterine balloon treatment group. The incidence of intraoperative complications was 3.2% in the hysteroscopic rollerball group and 0% in the thermal balloon group.

Conclusions.—Uterine balloon therapy is as effective as hysteroscopic rollerball ablation in the treatment of dysfunctional uterine bleeding. Uterine balloon therapy may be the safer of the 2 procedures.

▶ Although the actual amount of menstrual blood loss was not measured in this study, subjective assessment of the amount of blood loss showed a similar reduction in the large number of women treated by the 2 techniques in this randomized study. Learning how to use the thermal balloon system is easier than learning how to use rollerball endometrial ablation, especially for those who have not received training in operative hysteroscopy. Use of the thermal balloon system should result in a reduction in the number of hysterectomies performed because of excessive uterine blood loss without uterine disease.

D.R. Mishell, Jr., M.D.

Transvaginal Administration of Progesterone

Fanchin R, De Ziegler D, Bergeron C, et al (Hôpital Antoine Béclère, Clamart, France; Columbia Labs Inc, Paris; CERBA Lab, Cergy Pontoise, France)

Obstet Gynecol 90:396–401, 1997 12–10

Introduction.—The sequential administration of estradiol (E_2) and progesterone can induce normal secretory transformation of the endometrium in women with absent or inactive ovaries, enhancing the success of in vitro fertilization with oocyte donation. This finding suggested that an oocyte donation cycle could be used as an experimental model to study the hormonal control of endometrial morphology. The endometrial effects of 3 different doses of vaginally administered progesterone were examined in a study of 40 women without ovarian function.

Methods.—Study participants were aged 25–41 years; all had baseline hormonal levels within the menopausal range. The women received transdermal E_2 for 28 days at a dose from 0.1–0.4 mg/day and at a schedule designed to duplicate E_2 levels observed during the menstrual cycle. Progesterone was administered from a vaginal gel with controlled and sustained-release properties. In a double-blind manner, the women were assigned to 1 of 3 dose groups: progesterone gel (Crinone) 4%, 1.125 g of gel containing 45 mg of progesterone (group A, 14 women); progesterone gel 8%, 1.125 g of gel containing 90 mg of progesterone (group B, 13 women); and progesterone gel 8%, 2.250 g of gel containing 180 mg of progesterone (group C, 13 women). Plasma gonadotropins, estrone, E_2, and progesterone were measured and an endometrial biopsy was performed on day 20 or 24.

Results.—Plasma estrone and E_2 profiles during the 28-day cycle followed the normal menstrual cycle in all women. Mean progesterone levels (Fig 1) were lower in group A than in groups B or C. Both plasma follicle-stimulating hormone and luteinizing hormone decreased significantly during progesterone treatment. Secretory transformation in the glands and stroma was seen in all groups on days 20 and 24, respectively, and the distribution of estrogen and progesterone receptors was comparable to that of normal menstrual cycles.

Conclusion.—All 3 doses of transvaginally administered progesterone induced the secretory transformation of endometrial glands and stroma in these women without ovarian function. The concentration of progesterone (4% or 8%), rather than the actual dose delivered (90 or 180 mg), may control absorption and affect plasma levels in vaginal administration.

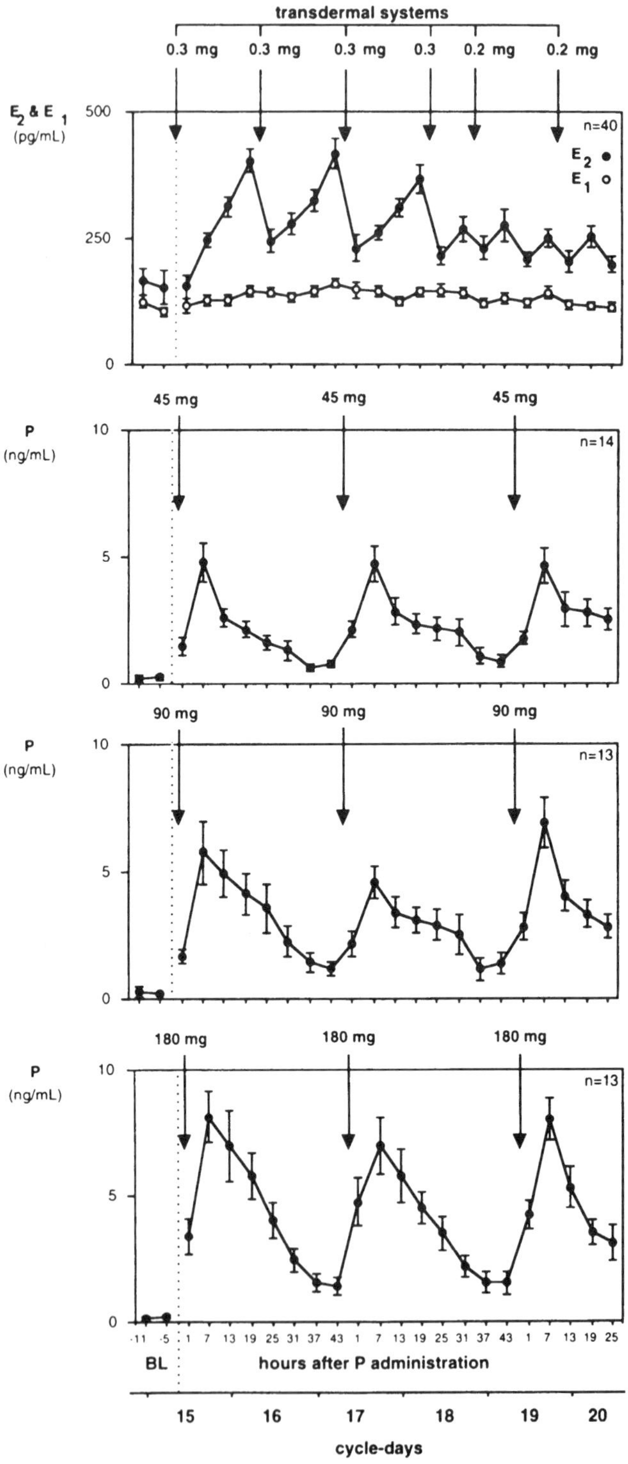

transdermal systems
0.3 mg
0.3 mg
0.3 mg
0.3
0.2 mg
0.2 mg
E2 & E1 (pg/mL)
500
250
0
n=40
E2 ●
E1 ○
45 mg
45 mg
45 mg
P (ng/mL)
10
5
0
n=14
90 mg
90 mg
90 mg
P (ng/mL)
10
5
0
n=13
180 mg
180 mg
180 mg
P (ng/mL)
10
5
0
n=13
-11 -5 1 7 13 19 25 31 37 43 1 7 13 19 25 31 37 43 1 7 13 19 25
BL
hours after P administration
15 16 17 18 19 20
cycle-days

(Continued)

Because plasma levels of progesterone remained low, findings suggest a direct transit into the uterus.

Randomized, Double-blind, Dose-ranging Study of the Endometrial Effects of a Vaginal Progesterone Gel in Estrogen-treated Postmenopausal Women

Ross D, Cooper AJ, Pryse-Davies J, et al (Menopause Clinic, King's College Hosp, London; Hammersmith Hosp, England)

Obstet Gynecol 177:937–941, 1997 12–11

Introduction.—Postmenopausal women who take systemic estrogens require concomitant progestogen treatment to prevent the increased risks of endometrial hyperplasia and carcinoma. Oral delivery of progesterone, however, yields poorly sustained plasma concentrations. In a randomized study, 31 estrogen-treated postmenopausal women were assessed for the endometrial effects of natural progesterone administered in a vaginal gel.

Methods.—The gel was designed to adhere to the vaginal epithelium, allowing sustained release of progesterone. Women recruited for the study had 1 year or more of amenorrhea or had received treatment for climacteric symptoms for 2 or more years. Treatment lasted for 3 cycles of 28 days each during which all women received conjugated estrogens tablets (Premarin) (0.625 mg daily) and sequential vaginal progesterone gel (Crinone). In the double-blind design, 15 women were allocated to gel containing 45 mg of progesterone and 16 to gel containing 90 mg of progesterone. One application of the gel was administered vaginally on days 17, 19, 21, 23, 25, and 27 of each cycle. The women were evaluated for endometrial histologic features, sex steroid hormone concentrations, and vaginal bleeding patterns.

Results.—Thirty-one of 41 histologic samples with adequate tissue for diagnosis were found to have secretory endometrium. There were no cases of hyperplasia and only 1 of proliferative endometrium (in the 45 mg progesterone group). Mean plasma progesterone concentrations (Table 3) were 4.6 ng/mL in the 45-mg progesterone group and 6.8 ng/mL in the 90 mg group. Data on vaginal bleeding were obtained from 19 women in cycle 2. The median duration of progesterone-associated bleeding was 6 days in both dosage groups, and vaginal bleeding was between spotting and light in both.

Conclusion.—Natural progesterone, administered vaginally as a bioadhesive gel, causes secretory transformation of the estrogenized endome-

---

FIGURE 1 (cont.)

FIGURE 1.—Plasma estradiol (E_2) and estrone (E_1) (**upper panel**) and progesterone (*P*) (**lower panels**) profiles in groups A (45 mg), B (90 mg), and C (180 mg) from days 15–20. Estrogen levels fluctuated in relation to changes of transdermal systems, but the E_2 to E_1 ratio remained greater than 1 throughout the observation interval. Overall mean progesterone levels were significantly lower in group A (2.4 ± 0.2 ng/mL) than in group B (3.6 ± 0.2 ng/mL) or C (3.4 ± 0.4 ng/mL) ($P < 0.005$). *Abbreviation: BL*, baseline. (Reprinted with permission from the American College of Obstetricians and Gynecologists, from Fanchin R, De Ziegler D, Bergeron C, et al: Transvaginal administration of progesterone. *Obstet Gynecol* 90:396–401, 1997.)

TABLE 3.—Plasma Progesterone Concentrations (Nanograms per Milliliter)

	Progesterone dose	
	45 mg	*90 mg*
Cycle 1		
No.	15	15
Mean and SE	4.6 (0.8)	6.2 (0.8)
Cycle 3		
No.	12	15
Mean and SE	3.6 (0.8)	6.8 (1.2)*

*$P < 0.05$.

(Reprinted with permission from the American College of Obstetricians and Gynecologists, from Ross D, Cooper AJ, Pryse-Davies J, et al: Randomized, double-blind, dose-ranging study of the endometrial effects of a vaginal progesterone gel in estrogen-treated postmenopausal women. *Obstet Gynecol* 177:937–941, 1997.)

trium in postmenopausal women. This method may cause fewer and less severe progestogenic side effects and have less impact on certain metabolic factors.

▶ The vaginal epithelium absorbs steroids and other substances very well with rapid transfer into the systemic circulation. After oral ingestion, natural steroids such as progesterone and estradiol are rapidly metabolized in the gut and liver and, thus, very large doses of these hormones need to be administered orally at frequent intervals to produce sustained physiologic levels in the circulation. Parenteral administration either transdermally or vaginally avoids the first pass of the steroids through the liver that occurs after oral administration. Estradiol is absorbed slowly through the skin and, thus, physiologic levels in the circulation can be maintained when the steroid is delivered through various types of adhesive patches. Progesterone, unfortunately, is absorbed very rapidly through the skin so sustained delivery of this hormone with the use of skin patches is not feasible. However, synthetic progestins have a slower rate of skin absorption and can be administered transdermally. The results of these 2 studies indicate that vaginal administration of natural progesterone in an adhesive gel results in sufficiently high blood levels to produce secretory transformation of an estrogen-primed endometrium. This effect was achieved with lower doses of progesterone in the circulation than occurs in the luteal phase of normal ovulatory cycles. This finding supports the existence of an intriguing first-pass effect to the uterus from the vagina. Because no arteries go from the vagina to the uterus, the mechanism for this effect, if it exists, remains unexplained at present.

D.R. Mishell, Jr., M.D.

Autoimmune Progesterone Dermatitis: Onset in a Woman Without Previous Exogenous Progesterone Exposure

Moody BR, Schatten S (Emory Univ, Atlanta, Ga)

South Med J 90:845–846, 1997 12–12

Introduction.—Autoimmune progesterone dermatitis is rare. Its clinical course can range from spontaneous remission to anaphylactic shock. Treatment includes suppression of ovulation with drugs or surgery. A woman with autoimmune progesterone dermatitis was successfully treated by oophorectomy.

Case Report.—Woman, 36, sought treatment for a facial rash that had occurred in 6 of the previous 9 months, but never before then. Two days before the office visit, the patient experienced burning and stinging in the face, with her entire face becoming beet red. In addition, her face, eyes, nose, lips, and chin had become swollen. The day of the office visit, her symptoms had begun to improve. The dermatitis had always occurred about 3 days before the onset of menses and resolved spontaneously within 7 days. She had had pruritic urticaria over her entire body from the fifth through ninth month of her second pregnancy. The patient also had painful dysmenorrhea and elected to have vaginal hysterectomy and bilateral salpingo-oophorectomy. At 1 year, she had no recurrence of facial urticaria.

Discussion.—Autoimmune progesterone dermatitis is a hypersensitivity reaction to increased levels of progesterone produced during the luteal phase of the menstrual cycle. Pruritus, urticaria, erythema multiforme, eczema, angioedema, and other papular and vesicular lesions can occur. The disease is exacerbated during the luteal phase of the menstrual cycle. Partial or complete remission occurs during or immediately after menses. Treatment involves suppression of ovulation and the luteal phase production of progesterone. Cyclic administration of conjugated estrogens, ethinyl estradiol, luteinizing hormone-releasing hormone agonists, tamoxifen, and danazol have been successfully used. Oophorectomy can provide definitive relief. It is important to recognize autoimmune progesterone dermatitis to avoid the rare possibility of anaphylactic shock.

► Autoimmune progesterone dermatitis is an extremely rare condition, especially if the woman has not had exposure to exogenous progesterone. Even though the condition is rare, clinicians should be aware that it can occur so that appropriate therapy to reduce progesterone levels can be undertaken. In addition to oophorectomy, exogenous estrogen, gonadotropin-releasing hormone agonists, tamoxifen, and danazol have each been used to successfully treat this condition.

D.R. Mishell, Jr., M.D.

13 Menopause

Rapid, Convenient Radioimmunoassay of Estrone Sulfate

Ranadive GN, Mistry JS, Damodaran K, et al (Diagnostic Systems Labs, Webster, Tex; Diagnostic Systems Labs, Toronto; Texas Tech Univ, Amarillo; et al)

Clin Chem 44:244–249, 1998 13–1

Background.—Estrone sulfate is a good marker of estrogenicity. Its serum concentrations are up to 20-fold higher than those of estrone or estradiol, it has slow metabolic clearance that is not affected by diurnal variation, and it does not bind to sex hormone-binding globulin. These authors developed a radioimmunoassay to quantitate estrone sulfate, and they describe reference ranges for men and for women pre- and postmenopause, during the menstrual cycle, and during pregnancy.

Methods.—Blood samples were drawn from numerous participants: men not taking medications; women not using oral contraceptives during the luteal and follicular phases of the menstrual cycle; women using oral contraceptives; postmenopausal women not receiving hormone replacement therapy (HRT); postmenopausal women receiving HRT; and pregnant women during the first, second, and third trimesters. For direct radioimmunoassay, the antiserum was created by conjugating estrone-3-sulfate-6-(O-carboxymethyl)oxime with bovine serum albumin and immunizing rabbits. The estrone sulfate tracer was created by iodinating a estrone-3-sulfate-6-(O-carboxymethyl)oxime histamine conjugate. Patient samples were incubated in polypropylene tubes with labeled estrone sulfate tracer (100 µL) and antiserum (100 µL) and shaken at room temperature for 3 hours. Then 1 mL of goat anti-rabbit immunoglobulin G was added as a precipitating reagent. After standing 10 minutes, samples were centrifuged for 15 minutes at 1,500*g*. The supernate was then decanted and radioactivity was counted for 1 minute.

Findings.—The dynamic range of the radioimmunoassay was 0.05–90 µg/L, and the detection limit was 0.009 µg/L. Interassay and intra-assay coefficients of variation were less than 10% on all samples run, and serum and plasma gave similar results. The antiserum was 100% cross-reactive with estrone sulfate, but less than 5% cross-reactive with estrone, unconjugated estrogens, and other related steroids. Excellent correlation (r = 0.99) was obtained between the results of this assay and those of a conventional assay that involves the hydrolysis of estrone sulfate and

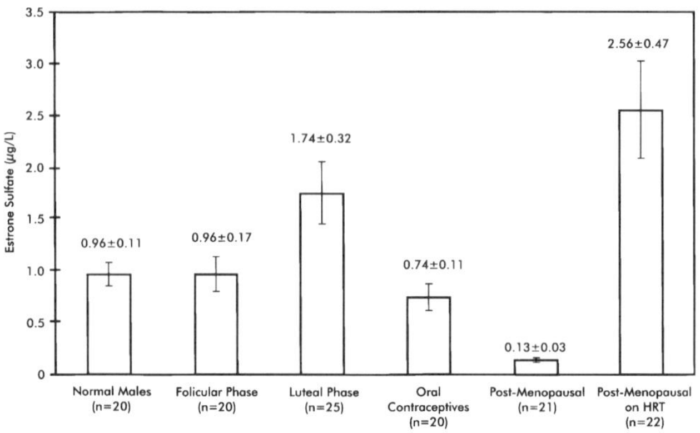

FIGURE 5.—Estrone sulfate concentrations (mean ± standard deviation) in different groups of samples. (Courtesy of Ranadive GN, Mistry JS, Damodaran K, et al: Rapid, convenient radioimmunoassay of estrone sulfate. *Clin Chem* 44:244–249, copyright 1998 The American Association for Clinical Chemistry [1–800–892–1400].)

indirect measurements of estrone. Mean estrone sulfate concentrations were as follows (Fig 5): men, 0.96 μg/L; women in the follicular phase, 0.96 μg/L; women in the luteal phase, 1.74 μg/L; women using oral contraceptives, 0.74 μg/L; postmenopausal women without HRT, 0.13 μg/L; postmenopausal women using HRT, 2.56 μg/L; pregnant women in the first trimester, 20 μg/L; pregnant women in the second trimester, 66 μg/L; and pregnant women in the third trimester, 105 μg/L.

Conclusions.—The radioimmunoassay described reliably measures estrone sulfate. It is simple to perform and has high sensitivity and reproducibility between and among runs. It does not require extensive sample pretreatment, and either serum or plasma can be used. This radioimmunoassay should prove helpful in determining the estrogenicity in women.

▶ Asymptomatic postmenopausal women frequently ask whether they need HRT. Women receiving HRT also are concerned about whether they are receiving too much or too little exogenous estrogen. It has been difficult to answer these questions by measuring estradiol or estrone levels in serum, because with oral therapy the levels vary greatly, according to the time after hormone ingestion when serum sample is obtained. The levels are generally low, and the biologically inactive estradiol, which is bound to sex hormone binding globulin, as well as the free form of estradiol are measured in most assays.

Development of an easily performed assay for estrogen sulfate, as described in this article, will provide clinicians with a means to determine the amount of biologic estrogens in the circulation of postmenopausal women receiving and not receiving HRT. This assay should have great clinical relevance.

D.R. Mishell, Jr., M.D.

Prevalence, 1-Year Incidence and Factors Associated With Urinary Incontinence: A Population-based Study of Women 50–74 Years of Age in Primary Care

Holtedahl K, Hunskaar S (Maison Suger, Paris)

Maturitas 28:205–211, 1998 13–2

Background.—Estimates of the incidence of urinary incontinence in women vary significantly. The reasons for this include varying definitions of urinary incontinence, variation in study populations, recall bias, unknown remission rates, and difficulties in classifying the type, severity, and impact of urinary incontinence.

Methods.—A random sample of 698 women between 50 and 74 were invited to receive 2 gynecologic examinations 1 year apart performed by their general physician. The request did not mention urinary incontinence. During the consultation, the women and their physicians completed a questionnaire. At 1-year follow-up, the incidence and remission rates of urinary incontinence were determined.

Results.—Of 507 respondents who received the first examination, 489 received the second examination 1 year later. The mean age of respondents was 60.7 years. Leakage of any kind was reported by 47.3% of women, 2 or more leakage episodes per month were reported by 30.6% of women, and incontinence according to the definition by the International Continence Society was reported by 18.9% of women. Three women who reported no leakage at the first examination reported that regular incontinence had developed during the following year. No cases of spontaneous remission were seen. Women who reported leakage had a mean weight of 71.5 kg and body mass index of 26.8 kg/m^2, and women who reported no leakage had a mean weight of 65.9 kg and body mass index of 24.6 kg/m^2. No association was seen between urinary incontinence and age, age at menopause, operations on cervix uteri, diagnosed cystourethrocoele and/or vaginal atrophy, municipality, smoking, gynecologic examination in the last 5 years, diabetes, previous diagnosis of cancer, reported urinary tract infection in the previous year, or current use of drugs such as diuretics, estriol, or hormone replacement therapy. The risk of being incontinent doubled when surgical subgroups in the regression model were replaced by the category of having had a previous gynecologic operation.

Discussion.—Among women between 50 and 74 years of age, approximately 1 in 5 may require treatment for urinary incontinence. Without treatment, urinary incontinence tends to be long-lasting, with little chance for remission. The condition is associated with high body weight, poor ability to contract the pelvic floor muscles, and previous gynecologic surgery.

▶ This prospective study indicates that about 20% of postmenopausal women aged 50–74 from an area of Norway have symptomatic and objective evidence of urinary incontinence. Women do not usually volunteer information about this problem. Therefore, clinicians should routinely question postmenopausal women about whether they have urinary incontinence. If the symptom is present, therapies should be offered to alleviate the problem, because spontaneous remission of urinary incontinence is extremely uncommon. Depending upon the frequency and severity of the urinary incontinence, either pelvic floor exercises, vaginal pessaries, or corrective surgical procedures can be offered to the woman.

D.R. Mishell, Jr., M.D.

Better Postural Balance in Elderly Women Receiving Estrogens

Naessen T, Lindmark B, Larsen H-C (Univ Hosp, Uppsala, Sweden)

Am J Obstet Gynecol 177:412–416, 1997 13–3

Background.—Bone mass decreases with age, as does the postural balance function as a result of decreased functional capacity in organs important in postural balance. The effect of long-term estrogen replacement therapy on postural balance function was studied.

Methods.—There were 16 women who were long-term users of 17β-estradiol implants 20 mg every 6 months, and 16 women who were age-matched nonusers of the implant. Static posturography on a computerized force platform was used to measure postural balance. Sway velocity was measured using data on forces and vectors from strain gauges.

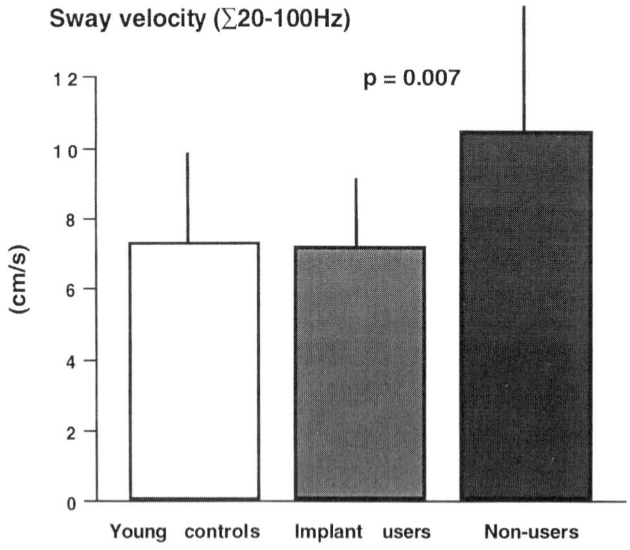

FIGURE 2.—Means and standard deviations for sway velocity (Σ20–100 Hz) in 16 long-term estrogen users (*shaded bar*), age-matched nonusers (*filled bar*), and 17 women in fertile age period, mean age 25 years (*open bar*) after provocation of balance function by blindfolding and disturbing the proprioception by increasing frequency of vibration stimulation to calf muscles (*P* values indicate tested differences between implant users and age-matched nonusers). (Courtesy of Naessen T, Lindmark B, Larsen, H-C: Better postural balance in elderly women receiving estrogens. *Am J Obstet Gynecol* 177:412–416, 1997.)

Results.—After blindfolding and disturbance of the proprioception by increasing frequency of vibration stimulation to calf muscles, women who used estrogen had significantly lower sway velocities than women who did not use estrogen for most separate frequencies and the frequencies 20–100 Hz combined. In women who used the implant, sway velocity values were low and similar to values seen in 17 heathy subjects in the fertile age period (Fig 2). Sway velocity was negatively correlated to serum estradiol and estradiol/sex hormone-binding globulin, and positively correlated to serum follicle-stimulating hormone for the frequencies 20–100 Hz combined and for peak vibration stimulation. This supported a causal relationship between estrogen and postural balance function.

Discussion.—These findings show that postural balance function is better in elderly women who have used estrogens for many years. This is the first report of a better postural balance function in older women who are long-term users of estrogens compared to nonusers of estrogens. If estrogen replacement therapy can improve postural balance function when started at an older age, it may lower the risk of fracture with only moderate effects on bone mass.

▶ The results of this observational study indicate that postmenopausal estrogen replacement helps to preserve postural balance function. This effect may help to reduce the fracture risk among postmenopausal women taking estrogen in addition to the known beneficial effect of estrogen upon bone density. If estrogen replacement rapidly improves postural balance in elderly women, administration of estrogen to women who are many years postmenopausal and already have osteoporosis may reduce their risk of fracture by reducing their risk of falling.

D.R. Mishell, Jr., M.D.

Postmenopausal Estrogen Replacement and Tooth Retention

Krall EA, Dawson-Hughes B, Hannan MT, et al (Tufts Univ, Boston; Boston Univ; Harvard Med School, Boston)

Am J Med 102:536–542, 1997 13–4

Background.—The incidence of tooth loss and edentulism increases with age, and approximately 50% of women older than 75 years are edentulous. Healthy women in late menopause and older men with higher levels of systemic bone mineral density tend to have more natural remaining teeth. Higher rates of bone mineral density loss after menopause are associated with a higher risk of tooth loss. This indicates that estrogen replacement therapy may increase tooth retention because it reduces or eliminates systemic bone loss. Two recent studies support this assumption by examining the relationship between history of estrogen use and tooth retention in elderly women.

Methods.—There were 488 elderly women participating in the Osteoporosis Study component of the Framingham Heart Study, begun in 1948

TABLE 2.—Comparison of Subjects by History of Estrogen Use

Ever Used Estrogen	No	Yes	P
Number	304	184	
Age (years)	81 ± 4	80 ± 4	0.02
Number of teeth (excluding third molars)	11.5 ± 10.2	13.7 ± 9.9	0.03
Incisors*	4.2 ± 3.5	4.9 ± 3.4	0.04
Canines†	2.1 ± 1.7	2.5 ± 1.7	0.03
Premolars‡	3.1 ± 3.1	3.7 ± 3.1	0.03
Molars§	2.0 ± 2.6	2.5 ± 2.7	0.07
Percent edentulous	33%	26%	0.13
Percent completed high school	70%	74%	0.33
Percent ever smoked	48%	53%	0.31
Percent currently smoke	15%	12%	0.38
Percent with any type of denture	75%	75%	0.87

*Central and lateral incisors in each jaw, maximum of 8 teeth.
†Maximum of 4 teeth.
‡Maximum of 8 teeth.
§First and second molars, maximum of 8 teeth.
(Reprinted by permission of the publisher, from Krall EA, Dawson-Hughes B, Hannan MT, et al: Postmenopausal estrogen replacement and tooth retention. *Am J Med* 102:536–542, Copyright 1997 by Excerpta Medica, Inc.)

to evaluate risk factors for heart disease. In the Framingham Heart Study, examinations are performed biennially. The number of teeth and their location were evaluated at the 23rd examination. Estrogen use had been documented at each examination since the early 1960s.

Results.—At the time of the dental evaluation, the subjects were between 72 and 95, and the median time since menopause was 31 years. The mean number of remaining teeth decreased with age in these women up to age 84, with a corresponding increase in edentulism. The number of remaining teeth and edentulism were associated with a history of smoking and less education. The percentage of women retaining a specific type of tooth was consistently greater in women who used estrogen than in those who did not use estrogen, except for second and third molars. After adjustment for age, smoking status, and level of education, the difference in mean number of teeth between women who used and did not use estrogen was the same. Among women who had smoked, women who used estrogen had an average of 2 more teeth than women who had not used estrogen, after adjustment for age and education. Among women who had never smoked, those who used estrogen also had an average of 2 more teeth than women who had not used estrogen (Table 2). In all women, the length of time a woman used estrogen predicted the number of remaining teeth. Compared to women who had not used estrogen, women who used estrogen for 1–4 years had 1.1 more teeth, women who used estrogen for 5–8 years had 1.5 more teeth, and those who used estrogen for more than 8 years had 3.6 more teeth. Use of estrogen for more than 8 years was associated with significantly greater retention of all types of teeth, except molars. The odds of being edentulous were reduced by 6% for each year of estrogen use, after adjustment for age, smoking, and education.

Discussion.—These findings show that elderly women who use estrogen retain significantly more teeth than women who do not use estrogen. Women who used estrogen longer had more natural remaining teeth. Different types of teeth were examined because each tooth has individual characteristics that affect the reasons for and chances of its being lost. The estrogen effect on different categories of teeth strengthens the assumption that the hormonal environment affects the risk of tooth loss. Long-term use of estrogen appears to both protect against tooth loss and lower the risk of edentulism.

▶ This is the third observational epidemiologic study reporting postmenopausal estrogen replacement therapy is associated with a protective effect against tooth loss. In this study, the number of teeth retained was directly related to the duration of estrogen use. This finding supports a causal relation between estrogen replacement and tooth retention. Women should be informed of this benefit of estrogen replacement, in addition to the well-known reduction in risk of cardiovascular disease and osteoporosis, to assist them in making a decision whether or not to use postmenopausal estrogen replacement.

D.R. Mishell, Jr., M.D.

The Effect of Estrogen on Blood Pressure in Hypertensive Postmenopausal Women

Sands RH, Studd JWW, Crook D, et al (Chelsea & Westminster Hosp, London; Wynn Inst for Metabolic Research, London; Royal Brompton Hosp, London)

J North Am Meno Soc 4:115–119, 1997 13–5

Background.—Most information sheets for estrogen replacement treatments caution use for hypertensive patients or state that hypertension is a contraindication. The effect of an oral estrogen on blood pressure and other cardiovascular risk markers (serum lipid and lipoprotein levels, coagulation, and endothelial cell function) was studied in hypertensive postmenopausal women.

Methods.—Twenty postmenopausal women with mild hypertension were enrolled in the randomized, placebo-controlled, crossover study. Eight weeks of active treatment followed by 8 weeks of placebo, or vice versa, was given. Active treatment consisted of 1 estrogen tablet containing 0.6 mg of estradiol, 0.27 mg of estriol, and 1.4 mg of estrone taken orally every day.

Findings.—Twenty-four-hour as well as day and night readings showed no significant changes in diastolic and systolic blood pressure while the women were taking estrogen. Mean 24-hour ambulatory blood pressure readings were 135.7 mm Hg/83.9 mm Hg at baseline, 131.7 mm Hg/83 mmHg during estrogen therapy, and 129.9 mm Hg/82.8 mm Hg during placebo. Serum levels of high-density lipoproteins and apolipoprotein AI

TABLE 2.—Summary of 24-Hour, Day, and Night Time Blood Pressure and Pulse Changes, From Baseline, for Patients Receiving Estrogen Treatment Compared With Those Receiving Placebo

	Hormonin			Placebo		
	Mean	(SD)	N	Mean	(SD)	N
24-hour						
Diastolic (mmHg)	−0.6	(5.3)	18	−1.1	(7.4)	19
Systolic (mmHg)	−2.6	(12.1)	18	−5.8	(12.3)	19
Pulse (bpm)	1.2	(14)	18	−.09	(8.8)	19
Day time						
Diastolic (mmHg)	0.7	(5.0)	18	−1.1	(8.6)	19
Systolic (mmHg)	−2.4	(13.2)	18	−7.3	(14)	19
Pulse (bpm)	2.9	(15.1)	18	0.1	(10.9)	19
Night time						
Diastolic (mmHg)	−6.0	(17.0)	18	−4.9	(19.6)	18
Systolic (mmHg)	−1.6	(14.0)	18	−0.0	(16.5)	18
Pulse (bpm)	−0.8	(11.1)	18	−2.3	(7.3)	18

Abbreviation: SD, standard deviation.

(Courtesy of Sands RH, Studd JWW, Warren JB, et al: The effects of estrogen on blood pressure in hypertensive postmenopausal women. *Menopause* 4:115–119, 1997.)

rose significantly by 0.1 mmol/L and 32 mg/dl, respectively, during estrogen treatment. Those of low-density lipoproteins and apolipoprotein B declined by 0.7 mmol/L and 5.5 mg/dl, respectively. Plasminogen was the only clotting factor significantly affected during active treatment, increasing by 13.6% (Table 2).

Conclusions.—Estrogens may be used safely in women with stable hypertension. No increase in ambulatory blood pressure was observed in the current series. Changes in other risk factors were beneficial, resembling those in normotensive postmenopausal women.

▶ Several longitudinal and cross-sectional studies have shown that administration of estrogen replacement therapy (ERT) to normotensive postmenopausal women does not affect their blood pressure in comparison with a control group receiving either no therapy or placebo. In this randomized, controlled trial, administration of ERT to a group of postmenopausal mildly hypertensive women also did not alter their mean systolic or diastolic blood pressure. In addition, beneficial changes in lipids and coagulant factors occurred with estrogen replacement in this group of women. The results of this study indicate that clinicians should not avoid use of ERT in postmenopausal hypertensive women. Because such women are at greater risk of developing cardiovascular disease than normotensive women, they should benefit from receiving ERT because of its demonstrated reduction in risk of developing a myocardial infarction.

D.R. Mishell, Jr., M.D.

Duration of Estrogen Replacement Therapy in Relation to the Risk of Incident Myocardial Infarction in Postmenopausal Women
Heckbert SR, Weiss NS, Koepsell TD, et al (Univ of Washington, Seattle)
Arch Intern Med 157:1330–1336, 1997 13–6

Introduction.—A decreased risk for first coronary heart disease events is said to be associated with estrogen replacement therapy in women after menopause. Little is known about whether the risk declines with increased duration of therapy. Estrogen is known to have procoagulant activity, to affect the endothelium and vascular smooth muscle, to favorably affect the lipid profile, decrease formation of new plaques, and stabilize existing plaques. A study of hormone replacement therapy in relation to a risk of cardiovascular disease in women was conducted.

Methods.—Medical records of 850 postmenopausal women aged 30–79 who had an incident fatal or nonfatal myocardial infarction during a 7-year period were reviewed, and telephone interviews were conducted with consenting survivors. They were compared with control postmenopausal women who did not have myocardial infarction (MI). An assessment was made of the use of estrogen or estrogen and progestin.

Results.—After adjustment for age, year of identification, diabetes mellitus, angina, and smoking, a longer duration of use of estrogen was inversely associated with a risk for MI among women who were currently using estrogen. There were 27% of women with MI who used estrogen replacement therapy at any time, and there were 33% of women without MI who used estrogen replacement therapy at any time. There was a 28% decrease in the risk of MI with the use of estrogens at any time. The odds ratio for MI was 1.00 for estrogen use of 0 years; 0.91 for estrogen use of less than 1.8 years; 0.70 for estrogen use of 1.8–4.2 years; 0.65 for estrogen use of 4.2–8.2 years; and 0.55 for estrogen use of 8.2 years or more. There was no evidence of decreasing risk with increasing duration of estrogen use among women who had used estrogen in the past.

Conclusion.—A reduced risk for first MI was associated with a long duration of hormone replacement therapy among women currently using estrogen. Those who had used estrogen for 8.2 years or more had a 45% reduction in risk for MI compared to those who had never used estrogen replacement therapy.

► The results of numerous observational epidemiologic studies indicate that use of postmenopausal estrogen replacement therapy is associated with a decreased risk of MI. It has been stated that because the women who elect to use estrogen may have a lower risk for having an MI than those who do not take estrogen replacement therapy, the protection associated with estrogen use may not be causally related to the use of this agent. The results of this study show that among women taking estrogen, the risk of having an MI decreased with increasing duration of estrogen use. These data support the assumption that estrogen itself protects against the development of MI by several systemic and local mechanisms.

D.R. Mishell, Jr., M.D.

Postmenopausal Estrogens and Risk of Myocardial Infarction in Diabetic Women

Kaplan RC, Smith NL, Heckbert SR, et al (Univ of Washington, Seattle; Fred Hutchinson Cancer Research Ctr, Seattle; Group Health Cooperative of Puget Sound, Seattle)

Diabetes Care 21:1117–1121, 1998 13–7

Background.—The effects of hormone replacement therapy (HRT) on the risk of myocardial infarction (MI) in women with diabetes has not been established. A case-control study of postmenopausal estrogen use and the risk of incident MI in diabetic women undergoing pharmacologic treatment was reported.

Methods.—Two hundred twelve postmenopausal, treated diabetic women who experienced a fatal or nonfatal MI incident between 1986 and 1994 made up the case group. One hundred twenty-two treated diabetic women with no previous MI constituted the control group. Estrogen use was determined from computerized pharmacy data and medical records. Adjustments were made for cardiovascular risk factors, which were determined from medical records, computerized pharmacy and laboratory data, and telephone interviews.

Findings.—Eight and one half percent of case subjects and 13.9% of control subjects were current users of estrogen. Current users had a relative risk (RR) of 0.51 for MI compared with those who had never used estrogen, after adjustment for age, study year, weight, angina, and duration of treated diabetes. Among current users, MI risk tended to decrease with each additional year of estrogen use. Past estrogen users—45.3% of case and 37.7% of control subjects—had an adjusted RR of 1.22.

Conclusions.—The use of postmenopausal estrogens does not appear to increase the risk of MI in diabetic women. In fact, sustained estrogen use may be beneficial.

▶ Diabetes mellitus, which occurs in from 4% to 7% of postmenopausal women, is a risk factor for MI. Estrogen replacement therapy has been shown in several observational studies to reduce the risk of MI. The results of this observational case-control study suggest that estrogen replacement given to postmenopausal women with diabetes mellitus probably reduces their risk of MI and certainly does not increase the risk. Diabetes mellitus is not a contraindication to the use of estrogen replacement, and estrogen appears to have a beneficial effect on the cardiovascular system in diabetic women.

D.R. Mishell, Jr., M.D.

Postmenopausal Hormone Use and Risk for Colorectal Cancer and Adenoma

Grodstein F, Martinez EM, Platz EA, et al (Harvard Med School, Boston)
Ann Intern Med 128:705–712, 1998 13–8

Background.—Epidemiologic evidence suggests that postmenopausal hormone therapy may be associated with a decreased risk of colorectal cancer. The relationship between postmenopausal hormone use and colorectal cancer risk was explored using data from the large, prospective Nurses' Health Study.

Study Design.—The Nurses' Health Study (NHS) originated in 1976 with 121,700 female registered nurses in 11 states completing health questionnaires. These questionnaires are updated every 2 years. This study group consisted of 29,264 women from the NHS who were postmenopausal in 1980 and 29,738 who joined as they became postmenopausal during the course of the 14-year study. This study included a total of 601,503 person-years of follow-up. Medical record review confirmed all cases of colorectal cancer or adenoma.

Findings.—From 1980 to 1994, 470 women in the study group had colorectal cancer and 838 had colorectal adenomas. Women who had never used hormones comprised 48.1%, current users, 28.3%, and past users, 23.6% of the total study time. Current use of postmenopausal hormone therapy was associated with a decreased risk for colorectal cancer (Table 1). There was no association between duration of hormone therapy and protection. There was no decreased risk detected for women who had taken hormones at least 5 years previously. Current use of postmenopausal hormone therapy was also associated with a decreased risk for large, but not small, adenomas.

Conclusions.—This large, prospective study indicated the risk for colorectal cancers and large adenomas was decreased by current postmenopausal hormone therapy. This protection receded after cessation of hormone therapy. There was no relation between duration of hormone therapy and reduction of risk.

▶ The results of this analysis of the large ongoing Nurses' Health Study provides additional data to that previously published, which indicates postmenopausal estrogen reduces the risk of colorectal cancer development. The Nurses' Health Study is a large observational study, and the results are consistent with other studies indicating that estrogen use by postmenopausal women reduces the risk of developing colorectal cancer by about 30%. Colorectal cancer is the third leading cause of cancer death among women in the United States Lung cancer is the most frequent cause of female cancer death, and breast cancer is second. There are several mechanisms whereby estrogen could reduce the incidence of this neoplasm, including changes in bile acid metabolism and alterations in steroid hormone receptors in the colorectal mucosa. Women should be informed about this

TABLE 1.—Relative Risk for Colorectal Cancer Among Women According to Postmenopausal Hormone Use, 1980-1994

Hormone Use	Patient-Years of Follow-up	Colorectal Cancer		Colon Cancer		Rectal Cancer	
		Cases *n*	RR (95% CI)	Cases *n*	RR (95% CI)	Cases *n*	RR (95% CI)
Never	289 589	262		203		59	
Current	170 170	90		69		21	
Age-adjusted			0.62 (0.49–0.79)		0.62 (0.47–0.81)		0.64 (0.39–1.06)
Multivariate-adjusted†			0.65 (0.50–0.83)		0.64 (0.48–0.85)		0.67 (0.40–1.12)
<5 years	75 299	30		20		10	
Age-adjusted			0.53 (0.36–0.78)		0.45 (0.29–0.72)		0.80 (0.40–1.59)
Multivariate-adjusted†			0.56 (0.39–0.83)		0.49 (0.31–0.77)		0.83 (0.42–1.64)
≥5 years	90 903	59		48		11	
Age-adjusted			0.69 (0.52–0.91)		0.71 (0.52–0.98)		0.59 (0.31–1.11)
Multivariate-adjusted†			0.72 (0.53–0.96)		0.75 (0.54–1.04)		0.59 (0.30–1.16)
Past	141 744	118		94		24	
Age-adjusted			0.82 (0.66–1.02		0.84 (0.65–1.08)		0.76 (0.47–1.23)
Multivariate-adjusted†			0.84 (0.67–1.05)		0.86 (0.67–1.11)		0.76 (0.47–1.24)
<5 years	99 458	77		61		16	
Age-adjusted			0.79 (0.61–1.03)		0.83 (0.62–1.12)		0.78 (0.44–1.38)
Multivariate-adjusted†			0.79 (0.61–1.03)		0.81 (0.60–1.08)		0.75 (0.43–1.31)
≥5 years	36 029	34		27		7	
Age-adjusted			0.88 (0.61–1.27)		0.89 (0.59–1.34)		0.84 (0.38–1.86)
Multivariate-adjusted†			0.90 (0.62–1.30)		0.91 (0.60–1.39)		0.83 (0.37–1.90)

*Information on duration of hormone use was missing for 8 cases (1 current user and 7 past users) and 10,225 person-years of follow-up (3,968 person-years of current use and 6,256 person-years of past use) RR = relative risk.

†Adjusted for age, body mass index, past use of oral contraceptives, family history of colorectal cancer, calcium intake, folate intake, methionine intake, red meat intake, aspirin use, alcohol intake, previous polyps, cigarette smoking, exercise, and age at menopause.

(Courtesy of Grodstein, F, Martinez EM, Platz EA, et al: Postmenopausal hormone use and risk for colorectal cancer and adenoma. *Ann Intern Med* 128:705–712, 1998.)

additional benefit of postmenopausal estrogen therapy when they are deciding whether to initiate such treatment.

D.R. Mishell, Jr., M.D.

Hormone Replacement Therapy and the Risk of Hospitalization for Venous Thromboembolism: A Population-based Study in Southern Europe

Varas-Lorenzo C, García-Rodríguez LA, Cattaruzzi C, et al (Novartis Pharmaceuticals, Barcelona; Centro Español de Investigación Farmacoepidemiológica, Madrid; Azienda Ospedaliera SM Misericordia, Udine, Italy; et al)

Am J Epidemiol 147:387–390, 1998 13–9

Background.—Recent American and British studies have reported that the use of oral hormone replacement therapy is associated with an increased risk of venous thromboembolism. This study examined the risk associated with transdermal hormone replacement therapy in a Southern European population.

Study Design.—The study population consisted of all women, aged 45–79 years, who had been residents of the Friuli-Venezia Giulia region of Italy since 1985. Women with a history of risk factors for thromboembolism and pregnant women were excluded. The study cohort consisted of 265,431 subjects who used hormone replacement therapy and were followed until thromboembolism, death, emigration, age of 80 years, or end of the study period in December 1995. The control group consisted of 10,000 randomly selected women who did not use hormone replacement therapy.

Findings.—Hospital record review identified 171 women with idiopathic incident cases of venous thromboembolism. The most important independent risk factors were a history of either varicose veins or superficial phlebitis and obesity. Users of hormone replacement therapy had a 2.3 times higher risk of venous thromboembolism than nonusers. This increased risk occurred only in the first year of therapy. The crude incidence rate in the population of women using hormone replacement therapy was 1.3/10,000 person-years. The overall case fatality rate was 1.8%.

Conclusion.—With the use of transdermal hormone replacement therapy, the risk of thromboembolism was increased almost threefold in a healthy southern European population in the first year of treatment. This translates to 2 additional cases of venous thromboembolism/10,000 women using hormone replacement therapy for 1 year.

► The results of this epidemiologic study are consistent with the other 4 epidemiologic studies published in 1996 and 1997, which showed that postmenopausal estrogen replacement therapy (ERT) increases the risk of the development of venous thrombosis or pulmonary embolism (VTE) about 2fold. In this study as well as that of Gutthann et al.,[1] the increase in risk occurs only in the first year of use.

In the previous studies, the majority of the users of ERT used oral preparations, whereas in this study, nearly 80% of the women used a transdermal preparation. For women without risk factors for VTE, the attributable risk of VTE with ERT is only about 1 extra event of VTE per 10,000 women per year—a small degree of risk for an individual woman.

D.R. Mishell, Jr., M.D.

Reference

1. 1998 Year Book of Obstetrics, Gynecology, and Women's Health, pp335–336.

Effect of Estrogen-Progestin Hormonal Replacement Therapy on Plasma Antithrombin III of Postmenopausal Women

Bonduki CE, Lourenço DM, Baracat E, et al (Universidade Federal de São Paulo, Brazil)

Acta Obstet Gynecol Scand 77:330–333, 1998 13–10

Introduction.—To relieve symptoms associated with climacterium, hormonal replacement therapy is increasingly recommended. The risk of cardiovascular disease, which increases in women after menopause, seems to be reduced with this therapy. The main inhibitor of blood coagulation is antithrombin III. An association between oral contraceptive drugs and thrombosis has been known for a long time. The effect of estrogen-progestin hormonal replacement therapy on antithrombin III levels in climacteric women was investigated by comparing the effects of oral to transdermal routes of estrogen administration.

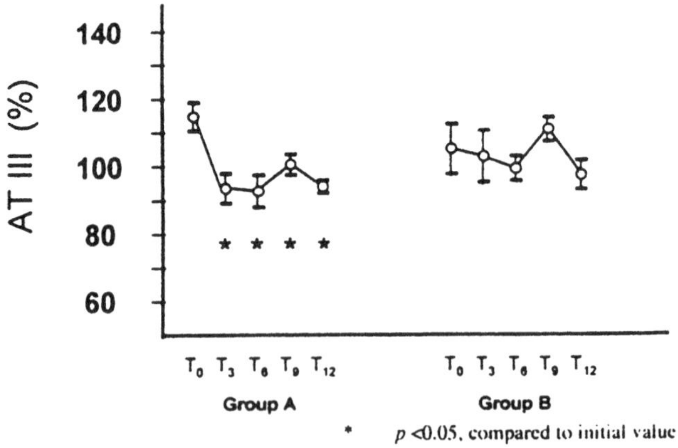

FIGURE 1.—Antithrombin III levels (mean ± standard error) during 1 year of hormone replacement therapy (T0–T12) with oral conjugated estrogen (group A) or transdermal 17 β-estradiol (group B). (Courtesy of Bonduki CE, Lourenço DM, Baracat E, et al: Effect of estrogen-progestin hormonal replacement therapy on plasma antithrombin III of postmenopausal women. *Acta Obstet Gynecol Scand* 77:330–333, copyright 1998 Munksgaard International Publishers Ltd., Copenhagen, Denmark.)

Methods.—There were 19 postmenopausal women, ages 40–65, in a prospective randomized study in which they received continuous daily oral equine conjugated estrogen at 0.625 mg or daily transdermal 17β-estradiol 50 μg. All women received medroxyprogesterone acetate at 5 mg/day for 14 days each month. Before and after 3, 6, 9, and 12 months of treatment, blood samples were obtained. Coagulation tests included prothrombin time, antithrombin II (functional method), thrombin time, partial activated prothrombin time, fibrinogen, factor V, euglobulin lysis time, and platelet count. Friedman analysis of variance and Mann-Whitney tests were used for statistical analysis.

Results.—In the group receiving daily oral equine conjugated estrogen, antithrombin III levels were reduced, but not in the group receiving daily transdermal 17β-estradiol (Fig 1). In other coagulation tests, no changes were detected. After hormonal administration, mean estradiol level was elevated in both groups.

Conclusion.—Oral conjugated estrogen replacement therapy reduces functional antithrombin III, but transdermal estradiol replacement therapy does not modify antithrombin III levels. In terms of coagulation, transdermal estradiol administration may be more beneficial than oral conjugated estrogen therapy, especially in women with predisposing factors to thrombosis.

► Before the publication of 4 epidemiologic studies in 1996, it was believed that the physiologic doses of postmenopausal estrogen replacement did not increase the risk of venous thrombosis and embolism (VTE), as the pharmacologic dose of estrogen in oral contraceptives did. However, each of these 4 studies showed that the risk of developing VTE was elevated twofold to threefold with the use of estrogen replacement therapy (ERT). The increase in risk was confined mainly to the first year of ERT. The increased risk of VTE in ERT users probably occurs mainly in women with hereditary thrombophilic disorders, such as activated protein C resistance. The results of this small study indicate that oral estrogen is associated with a decrease in levels of the coagulation inhibitor antithrombin III, while transdermal estrogen produces no change in this factor. This difference is probably caused by lack of a first-pass effect upon the liver with transdermal administration of estrogen.

D.R. Mishell, Jr., M.D.

Breast Cancer and Hormone Replacement Therapy: Collaborative Reanalysis of Data From 51 Epidemiological Studies of 52,705 Women With Breast Cancer and 108,411 Women Without Breast Cancer

Beral V, for the Collaborative Group on Hormonal Factors in Breast Cancer (Radcliffe Infirmary, Oxford; American Cancer Society; Emory Univ, Atlanta; et al)

Lancet 350:1047–1059, 1997 13–11

Introduction.—To replace the cyclic production of ovarian hormones that normally ceases at the menopause, various estrogens and progestogens have been prescribed for almost 50 years. In many epidemiologic studies, the relation between the risk of breast cancer and the use of hormone replacement therapy has been investigated. A reanalysis of the published data was conducted.

Methods.—The reanalysis included data from 52,705 women with breast cancer and 108,411 women without breast cancer from 21 countries, although most were from North America or Europe. Of 53,865 postmenopausal women, 17,830 (33%) used hormone replacement therapy at some time. At first use, the median age was 48 years. Hormone replacement therapy was used by 34% of ever-users for 5 years or longer.

Results.—For each year of use of hormone replacement therapy, the relative risk of having a diagnosis of breast cancer increased by a factor of

Duration of use and time since last use	Cases/Controls	RR (FSE)*	RR and 99% FCI*
Never-user	12467/23568	1.00 (0.021)	
Last use <5 years before diagnosis			
Duration <1 year	368/860	0.99 (0.085)	
Duration 1-4 years	891/2037	1.08 (0.060)	
Duration 5-9 years	588/1279	1.31 (0.079)	
Duration 10-14 years	304/633	1.24 (0.108)	
Duration ≥15 years	294/514	1.56 (0.128)	
Last use ≥5 years before diagnosis			
Duration <1 year	437/890	1.12 (0.079)	
Duration 1-4 years	566/1256	1.12 (0.068)	
Duration 5-9 years	151/374	0.90 (0.115)	
Duration ≥10 years	93/233	0.95 (0.145)	

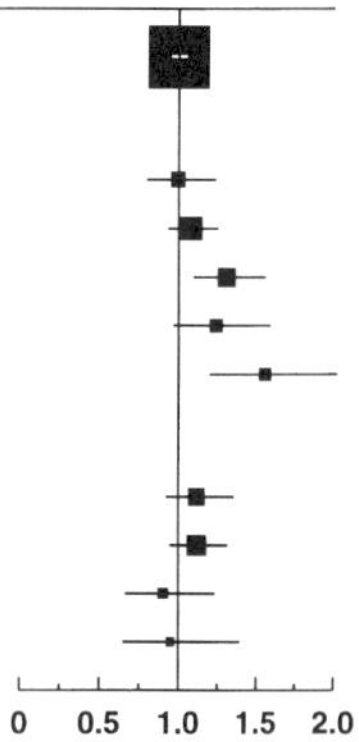

FIGURE 5.—Relative risk (RR) of breast cancer for duration of use within categories of time since last use of hormone replacement therapy. *Note*: Floated SE (*FSE*) and confidence interval (*FCI*) calculated from floated variance for each exposure category. Any comparison between groups must take variation in each estimate into account. Each analysis is based on aggregate data from all studies. *Black squares* indicate relative risk, area of which is proportional to amount of information contributed (i.e., to inverse of variance of logarithm of relative risk). *Lines* indicate 99% FCI (lines are white when 99% FCI are so narrow as to be entirely within width of square). "Last use within 5 years before diagnosis" includes current users. *Relative to never-users, stratified by study, age at diagnosis, time since menopause, body mass index, parity, and the age a woman was when her first child was born. (Courtesy of Beral V, for the Collaborative Group on Hormonal Factors in Breast Cancer: Breast cancer and hormone replacement therapy: Collaborative reanalysis of data from 51 epidemiological studies of 52,705 women with breast cancer and 108,411 women without breast cancer. *Lancet* 350:1047–1059, 1997. Copyright by the Lancet Ltd, 1997.)

Extent of tumour spread	HRT ever-users/never-users	RR (FSE)*	RR and 99% FCI*
Localised to breast	1387/4104	1.00 (0.056)	
Spread to axillary lymph nodes only	940/2827	0.82 (0.060)	
Metastatic beyond breast and lymph nodes	98/312	0.54 (0.173)	

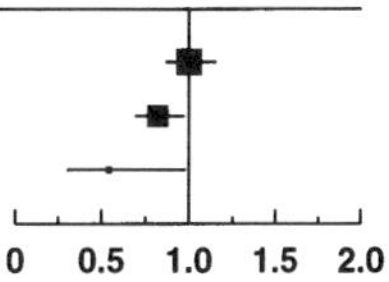

FIGURE 7.—Analysis relating extent of tumor spread among women with breast cancer to ever-use of hormone replacement therapy. *Note*: Floated SE (*FSE*) and confidence interval (*FCI*) calculated from floated variance for each exposure category. Any comparison between groups must take variation in each estimate into account. Each analysis based on aggregate data from all studies. *Black squares* indicate relative risk, area of which is proportional to amount of information contributed (i.e., to inverse of variance of logarithm of relative risk). Lines indicate 99% FCI (lines are white when 99% FCI are so narrow as to be entirely within width of square). *Relative probability that a woman with breast cancer is an ever-user rather than a never-user. Relative to women with localized disease, stratified by study, age at diagnosis, time since menopause, body mass index, parity, and the age a woman was when her first child was born. *Abbreviations: HRT*, hormone replacement therapy; *RR*, relative risk. (Courtesy of Beral V, for the Collaborative Group on Hormonal Factors in Breast Cancer: Breast cancer and hormone replacement therapy: Collaborative reanalysis of data from 51 epidemiological studies of 52,705 women with breast cancer and 108,411 women without breast cancer. *Lancet* 350:1047–1059, 1997. Copyright by the Lancet Ltd, 1997.)

1.023 among current users of hormone replacement therapy or those who stopped using it 1–4 years previously (Fig 5). For women who used hormone replacement therapy 5 years or longer, the relative risk was 1.35. The relative risk of breast cancer increases by a factor of 1.028 for each year older at menopause among never-users of hormone replacement therapy. There was no significant excess of breast cancer overall 5 or more years after cessation of hormone replacement therapy. Tumors in ever-users were less likely to have spread to axillary lymph nodes or to more distant sites than to be localized to the breast when compared with tumors in never-users (Fig 7) For women of lower weight or body mass index, the relative risk of breast cancer increased among those associated with long duration of use in current and recent users. The cumulative incidence of breast cancer between the ages of 50 and 70 years in never-users of hormone replacement therapy in North America and Europe is about 45 per 1,000 women. Among women who used hormone replacement therapy at age 50 and used it for 5 years, the cumulative excess numbers of breast cancers diagnosed per 1,000 was 2; for those who used it for 10 years, the excess number was 6, and for those who used hormone replacement therapy for 15 years, the excess number was 12. It is not known whether mortality from breast cancer is affected by hormone replacement therapy.

Conclusion.—In women using hormone replacement therapy, the risk of having breast cancer diagnosed is increased, and the risk increases with increasing duration of use. After cessation of use of hormone replacement therapy, this effect is reduced. After about 5 years, the effect largely, if not wholly, disappeared. There is a possibility that results could be biased because women taking hormone replacement therapy may have more opportunities for diagnosis.

► This large reanalysis of the existing published data regarding the use of hormone replacement therapy (HRT) and breast cancer has many interesting findings. The finding of an increased risk of diagnosis of breast cancer in users of HRT compared with nonusers only occurred in current and recent HRT users. Women who had used HRT for up to 10 or more years and stopped using it more than 5 years previously had no change in the risk of breast cancer diagnosis compared to women who never used HRT. In addition, the increased risk of diagnosis of breast cancer in current or recent HRT users was limited to localized disease. Users of HRT had a decreased risk of diagnosis of breast cancer that had spread to the axillary lymph nodes or beyond. These findings are very similar to the large reanalysis of data investigating the risk of breast cancer to use of oral contraceptives,[1] which also found an increased risk of diagnosis only in current users not in past users. Other large studies of HRT use and breast cancer risk also found an increased risk of breast cancer diagnosis only in long-term current users of HRT, not in past users. As the authors themselves point out, these results could be attributable to diagnostic bias, as women taking HRT have been reported to have an increased rate of diagnostic surveillance, particularly screening mammography, compared to non-HRT users. Another possibility is that estrogen promotes the growth of early subclinical cancers making their diagnosis more likely when the disease is localized. The data in this analysis argue against estrogen initiating breast cancer by changing a normal cell to a cancer cell because the increased risk of breast cancer was no longer evident 5 or more years after the women had stopped HRT, even with prior long-term use. If estrogen use actually caused breast cancer to develop, given the long time between initiation of the malignancy and clinical detection of the tumor, one would expect the increased risk to be present in both current and past users.

D.R. Mishell, Jr., M.D.

Reference

1. 1997 Year Book of Obstetrics, Gynecology, and Women's Health, p 377.

The Role of Hormone Replacement Therapy in the Risk for Breast Cancer and Total Mortality in Women With a Family History of Breast Cancer

Sellers TA, Mink PJ, Cerhan JR, et al (Univ of Minnesota, Minneapolis; Univ of Iowa, Iowa City)
Ann Intern Med 127:973–980, 1997 13–12

Background.—One important risk factor for breast cancer is a family history of the disease. It is important for physicians to know how to advise patients with a family history of breast cancer about the use of hormone replacement therapy. Various studies of the association of hormone replacement therapy and risk of breast cancer have reported inconsistent

TABLE 2.—Association of Use of Hormone Replacement Therapy With Risk for Postmenopausal Breast Cancer by Family History of Breast Cancer

Use of Hormone Replacement Therapy	No Family History of Breast Cancer			Family History of Breast Cancer		
	Cases *n*	Age-Adjusted Incidence Rate per 10,000 Person-Years (95% CI)	Multivariate-Adjusted Relative Risk (95% CI)*	Cases *n*	Age-Adjusted Incidence Rate per 10,000 Person-Years (95% CI)	Multivariate-Adjusted Relative Risk (95% CI)*
Never	528	36 (32–39)	1.00 (reference)	97	46 (36–55)	1.00 (reference)
Former (duration ≤ 5 years)	202	37 (31–42)	1.01 (0.85–1.20)	45	54 (38–70)	1.19 (0.81–1.73)
Former (duration > 5 years)	27	29 (17–40)	0.80 (0.53–1.19)	8	51 (14–87)	1.17 (0.55–2.47)
Current (duration ≤ 5 years)	41	46 (31–61)	1.31 (0.94–1.83)	7	70 (17–122)	1.37 (0.59–3.18)
Current (duration > 5 years)	67	41 (31–51)	1.13 (0.86–1.50)	13	61 (28–94)	1.35 (0.72–2.53)

*Adjusted for age, age at menarche, age at menopause, type of menopause, age at first live birth, waist-to-hip ratio, body mass index at 18 years of age, education level, and alcohol use.
Abbreviation: CI, confidence interval.

(Courtesy of Sellers TA, Mink PJ, Cerhan JR, et al: The role of hormone replacement therapy in the risk for breast cancer and total mortality in women with a family history of breast cancer. *Ann Intern Med* 127:973–980, 1997.)

TABLE 3.—Association of Use of Hormone Replacement Therapy With Total Mortality by Family History of Breast Cancer

Use of Hormone Replacement Therapy	No Family History of Breast Cancer			Family History of Breast Cancer		
	Cases *n*	Age-Adjusted Mortality Rate per 10,000 Person-Years (95% CI)	Multivariate-Adjusted Relative Risk (95% CI)*	Cases *n*	Age-Adjusted Mortality Rate per 10,000 Person-Years (95% CI)	Multivariate-Adjusted Relative Risk (95% CI)*
Never	1140	70 (65–74)	1.00 (reference)	194	80 (69–92)	1.00 (reference)
Former (duration ≤ 5 years)	408	63 (57–70)	0.86 (0.76–0.97)	56	65 (47–82)	0.71 (0.51–0.98)
Former (duration > 5 years)	62	58 (42–73)	0.76 (0.57–1.00)	9	82 (23–141)	0.59 (0.30–1.16)
Current (duration ≤ 5 years)	51	62 (44–80)	1.00 (0.75–1.35)	2	22 (–8 to 52)	0.24 (0.06–0.97)
Current (duration > 5 years)	91	51 (40–61)	0.84 (0.67–1.06)	11	46 (19–74)	0.55 (0.28–1.07)

*Adjusted for age, waist-to-hip ratio, body mass index, alcohol use, physical activity, pack-years of smoking, marital status, hypertension, diabetes, and type of menopause.

Abbreviation: CI, confidence interval.

(Courtesy of Sellers TA, Mink PJ, Cerhan JR, et al: The role of hormone replacement therapy in the risk for breast cancer and total mortality in women with a family history of breast cancer. *Ann Intern Med* 127:973–980, 1997.)

results. Another important issue is the effect of hormone replacement therapy on risk of death from breast cancer. When analyzing the benefits and risks of hormone replacement therapy in women with a family history of breast cancer, all-cause mortality should be examined.

Methods.—In a prospective cohort study, a population-based random sample of 41,837 women who had completed and returned a questionnaire was analyzed. All the women were between 55 and 69 years of age. Outcome measures included incidence and relative risk of breast cancer and total mortality during a follow-up period of 8 years.

Results.—Among the cohort of women at risk, 12.2% reported family histories of breast cancer. Among those with family history of breast cancer, women who had been using hormone replacement therapy for at least 5 years developed breast cancer at an annual age-adjusted rate of 61 cases per 10,000 person-years (Table 2). However, this rate was not significantly higher than the rate in women who had never received hormone replacement therapy. Total mortality was significantly lower in the women with a family history of breast cancer who received hormone replacement therapy than in women who never used hormone replacement therapy; this included total cancer-related mortality. For women who had been using hormone replacement therapy for at least 5 years, the age-adjusted annual mortality rate was 46 deaths per 10,000 person-years, which was about half the mortality rate in women who had never used hormone replacement therapy (Table 3).

Discussion.—These findings suggest that hormone replacement therapy is not associated with a significantly higher risk of breast cancer in postmenopausal women, and that women with family history of breast cancer who have used hormone replacement therapy have lower overall mortality. The results of this and similar studies may help physicians and patients with a family history of breast cancer make informed decisions about using hormone replacement therapy.

▶ The major concern of postmenopausal women in the United States in regard to use of estrogen replacement therapy (ERT) is the common misperception that exogenous estrogen acts as a carcinogen and causes the development of breast cancer. This concern is enhanced among postmenopausal women with a family history of breast cancer because they have a greater risk of developing this feared disease. The results of this large follow-up study of postmenopausal women living in Iowa should alleviate these concerns. First, in contrast to the findings of the follow-up Nurses' Health Study, analysis of questionnaires of nearly 41,000 women found that there was no significantly increased risk for the diagnosis of breast cancer among current long-term (more than 5 years) users of ERT compared to nonusers adjusted for age and other risk factors, even those with a family history of breast cancer. This lack of an increased risk of breast cancer diagnosis among ERT users occurred despite the fact that estrogen users were more likely to have screening mammograms than non-users. Secondly, for current long term estrogen users who developed breast cancer, their chances of dying were less than among women of the same age who developed breast cancer and were not taking ERT. The magnitude of the decreased risk of mortality among ERT users was greater among women with a family history of breast cancer (45%) than those without such a history (16%). These data indicate that women with a family history of breast cancer should not be concerned about the use of ERT with its many short-term and long-term health benefits.

D.R. Mishell, Jr., M.D.

Evista

Effects of Raloxifene on Bone Mineral Density, Serum Cholesterol Concentrations, and Uterine Endometrium in Postmenopausal Women

Delmas PD, Bjarnason NH, Mitlak BH, et al (Hôpital Edouard Herriot, Lyons, France; Ctr for Clinical and Basic Research, Ballerup, Denmark; Lilly Corp Ctr, Indianapolis, Ind)

N Engl J Med 337:1641–1647, 1997 13–13

Introduction.—The incidences of osteoporosis and of cardiovascular disease increase in women after menopause. Raloxifene, a nonsteroidal

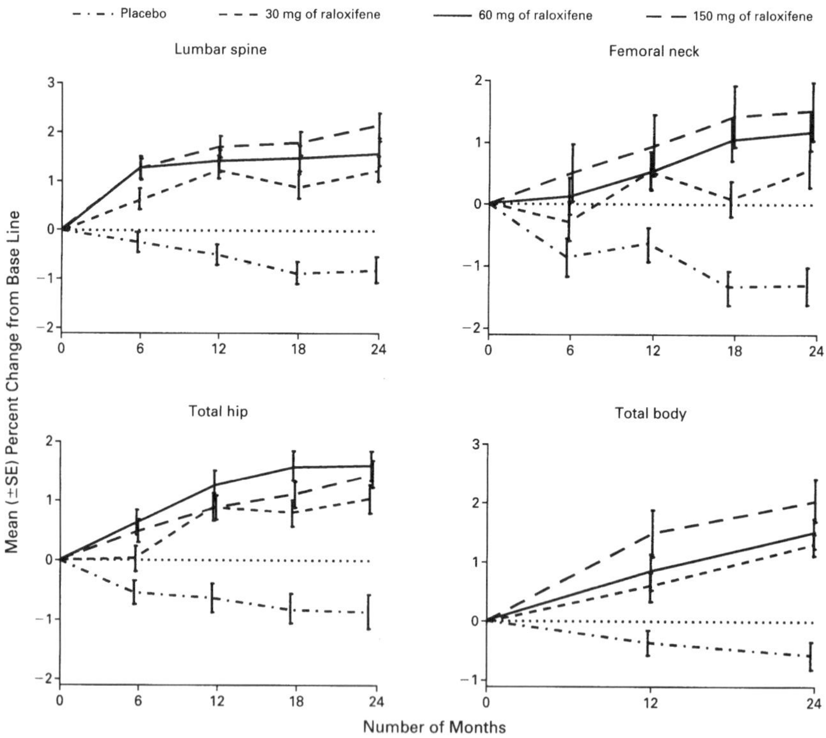

FIGURE 2.—Mean percent change in bone mineral density in postmenopausal women given raloxifene or placebo for 2 years. (Reprinted by permission of *The New England Journal of Medicine*. Delmas PD, Bjarnason NH, Mitlak BH, et al: Effects of raloxifene on bone mineral density, serum cholesterol concentrations, and uterine endometrium in postmenopausal women. *N Engl J Med* 337:1641–1647, copyright 1997, Massachusetts Medical Society. All rights reserved.)

benzothiphene that inhibits the growth of estrogen-receptor-dependent, dimethylbenzanthracene-induced mammary tumors and reduces the occurrence of nitrosomethylurea-induced mammary tumors in rats has been classified as a selective estrogen-receptor modulator. Previous studies show that administration of raloxifene decrease bone turnover and lower serum cholesterol concentrations. The 24-month interim results of a long-term, multicenter, placebo-controlled, double-blind study are reported.

Methods.—The effect of raloxifene on bone mineral density, serum lipid concentration, and endometrial thickness was studied in 601 postmenopausal women. For 24 months, the women were randomly assigned to receive placebo, or 30 g, 60 g, or 150 g of raloxifene.

Results.—Women receiving placebo had decreases in bone mineral density, whereas women receiving each dose of raloxifene had significant increases from baseline values in bone mineral density of the lumbar spine, hip, and total body. Between the women receiving 60 mg of raloxifene per day and those receiving placebo, the mean difference in the change in bone mineral density at 24 months was 2.4%±0.4% for the lumbar spine, 2.4%±0.4% for the total hip, and 2.0%±0.4% for the total body. In all the raloxifene groups, serum concentrations of total cholesterol and low-density lipoprotein cholesterol decreased, but there was no change in serum concentrations of high-density lipoprotein cholesterol and triglycerides (Fig 2). In all groups, the endometrial thickness was similar at all times during the study. The women receiving placebo and raloxifene similarly reported that they received hot flashes or vaginal bleeding.

Conclusion.—Bone mineral density is increased with daily therapy with raloxifene, which also lowers serum concentrations of total and low-density lipoprotein cholesterol, and does not stimulate the endometrium.

Effects of Raloxifene on Serum Lipids and Coagulation Factors in Healthy Postmenopausal Women

Walsh BW, Kuller LH, Wild RA, et al (Brigham and Women's Hosp, Boston; Univ of Pittsburgh, Pa; Univ of Oklahoma, Oklahoma City; et al)

JAMA 279:1445–1451, 1998 13–14

Background.—Although estrogen replacement therapy protects postmenopausal women from osteoporosis and heart disease, it also increases the risk of both breast and endometrial cancer. Raloxifene, a selective estrogen receptor modulator, has estrogen-antagonistic effects on breast and uterine tissue and estrogen-agonistic effects on bone and cholesterol. A double-blind, randomized, multisite, parallel trial was performed to determine the effects of 60 mg/day and 120 mg/day of raloxifene on cardiovascular risk factors in postmenopausal women.

Methods.—The study group consisted of 390 healthy postmenopausal women, aged 45 to 72 years, who were randomly assigned in a blinded fashion to 60 mg/day of raloxifene, 120 mg/day of raloxifene, hormone replacement therapy (HRT), or placebo for 6 months. Lipid levels and coagulation parameters were compared at baseline and at 3 and 6 months of treatment.

Results.—At baseline, there were no significant differences in lipoprotein levels among these 4 treatment groups. Low-density lipoprotein cholesterol levels were lowered 12% with either raloxifene dosage and 14% with HRT. High-density lipoprotein cholesterol levels were not affected by raloxifene but increased 10% with HRT. High-density lipoprotein-2 levels increased 15% to 17% with the 2 raloxifene doses and 33% with HRT. Triglyceride levels were not affected by raloxifene but increased 20% with HRT. Apolipoprotein A-I levels increased 5% with raloxifene and 12% with HRT. Lipoprotein(a) levels were lowered 7% to 8% with raloxifene and 19% with HRT. At baseline, there were no significant differences in coagulation factors among the treatment groups. Fibrinogen levels were lowered by 10% and 12% with the 2 raloxifene dosages but were unchanged by HRT. Plasminogen activator inhibitor–1 levels were not changed by raloxifene but were reduced 19% by HRT. Hot flashes were the most common adverse effect with raloxifene, whereas vaginal bleeding was the most common adverse effect with HRT. Significantly more patients discontinued treatment in the HRT group than in the raloxifene group.

Conclusion.—This double-blind, placebo-controlled, randomized clinical trial of the selective estrogen receptor modulator, raloxifene, demonstrated that raloxifene had a beneficial effect on several biochemical markers of cardiovascular risk: reducing levels of low-density lipoprotein–C, fibrinogen, and lipoprotein(a), and raising high-density lipoprotein–2 C levels in post-menopausal women. In contrast to HRT, raloxifene treatment had no effect on high-density lipoprotein–C and plasminogen activator inhibitor–1 levels. The effects of raloxifene treatment on cardiovascular risk in postmenopausal women should be investigated in further clinical trials.

Lack of Effect of Raloxifene on Coronary Artery Atherosclerosis of Postmenopausal Monkeys

Clarkson TB, Anthony MS, Jerome CP (Wake Forest Univ, Winston-Salem, NC)

J Clin Endocrinol Metab 83:721–726, 1998 13–15

Introduction.—The health and well-being of postmenopausal women has greatly benefited from postmenopausal estrogen replacement, which reduces coronary heart disease, prevents bone loss and fractures, and perhaps reduces the occurrence of Alzheimer's disease. The compliance rate among postmenopausal women is about 10% or less, however, because of a fear of breast cancer. Gonadal hormone substitutes with estradiol's beneficial effects are being sought. Estrogen agonist effects on bone and cholesterol metabolism have been found with raloxifene, which also has estrogen antagonist effects on mammary gland and uterus. It is still

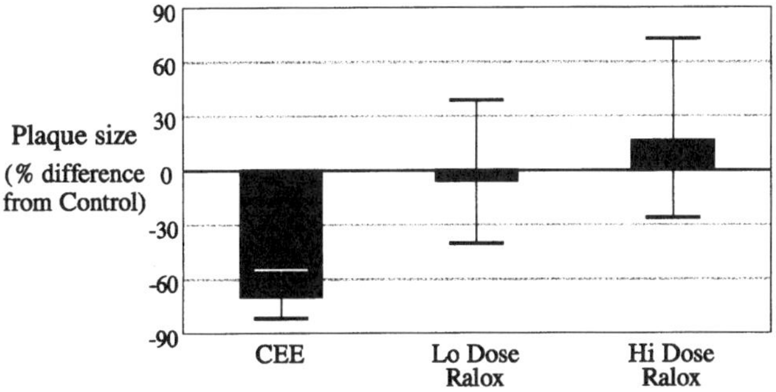

FIGURE 4.—Extent of coronary artery atherosclerosis (mean intimal area), expressed as the percent difference from the placebo-treated ovariectomized group, using adjusted mean ± standard error of the mean. Atherosclerosis was measured as the average of 3 coronary arteries, with 5 blocks per artery. (Courtesy of Clarkson TB, Anthony MS, Jerome CP: Lack of effect of raloxifene on coronary artery atherosclerosis of postmenopausal monkeys. *J Clin Endocrinol Metab* 83:721–726, 1998. Copyright The Endocrine Society.)

unknown whether selective estrogen receptor modulators, such as raloxifene, have the estrogen agonistic effect of inhibiting coronary artery atherogenesis. The lack of an estrogen agonistic effect in the diminution of diet-induced coronary artery atherosclerosis of surgically postmenopausal cynomolgus monkeys was reported.

Methods.—A moderately atherogenic diet was given to ovariectomized (surgically postmenopausal) cynomolgus monkeys, who were then given either a placebo, conjugated equine estrogen at a dose that mimicked that of 0.625 mg/day in women, raloxifene at 1 mg/kg/day, or raloxifene at 5 mg/kg/day.

Results.—Plasma lipid concentrations among the monkeys receiving raloxifene were generally comparable to those reported in postmenopausal women receiving raloxifene, with reductions in low-density lipoprotein cholesterol concentrations and no significant effects on high-density lipoprotein cholesterol. An estrogen agonist effect on coronary arteries was not found with raloxifene. A 70% reduction in coronary artery plaque size, relative to that in the placebo group, was found in the group treated with conjugated equine estrogens. Coronary artery plaque size was not affected by either the low or the high dose of raloxifene. There was 2 times more atherosclerosis in the low-dose raloxifene group and 3 times more atherosclerosis in the high-dose group than in the conjugated equine estrogen group (Fig 4).

Conclusion.—No evidence that raloxifene has an estrogen agonistic effect on coronary arteries was found in this animal model, despite a moderately beneficial effect on plasma lipid concentrations. Estrogens may have multiple mechanisms of action, including antioxidant effects on lipoprotein and direct effects on the artery wall.

▶ (Abstracts 13–13–13–15) Raloxifene, like clomiphene citrate and tamoxifen, is one of a group of agents called selective estrogen receptor modulators. Each of these agents has estrogenic agonist actions in certain tissues and antagonist actions in others. Raloxifene, like estrogen, causes a slight increase in bone density in postmenopausal women. However, unlike estrogen, raloxifene does not stimulate breast or endometrial tissue. Also, unlike estrogen, raloxifene also does not have a beneficial effect upon vasomotor symptoms or vaginal atrophy. Because estrogen use has been shown to increase the risk of endometrial cancer and to increase the diagnosis of breast cancer in long-term current users, it has been suggested that raloxifene be used instead of estrogen to prevent the development of osteoporosis among women at high risk for breast cancer. Clinicians should be aware that there is a difference between the effects of agents upon risk markers, such as bone density, and upon clinical events, such as fracture. Data from several observational studies have shown that estrogen replacement therapy reduces the risks of developing vertebral and hip fracture as well as myocardial infarction.

Although data indicate that raloxifene prevents a decrease in bone density in postmenopausal women, there are no data available regarding risk of fracture with this agent compared with placebo. Estrogen and alendronate have each been shown to reduce fracture risk among women with established osteoporosis. There are no published data regarding the effect of raloxifene on women with pre-existing osteoporosis. The product labeling for raloxifene states that the indication for use is prevention of osteoporosis, not treatment of established osteoporosis. A beneficial effect upon risk markers does not always mean that there is also a beneficial effect upon clinical events. Even though raloxifene has a beneficial effect upon some risk markers for athersclerosis, such as changes in total cholesterol and low-density lipoprotein-cholesterol, the elegant studies in postmenopausal monkeys indicate that raloxifene, unlike estrogen, does not retard the development of coronary artery atherosclerosis. Clinicians should wait for data regarding the effect of raloxifene upon the clinical events of fracture and myocardial infarction before offering raloxifene to women instead of recommending estrogen replacement therapy, with its demonstrated effectiveness against fractures and myocardial infarction.

D.R. Mishell, Jr., M.D.

fosamax

Prevention of Bone Loss With Alendronate in Postmenopausal Women Under 60 Years of Age

Hosking D, for the Early Postmenopausal Intervention Cohort Study Group (Univ of Nottingham, England)

N Engl J Med 338:485–492, 1998 13–16

Background.—Osteoporosis is a common cause of morbidity among postmenopausal women. Estrogen replacement is the accepted therapy for osteoporosis, but not all postmenopausal women can receive estrogen therapy. Biophosphonates, such as alendronate, also inhibit bone resorption and increase bone mineral density in women with osteoporosis. The safety and efficacy of alendronate was compared with estrogen replacement therapy in a large international study of postmenopausal women.

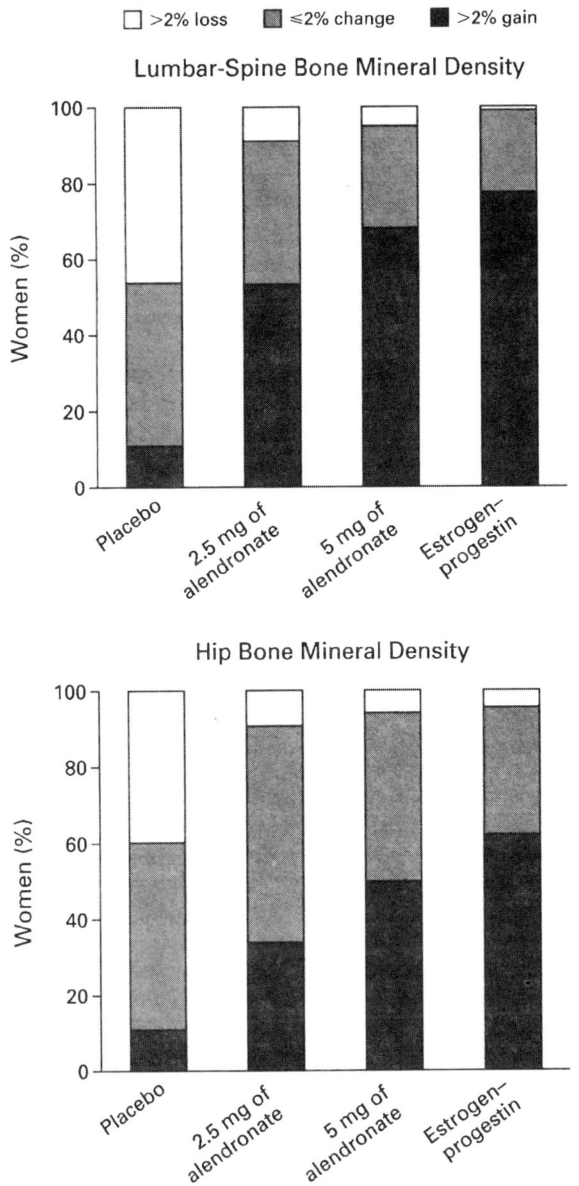

FIGURE 2.—Proportion of women with a loss of more than 2%, a change of 2% or less, or a gain of more than 2% in bone mineral density of the lumbar spine and hip after 2 years of treatment with placebo, 2.5 mg or 5 mg of alendronate or estrogen-progestin. Results for the 2 strata were combined according to treatment. (Reprinted by permission of *The New England Journal of Medicine* courtesy of Hosking D, for the Early Postmenopausal Intervention Cohort Study Group: Prevention of bone loss with alendronate in postmenopausal women under 60 years of age. *N Engl J Med* 338:485–492,

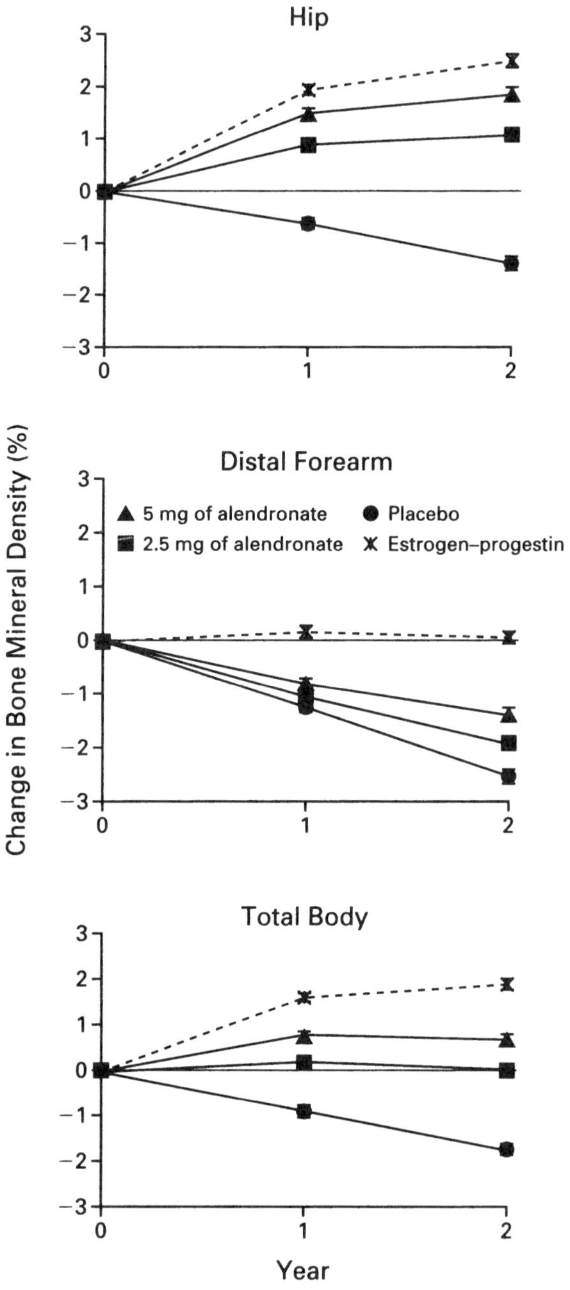

FIGURE 3.—Mean (± standard error) change from baseline in the bone mineral density of the hip, distal forearm, and total body after 1 and 2 years of treatment with placebo, 2.5 mg or 5 mg of alendronate or estrogen-progestin. Results for the 2 strata were combined according to treatment. (Reprinted by permission of *The New England Journal of Medicine* courtesy of Hosking D, for the Early Postmenopausal Intervention Cohort Study Group: Prevention of bone loss with alendronate in postmenopausal women under 60 years of age. *N Engl J Med* 338:485–492, copyright 1998, Massachusetts Medical Society. All rights reserved.)

Methods.—The study group consisted of 1,609 healthy postmenopausal women, aged 45 to 59, from 4 centers. Bone mineral density of the lumbar spine, hip, forearm, and total body was assessed by dual energy x-ray absorptiometry at baseline and after 1 and 2 years of treatment. Women were randomly assigned to treatment with 2.5 mg or 5 mg of alendronate, placebo, or open-label estrogen-progesterone. Participants were examined at clinics every 3 months.

Results.—Lumbar spine bone mineral density decreased continually in the placebo group but increased significantly in both alendronate groups. Most of the gain in density occurred in the first year of treatment, but significant gains occurred in the second year also. The gains in bone mineral density were significantly greater at the higher dosage. The changes in bone mineral density of the hip were similar to those of the spine (Fig 2). The loss of bone mineral density of the distal forearm was decreased by treatment with alendronate (Fig 3). Over the 2 years of this study, total body bone mineral density decreased in the placebo group, did not change significantly in the group receiving 2.5 mg daily of alendronate, and increased in the group given 5 mg daily of alendronate as well as in the estrogen-progestin group.

Conclusion.—This large international study found that daily alendronate therapy increased bone mineral density in postmenopausal women under the age of 60. Alendronate is a safe and effective alternative to estrogen replacement therapy in postmenopausal women who wish to maintain bone mass to reduce fracture risk.

▶ Earlier studies have shown that ingestion of the biophosphonate alendronate in doses of 5 or 10 mg/day reduces the risk of subsequent fractures in women with established osteoporosis. The results of this study demonstrate that 5 mg of alendronate daily will prevent the development of osteoporosis in most postmenopausal women. Both this study and studies of women with established osteoporosis indicate that alendronate does not prevent bone loss or reduce fracture risk to a greater extent than estrogen replacement therapy. Alendronate is expensive, difficult to ingest, and does not have the other health benefits of estrogen replacement therapy. Nevertheless, in women at risk for the development of osteoporosis and those with established osteoporosis who have contraindications for use of estrogen replacement therapy, alendronate is a useful alternative.

D.R. Mishell, Jr., M.D.

Fosamax

Alendronate Prevents Postmenopausal Bone Loss in Women Without Osteoporosis: A Double-Blind, Randomized, Controlled Trial

McClung M, for the Alendronate Osteoporosis Prevention Study Group (Providence Health System, Portland, Ore, et al)

Ann Intern Med 128:253–261, 1998 13–17

Background.—Preventing the bone loss that accompanies menopause and aging and maintaining the normal microarchitecture of bone are important goals in the prevention of osteoporosis and fractures. The safety and efficacy of alendronate in preventing postmenopausal bone loss were assessed.

Methods.—Four hundred forty-seven women who had begun menopause 6–36 months before entry into the study were included in the 3-year, double-blind, randomized, placebo-controlled trial. By random assignment, patients received oral placebo, oral alendronate (1, 5, or 10 mg/day), or oral alendronate (20 mg/day) for 2 years. In the third year, all women took placebo.

Findings.—Alendronate dosages of 5, 10, and 20 mg/day increased bone mineral density from baseline by 1% to 4% at the lumbar spine, femoral neck, and trochanter. These dosages also increased total body bone mineral density by 0.3% to 1%. Women given placebo had losses of 2% to 4% at these sites. At 1 mg/day, alendronate attenuated the bone mineral losses compared with placebo. Alendronate reduced bone resorption markers to a new steady state by 3 months and bone formation markers by 6–12 months. The quality of bone remained normal. The safety and tolerability of alendronate at all dosages tested were comparable to those of placebo.

Conclusions.—Alendronate at dosages of 5 mg/day or greater given to early postmenopausal women for 3 years can prevent the loss of bone mineral density at the spine and hip as well as in the total body. This agent appears to be a safe, effective nonhormonal option for preventing bone loss in such women.

▶ Alendronate has been shown to reduce the incidence of new fractures in women with established osteoporosis. Therefore, it is currently being used as therapy for women who have osteoporosis. The results of this prospective randomized clinical trial indicate that ingestion of 5 mg/day or more of alendronate by women in early menopause without osteoporosis prevents bone loss in both the spine and hip as well as in the total skeleton. Alendronate does not prevent bone loss in women with and without osteoporosis to a greater extent than estrogen replacement. Because estrogen has many other health benefits and is better tolerated than alendronate, estrogen should be the preferred therapy to prevent bone loss in women with and without osteoporosis. However, if a woman has contraindications to the use of estrogen, alendronate can be used for at least 3 years to prevent postmenopausal bone loss as well as reduce recurrent fractures in women with established osteoporosis.

D.R. Mishell, Jr., M.D.

Intrauterine Administration of Levonorgestrel 5 and 10 μg/24 Hours in Perimenopausal Hormone Replacement Therapy: A Randomized Clinical Study During One Year

Wollter-Svensson L-O, Stadberg E, Andersson K, et al (Univ Hosp, Uppsala, Sweden; Univ of Göteborg, Sweden)

Acta Obstet Gynecol Scand 76:449–454, 1997 13–18

Background.—Studies have shown that 20 μg/24 hr of levonorgestrel released continuously from an intrauterine system (IUS) in combination with oral estradiol induces atrophia of the endometrium and causes amenorrhea in most peri- and postmenopausal women. The required dosage of progestogen is lower when given by an IUS than when given orally. The effect of 5 and 10 μg/24 hr of IUS-delivered levonorgestrel on endometrium and bleeding patterns as well as its safety and acceptability when combined with oral or transdermal estradiol in perimenopausal women were investigated.

Methods and Findings.—One hundred twelve perimenopausal women with vasomotor symptoms were enrolled in the prospective, randomized, single-blind study. Twelve of the 108 women starting the study discontinued, most commonly because of frequent bleeding. A total of 96 women were followed up for 12 months. All but 1 woman receiving either the 5 or 10 μg dose had nonproliferative endometrium after 12 months. None of the women had hyperplasia. Irregular bleeding occurred in the first months of treatment but declined after 6 months. At the end of the 12-month

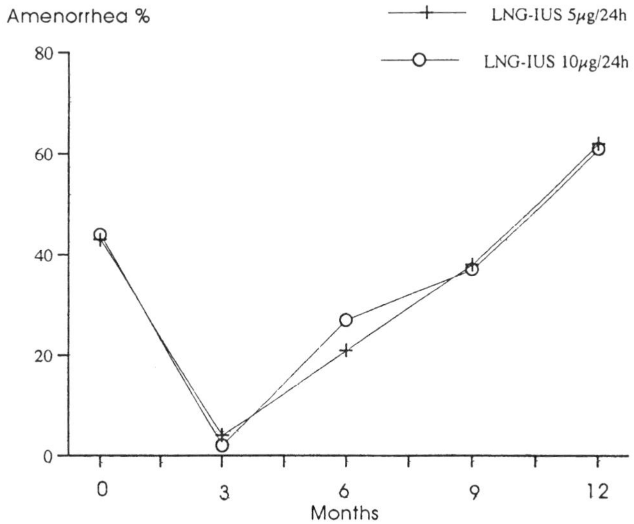

FIGURE 2.—Percentage of women with amenorrhea, defined as no bleeding or spotting during the preceding 90 days. (Courtesy of Wollter-Svensson L-O, Stadberg E, Andersson K, et al: Intrauterine administration of levonorgestrel 5 and 10 μg/24 hours in perimenopausal hormone replacement therapy: A randomized clinical study during one year. *Acta Obstet Gynecol Scand* 76:449–454, 1997. Copyright 1997 Munksgaard International Publishers Ltd., Copenhagen, Denmark.)

study, 62% of the women receiving the 5 μg dose and 61% receiving 10 μg were amenorrheic. The 2 dosages of levonorgestrel did not have different effects on bleeding patterns (Fig 2).

Conclusions.—The IUS release of 5 or 10 μg/24 hr of levonorgestrel appears to minimize the progestogenic side effects while effectively preventing endometrial stimulation by estrogen treatment in perimenopausal women receiving hormone replacement therapy. These findings, along with previously reported data, underscore that intrauterine levonorgestrel exerts a marked local effect on the endometrium and that the dose needed is much lower than that used in oral administration.

► Administration of estrogen without progestin to postmenopausal women with a uterus increases their risk of developing endometrial cancer. When a progestin is also administered, the excess risk of endometrial cancer associated with use of estrogen alone is no longer present. However, the use of oral progestin is frequently associated with the development of adverse side effects such as mood changes and weight gain. The administration of progesterone locally in the endometrial cavity together with systemic estrogen prevents the development of endometrial proliferation and hyperplasia, without the development of progestogenic side effects. Although intrauterine systems releasing 20 μg/day of levonorgestrel have been developed for contraceptive use, the results of this study indicate that a smaller device releasing only 5 μg/day of levonorgestrel is sufficient to suppress the endometrial proliferation produced by systemic estrogen replacement. When these devices are manufactured and marketed they can be used in combination with oral or transdermal estrogen instead of systemic progestins.

D.R. Mishell, Jr., M.D.

Herbal Therapies for Perimenopausal and Menopausal Complaints

Israel D, Youngkin EQ (St David's Med Ctr, Austin, Tex; Florida Atlantic Univ, Boca Raton)

Pharmacotherapy 17:970–984, 1997 13–19

Introduction.—Hormone replacement therapy (HRT) is frequently offered to women with menopause-related complaints, but many cannot or will not take HRT. Some women decide to try herbal therapies, either alone or with prescribed agents, with the belief that herbal treatment is "natural" and safe. The lay media claims, adverse effects, and scientific evidence for efficacy of a number of herbal remedies were reviewed.

General Concepts and Safety Concerns.—Many herbs are known to have medicinal effects and must be considered drugs, even though they are sold in health food and grocery stores and cannot be claimed to prevent or treat disease. Herbal preparations vary considerably from one product to another in the amount of drug contained, and a lack of standards means that quality is also variable. Products may be adulterated and cause adverse effects.

Herbal Remedies for Menopausal Symptoms.—Numerous herbs have been recommended for hot flashes, menstrual irregularities, dyspareunia, vaginal and urinary complaints, insomnia, mood alterations, memory and concentration difficulties, and changes in libido. A significant concern is that some herbal therapies may have estrogenic properties, thus carrying the same dangers as estrogen therapy. And because the combination of herbs and certain prescribed medications may cause serious illness, women should check with their physician before taking any herbal or natural substance.

Herbal Therapies.—Many herbs promoted in the lay media are not recommended for the treatment of menopausal symptoms because scientific evidence of their efficacy is lacking. And in many instances, these herbs may cause adverse effects. Among such herbs are agrimony, angelica, catnip, chamomile, damiana, dandelion, dong quai, fenugreek, gotu kola, hops, licorice, life root, sage, sarsaparilla, and skullcap. Germany's Commission E, which reviewed the safety and use of more than 1,400 herbal drugs, found some benefits from balm tea, black cohosh, chaste tree berry extract, ginkgo, ginseng, passion flower, St. John's wort, and valerian. Only 1 of the 24 herbs discussed, however, is approved by the United States Food and Drug Administration.

Conclusion.—Because women are using herbs to self-manage menopausal complaints, it is important that they be provided with accurate information about potential toxicity and drug interactions.

▶ This review provides clinicians with an excellent compilation of the claims made in the lay media regarding the benefits of most of the alternative medicines used by women. Of greater importance is a summation of the scientific evidence regarding the efficacy and adverse effects of these agents. Clinicians should have a copy of the full article in their office to counsel their patients regarding the use of these agents.

D.R. Mishell, Jr., M.D.

Does Dong Quai Have Estrogenic Effects in Postmenopausal Women? A Double-blind, Placebo-controlled Trial

Hirata JD, Small R, Sweirsz LM, et al (Kaiser Permanente Med Ctr, Oakland and Richmond, Calif)

Fertil Steril 68:981–986, 1997 13–20

Background.—Alternative therapy is very popular in the United States, yet many of these treatments have not been examined scientifically for effectiveness. This study examines the effect of dong quai, a Chinese herbal remedy used to treat symptoms associated with menopause, to determine if this herbal therapy has an effect on the internal production of estradiol or estrone as determined by examination of vaginal and endometrial linings.

Method.—Seventy-one postmenopausal women who were screened for various medical conditions and who exhibited frequent night sweats or vasomotor flushes were given randomized dong quai or placebo treatment. Dong quai recipients took the equivalent of 4.5 g of the root per day. The women were examined at 6, 12, and 24 weeks. All of these visits included endometrial ultrasonography. At the initial visit and at 12 weeks, blood pressure serum estrogen levels and vaginal cells were evaluated. At week 24, blood pressure and weight were also measured. If a more than 5-mm endometrial thickness was determined through endometrial ultrasonography at the final visit, endometrial biopsy was performed. Participants kept journals to record the vasomotor episodes they experienced and were also evaluated using the Kupperman index, which ranks menopausal symptom complaints as nonexistent, mild, or severe. Significance of difference between the placebo and dong quai groups was determined using *t* and chi-squared tests.

Results.—Table 1 in the original article shows the baseline characteristics of test subjects. Six women receiving placebos dropped out of the study before test completion as did 4 receiving dong quai. Participants could not accurately tell whether they were taking the placebo or the actual drug. All women reported mild side effects including burping, headaches, and gas. Statistically significant differences were not recorded in any of the test categories: vaginal maturation index, frequency of vasomotor flushes, endometrial thickness, or Kupperman index.

Conclusion.—This test suggests that dong quai administered in isolation does not relieve menopausal symptoms any more readily than a placebo. Endometrial proliferation did not occur as a result of administering dong quai. Hence, the herbal therapy does not seem to increase the production of estradiol or estrone.

▶ Many postmenopausal women do not wish to take estrogen replacement therapy despite its many benefits because they believe that taking supplemental estrogen is not natural and that exogenous estrogen will cause breast cancer. These concerns have led to an increased use of more natural substances by perimenopausal women to relieve menopausal symptoms and provide them with more energy. These agents have been called "alternative medicines." A recent survey indicated that about 34% of U.S. adults used 1 or more alternative therapies in the prior year. Dong quai is an herbal medium that has been used in China for more than 2,000 years for symptoms associated with menopause: nervousness, dizziness, insomnia, and forgetfulness. This well-done randomized clinical trial conclusively demonstrates that dong quai has no estrogenic effects and does not improve symptoms associated with menopause more than a placebo does. Patients need to be informed that dong quai does not provide the same health benefits as estrogen replacement.

D.R. Mishell, Jr., M.D.

14 Infertility

Impaired Fecundity in the United States: 1982–1995

Chandra A, Stephen EH (Natl Ctr for Health Statistics, Hyattsville, Md; Georgetown Univ, Washington, DC)

Fam Plann Perspect 30:34–42, 1998 14–1

Objective.—The number of women seeking help for fecundity problems increased from the 1980s to 1995, possibly because many were in older age groups. This trend was analyzed.

Methods.—Data on the prevalence of infertility and the receipt of related medical help were obtained from the 1982, 1988, and 1995 National Survey of Family Growth (NSFG). "Impaired fecundity" applies to women who are not sterile but cannot conceive after 3 years of trying or are unable to carry a pregnancy to term.

Results.—Among women aged 15–44, the prevalence of impaired fecundity was 8% in 1982 and 1988 and 10% in 1995. Among married women, it was 11% in 1982 and 1988 and 13% in 1995 (Table 1). There were 1.1 million more women with impaired fecundity in 1995 than anticipated by 1988 rates. The percentage of childless women aged 35–44 with impaired fecundity was 37% in 1995 and 24% in 1982, probably because of delayed marriage and childbearing patterns and the fact that the baby boomers were in the oldest reproductive group. Impaired fecundity among college-educated women increased from 15% in 1982 to 23% in 1995. Even if impaired fecundity rates had been the same in 1995 as in 1982, the number of women reporting impaired fertility would be increased because the number of women in their reproductive years had increased, but the rates were 20% in all age, parity, marital status, education, income, and race and ethnic subgroups. Childless women were more likely than women with children to report impaired infertility. The incidence of impaired fertility increased with age and history of pelvic inflammatory disease, with married women being twice as likely as unmarried women to report impaired fertility. Receipt of infertility services increased by 40% by 1995 to 2.7 million over 1.8 million in 1982. Women seeking services were older, married, better educated, white, and wealthier.

Conclusion.—The number of women seeking help for impaired fecundity increased by nearly 30% from 1982 to 1995, primarily because there were more women in the childbearing group. Women with primary im-

TABLE 1.—Percentage Distribution of U.S. Women Aged 15–44 years by Fecundity Status

Fecundity status	All women 1982 (N=7,969)	1988 (N=8,450)	1995 (N=10,847)	Married women 15–44 1982 (N=3,551)	1988 (N=4,031)	1995 (N=5,291)
Surgically sterile	**25.3 (0.8)**	**28.0 (0.6)**	**27.3 (0.5)**	**38.8 (1.4)**	**42.4 (1.0)**	**40.7 (0.7)**
For contraceptive reasons	17.5 (0.7)	23.3 (0.6)	24.2 (0.5)	27.8 (1.3)	36.2 (0.9)	36.7 (0.7)
For noncontraceptive reasons	7.8 (0.5)	4.7 (0.3)	3.1 (0.2)	11.0 (0.9)	6.2 (0.5)	4.1 (0.3)
Impaired fecundity	**8.4 (0.5)**	**8.4 (0.4)**	**10.2 (0.3)**	**10.8 (0.9)**	**10.7 (0.6)**	**12.9 (0.5)**
Nonsurgically sterile	1.7 (0.3)	1.4 (0.2)	1.7 (0.2)	2.0 (0.4)	1.6 (0.2)	2.0 (0.2)
Subfecund	5.6 (0.4)	5.7 (0.3)	7.7 (0.3)	6.7 (0.7)	6.8 (0.5)	9.4 (0.5)
Long interval without conception	1.1 (0.2)	1.3 (0.2)	0.9 (0.1)	2.1 (0.4)	2.3 (0.3)	1.6 (0.2)
Fecund	**66.3 (0.9)**	**63.6 (0.7)**	**62.5 (0.6)**	**50.3 (1.5)**	**46.9 (1.0)**	**46.4 (0.8)**
Total	100.0	100.0	100.0	100.0	100.0	100.0

Note: Standard errors appear in parentheses.
(Reproduced with the permission of the Alan Guttmacher Institute from Chandra A, Stephen EH: Impaired fecundity in the United States: 1982–1995. *Fam Plann Perspec* 30:34–42, 1998.)

paired fecundity were more likely than women with secondary impaired fecundity to seek help and were more likely to be childless.

▶ The data accumulated in the 3 national surveys of family growth conducted in 1982, 1988, and 1995 provide much information regarding the problems of infertility and impaired fecundability. The data indicate that although the age-specific rate of infertility did not change in this time, there was about a 30% increase in the number of infertile women in the United States between 1988 and 1995. The increased percentage of infertile women (from 8% to 10%) in this period represents an increase of about 1.6 million women with impaired fecundity.

This increase is the result of 2 factors. First, there is a greater number of women in the oldest reproductive age group (35–44) and, secondly, more women are delaying the planned birth of their first or subsequent child until they are older and less fecund. About 44% of infertile women in the United States seek medical assistance for their fertility problems. ICSI

Fortunately, with the assistance of in vitro fertilization and intracytoplasmic sperm injection, a higher percentage of infertile couples can now conceive than could do so in 1988. Unfortunately, the cost of such therapy remains high and is usually not reimbursed by third party payers.

D.R. Mishell, Jr., M.D.

How to Use Chlamydia Antibody Testing in Subfertility Patients

Land JA, Evers JLH, Goossens VJ (Academisch Ziekenhuis Maastricht, The Netherlands)

Hum Reprod 13:1094–1098, 1998 14–2

Objective.—*Chlamydia* infections can lead to compromised tubal function resulting in subfertility. Screening for tubal factor subfertility using *Chlamydia* antibody testing (CAT) has led to varied results. The implications of varying cutoff levels and definitions of tubal pathology on the clinical impact of CAT in a subfertile population were prospectively evaluated.

Methods.—CAT is a routine procedure for all female patients undergoing fertility testing. All patients had laparoscopy, the value of which was used as the standard for comparison with the CAT results.

Results.—There were 253 patients with analytical data. The *Chlamydia* IgG antibody titer was less than 8 in 127 patients, 8 in 19 patients, 16 in 17 patients, 32 in 20 patients, 64 in 17 patients, 128 in 13 patients, 256 in 7 patients, 512 in 5 patients, 1,024 in 1 patient, and 2,048 in 1 patient. Increasing the cutoff levels of IgG titers improved specificity and positive likelihood ratio (LR+) but decreased sensitivity and negative LR (LR−). Therefore CAT could predict a subgroup of patients with severe, distal tubule pathology with an accuracy that agrees with literature results. Statistically, the optimum cutoff point is 16. CAT cannot predict proximal tubal occlusion, which is typically not caused by *C. trachomatis*.

Conclusion.—Using a cutoff point of 16, CAT can be used as an inexpensive screening test for tubal factor infertility.

The Role of Transvaginal Ultrasonography in the Detection of Pelvic Pathologies in the Infertility Workup

Ubaldi F, Wisanto A, Camus M, et al (Dutch-Speaking Brussels Free Univ, Belgium; European Hosp, Rome, Italy; Virga Jesse Hosp, Hasselt, Belgium)
Hum Reprod 13:330–333, 1998 14–3

Objective.—Transvaginal ultrasonography (TVUS) has made it possible to identify pelvic pathologies that can lead to infertility. How TVUS compares with laparoscopy, the gold standard for infertility workup, was assessed prospectively. The predictive value of TVUS in differentiating the normal from the pathologic pelvis was analyzed.

Methods.—Between February 1994 and April 1995, 133 premenopausal women, aged 21–41, underwent TVUS before laparoscopy for infertility, chronic pelvic pain, or adnexal masses. Scans were defined as normal when the uterus showed normal morphology with no contour or positional abnormalities, adnexa were anatomically normal, and no ovarian masses, hydrosalpinges, or other pathologies were present.

Results.—Ultrasound scans were normal in 57 (43%) patients and laparoscopy was normal in 45 (78.9%) of the 57 patients. The 12 false-negative patients with normal ultrasound scans had minimal endometriosis (n = 6), filmy adnexal adhesions (n = 4), omental-to-bowel adhesions (n = 1), and hydrosalpinx (n = 1). Ultrasound was abnormal in 76 (57%) patients. Laparoscopy also was abnormal in 75 (56%) of these patients. In the remaining patients, the TVUS diagnosis of adhesions was not confirmed at surgery. The sensitive, specificity, and positive and negative predictive values of TVUS were 86.2%, 97.8%, 98.6%, and 78.8%, respectively. The agreement between TVUS and laparoscopy was 90.2%. Nine of the 13 TVUS-diagnosed endometriomas were confirmed by histopathology. The 4 false-positive diagnoses were found by laparoscopy and pathology to be hemorrhagic cysts (n = 2), hydrosalpinx, and dermoid cyst. The efficiency of TVUS as a screening technique was 96.4% with a sensitivity, specificity, and positive and negative predictive values of 90%, 96.7%, 75%, and 99.1%, respectively. The sensitivity, specificity, positive and negative predictive values, and efficiency of TVUS for screening pelvic adhesions were 61.1%, 98.2%, 84.6%, 94.1%, and 93.2%, respectively. The false-negative and false-positive results did not appear to be operator dependent. Although pelvic sonography cannot be used to detect endometriosis, classifying the 6 minimal endometriosis diagnoses as normal resulted in an efficiency, sensitivity, specificity, and positive and negative predictive values of 94.7%, 92.5%, 98.6%, 98.6%, and 89.4%, respectively.

Conclusion.—TVUS can accurately diagnose pelvic pathologies with the exception of filmy adhesions. Laparoscopy can be postponed in younger patients with patent tubes (as demonstrated with hydrosalpingography) and negative TVUS.

► These 2 studies (Abstracts 14–2 and 14–3) demonstrate that determination of whether chlamydia antibodies are present in the serum and performance of pelvic sonography should be part of the initial infertility evaluation. If no antibodies are present, the hysterosalpingogram is normal, and pelvic sonography does not reveal any abnormalities, it is unlikely that sufficient pelvic abnormalities will be present to cause infertility. Therefore, it is not cost-effective to perform a diagnostic laparoscopy as part of the infertility evaluation if the 3 tests mentioned above are normal. If the semen analysis contains a sufficient number of motile sperm, infertile women without evidence of pelvic pathology, as determined by these 3 tests, should be treated with several cycles of controlled ovarian hyperstimulation and intrauterine insemination before considering use of diagnostic laparoscopy. It is very unlikely that laparoscopy will detect pathologic entities of sufficient severity to be a cause of the infertility.

D.R. Mishell, Jr., M.D.

Transvaginal Hydrolaparoscopy as an Outpatient Procedure for Infertility Investigation

Gordts S, Camp R, Rombauts L, et al (Leuven Inst for Fertility and Embryology, Belgium)

Hum Reprod 13:99–103, 1998 14–4

Objective.—Diagnostic laparoscopy is not an innocuous procedure, and minilaparoscopy has visualization problems when investigating infertility in women without obvious pelvic pathology. The performance of a new technique called transvaginal hydrolaparoscopy for exploration of the tubo-ovarian structure was evaluated in infertile women with no obvious pelvic pathology.

Technique.—Transvaginal hydrolaparoscopy was performed in 28 women to exclude endometriosis and adhesions of the tubo-ovarian structures. The women were placed in the dorsal decubitus position so they could view the procedure on a video screen. The central posterior fornix was infiltrated with 1–2 mL of 1% lidocaine:adrenaline (1:100,000). A tenaculum was placed in the posterior lip, and the cervix was lifted. A Veress needle was introduced about 1.5 cm below the cervix, and approximately 100 mL of 37°C saline with 1% lidocaine (1/100) was instilled into the pouch of Douglas. A 3-mm blunt trocar was inserted into a stab incision in the posterior fornix. A 2.7-mm diameter semirigid endoscope was inserted to visualize the posterior wall of the uterus, and, by rotation and deeper insertion, the tubo-ovarian structures.

Approximately 400 mL of saline was left in situ and the vaginal fornix was left to close, spontaneously.

Results.—Laparoscopic and transvaginal hydrolaparoscopic findings were similar in the first 7 patients. Access to the Douglas pouch was not possible in 3 patients as a result of extensive adhesions that were later confirmed laparoscopically. Tubal patency was tested using transcervical dye hydrotubation with methylene blue. Ovarian endometriosis in 4 patients, adhesions in 7, and small pedunculated fibromas were observed by moving the optic around the ovary. These lesions were not detected by vaginal sonography. One patient had pain from a hemorrhage at the puncture site. There were no other complications. This procedure is contraindicated when there is obstruction of Douglas by the rectum or a prolapsed tumor, which are usually ruled out by bimanual examination and transvaginal ultrasound.

Conclusion.—Transvaginal hydrolaparoscopy can diagnose ovarian endometriosis, adhesions, and pedunculated fibromas and also include hysteroscopy and dye hydrotubation in less than 1 hour in an outpatient setting, thus reducing the cost and complexity of pelvic endoscopic examination.

► It would be useful to have a technique whereby the pelvis can be visualized in infertile women without the need of insufflating CO_2 into the peritoneum and without general anesthesia. Transvaginal hydrolaparoscopy promises to be less expensive and safer than routine diagnostic laparoscopy. With continued experience, it may be possible to perform this procedure in a clinic setting and thus avoid the use of an operating facility.

D.R. Mishell, Jr., M.D.

Treatment for Infertility and Risk of Invasive Epithelial Ovarian Cancer

Parazzini F, Negri E, La Vecchia C, et al (Istituto di Ricerche Farmacologiche 'Mario Negri', Milan, Italy; Centro di Riferimento Oncologico, Pordenone, Italy; Universîtà delgi Studi di Milano, Italy; Instituto Nazionale Tumori, Italy; et al)

Hum Reprod 12:2159–2161, 1997 14–5

Background.—Research suggests that women who have been treated for infertility may be at increased risk for invasive and borderline ovarian cancer. Data from an Italian case-control study were analyzed to further investigate the relationship between fertility drug use and ovarian cancer risk.

Methods.—Nine hundred seventy-one women aged younger than 75 years with recently diagnosed, histologically confirmed invasive epithelial ovarian cancer formed the case group. The control group consisted of 2,758 women without ovarian cancer.

TABLE 2.—Distribution of Ovarian Cancer Patients and Controls According to Use of Fertility Drugs and Selected Covariates

	Ovarian cancer	Controls	OR (95% CI)*
Fertility drug use (total series)			
No	966	2,692	1†
Yes	5	11	1.1 (0.4–3.3)
Duration of use of fertility drug use (cycles)†			
<6	1	3	0.7 (0.1–7.9)
≥6	4	7	1.0 (0.2–3.8)
Aged <50 years			
No	349	1,111	1†
Yes	3	7	1.3 (0.3–4.9)
Aged ≥50 years			
No	617	1,581	1†
Yes	2	4	0.9 (0.2–6.3)

Note: In some cases the sum does not add up to the total because of missing values.
*OR (*odds ratio*) estimated from a multiple logistic model including terms for age, education, parity, oral contraceptive use, and the above variables.
Abbreviation: CI, confidence interval.
†Reference category (i.e., referent group for the computation of odds ratios).
(Courtesy of Parazzini F, Negri E, La Vecchia C, et al: Treatment for infertility and risk of invasive epithelial ovarian cancer. *Hum Reprod* 12:2159–2161, 1997, reprinted by permission of Oxford University Press. Copyright European Society for Human Reproduction and Embryology.)

Findings.—Fertility drug use was reported by 0.5% of the case group and 0.4% of the control group. Compared with women who had never used fertility drugs, fertility drug users had an odds ratio (OR) of 1.1 for ovarian cancer. The ORs were 0.7 and 1.0 among women who had used fertility drugs for less than 6 and for 6 or more cycles, respectively. In an analysis of the 14 case patients and 45 control subjects reporting problems in conceiving, the risk of ovarian cancer was 0.5 for those who had taken fertility drugs. In an analysis of nulliparous women only, the estimated OR for ovarian cancer for any fertility drug use was 0.6 (Table 2).

Conclusion.—Fertility drug use is apparently not associated with an increased risk of invasive epithelial ovarian cancer. Although this analysis is limited by its low statistical power, these findings should be reassuring for women using fertility drugs.

▶ The results of 1 case-control and 1 cohort study[1-2] performed in the United States suggested that the use of drugs to treat infertility may be associated with an increased risk of the development of epithelial ovarian cancer. However, several other epidemiologic studies did not confirm that infertility drugs were a risk factor for development of invasive ovarian cancer. Nevertheless, infertile women are still concerned about a possible relation between use of agents that induce ovulation and an increased risk of ovarian cancer.

This study analyzed data from nearly 1,000 women with ovarian cancer and 2,758 controls and found no association between use of fertility drugs and development of ovarian cancer. Unfortunately, only 16 women in this study used fertility drugs. The low statistical power of this small number of women limits the value of the conclusions of this study. Nevertheless, the results provide additional data indicating the lack of a strong association between the use of fertility drugs and the development of ovarian cancer.

D.R. Mishell, Jr., M.D.

References

1. Rossing MA, Daling JR, Weiss NS, et al: Ovarian tumors in a cohort of infertile women. *N Engl J Med* 331:771–776, 1994.
2. Whittemore AS, Harris R, Intyre J, et al: Characteristics relating to ovarian cancer risk: Collaborative analysis of 12 U.S. case-control studies. II. Invasive epithelial ovarian cancers in white women. *Am J Epidermiol* 136:1184–1203, 1992.

Laparoscopic Surgery in Infertile Women With Minimal or Mild Endometriosis

Marcoux S, and the Canadian Collaborative Group on Endometriosis (Universitaire de Quebec, et al)
N Engl J Med 337:217–222, 1997 14–6

Background.—Infertile women are often found to have minimal or mild endometriosis, which is commonly treated by resection or ablation of the lesions. Whether such treatment improves fertility has not been established. The value of laparoscopic surgery in enhancing fecundity in infertile women with minimal or mild endometriosis was investigated in a randomized, controlled study.

Methods.—Three hundred forty-one infertile women, aged 20 to 39, with minimal or mild endometriosis were assigned to resection or ablation of visible endometriosis or diagnostic laparoscopy only. Follow-up data were collected for 36 weeks after laparoscopy or for up to 20 weeks of pregnancy.

Findings.—Of the 172 women undergoing resection or ablation of endometriosis, 50 (30.7%) conceived and had pregnancies that continued for 20 weeks or longer. Of the 169 women in the diagnostic laparoscopy group, 29 (17.7%) conceived and had pregnancies that continued for 20 weeks or longer. The fecundity rates were 4.7 and 2.4 per 100 person-months, respectively. Fetal losses occurred in 20.6% and 21.6% of the recognized pregnancies in the 2 groups, respectively. Four minor complications occurred—3 in the surgery group and 1 in the control group. These were intestinal contusion, slight tearing of the tubal serosa, difficult pneumoperitoneum, and vascular trauma.

Conclusions.—Compared with laparoscopy alone, resection or ablation of minimal or mild endometriosis increases the likelihood of pregnancy in infertile women. One in 8 women with minimal or mild endometriosis can be expected to benefit from this procedure. Furthermore, laparoscopic surgery performed at the same time as diagnostic laparoscopy prolongs the procedure by only a few minutes, involves few risks, and can be done on an outpatient basis.

► Other studies in which progestins or gonadotropin-releasing hormone analogues were given to women with mild endometriosis showed that suppression of the disease did not enhance pregnancy rates. Therefore, the results of this study are somewhat surprising. Since the monthly fecundity rate after laparoscopic resection of endometriosis was only 6% compared with the 15% rate reported with the use of controlled ovarian hyperstimulation and intrauterine insemination, I do not believe that these results justify laparoscopy in all women with unexplained infertility. Women with ovulatory cycles and a normal hysterosalpingogram, whose partners have an adequate number of motile sperm, should be initially treated with controlled ovarian hyperstimulation and intrauterine insemination, with a 15% per cycle pregnancy rate, instead of a laparoscopy to determine whether mild endometriosis is present so that it can be treated and have a 6% per cycle pregnancy rate.

D.R. Mishell, Jr., M.D.

Randomized Controlled Trial of Superovulation and Insemination for Infertility Associated With Minimal or Mild Endometriosis

Tummon IS, Asher LJ, Martin JSB, et al (Univ of Western Ontario, London, Canada; McGill Univ, Montréal)

Fertil Steril 68:8–12, 1997 14–7

Background.—Untreated women with infertility associated with minimal or mild endometriosis have a 36-month cumulative live birth rate of 0.20. There have been few controlled studies evaluating the effectiveness of superovulation and intrauterine insemination. Also, many trials have used active treatment controls that have not been shown to be effective. The efficacy of superovulation and intrauterine insemination vs. no treatment for infertility resulting from minimal or mild endometriosis was evaluated.

Methods.—There were 53 couples who were treated by superovulation with intrauterine insemination, and 50 couples who received no treatment. Ovarian stimulation began on menstrual day 3 with daily injection of follicle-stimulating hormone. A final trigger to ovulation was given by injection of 5,000 IU of human chorionic gonadotropin when at least one follicle was greater than 1.8 cm in greatest diameter. Intrauterine insemination was performed 20 hours later.

Results.—Live birth occurred after 14 of 127 treatment cycles and 4 of 184 control cycles. Superovulation with intrauterine insemination resulted in 11 singleton, 2 twin, and 1 triplet births. Four couples who received no treatment had a singleton birth. The odds ratio of a live birth was 5.6 in favor of superovulation with intrauterine insemination compared to no treatment. After 4 cycles of superovulation with intrauterine insemination, there were 30% cumulative live births; after 4 cycles of no treatment, there were 10% cumulative live births (Fig 1).

Discussion.—These results show that superovulation with intrauterine insemination improved the live birth rate in women with infertility asso-

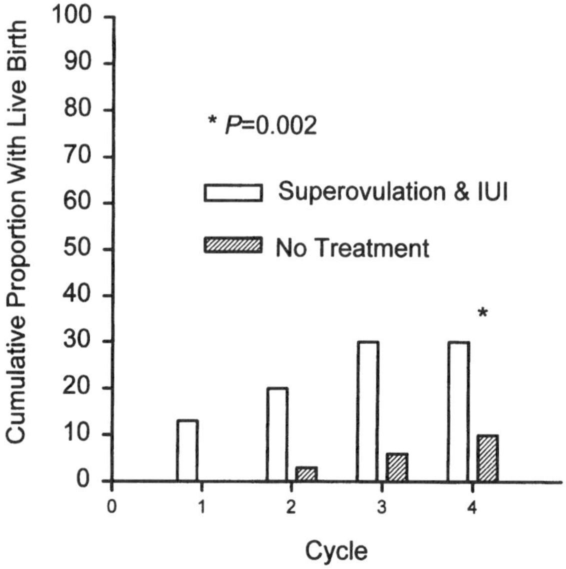

FIGURE 1.—Cumulative proportion of patients with live birth. *Abbreviation*: *IUI*, intrauterine insemination. (From Tummon IS, Asher LJ, Martin JSB, et al: Randomized controlled trial of superovulation and insemination for infertility associated with minimal or mild endometriosis. *Fertil Steril* 68:8–12, 1997. Reproduced with permission of the publisher, the American Society for Reproductive Medicine.)

ciated with minimal or mild endometriosis compared to no treatment. Both the crude live birth rate calculated per treatment cycle and proportional hazard analysis showed superior results from superovulation with intrauterine insemination.

▶ Performance of randomized controlled trials with a no-treatment arm in the field of infertility are of great scientific benefit but, unfortunately, are infrequently done. The results of this randomized controlled trial of a large group of infertile women with no etiologic factor for their infertility other than the presence of minimal or mild pelvic endometriosis provide evidence that controlled ovarian hyperstimulation and intrauterine insemination is an effective therapy. The odds ratio for a live birth was 5.6 times higher when this treatment was performed compared with no therapy. It has not been shown that mild pelvic endometriosis is a cause of infertility, as treatment of the lesions medically or surgically does not lead to increased fecundity. It is likely that women with mild pelvic endometriosis have impaired fecundity resulting from some other unexplained cause. It has been shown in other studies that treatment of unexplained infertility with controlled ovarian hyperstimulation and intrauterine insemination results in significantly greater pregnancy rates than appropriately timed sexual intercourse. Therefore, this therapy should be the initial treatment in all couples with unexplained infertility as well as those in women with mild pelvic endometriosis that does not involve the oviducts.

D.R. Mishell, Jr., M.D.

Comparison of Intrauterine Insemination With Timed Intercourse in Superovulated Cycles With Gonadotropins: A Meta-Analysis

Zeyneloglu HB, Arici A, Olive DL, et al (Yale Univ, New Haven, Conn)

Fertil Steril 69:486–491, 1998 14–8

Objective.—Although the treatment of choice for unexplained infertility is superovulation with gonadotropins and intrauterine insemination (IUI), some women still fail to conceive. There is a dearth of large randomized studies evaluating the effect of adding IUI. The benefit of IUI in combination with superovulation with gonadotropins in the treatment of couples with unexplained infertility was compared with timed intercourse combined with superovulation with gonadotropins.

Methods.—A meta-analysis was performed on studies involving random allocation of infertile couples, with unexplained infertility of at least 2 years, to either superovulation with gonadotropins with IUI using the husband's sperm or superovulation with gonadotropins combined with timed intercourse. Couples had to have confirmed spontaneous ovulation, diagnostic laparoscopy revealing tubal patency, and 2 normal semen analyses. The outcome was clinical pregnancy.

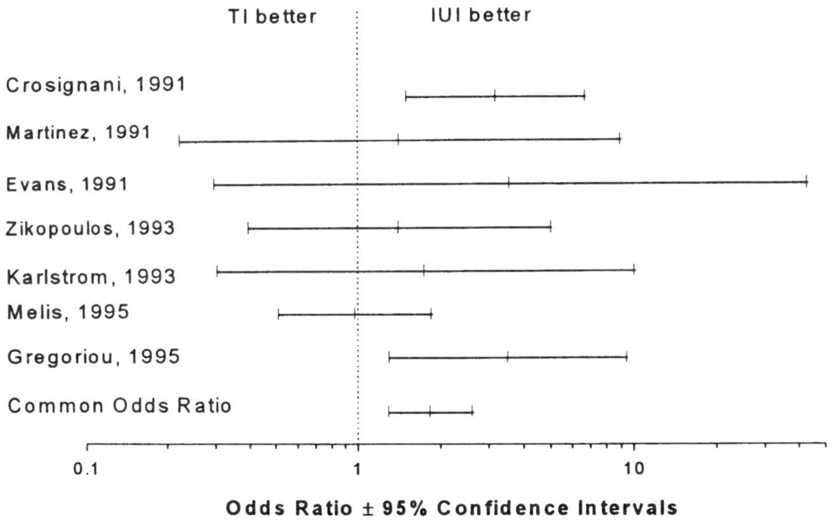

FIGURE 1.—The odds ratio of the studies included in the meat-analysis. *Abbreviation*: *TI*, timed intercourse. (Courtesy of Zeyneloglu HB, Arici A, Olive DL: Comparison of intrauterine insemination with timed intercourse in superovulated cycles with gonadotropins: A meta-analysis. *Fertil Steril* 69:486–491, 1998. Reprinted with permission of the publisher, the American Society for Reproductive Medicine.)

Results.—The 7 studies included involved 980 cycles. There were 49 (11.4%) pregnancies in 431 cycles of timed intercourse, and 110 (20.0%) pregnancies in 549 cycles of IUI. The odds ratio of 1.84 for IUI vs. timed intercourse was significant (Fig 1). The use of IUI did not significantly increase the number of multiple fetuses (odds ratio, 1.59).

Conclusion.—The use of IUI with superovulation increases the chances of pregnancy in couples with unexplained infertility.

▶ This meta-analysis combined results of 7 randomized clinical trials comparing the use of timed intercourse to intrauterine insemination in couples with unexplained infertility who were also treated with gonadotropins for controlled ovarian hyperstimulation. The use of intrauterine insemination increased the per-cycle pregnancy rate nearly 2-fold, from 11% to 20%. The results of this study add additional data to confirm the belief that the initial therapy for unexplained infertility should be controlled ovarian hyperstimulation together with intrauterine insemination of spermatozoa that have been separated from the seminal fluid.

D.R. Mishell, Jr., M.D.

A Randomized, Prospective Analysis of Five Sperm Preparation Techniques Before Intrauterine Insemination of Husband Sperm

Carrell DT, Kuneck PH, Peterson CM, et al (Univ of Utah, Salt Lake City)

Fertil Steril 69:122–126, 1998 14–9

Objective.—There are a variety of sperm preparation techniques used before intrauterine insemination (IUI) designed to increase the pregnancy rate. Five sperm preparation techniques before IUI with husband sperm were compared prospectively: sperm washing, swim-up, swim-down, refrigeration/heparin incubation, and Percoll gradient centrifugation.

Methods.—A total of 363 patients with a wide range of unexplained male- and/or female-related disorders, randomly underwent homologous artificial insemination 36 hours after spontaneous LH surge or 36 hours after injection of hCG. If pregnancy did not occur, the sperm preparation technique was changed for the next cycle. Patients with oligoasthenozoospermia were not included. Ovulation was induced with clomiphene citrate on days 5 to 9 of the cycle. Patients receiving gonadotropin stimulation were given 1 to 4 vials daily beginning on cycle day 3.

Results.—There were 898 inseminations performed, a mean of 2.5 inseminations per participant, 2.0 inseminations per successful pregnancy, and 2.6 inseminations per miscarriage. On day 14 after an insemination, 107 (29.5%) patients had a positive hCG level, and 87 (23.9%) had live births. The pregnancy rate was highest and the miscarriage rate lowest with the swim-up technique (Table 1). The ongoing pregnancy rate was highest for the gonadotropin-stimulated cycles (Table 2). Almost half (46%) of patients who achieved pregnancy became pregnant after the first insemination.

TABLE 1.—Pregnancy Rates After 898 Inseminations With Five Sperm Preparation Techniques

Patient group	Wash	Swim-up	Percoll gradient	Swim-down	Refrigeration/heparin	All
Chemical pregnancy*	8.9 (14/157)	14.7 (29/197)	16.1 (33/204)	7.7 (15/195)†	11.0 (16/145)	11.9 (107/898)
Miscarriage§	21.4 (3/14)	10.3 (3/29)	21.2 (7/33)	20.0 (3/15)	25.0 (4/16)	18.7 (20/107)
Delivery‖	7.0 (11/157)†‡	13.2 (26/197)	12.7 (26/204)	6.1 (12/195)†‡	8.3 (12/145)	9.7 (87/898)

*Values represent percent pregancy rate (no. of pregnancies/no. of inseminations).
†$P < 0.05$ (compared with swim-up and Percoll treatments).
‡$P < 0.10$ (compared with swim-up and Percoll treatments).
§Values represent percent of miscarriages (no. of miscarriages/no. of inseminations).
‖Values represent percent of deliveries (no. of deliveries/no. of inseminations).
(From Carrell DT, Kuneck PH, Peterson CM, et al: A randomized, prospective analysis of five sperm preparation techniques before intrauterine insemination of husband sperm. *Fertil Steril* 1998, 69:122–126. Reproduced with permission of the publisher, the American Society for Reproductive Medicine.)

TABLE 2.—Pregnancy Rates After Insemination in Subgroups of Ovarian Stimulation Treatment

Pregnancy	Natural	Clomiphene citrate	Gonadotropin
Chemical pregnancy*	7.7 (15/196)	15.8 (16/101)†	12.6 (76/601)†
Miscarriage‡	20.0 (3/15)	18.8 (3/16)	18.4 (14/76)
Delivery§	6.1 (12/196)	12.9 (13/101)†	10.3 (62/601)†

*Values represent percent pregnancy rate (no. of pregnancies/no. of inseminations).
†$P < 0.05$ (compared with natural cycles).
‡Values represent percent of miscarriages (no. of miscarriages/no. of inseminations).
§Values represent percent of deliveries (no. of deliveries/no. of inseminations).
(From Carrell DT, Kuneck PH, Peterson CM, et al: A randomized, prospective analysis of five sperm preparation techniques before intrauterine insemination of husband sperm. *Fertil Steril* 1998, 69:122–126. Reproduced with permission of the publisher, the American Society for Reproduction Medicine.)

Conclusion.—The Percoll gradient and swim-up sperm preparation techniques yielded the highest pregnancy rates, particularly after ovarian stimulation.

► At least 2 randomized clinical trials have shown that in groups of women with unexplained infertility the use of controlled ovarian hyperstimulation with clomiphene citrate followed by intrauterine insemination results in enhanced fecundity rates compared with nonstimulated cycles with and without intrauterine insemination. Stimulation with hMG followed by intrauterine insemination has also been shown to enhance fecundity rates in comparison with control groups of women with unexplained infertility. Although ovarian stimulation was not randomly compared with no stimulation in this study, the results show that stimulation resulted in nearly twice the pregnancy rate and delivery rate compared with nonstimulated cycles. Furthermore, pregnancy rates were higher when clomiphene citrate was used for stimulation than when hMG was used. In addition, the study demonstrated that for men with a normal amount of motile sperm, separation of the spermatozoa from the seminal fluid by the swim-up or density gradient technique results in a significantly greater pregnancy rate than a single 2-step wash. Therefore, the data obtained in this study support the belief that couples with unexplained infertility in whom the woman is ovulating and has patent oviducts and the man has a normal semen analysis are best initially treated with clomiphene citrate followed by sperm separation with the swim-up or density gradient technique. A pregnancy rate of about 15% per treatment cycle should be expected if the woman is under age 35.

D.R. Mishell, Jr., M.D.

Intrauterine Insemination After Ovarian Stimulation With Clomiphene Citrate: Predictive Potential of Inseminating Motile Count and Sperm Morphology

Ombelet W, Vandeput H, Van de Putte G, et al (Genk Inst for Fertility Technology, Belgium; Univ of Leuven; Tygerberg Hosp, South Africa)

Hum Reprod 12:1458–1463, 1997 14–10

Introduction.—The use of homologous intrauterine insemination (IUI) after clomiphene citrate (CC) stimulation can be considered a first-step procedure in selected cases of subfertility. The influence of the inseminating motile count (IMC) and sperm morphological characteristics on the success rate in CC-IUI cycles was studied retrospectively.

Methods.—Over a 64-month period, 373 subfertile couples underwent homologous artificial insemination combined with CC stimulation during 792 treatment cycles. All patients had undergone an infertility workup, which determined that a male factor only was involved in 55.1% of couples and a male plus female factor in 32.4%; subfertility was idiopathic in 7.8%. Semen was analyzed according to World Health Organization guidelines, but stricter criteria were used for sperm morphology. The cutoff level for normality was 10%. A double insemination was performed in 82.3% of cycles. Inseminations were timed for 14–18 and 36–40 hours after CC-human chorionic gonadotropin. Spermatozoa were prepared by the conventional swim-up technique.

Results.—Pregnancy was achieved in 116 of 373 couples. The first cycle was the most successful, with a pregnancy rate of 18.5% and a baby take-home rate of 12.6%. After 3 cycles, the cumulative cycle fecundity and baby take-home rate per couple were 30.6% and 21.1%, respectively. When the study population was classified into subgroups according to IMC, sperm morphological features were a valuable prognostic factor in group 1 (less than 1×10^6 motile spermatozoa recovered after washing). No pregnancies occurred in this group (Table 2) when the morphology score was less than 4%. For subgroups 2, 3, and 4, sperm morphologic characteristics were not predictive of IUI outcome. The rate of miscarriage (31.9%) was equally distributed among the 4 subgroups. Multiple births (both twins) occurred in only 2 of 79 births.

Conclusion.—In a selected group of patients with normal ovarian response after CC stimulation, IUI combined with CC-human chorionic gonadotropin can provide a very safe and inexpensive first-line treatment, provided that IMC is greater than 1×10^6 spermatozoa. When less than 1×10^6 spermatozoa are present, CC-IUI can be effective if the sperm morphology score is 4% or greater.

► The results of this large retrospective study indicate that controlled ovarian hyperstimulation (COH) utilizing CC followed by IUI is effective for treating infertility associated with oligospermia as well as for unexplained infertility. Several important conclusions that can be made by analysis of the data in this study. First, with the use of CC COH followed by IUI, the cycle

TABLE 2.—Cycle Fecundity and Baby Take-home Rate in the Different Inseminating Motile Count Subgroups (1, 2, 3, 4), According to the Cycle Number (χ^2 Statistics for Differences Among Subgroups)

IMC Cycle number	Subgroup 1			Subgroup 2			Subgroup 3			Subgroup 4			Total		
	n	CF	BTH	*n*	CF	BTH	*n*	CF	BTH	*n*	CF	BTH	*n*	CF	BTH
1	56	4 (7.1)*	3 (5.4)*	37	5 (13.5)	3 (8.1)	156	29 (18.6)	19 (12.2)	124	31 (25.0)*	22 (17.7)*	373	69 (18.5)	47 (12.6)
2	52	5 (9.6)	3 (5.8)	31	6 (19.4)	4 (12.9)	125	17 (13.6)	13 (10.4)	92	9 (9.8)	7 (7.6)	300	37 (12.3)	27 (9.0)
3	13	1 (7.7)	1 (7.7)	12	1 (8.3)	1 (8.3)	37	3 (8.1)	2 (5.4)	20	3 (15.0)	1 (5.0)	82	8 (9.8)	5 (6.1)
4 or more	7	0	0	6	1 (8.3)	0	15	1 (6.7)	0	9	0	0	37	2 (5.4)	0
	128	10 (7.8)†	7 (5.5)†	86	13 (15.1)	8 (9.3)	333	50 (15.0)	34 (10.2)	245	43 (17.6)†	30 (12.2)†	792	116 (14.6)	79 (10.0)

Note: Subgroups are defined by number of motile spermatozoa recovered after washing. Subgroup 1: $<1 \times 10^6$; subgroup 2: $\geq 1-<2 \times 10^6$; subgroup 3: $\geq 2-<10 \times 10^6$; subgroup 4: $\geq 10 \times 10^6$. Figures in parenthesis are percentages.

*Cycle 1, subgroup 1 vs. subgroup 4; $P < 0.05$ for CF and BTH.

†All cycles, subgroup 1 vs. subgroup 4; $P < 0.05$ for CF and BTH.

Abbreviations: IMC, inseminating motile count; *CF*, cycle fecundity; *BTH*, baby take-home rate.

(Courtesy of Ombelet W, Vandeput H, Van de Putte G, et al: Intrauterine insemination after ovarian stimulation with clomiphene citrate: Predictive potential of inseminating motile count and sperm morphology. *Hum Reprod* 12:1458–1463, 1997. Reprinted by permission of Oxford University Press, copyright European Society for Human Reproduction and Embryology.)

fecundability rate is about 15% as long as more than 1 million motile sperm are available for insemination after the separation procedure. If at least 4% or more of the spermatozoa have normal morphological characteristics, the same fecundability rate occurs with treatment. Second, if the motile sperm count after separation was between 100,000 and 1,000,000, a similar 15% cycle fecundability rate was observed as long as less than 4% of the spermatozoa had abnormal morphological characteristics, according to the strict criteria described by Kruger. The cumulative pregnancy rate after 3 cycles of COH + IUI was more than 30% and there was a low incidence of multiple gestation and no instance of moderate or severe ovarian hyperstimulation. Clinicians can perform COH with CC followed by IUI in their office to enhance the pregnancy rates of couples with unexplained infertility as well as those whose male partner has a mild degree of oligospermia.

D.R. Mishell, Jr., M.D.

The Effectiveness of Intrauterine Insemination in Couples With Sterility Caused by Male Infertility With and Without a Female Hormone Factor

Rammer E, Friedrich F (Gen Public Hosp, Horn, Austria)

Fertil Steril 69:31–36, 1998 14–11

Background.—Sterility caused by both male and female factors is addressed by intrauterine insemination (IUI) coupled with hormone treatment for the woman and special preparation of the man's semen. The results of the combined methods were studied retrospectively and assessed with respect to various causes of sterility attributed to the male factor both with and without a female hormone factor.

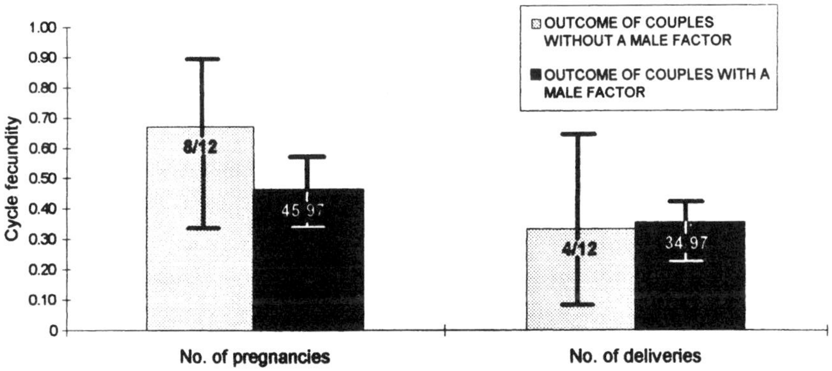

FIGURE 1.—Outcome of inseminations in couples without (□) and with (■) a male factor. Data are presented as fecundity (delivery) rate ± 95% CI. Values at the top of the bars represent the number of pregnancies (deliveries)/number of cycles. Fecundity rate and delivery rate are not significantly different in the two groups. (From Rammer E, Friedrich F: The effectiveness of intrauterine insemination in couples with sterility due to male infertility with and without a women's hormone factor. *Fertil Steril* 1998; 69:31–36. Reproduced with permission of the publisher, the American Society for Reproductive Medicine.)

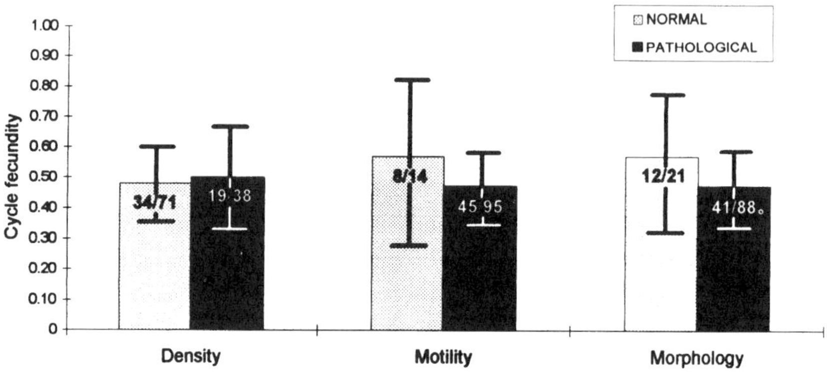

FIGURE 3.—Comparison of the fecundity cycle with respect to normal (□) and pathologic (■) sperm density, motility, and morphology. Data are presented as fecundity rate ± 95% CI. Values at the top of the bars represent the number of pregnancies/number of cycles. (From Rammer E, Friedrich F: The effectiveness of intrauterine insemination in couples with sterility due to male infertility with and without a women's hormone factor. *Fertil Steril* 1998; 69:31–36. Reproduced with permission of the publisher, the American Society for Reproductive Medicine.)

Methods.—IUI was used for 78 couples who had wanted children for 2 to 10 years. The principal causes of infertility were the women's hormone factor (elevated DHEAS, T, or FSH levels) and the men's reduced sperm motility in addition to their pathologic sperm forms or the reduced motility, reduced density, and pathologic forms of their sperm with or without the women's hormone factor. Couples were treated for 114 cycles, IUI was used 109 times with 1 insemination for each cycle, and women were stimulated with hMG for 103 cycles. IUI was used when no fallopian tube factor was present, and the man's sperm density was greater than 1×10^6 mL. When the leading follicle was 1.8 cm, ovulation was induced by an intramuscular injection of 10,000 IU hCG. After 24 hours, insemination was performed with sperm prepared by Percoll gradient centrifugation.

Results.—Of the 76 women inseminated, 46 (60.5% conceived and 35 (76.1%) delivered at least 1 child. Of 109 inseminations, 53 (48.6%) resulted in pregnancy and 18 (34.9%) led to deliveries. There were 28 (73.7%) single births and 10 (26.3%) multiple births (9 sets of twins (23.77%) and 1 set of triplets (2.6%). Fourteen (43.8%) pregnancies and 10 (71.4%) deliveries resulted from 32 inseminations in women with a hormone factor. In women without a hormone factor, 77 inseminations resulted in 39 pregnancies (50.6%) and 28 (71.8%) deliveries. A high percentage of pregnancies was possible in couples with a causative male factor, in cases of reduced motility and triple pathology, with and without a woman's hormone factor (Fig 1). Equal success was realized where sperm density, motility, and morphology were poor (Fig 3). Where the percentage of fast motile sperm was less than 10%, 34 inseminations yielded 15 (44.1%) pregnancies. Results were equally good in men with low sperm density and a low percentage of normal sperm forms. Even when infertility was the result of a causative male factor with and without the woman's hormone factor or in cases of oligoasthenoteratozoospermia, this technique resulted in a high percentage of live births.

Conclusion.—IUI coupled with specific treatment for both women and men results in a high percentage of live births in couples with male factor both with and without the female hormone factor.

▶ This report is a retrospective analysis of treatment with controlled ovarian hyperstimulation with hMG and intrauterine insemination among couples in whom some of the women were anovulatory, and some of the men had abnormalities in 1 or more of the variables analyzed in the semen analysis (concentration, motility, or morphology). The results indicate that as long as ovulation could be induced and at least 1 million sperm were present in the pretreatment ejaculate, a high rate of pregnancy and live births were achieved in each treatment cycle. Thus, in addition to treatment of unexplained infertility, the use of controlled ovarian hyperstimulation and IUI can achieve a high rate of pregnancy in couples in whom anovulation and either oligo (few) astheno (abnormal motility), or terato (abnormal morphology), in spermia are also present.

D.R. Mishell, Jr., M.D.

The Role of In Vitro Fertilization and Intracytoplasmic Sperm Injection in Couples With Unexplained Infertility After Failed Intrauterine Insemination

Ruiz A, Remohí J, Minguez Y, et al (Instituto Valenciano de Infertilidad, Spain; Valencia Univ, Spain)

Fertil Steril 68:171–173, 1997 14–12

Introduction.—An acceptable method for treating infertility of different causes is intrauterine insemination in combination with ovarian stimulation. In in vitro fertilization (IVF) cycles performed for unexplained infertility, reduced fertilization and cleavage rates have been documented, suggesting gamete defects in such couples. Clinicians have had a powerful tool to overcome fertilization problems with the introduction of intracytoplasmic sperm injection for the treatment of male infertility. In couples with unexplained infertility who failed to conceive with standard intrauterine insemination, the value of intracytoplasmic sperm injection was studied. During the first attempt of IVF in couples with unexplained infertility, intracytoplasmic sperm injection and routine in vitro fertilization were applied randomly on sibling oocytes.

Methods.—There were 7 couples with mild endometriosis and 63 with unexplained infertility who had IVF after 4 failed intrauterine insemination cycles. There was a randomization of sibling oocytes into standard intracytoplasmic sperm injection or conventional IVF. In IVF and intracytoplasmic sperm injection-inseminated oocytes, fertilization, cleavage, and embryo quality were compared.

Results.—In conventional IVF, the fertilization rate was 54% and in intracytoplasmic sperm injection, the fertilization rate was 60.4%. This was not a significant difference. There was no difference in embryo quality in the 2 groups. When conventional IVF was used, fertilization failed to occur in 8 of 70 couples (11.4%). In intracytoplasmic sperm injection-inseminated oocytes, there was no total fertilization failure.

Conclusion.—There is an 11.4% chance of fertilization failure that can be overcome easily by using intracytoplasmic sperm injection in at least some oocytes in couples with unexplained infertility and mild endometriosis failing to conceive with intrauterine insemination. In most couples, however, intracytoplasmic sperm injection is not superior to IVF as an insemination technique. When counseling patients, these data should be used. Fertilization rates are not increased in couples with unexplained infertility having IVF with intracytoplasmic sperm injection.

► The initial treatment for unexplained infertility is controlled ovarian hyperstimulation followed by intrauterine insemination. If pregnancy does not occur after 4–6 cycles of this therapy, the couple is usually advised to undergo IVF. A certain proportion of couples with unexplained infertility do not conceive because fertilization does not occur even under in vitro conditions. In this study, fertilization failed to occur with in vitro fertilization in about 10% of the couples who failed to conceive after treatment with 4 cycles of controlled ovarian hyperstimulation plus intrauterine insemination. It does not appear to be cost-effective to routinely perform intracytoplasmic sperm injection in the initial IVF cycle utilized in these couples as fertilization will occur in 90% of these cycles. If fertilization does not occur with routine IVF, then intracytoplasmic sperm injection should be performed in a subsequent treatment cycle.

D.R. Mishell, Jr., M.D.

Assisted Reproductive Technology in the United States and Canada: 1995 Results Generated From the American Society for Reproductive Medicine/Society for Assisted Reproductive Technology Registry

Zeitz J, for the Society for Assisted Reproductive Technology and the American Society for Reproductive Medicine (American Society for Reproductive Medicine, Birmingham, Ala)

Fertil Steril 69:389–398, 1998 14–13

Introduction.—The procedures and outcomes of assisted reproductive technology activities initiated in the United States and Canada in 1995 were summarized from data voluntarily reported by 281 programs.

Data.—Cycle-specific data were obtained retrospectively for procedures performed in 1995. Main outcome measures were pregnancy, ectopic pregnancy, abortion, stillbirth, delivery, and congenital abnormality.

Results.—In 1995, the 281 participating programs reported 59,142 initiated cycles of assisted reproductive technology treatment. Of these, 41,087 were in vitro fertilization with 22.5% deliveries per retrieval. Of in vitro fertilization procedures, 5,052 involved intracytoplasmic sperm injection, 3,741 were cycles of gamete intrafallopian transfer, and 1,078 were cycles of zygote intrafallopian transfer. There were 3,555 reported donor oocyte and 200 cycles of in vitro fertilization for host uterus, as well as 8,453 cryopreserved embryo thaw procedures with embryos generated from the woman's own oocytes and 1,028 cryopreserved embryo thaw procedures of embryos generated from donated oocytes. These procedures resulted in 11,631 reported deliveries. Of the 41,087 in vitro fertilization procedures, 85.8% led to a retrieval; the overall cancellation rate was 14.2%. Of the 35,269 retrievals, 90.1% led to transfers. These resulted in 9,760 clinical pregnancies.

Overall, the pregnancy rate was 23.7% per initiated cycle, 27.7% per retrieval, and 30.7% per transfer. There were 7,939 reported deliveries: 19.3% deliveries per initiated cycle, 22.5% per retrieval, and 25.0% per transfer. Of clinical pregnancies, 18% were lost. There were 259 reported ectopic pregnancies (2.6% of intrauterine pregnancies established and 0.8% of in vitro fertilization transfers). Of deliveries overall, 63.4% were singleton, 29.6% were twins, 6.4% were triplets, and 0.6% were multiple deliveries of 4 or more. There were 1,659 pregnancies established with embryos fertilized by intracytoplasmic sperm injection. Of the 5,638 initiated cycles, 5,428 retrievals, and 5,248 transfers of embryos after intracytoplasmic sperm injection, 1,350 deliveries resulted. Pregnancy loss was 18.6%; there were 1,901 normal infants and 25 infants with structural or functional abnormalities. Seventeen ectopic pregnancies occurred. Of 41,087 initiated in vitro fertilization cycles, 5,052 involved intracytoplasmic sperm injection. The pregnancy rate was 28.9% per initiated cycle, 29.0% per retrieval, and 31.3% per embryo transfer (ET) (compared with 23.0% per initiated cycle, 27.5% per retrieval, and 30.6% per ET for cycles without intracytoplasmic sperm injection).

The delivery rate for in vitro fertilization cycles using intracytoplasmic sperm injection was 23.5% per initiated cycle, 23.5% per retrieval, and 25.4% per ET (compared with 18.7% per initiated cycle, 22.3% per retrieval, and 24.9% per ET for cycles without intracytoplasmic sperm injection). The clinical pregnancy rate for donor cycles using intracytoplasmic sperm injection was 39.3% per ET. The delivery rate was 36.2% per ET (compared with a 43.7% pregnancy rate and 33.7% delivery rate for cycles without intracytoplasmic sperm injection). Among all cycles of gamete intrafallopian transfer, there were 1,142 clinical pregnancies, or a pregnancy rate of 30.5% per initiated cycle, 34.4% per retrieval, and 34.9% per gamete transfer.

Discussion.—In assisted reproductive technology, age continues to have a dominant effect, with significantly lower success rates in each age bracket. Male factor infertility seems to have a more limited effect on outcome than in previous years. An increase in the number of programs reporting data was seen, as well as an increase in the number of cycles of assisted reproductive technology. The number of couples receiving oocyte donation treatment and embryo cryopreservation continues to increase.

▶ This activity report of treatment with assisted reproductive technologies in the United States for the year 1995 is the first year in which data from individual patients were compiled in a central depository instead of the individual clinics. Analysis of the data shows close similarities between the outcome of assisted reproductive technologies in 1995 and that obtained in prior years. The main difference between the 1995 results and those completed earlier is the enhanced success for treatment of problems of male infertility with the use of intracytoplasmic sperm injection. Intracytoplasmic sperm injection was used in 12.3% of in vitro fertilization (IVF) cycles in the United States in 1995 and was associated with a 23.5% rate of delivery per ovum retrieval, slightly higher than the 22.5% delivery rates when IVF was performed for other causes of infertility. The information in this report, as well as data from each clinic, should be available for couples wishing to undertake these expensive methods of infertility therapy.

D.R. Mishell, Jr., M.D.

Low Pregnancy Rate Is Achieved in Patients Treated With Intracytoplasmic Sperm Injection Due to Previous Low or Failed Fertilization in In-Vitro Fertilization

Tomás C, Orava M, Tuomivaara L, et al (Univ of Oulu, Finland; The Family Federation of Finland, Oulu)

Hum Reprod 13:65–70, 1998 14–14

Objective.—The high fertilization rates with intracytoplasmic sperm injection (ICSI) make this the technique of choice for couples with infertility caused by severe sperm defects and for couples with failed or low fertilization in previous in vitro fertilization (IVF) treatments. Subgroups of patients suitable for ICSI were identified and treatment results of fertilization, cleavage, implantation, and pregnancy rates were compared.

Methods.—ICSI was performed in 65 couples with failed fertilization or a low fertilization rate (less than 25%) in previous IVF treatments and a normal spermiogram, and in 219 couples with severe male factors.

Results.—Mature oocyte numbers, fertilization rate, and cleavage rate were similar for the 2 groups. A total of 2,726 oocytes were collected, 2,087 were micro-injected, and 1,355 were fertilized. The pregnancy rate per embryo transferred was significantly lower in the failed or low fertilization group than in the male factor group (19.6% vs. 33.5%). Although the cleavage rate and morphologic quality of the embryos transferred were similar, the implantation rate was significantly lower in the failed or low fertilization group compared with the male factor group (9.6% vs. 19.5%). In patients younger than 36, 18% of failed- or low-fertilization patients and 34% of male factor patients became pregnant. In patients more than 36, the rates were 24% and 30%.

Conclusion.—Patients with failed or low fertilization rates have significantly lower pregnancy rates after ICSI than male factor patients. This result indicates that oocyte defects decrease embryo development or implantation and can be helped only by oocyte donation.

▶ This interesting study indicates that when ICSI is performed for abnormalities in the semen analysis, the pregnancy rate per embryo transfer after in vitro fertilization (IVF) is about 33%. However, when ICSI followed by IVF is performed for failed fertilization in a prior IVF attempt, the pregnancy rate per embryo transfer is only about 20%. The incidence of fertilization and embryo transfer was similar in the 2 groups studied, indicating that failure of fertilization with IVF is frequently caused by a problem in the oocyte that persists after IVF. Because of the 20% pregnancy rate per cycle when ICSI-IVF is performed for prior IVF fertilization failure, this therapy is still valuable. However, if pregnancy does not occur after several treatment cycles, consideration should be given to the use of donor oocytes.

D.R. Mishell, Jr., M.D.

The Effect of Female Age and Ovarian Reserve on Pregnancy Rate in Male Infertility: Treatment of Azoospermia With Sperm Retrieval and Intracytoplasmic Sperm Injection

Silber SJ, Nagy Z, Devroey P, et al (St Luke's Hosp, St Louis; Dutch-Speaking Free Univ, Brussels, Belgium)

Hum Reprod 12:2693–2700, 1997 14–15

Background.—In patients with male infertility who are undergoing assisted reproduction procedures, factors other than spermatozoa may be the major determinants of success. The effects of the partner's age and ovarian reserve on the success rates of assisted reproduction performed for azoospermia were studied.

Methods.—Two hundred forty-nine consecutive couples with male infertility caused by azoospermia underwent microsurgical epididymal sperm aspiration or testicular sperm extraction with intracytoplasmic sperm injection (ICSI). One hundred eighty-six men had irreparable obstructive azoospermia. Sixty-three had nonobstructive azoospermia caused by testicular failure.

Findings.—Neither fertilization nor pregnancy was affected by the pathology, source, quantity, or quality of the spermatozoa. Maternal age and ovarian reserve did not affect fertilization or embryo cleavage but dramatically influenced embryo implantation, pregnancy rates, and delivery rates. Women in their 20s had a 46% live delivery rate per cycle, compared with 34% for women aged 30–36 and 13% for those aged 37–39. Women aged 40 or older had a live delivery rate per cycle of only 4%. Number of eggs retrieved affected pregnancy and delivery rates to a lesser degree than maternal age. Sufficient spermatozoa could be retrieved to perform ICSI, with normal fertilization and embryo cleavage, from virtually all men with obstructive azoospermia and 62% of men with nonobstructive azoospermia caused by germinal failure.

Conclusions.—The success of microsurgical epididymal sperm aspiration-ICSI and testicular sperm extraction-ICSI for male infertility is limited by the partner's age and possibly ovarian reserve. Live delivery rates of 42% per cycle are readily achieved when the woman is younger than 37 and when 9 or more eggs are retrieved.

Effect of Parental Age on Fertilization and Pregnancy Characteristics in Couples Treated by Intracytoplasmic Sperm Injection

Spandorfer SD, Avrech OM, Colombero LT, et al (The New York Hosp-Cornell Univ)

Hum Reprod 13:334–338, 1998 14–16

Background.—Maternal age is known to adversely affect fecundity, with an increase in sterility beginning at the age of 35. This rise increases sharply after the age of 39, and after the age of 44, women are almost completely unable to conceive. This trend has also been observed in women undergoing assisted reproductive technologies. The current study determined the influence of maternal and paternal age on gamete characteristics and pregnancy outcomes in intracytoplasmic sperm injection (ICSI) cycles.

Methods and Findings.—Eight hundred twenty-one consecutive patients undergoing ICSI were analyzed retrospectively. Semen volume showed a significant linear decline with paternal aging, although concentration, motility, and morphology of the spermatozoa were unaffected. Advancing maternal age was associated with a significant decline in the number of oocytes retrieved and in the number of mature oocytes obtained. The occurrence of digyny increased with parental aging, although there was no difference in single or bipronuclear fertilization. Older women had a reduced incidence of single pronucleus formation and increased digyny. However, maternal aging did not affect the percentage of oocytes undergoing 2-pronuclear fertilization. Paternal age did not influence pregnancy outcomes, whereas maternal age did. In a subgroup of couples in which the female partner was younger than 35, the age of the male partner did not affect ICSI pregnancy outcome.

Conclusions.—Advancing paternal age does not appear to affect clinically meaningful semen characteristics. In addition, it is not associated with lower pregnancy rates. However, the association between advancing maternal age and compromised outcome after ICSI treatment was confirmed in this study.

▶ The results of these 2 studies (Abstracts 14–15 and 14–16) show that maternal age is a major factor affecting embryo implantation and viable birth rate (but not fertilization) when ICSI is performed with ejaculated sperm as well as with sperm aspirated from the epididymis or extracted from the testes of men with azoospermia. Thus, increasing maternal age, but not advanced paternal age, reduces the chance of a viable pregnancy in couples with male cause of infertility. Infertile couples should be counseled accordingly.

D.R. Mishell, Jr, M.D.

In Vitro Fertilization in Women Over 40 Years of Age: A Study on Retrospective Data for Eight Years

Bongain A, Castillon JM, Isnard V, et al (Hôpital l'Archet, Nice, France)
Eur J Obstet Gynecol Reprod Biol 76:225–231, 1998 14–17

Background.—The number of older women wishing to become pregnant is increasing. In France, the percentage of in vitro fertilization (IVF) performed in women over 40 rose from 7.8% in 1987 to 11.1% in 1991. In the current study, the outcomes of IVF attempts in women older than 40 years were compared with those in younger women.

Methods.—Data on women undergoing IVF at 1 center between 1987 and 1995 were analyzed retrospectively. One hundred ninety-four IVF attempts in women older than 40 were compared with 209 IVF attempts in women of 35 or younger. Mean ages were 40.9 years and 29.3 years, respectively.

Findings.—Duration of follicle stimulation and number of ampules did not differ significantly in the 2 groups. Serum estradiol levels were 1,435.8 pg/mL in the older group and 2,020.8 pg/mL in the younger group, a significant difference. Other significant differences were number of oocytes (4.6 and 7.3, respectively), number of embryos (1.7 and 2.8, respectively), and percentage of full-term deliveries (3.6% and 13.4%, respectively). In a long protocol compared with a short one, the older group had better oocyte retrieval (5.3 compared with 3.3), but the rate of embryo transfer (1.9 and 1.3, respectively) and full-term deliveries (4.2% and 2.9%, respectively) did not differ significantly.

Conclusions.—Women older than 40 who desire to become pregnant should be told of the low success rate. In light of this low success rate and the great emotional and financial investment required for IVF, couples and health care providers must carefully consider the indications for such treatment.

► The results of this study from a single center confirm the results of other studies, which show that the chance of having a viable pregnancy following use of IVF in women more than 40 years of age is less than 5% per initiated cycle. This rate is much less than the 13.4% rate found in the same clinic during the same time in women who were 35 years of age or younger. Women over 40 should be told about the poor likelihood of success with IVF and informed that improved rates can be achieved with the use of donor oocytes. However, many women over 40 do not wish to use donor oocytes.

They should be thoroughly counseled about the poor likelihood of a viable birth with IVF before investing the time and effort this procedure requires.

D.R. Mishell, Jr., M.D.

Intracytoplasmic Sperm Injection in Obstructive and Non-obstructive Azoospermia

Mansour RT, Kamal A, Fahmy I, et al (Egyptian IVF-ET Ctr, Cairo; Cairo Univ, Egypt)
Hum Reprod 12:1974–1979, 1997 14–18

Background.—In the past, infertility has been considered untreatable in patients with obstructive azoospermia from congenital absence of the vas deferens (CAVD) and in those in whom reconstructive surgery has failed. However, intracytoplasmic sperm injection (ICSI) has significantly improved outcomes in such patients. The results were reported of ICSI in the treatment of obstructive vs. nonobstructive azoospermia, acquired obstructive azoospermia vs. congenital obstruction from CAVD, and epididymal vs. testicular spermatozoa in obstructive azoospermia.

Methods.—Data on 106 consecutive ICSI cycles done in 103 patients with nonobstructive azoospermia and on 135 cycles in 119 patients with obstructive azoospermia were analyzed. In the obstructive group, epididymal spermatozoa were used in 44 cycles and testicular spermatozoa in 91.

Findings.—The fertilization and pregnancy per cycle rates were 59.5% and 27.3%, respectively, using epididymal spermatozoa; 54.4% and 31.9%, respectively, using testicular spermatozoa in obstructive cases; and 39% and 11.3%, respectively, in nonobstructive cases. In acquired cases, the fertilization and pregnancy per cycle rates were 56.6% and 37%,

TABLE 3.—Outcome of Intracytoplasmic Sperm Injection for Patients With Obstructive and Nonobstructive Azoospermia

	Obstructive			Non-obstructive	Total
	Epididymal*	Testicular*	Total	testicular	
No. of ICSI cycles	44	91	135	106	241
No. of injected oocytes (MII)	471	955	1,426	754	2,180
No. of fertilized oocytes (2PN)	280	519	799	294	1,093
Fertilization rate (%)	59.5	54.4	56†	39†	50.1
No. of ICSI cycles reaching embryo transfer stage (%)	44 (100)	91 (100)	135 (100)	79 (74.5)	213 (88.4)
No. of clinical pregnancies	12	29	41	12	53
Clinical pregnancy rate					
per cycle (%)	27.3	31.9	30.4†	11.3†	22
per embryo transfer (%)	27.3	31.9	30.4	15.2	24.9

*There were no significant differences between the testicular and epididymal groups of the obstructive azoospermia cycles.
†Values with the same superscript were significantly different (*P* less than 0.05).
Abbreviations: ICSI, intracytoplasmic sperm injection; *MII,* metaphase II; *PN* pronuclear.

respectively. In CAVD cases, these rates were 55.2% and 20.4%, respectively (Table 3).

Conclusion.—In patients with obstructive azoospermia, ICSI with surgically retrieved spermatozoa resulted in a 56% fertilization rate per cycle and a 30.4% pregnancy rate per cycle. In patients with nonobstructive azoospermia, these rates were 39% and 11.3%, respectively. Spermatozoa for ICSI could be found in 67% of cycles involving nonobstructive azoospermia. The fertilization and pregnancy rates associated with the use of testicular spermatozoa in obstructive cases were significantly greater than in nonobstructive cases.

► Infertile men with no sperm in their ejaculate were previously considered sterile. However, by combining 2 recently developed techniques, testicular sperm extraction (TESE) and ICSI, infertile males with azoospermia now have the possibility of achieving impregnation. Various centers have reported various rates of pregnancy with the use of these 2 techniques in men with azoospermia caused by obstruction of the vas deferens as well as those with nonobstructive azoospermia. In this study, the pregnancy rate per treatment cycle was about 30% for obstructive azoospermia and 11% for nonobstructive azoospermia. More widespread development of expertise in the technique of performing testicular sperm extraction will present a greater opportunity for men with azoospermia to achieve fertility.

D.R. Mishell, Jr., M.D.

Intracytoplasmic Injection of Fresh and Cryopreserved Testicular Spermatozoa in Patients With Nonobstructive Azoospermia—A Comparative Study

Friedler S, Strassburger D, Raziel A, et al (Assaf Harofeh Med Ctr, Zerifin, Israel)

Fertil Steril 68:892–897, 1997 14–19

Objective.—The ability to use cryopreserved testicular tissue for sperm extraction is of benefit to patients with obstructive azoospermia and to those with nonobstructive azoospermia who may have small testicles and who may run the risk of decreased testicular function after repetitive biopsies. Results of intracytoplasmic sperm injection (ICSI) using cryopreserved testicular spermatozoa of patients with nonobstructive azoospermia selected by rigorous criteria, and a comparison of outcome with that of ICSI using fresh testicular sperm are presented.

Methods.—Testicular sperm extraction was performed on 41 patients and was successful in 18. Sperm from 14 patients were cryopreserved.

Results.—Spouses of 6 (33.3%) of the 18 patients became pregnant during the testicular sperm extraction plus ICSI cycle. ICSI was performed using 9 of the 14 cryopreserved testicular sperm samples. All 9 contained testicular sperm. There was no significant difference in outcome between fresh and cryopreserved spermatozoa. Testicular sperm were successfully

TABLE 3.—Outcome of Intracytoplasmic Sperm Injection of Fresh or Cryopreserved-Thawed Testicular Spermatozoa in 18 Patients With Nonobstructive Azoospermia

	Spermatozoa used for ICSI	
	Fresh	Cryopreserved-thawed
No. of patients	18	9
No. of ICSI cycles	25	14
No. of injected oocytes	261	124
Mean no. (±SD) per cycle	8.4 ± 3.7*	8.8 ± 5.5*
No. of fertilized oocytes (%)	122 (47)†	54 (44)†
No. of cleaved embryos (%)	115 (93)†	48 (89)†
No. of embryo transfers	23	11
Mean no. (±SD) of transferred embryos/ET	3.2 ± 1.3*	3.4 ± 1.7*
Embryo quality (%)		
Excellent	24	19
Good	53	57
Fair	21	19
Poor	3	5
Implantation rate (%)	8/91 (9)†	4/37 (11)†
Clinical PR/ET (%)	6/23 (26)†	3/11 (27)†
Delivery or ongoing PR/ET (%)	5/23 (22)‡	1/11 (9)‡

Note: There were no statistically significant differences between fresh and cryopreserved spermatozoa in all variables measured.

* Student's *t*-test.

† χ^2 test

‡ Fisher's exact test.

(From Friedler S, Strassburger D, Raziel A, et al: Intracytoplasmic injection of fresh and cryopreserved testicular spermatozoa in patients with nonobstructive azoospermia—a comparative study. *Fertil Steril* 1997 68:892–879. Reproduced with permission of the publisher, the American Society for Reproductive Medicine.)

retrieved in 25 (52.1%) of 48 procedures and allowed 25 ICSI cycles to be performed. There were no significant differences in parameters measured in these cycles when compared with 14 ICSI cycles performed using cryopreserved sperm (Table 3). The implantation rate and ongoing pregnancy rates were lower for the cryopreserved sperm than for the fresh sperm but not significantly so. The pregnancy rate was 50% (9 of 18). Another 5 patients have cryopreserved testicular sperm cryopreserved for future use. Of the pregnancies achieved using cryopreserved sperm, 1 twin and 1 single pregnancy out of 3 pregnancies ended in a first trimester spontaneous abortion. The delivery or ongoing pregnancy rate was 22% using fresh sperm and 9% using cryopreserved sperm for a cumulative ongoing pregnancy rate of 24%.

Conclusion.—In this carefully selected group of patients with nonobstructive azoospermia, no significant difference was noted in any variables measured or in outcome using fresh versus cryopreserved sperm.

► This is the first set of data in which intracytoplasmic sperm injection (ICSI) was performed with cryopreserved and thawed spermatozoa obtained from testicular biopsy specimens of men with nonobstructive azoospermia. The rate of fertilization of oocytes and resultant embryo quality were similar in the ova injected with fresh and cryopreserved testicular sperm as were the implantation rates and clinical pregnancy rates; however, only 1 of the women whose ova were injected with cryopreserved testicular sperm had an ongoing pregnancy. More data are needed, therefore, to determine whether cryopreserving of testicular sperm will avoid the need of performing repetitive testicular biopsies when a viable birth does not result from the initial ICSI procedure in which sperm obtained from the biopsy specimen are injected into ova.

D.R. Mishell, Jr., M.D.

Successful Testicular Sperm Extraction (TESE) in Spite of High Serum Follicle Stimulating Hormone and Azoospermia: Correlation Between Testicular Morphology, TESE Results, Semen Analysis and Serum Hormone Values in 103 Infertile Men

Jezek D, Knuth UA, Schulze W (Zagreb Med School, Croatia; Gemeinschaftspraxis, Hamburg, Germany; Universitäts-Krankenhaus Eppendorf, Hamburg, Germany)

Hum Reprod 13:1230–1234, 1998 14–20

Objective.—A new testicular spermatozoa extraction (TESE) process has been proposed that involves enzymatic treatment of the testicular tissue with a mild concentration of collagenase, instead of mechanical mincing. The effectiveness of this process in achieving successful sperm retrieval in men with azoospermia or severe oligospermia was assessed.

Methods.—Bilateral tissue specimens were obtained from 108 men with proven azoospermia or oligospermia. Specimens were evaluated histologically and cryopreserved. Tissue from the middle biopsy layer was incubated with 0.8 mg of collagenase, type A1, and 0.2 μg of trypsin inhibitor for 2 hours and centrifuged. The pellet was TESE-tested using a light microscope (×400).

Results.—Complete data are presented for 103 patients, 64 (62.1%) of whom had azoospermia, 29 (28.2%) had severely reduced number of normal spermatozoa, and 10 had mostly nonmotile spermatozoa. Serum follicle-stimulating hormone (FSH) levels were elevated in 62 men, including 58% of azoospermic men and 64% of severely oligospermic men. Biopsy material had pathologic changes in seminiferous tubules and interstitial tissue with scores of 1 to 10. The majority of tubules were classified as "mixed atrophy" with seminiferous tubules showing degeneration alternating with regions of intact spermatogenesis. TESE was successful in 82 men, 64 (78%) of them azoospermic. Although 96.2% of azoospermic men with normal FSH levels had positive TESE results, 62% of azoospermic men with elevated FSH levels also had positive TESE results. The risk of negative TESE results increased when only primary spermatocytes or spermatogonia or Sertoli's cells; tubular sclerosis; or general reduction of tubular diameter and/or increased lamina propria thickness were present. Men with tubules containing mature spermatids with normal diameter and a regular thickness of the lamina propria had the best chance of a positive

TESE result. Because of the differences between right and left testes in half the patients, bilateral testicular biopsy is recommended.

Conclusion.—The new TESE concept is effective for retrieving viable spermatozoa. There is a correlation between histologic analysis and TESE outcome that is useful for diagnosing and predicting the success of treatment of male-factor infertility.

► The management of male infertility has been remarkably enhanced with the use of intracytoplasmic sperm injection. Recently, techniques have been developed to recover spermatozoa directly from testicular tissue when there are no or very few spermatozoa in the ejaculated specimen. The results of this study indicate that the likelihood of retrieval of spermatozoa from testicular tissue of men with azoospermia and normal FSH levels is nearly 100%. Furthermore, even if the FSH levels are markedly elevated, there is at least a 50% likelihood that spermatozoa can be retrieved from the testes and used to perform an intracytoplasmic sperm injection procedure. Thus the presence of a combination of azoospermia and an elevated FSH level is not a contraindication for performing a testicular sperm extraction procedure.

D.R. Mishell, Jr., M.D.

An Improved Treatment Procedure for Testicular Biopsy Specimens Offers More Efficient Sperm Recovery: Case Series

Nagy ZP, Devroey P, Verheryen G, et al (Dutch-speaking Brussels Free Univ, Belgium)

Fertil Steril 68:376–379, 1997 14–21

Objective.—Microinjection of ejaculated, epididymal, and testicular spermatozoa yields about the same fertilization rate, embryo quality, and pregnancy rate. Recovery of sperm cells from testicular biopsy specimens, especially in the presence of nonobstructive azoospermia, was difficult. A report of an improved procedure for testicular biopsy specimens based on the elimination of red blood cells to facilitate recovery of spermatozoa for intracytoplasmic sperm injection (ICSI) is presented.

Methods.—Testicular tissue from 15 men with nonobstructive azoospermia and 5 with obstructive azoospermia was recovered under general anesthesia by making an incision in the scrotal skin and through the peritoneal tunica vaginalis. An incision was made in the tunica albuginea. A piece of extruding testicular tissue was excised and placed in a Petri dish containing HEPES-buffered Earle's medium with 2.25% human serum albumin solution. The tissue was diced and squeezed, and the medium containing the tissue was centrifuged. When few motile spermatozoa were collected after a long search time, the pellet was treated with erythrocyte lysing buffer. Six motile sperm cells were collected, and the ICSI procedure was performed. Another 15 cycles were performed using the erythrocyte lysing buffer because virtually no spermatozoa were seen after shredding. Nonobstructive azoospermia was the reason for ICSI.

Results.—In case series I, no sperm were found in 8 of the 15 cycles even after using erythrocyte lysing buffer and searching for 60 to 120 minutes. At least 1 spermatozoon was found in the other 7 cases. Ten embryos were transferred, and 1 pregnancy resulted. In case series II, 5 cycles were performed. Spermatozoa were collected by the conventional method, and after treatment with erythrocyte lysing buffer, oocytes were injected with conventionally collected sperm (n = 27) and with treated sperm (n = 27). There were 25 and 24 intact oocytes, respectively, after microinjection. Respective fertilization rates (68% and 83%) and embryo development rates (89% and 87%) were similar between the 2 groups. Removal of erythrocytes improved the yield and shortened the collection time of spermatozoa. In the cases of nonobstructive azoospermia, spermatozoa recovery probably would not have been possible without using the erythrocyte lysing buffer.

Conclusion.—Treatment of testicular biopsy specimens with erythrocyte lysing buffer enhanced spermatozoa recovery and decreased recovery time, particularly for patients with nonobstructive azoospermia.

▶ Men with nonobstructive azoospermia were considered to be sterile until the techniques of ICSI and testicular epididymal sperm aspiration were developed in Van Steirteghem's clinic a few years ago. It is difficult to obtain spermatozoa from some men with azospermia and elevated follicle-stimulating hormone levels after a small amount of testicular tissue is excised. The technique of erythrocyte lysing buffer treatment appears to enhance the ability to retrieve sperm from the testicular biopsy specimens of some men with nonobstructive azoospermia.

D.R. Mishell, Jr., M.D.

Birth of Infant After Transfer of Anucleate Donor Oocyte Cytoplasm Into Recipient Eggs

Cohen J, Scott R, Schimmel T, et al (Saint Barnabas Med Ctr, Livingston, NJ; Tel Hashomer Hosp, Tel-Aviv, Israel)

Lancet 350:186–187, 1997 14–22

Introduction.—Transfer of ooplasm from a normal donor egg has been performed in animals and has successfully restored normal developmental potential to eggs with ooplasm deficiencies.

Case Report.—Woman, 39, had 6.5 years of infertility and had not conceived because of inadequate embryo development in 4 attempts at assisted conception and embryo transfer. This occurred in spite of changes in follicular stimulation protocol, in vitro coculture of embryos with helper cells, assisted hatching, and fragment removal. The woman and her husband consented to cytoplasm transfer with ooplasm from donor eggs transferred to the woman's eggs at the same time that conventional egg donation with spare donor eggs was performed.

Technique.—Leuprorelin and gonadotropin stimulation were used for simultaneous ovarian stimulation in the patient and egg donor. Spermatozoa were immobilized individually, and one was sucked into a micropipette before aspiration of the donor ooplasm. The ooplasm filled 500 μm of the micropipette and was removed from the egg pole opposite the polar body to avoid the oocyte metaphase spindle. The aspirated ooplasm and sperm cell were put in the patient's egg close to its metaphase spindle. Fourteen patient eggs were treated with 7 donor eggs. As a control, 6 untreated patient eggs were injected with the husband's sperm. The remainder of the donor eggs were injected with the husband's sperm. The resulting cleaved embryos were frozen. Signs of fertilization or activation were seen in 9 of the patient's 14 treated eggs. Cleavage occurred in 8 of these eggs and 6 of the 8 had more normal morphological characteristics and rate of development than the control embryos and embryos in prior treatment cycles. Fragments from 4 of the treated embryos were removed and transferred transcervically. This resulted in a confirmed singleton pregnancy.

Discussion.—After comparison of nuclear and mitochondrial DNA fingerprinting profiles from aspirated aminocytes and the parents and egg donor, an XX fetus with nuclear characteristics matching those of the parents was confirmed. Although there is little information about the pathophysiology of the human oocyte, this procedure may be valuable in assisted human conception.

▶ Many older infertile women do not wish to become pregnant utilizing fertilized donor eggs because the offspring will have genes from the egg donor, not the recipient. In this unique case report, transfer of the ooplasm but not the nucleus of the egg of a 27-year-old donor into the egg of a 39-year-old woman for whom 4 previous attempts at assisted reproduction had failed, resulted in a viable pregnancy, with an infant whose genetic characteristics matched those of the parents, not the egg donor. Additional studies are needed to confirm the results of this single case report. If the results can be confirmed, another advance in the science of assisted human reproduction will have been achieved.

D.R. Mishell, Jr., M.D.

15 Contraception

Trends in Contraceptive Use In the United States: 1982–1995

Piccinino LJ, Mosher WD (Natl Ctr for Health Statistics, Hyattsville, Md)

Fam Plann Perspect 30:4–10 & 16, 1998 15–1

Objective.—Trends in contraceptive use between 1982 and 1995 were described and subgroup changes identified.

Methods.—Data were taken from the 1982 (N = 7,969), 1988 (N = 8,450), and 1995 (N = 10,847) National Survey of Family Growth and expressed as weighted national estimates.

Contraceptive Use.—The number of 15- to 44-year-old women using contraceptives was 56% in 1982, 60% in 1988, and 64% in 1995. Nonusers in 1995 were sterile because of hysterectomy (5%); were pregnant, postpartum, or trying to become pregnant (9%); never had intercourse (11%); not sexually active in the previous 3 months (6%); or were having unprotected sex (5%).

Overall Trends.—In 1982, 1988, and 1995, 30, 35, and 39 million women, respectively, were using contraceptives (Table 2). Female sterilization increased most among Hispanics. Pill use declined among Hispanic and black women but remained stable among white women. Condom use increased faster among blacks and Hispanics than among whites and was approximately 20% in all 3 groups in 1995. Use of the IUD declined dramatically among Hispanics to 2% in 1995, compared with 1% for whites and blacks. In 1995, 3% of white women aged 20–24 and 45% of white women aged 40–44 used female sterilization, whereas pill use was 57% and 6%, respectively. Women younger than 30 years, women never married, women with 1 year or less of college education, and those who intended to have more children used the pill. Women in their 30s and 40s, formerly married women, those with the least amount of education, and Hispanic and black women preferred female sterilization. Pill use declined most among teenagers (from 59% in 1988 to 44% in 1995) and among women aged 20–24 years (from 68% to 52%).

Condom use increased in all groups but particularly in women in their 20s. Pill use declined most sharply among never married women (from 59% in 1988 to 44% in 1995). Contraceptive use among currently married white women changed little. Female sterilization increased among black women (from 37% to 54% from 1982–1995), whereas pill use declined from 25% to 19%.

TABLE 2.—Percentage Distribution and Number of Contraceptive Users Aged 15–44 Years, by Current Method

Method	1982		1988		1995	
	%	No.	%	No.	%	No.
Sterilization	34.1	10,295	39.2	13,686	38.6	14,942
Female	23.2	6,998	27.5	9,614	27.7	10,727
Male	10.9	3,298	11.7	4,069	10.9	4,215
Pill	28.0	8,431	30.7	10,734	26.9	10,410
Implant	na	na	na	na	1.3	515
Injectable	na	na	na	na	3.0	1,146
IUD	7.1	2,153	2.0	703	0.8	310
Diaphragm	8.1	2,436	5.7	2,000	1.9	720
Male condom	12.0	3,608	14.6	5,093	20.4	7,889
Foam	2.4	711	1.1	371	0.4	161
Per. abstinence	3.9	1,166	2.3	806	2.3	883
Withdrawal	2.0	588	2.2	778	3.0	1,178
Other*	2.5	754	2.1	733	1.3	508
Total	100.0	30,142	100.0	34,912	100.0	38,663
Sample n	na	4,242	na	5,176	na	7,145

*"Other" consists of douche, sponge, jelly or cream alone, and other methods.
Abbreviation: na, not applicable.
(Reproduced with the permission of the Alan Guttmacher Institute from Piccinino LJ, Mosher WD: Trends in contraceptive use in the United States: 1982–1995. *Fam Plann Perspect* 30:4–10 & 16, 1998.)

Diaphragm use declined among never married women from 17% to 1% and male condom use increased from 14% to 30%. Formerly married women preferred sterilization. About half of childless white women using contraceptives used the pill. Diaphragm use among this group declined. Half the white women with 12 years of education used female sterilization in 1995 vs. 16% of those with a college education. For black women, the percentages were 65% and 32%, respectively. Pill use among the least and most educated white women in 1995 was 13% and 33%, respectively. Almost all users of multiple methods used the condom.

Conclusion.—Condom use increased particularly among younger, black, Hispanic, and never married women but not among married couples. Pill and diaphragm use declined. Condom use, implants, and injectables declined among never married black women. Effects on contraception of delayed marriage and childbearing, and racial and ethnic diversity should be studied.

► The data accumulated from the 3 national surveys on family growth conducted in the United States in 1982, 1988, and 1995 provide useful information regarding the methods of contraception used by women in this country. It is encouraging to observe that overall contraceptive use has increased from 56% to 64% in women in the reproductive years 15–44, and that only 5% of sexually active women who did not wish to conceive were not using a method of contraception. However, it is disconcerting to learn that of the contraceptive users, only 70% were using the most effective methods, whereas 30% used methods with high typical failure rates. Because many sexually active women in the United States do not use the most effective methods of contraception, there is a very high incidence of both unintended pregnancies and elective abortions in this country, in contrast to the lower rates in both Canada and Western European countries.

D.R. Mishell, Jr., M.D.

Unintended Pregnancy in the United States
Henshaw SK (Alan Guttmacher Inst, New York)
Fam Plann Perspect 30:24–29 & 46, 1998 15–2

Background.—The United States has a relatively high rate of unintended pregnancy. The 1995 National Survey of Family Growth (NSFG) provides data on births for a cohort of 10,847 American women, aged 15 to 44 years, during the preceding 5 years. These data were used to examine the prevalence of unintended pregnancy over time and its effect on the abortion and birth rates.

Study Design.—Data from the 1995 NSFG and other sources were used to estimate unintended pregnancies for 1994. Unintended pregnancies was defined as the sum of abortions and births reported to be unintended.

Findings.—Excluding miscarriages, there were a total of 5.38 million pregnancies, composed of 3.95 million births and 1.43 million abortions in 1994 in the United States. It was estimated that there were 2.65 million unintended pregnancies, which was 49% of the pregnancies for the year. Of those women who had an unintended pregnancy, 54% had an abortion and 46% carried the pregnancy to term. About half of these women had been using contraception when they became pregnant. The unintended pregnancy rate was highest for teenagers, unmarried women, poor women, and black women. The rates of both unintended births and abortions fell from 1987 to 1994. In 1994, teenagers were the least likely age group to end an unintended pregnancy with abortion. Approximately 48% of all American women aged 15 to 44 years have had an unintended pregnancy.

Conclusion.—In the United States in 1994, approximately half of all pregnancies were unintended. Only about half of these pregnancies were terminated by abortion. Between 1987 and 1994, the rate of unintended pregnancy decreased, presumably because of better contraception. Further reduction in the high rate of unplanned pregnancy can only be achieved by reducing risky behavior and promoting effective contraception use.

▶ This article provides a great amount of information about the extent and consequences of unintended pregnancies among U.S. women in 1994. The information is derived from analysis of data obtained in the 1995 NSFG which were accumulated after interviewing 10,847 civilian women aged 14 to 44 years.

The information in the article is both important and disturbing. About half of the 6 million pregnancies occurring in the United States (3 million) were unintended and about half of these, or 1.4 million, ended in elective abortion. This abortion rate is higher than that found in all other Western European countries, Australia, and Canada. Among the women surveyed who had an unintended pregnancy, more than half (53%) reported that they had used a method of contraception in the month they conceived. Only about 55% of women of reproductive age in the United States use effective methods of contraception.

To reduce the rate of unintended pregnancies, effective methods of contraception need to be more accessible, affordable, and acceptable. Clinicians should strongly encourage sexually active women not wishing to conceive to use effective methods of contraception and to have a package of emergency contraceptive pills readily available.

D.R. Mishell, Jr., M.D.

Blood Pressure in Women Using Oral Contraceptives: Results From the Health Survey For England 1994

Dong W, Colhoun HM, Poutler NR (Univ College London)

J Hypertens 15:1063–1068, 1997 15–3

Background.—Several studies have suggested that blood pressure is increased in women who take oral contraceptives. However, the magnitude of this effect and the influence of specific oral contraceptive preparation are unknown. The effects of taking oral contraceptives on blood pressure were studied.

Methods.—Using data from the Health Survey for England (a cross-sectional survey of a stratified random sample of English adults), the study included a representative sample of 3,545 premenopausal women. Of these, 892 women were currently using oral contraceptives. The women completed a detailed interview regarding their menopausal status, oral contraceptive use, antihypertensive drug use, and other sociodemographic factors. Height, weight, and blood pressure were measured. The effects of oral contraceptive use on systolic and diastolic blood pressure were evaluated, with adjustment for potential confounding factors.

Results.—Mean age-adjusted blood pressure was 125/70 mm Hg for women who used oral contraceptives vs. 123/68 mm Hg for those who did not. The mean difference was 2.3 mm Hg for systolic and 1.6 mm Hg for diastolic blood pressure. Blood pressure was higher for users of oral contraceptives even after adjustment for body mass intake, alcohol use, physical activity, and blood pressure treatment. Oral contraceptives containing progestogen only were not associated with increased blood pressure.

Conclusions.—Women who are current users of oral combined contraceptives have slightly but significantly higher blood pressures than those who do not use oral contraceptives. At the population level, a difference of this magnitude could have a significant impact. Women should have their blood pressure checked before oral contraceptives are prescribed and rechecked regularly during oral contraceptive use.

► The original oral contraceptive formulations which contained much higher doses of both types of steroids than are present in currently used formulations, and were associated with an increase in blood pressure in many individuals. The results of this large cross sectional survey indicates that use of oral contraceptives containing low doses of estrogen are still associated with a slight increase in mean blood pressure. Because some women receiving these types of oral contraceptives develop a moderate increase in blood pressure, it is important to monitor blood pressure before and a few months after patients begin using all types of combination oral contraceptives, as well as annually (at least) while these medications are being used.

D.R. Mishell, Jr., M.D.

Use of Low-dose Oral Contraceptives and Stroke in Young Women

Schwartz SM, Siscovick DS, Longstreth WT Jr., et al (Univ of Washington, Seattle)

Ann Intern Med 127:596–603, 1997 15–4

Introduction.—In the 1970s, research showed that women who used oral contraceptives containing more than 50 µg of ethinyl estradiol had a higher risk for stroke as well as myocardial infarction. Since then, oral contraceptives have contained less than 50 µg of ethinyl estradiol, and data on increased risk of stroke among oral contraceptive users are conflicting. It was not known whether there was a difference in risk of stroke between low-dose oral contraceptives containing the norethindrone-type of progestins or norgestrel-type progestins. One theory is that the levonorgestrel component of oral contraceptives may offset the cardiovascular benefits from low doses of estrogen. Whether use of low-dose oral contraceptives influenced the risk for stroke was investigated in a population-based case-control study.

Methods.—In-person interviews were conducted with 60 women with ischemic stroke, 102 women with hemorrhagic stroke, and 11 women with other types of stroke. They were compared with 485 control subjects. All of the women were between the ages of 18 and 44 years. Interviews concerned the time period that oral contraceptives were used before the first stroke.

Results.—The estimated incidence of hemorrhagic stroke per 100,000 women was 6.4 and for ischemic stroke per 100, 199 women was 4.3. For hemorrhagic stroke, current users of oral contraceptives had an estimated odds ratio of 0.93 compared to women who had never used oral contraceptives. For ischemic stroke, the odds ratio was 0.89. Current users of oral contraceptives had an odds ratio of 1.41 for hemorrhagic stroke compared to past users of oral contraceptives. For ischemic stroke, the odds ratio for current users was 1.37. Past users of oral contraceptives had an odds ratio of 0.59 for hemorrhagic stroke compared to never-users, and an odds ratio of 0.57 for ischemic stroke. There was an elevated odds ratio for hemorrhagic stroke in current users of low-dose oral contraceptives containing norgestrel or levonorgestrel. The odds ratio for aneurysmal bleeding associated with current use of low-dose oral contraceptives containing norgestrel or levonorgestrel was 4.46 among patients with hemorrhagic stroke.

Conclusion.—Among current users of oral contraceptives, the overall risk for stroke and type of stroke was not increased. To clarify the relationship between current use of norgestrel-containing oral contraceptives and hemorrhagic stroke and the relation of risk for stroke to past use of oral contraceptives, further larger studies are needed.

► Studies performed in the 1970s showed that use of high-dose oral contraceptives may have increased the risk of stroke in women. This large case-control study provides additional data to results published from another U.S. population group,[1] which indicate that use of low-dose oral contraceptives does not increase the risk of either an ischemic or hemorrhagic stroke. The incidence of stroke is very low in young women but is increased in women who have hypertension. There are data from some studies indicating that use of oral contraceptives by hypertensive women may further enhance their risk of having a stroke. Although the data from this study did not show an increased risk of stroke among hypertensive women who used oral contraceptives, it is still good practice to not prescribe oral contraceptives to women whose hypertension cannot be controlled with medication.

D.R. Mishell, Jr., M.D.

Reference

1. Petti DB, Sidney S, Bernstein A, et al: Stroke in users of low-dose oral contraceptives. *N Engl J Med* 335:8–15, 1996. (1997 YEAR BOOK OF OBSTETRICS, GYNECOLOGY, AND WOMEN'S HEALTH, p. 375.)

Oral Contraceptives and Ovulatory Causes of Delayed Fertility

Chasan-Taber L, Willett WC, Stampfer MJ, et al (Harvard Med School, Boston; Harvard School of Public Health, Boston)
Am J Epidemiol 146:258–265, 1997 15–5

Background.—Women who discontinue use of oral contraceptives take longer to regain fertility than women who use other methods of contraception. It is unclear if this is related to the length of time a woman uses oral contraceptives or her age at first use. This article investigates the association between length of use of oral contraceptives, age at first use, and impaired fertility because of ovulatory disorder.

Methods.—A nested, case-control study was conducted within the Nurses' Health Study II, which began in 1989 and included more than 116,000 female registered nurses living in 14 states in the United States. Baseline information on medical history, use of oral contraceptives, parity, and menstrual patterns during adolescence was obtained through a questionnaire in 1989. Follow-up information was obtained in 1991 and 1993.

In the current study, the study group consisted of 1,917 married nurses without previous pregnancy who were unable to become pregnant for at least 1 year and in whom primary ovulatory infertility was later diagnosed. The control group consisted of 44,521 married parous nurses with no history of infertility and no pregnancies lasting less than 6 months.

Results.—On the baseline questionnaire in 1989, 18.3% of respondents reported that they had tried to become pregnant for more than 1 year without success. A greater percentage of study subjects than control subjects had used oral contraceptives before the outcome event. The mean duration of oral contraceptive use was 3.3 years for study subjects and 3.25 years for control subjects. The mean age at first use of oral contraceptives was 20 years for study subjects and 20.2 years for control subjects.

Discussion.—After allowing for 2 years of suppressed fertility after discontinuing use of oral contraceptives, and excluding women with menstrual or hormonal disorders, a small, nonsignificant increased risk of ovulatory causes of delayed fertility for women who had ever used oral contraceptives was observed. The multivariate relative risk of a woman having an ovulatory cause of delayed fertility was 1.2 for women who had ever used oral contraceptives. No significant trend of higher risk was found with longer use of oral contraceptives or younger age at first use. That 88% of study subjects reported a pregnancy by 1993 indicates no impairment of absolute fertility.

► The data from this large cohort study indicate, after correction for several possible confounding factors, that use of oral contraceptives does not result in a significantly increased risk of anovulation as a cause of infertility. Furthermore, the risk of ovulatory causes of infertility is not related to increased duration of oral contraceptive use or younger age at first use. It is of interest that nearly 90% of the women with ovulatory causes of infertility in this study eventually conceived with therapy.

D.R. Mishell, Jr., M.D.

Ovarian Function During the Use of a Single Contraceptive Implant: Implanon Compared With Norplant

Mäkäräinen L, van Beek A, Tuomivaara L, et al (Univ of Oulu, Finland; NV Organon, Oss, The Netherlands; Växjö Hosp, Sweden)

Fertil Steril 69:714–721, 1998 15–6

Background.—Norplant (levonogestrel) is a 6-capsule commercially available contraceptive implant. Implanon is a single–rod contraceptive implant containing etonogestrel (3–ketodesogestrel). The efficacy of Implanon was compared to Norplant in a group of healthy, fertile women.

Methods.—The study group consisted of 32 women, aged 18–40, from 1 Swedish and 1 Finnish clinic, who were randomized to receive either Implanon or Norplant. This prospective study was conducted for 2 years

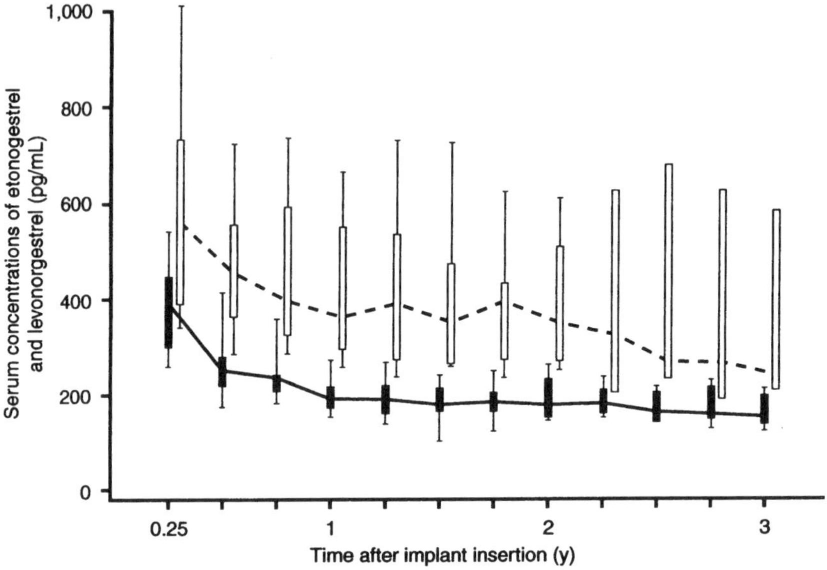

FIGURE 2.—Serum concentrations of etonogestrel (-) and levonorgestrel (□) from 3 months after implant insertion. Boxes represent the P25 to P75 range; T bars represent the minimum and maximum concentrations. Mean values are corrected. (Courtesy of Mäkäräinen L, van Beek A, Tuomivaara L, et al: Ovarian function during the use of a single contraceptive implant: Implanon compared with norplant. *Fertil Steril* 69:714–721, 1998. Reprinted by permission from the American Society for Reproductive Medicine.)

in Sweden and 3 years in Finland. Participants were assessed during the first 4 weeks and then after 6, 12, 18, 24, 30, 33, and 36 months. They were reevaluated just before implant removal and 6 weeks after implant removal. Ovulation, follicular development, endometrial thickness, and serum concentrations of 17β-estradiol and progesterone were assayed. Time to removal and complications were noted.

Results.—An increase in serum etonogestrel was detected within 8 hours of implantation of Implanon. After removal, serum concentrations dropped below the limit of detection (Fig 2). There were no pregnancies with either contraceptive device throughout the study period. Ovulation occurred after 18 months on Norplant and after 30 months on Implanon. Follicular cysts occurred in both groups, but were more common with Norplant. Estradiol concentrations increased during implant use. Amenorrhea did not occur in the Norplant group, but amenorrhea and infrequent bleeding was common in the Implanon group. Contraceptive use was stopped due to bleeding pattern in 37.5% of the Implanon group and 12.5% of the Norplant group. The average endometrial thickness was less than 4 mm from month 12 to removal with Implanon. The average time necessary for removal of Implanon was approximately 6 minutes, while the average time necessary for removal of Norplant was approximately 18 minutes. Ovulation resumed rapidly after the removal of either type of implant.

Conclusions.—The subdermal contraceptive implant, Implanon, was compared to Norplant in a prospective clinical study involving 32 healthy Finnish and Swedish women. The results of this study indicate that Implanon is effective within 8 hours after implantation and successfully inhibits ovulation for 3 years. Implanon, a single rod, can be inserted and removed much faster and easier than Norplant, which consists of 6 capsules.

▶ Subdermal implants of capsules or rods containing contraceptive progestins are an effective long-lasting method of contraception. As with other contraceptive steroid agents containing a progestin without estrogen, their major problem is unpredictable and irregular uterine bleeding. The first subdermal implant, Norplant, requires insertion of 6 capsules to achieve sufficiently high circulating levels of levonorgestrel to prevent pregnancy. A more recently developed implant containing 2 rods of polysiloxane releasing levonorgestrel produces similar circulating levels of levonorgestrel as Norplant, and is also effective for 5 years. Both techniques require a small skin incision before insertion. A single implant that releases the progestin etonogestrel, as shown in this study, is effective for 3 years and does not require an incision before insertion. Removal of a single implant is quicker and easier than removal of 2 rods or 6 capsules. Ongoing studies with this contraceptive method are promising and, hopefully, it will be marketed in the near future.

D.R. Mishell, Jr., M.D.

Introductory Study of the Once-a-Month, Injectable Contraceptive Cyclofem in Brazil, Chile, Colombia, and Peru

Hall P, Bahamondes L, Diaz J, et al (World Health Organization, Geneva; Universidade Estadul de Campinas, Brazil)

Contraception 56:353–359, 1997 15–7

Background.—A World Health Organization introductory trial of the injectable, once-a-month contraceptive, Cyclofem, was conducted in Brazil, Chile, Colombia, and Peru to obtain data for registration in these 4 countries. The results of this trial were reported.

Methods.—The study group consisted of 3,183 healthy women, 18 to 40 years of age, with at least 1 previous pregnancy. The first injection was provided up to the fifth day of the menstrual cycle and subsequent injections were provided every 30 ± 3 days.

Results.—During the first year of the trial, 21,912 woman-months accrued. There were no pregnancies. The discontinuation rate for amenorrhea varied from 3.4 in Brazil to 8.1/100 in Colombia. The continuation rate varied from 42.3 in Columbia to 52.0 in Chile (Table 4). Continuing to the second year of the trial, a total of 29,676 woman-months accrued. No pregnancies occurred. The discontinuation rates were lower than in the first year, except for personal reasons, which had the same rate both years (Table 5).

TABLE 4.—Cumulative Gross Rates by Reasons for Discontinuation and Continuation up to 1 Year of Use of Cyclofem in 4 Countries

Reasons	Brazil	Chile	Colombia	Peru
Pregnancy	0.0	0.0	0.0	0.0
Amenorrhea	3.4	6.7	8.1	6.4
Menstrual disturbances	9.2	5.1	7.7	8.9
Other medical	7.8	19.7	26.3	20.5
Desire for pregnancy	5.5	8.5	7.6	3.9
Other personal	23.5	17.2	20.9	21.4
Other causes	13.2	3.5	7.3	1.0
All reasons	49.2	48.0	57.7	49.3
Lost to follow-up	4.7	10.2	2.3	24.3
Continuation rate	50.8	52.0	42.3	50.7
Woman-years	186	747	367	526
Women at beginning	369	1,114	600	1,100

(Reprinted by permission of the publisher from Hall P, Bahamondes L, Diaz J, et al: Introductory study of the once-a-month, injectable contraceptive Cyclofem in Brazil, Chile, Colombia, and Peru. *Contraception* 56:353–359, copyright 1997 by Elsevier Science Inc.)

Conclusion.—This large, multicenter, international study demonstrated that the injectable, once-a-month contraceptive, Cyclofem, is safe and effective. The data collected during this trial were submitted to national regulatory authorities, and registration was obtained in all 4 participating countries. Cyclofem can improve the quality of care by providing women with another contraceptive option.

TABLE 5.—Cumulative Gross Rates by Reasons for Discontinuation and Continuation up to 2 Years of Use of Cyclofem in 4 Countries

Reasons	Brazil	Chile	Colombia	Peru
Pregnancy	0.0	0.0	0.0	0.0
Amenorrhea	5.3	9.0	10.9	13.2
Menstrual disturbances	12.8	7.3	9.4	12.1
Other medical	9.4	29.2	36.0	29.7
Desire for pregnancy	10.3	12.5	18.3	9.9
Other personal	51.3	26.7	35.4	34.8
Other causes	39.8	4.0	10.7	3.1
All reasons	80.6	63.2	75.7	69.5
Lost to follow-up	7.3	16.0	3.5	33.8
Continuation rate	19.4	36.8	24.3	30.5
Women-years	230	1,066	527	650
Women at beginning	92	498	248	253

(Reprinted by permission of the publisher from Hall P, Bahamondes L, Diaz J, et al: Introductory study of the once-a-month, injectable contraceptive Cyclofem in Brazil, Chile, Colombia, and Peru. *Contraception* 56:353–359, copyright 1997 by Elsevier Science Inc.)

▶ In the United States, women have the choice of 4 effective, reversible methods of contraception: oral contraceptives, the intrauterine device, the long-acting progestin implant, and injectable progestin. In addition, they have the option of undergoing tubal sterilization or their partner can have a vasectomy. Only about 55% of reproductive age women currently use one of these effective methods of contraception. About half the 6 million pregnancies that occur annually in the United States are unwanted, and half of these occur among women using some type of contraception. It would be useful for women in the United States and elsewhere to have an additional effective method of contraception.

The once-a-month injectable combination of the natural estrogen, estradiol, and the nonandrogenic progestin, medroxyprogesterone acetate, is extremely effective. The pregnancy rate in this 2-year, 4-country study was zero. Bleeding patterns are very acceptable and the method is rapidly reversible. This method of contraception will soon become available for use in the United States as a multicenter, phase III clinical trial is nearing completion. It will be beneficial for women in the United States to have an additional effective, reversible method of contraception to use if they wish to do so.

D.R. Mishell, Jr., M.D.

Long-term Reversible Contraception: Twelve Years of Experience With the TCu380A and TCu220C

Rowe PJ, for United Nations Development Programme/United Nations Population Fund/World Health Organization/World Bank, Special Programme of Research, Development, and Research Training in Human Reproduction (World Health Organization, Geneva)

Contraception 56:341–352, 1997 15–8

Background.—Nonhormonal fertility regulation methods that are effective for more than a few years and do not require repeated clinic attendance would be useful for many women. This report summarizes the safety and efficacy data from 2 long-term, international, multicentered (24 centers), randomized clinical trials of the intrauterine devices, TCu220C and TCu380A.

Methods.—The study group consisted of 3,277 women recruited for the TCu220C device and 1,396 women recruited for the TCu380A device between 1981 and 1986. Excluded were nulliparous women; those with a history of pelvic inflammatory disease since their last pregnancy; those with less than 6 weeks since parturition or abortion; women with a history of ectopic pregnancy; and those with recent sexually transmitted disease, undiagnosed genital tract bleeding, congenital genital tract malformation, genital tract malignancy, uterine fibromyomas associated with menstrual disorders, anemia, or a history of hydatiform mole. The volunteers returned for follow-up at 3, 6, and 12 months and then yearly until the devices had been used for 12 years.

TABLE 4.—Cumulative Net Probabilities of Discontinuation, Standard Error per 100 Women, and Significance of Differences Between Devices

	TCu380A		Study 1 TCu220C			Study 2 TCu220C		Studies 1 & 2* TCu220C	
	Rate	SE	Rate	SE	P	Rate	SE	Rate	SE
Total pregnancies	2.2	(0.6)	5.8	(0.9)	0.001	8.9	(0.9)	7.6	(0.7)
Intrauterine	1.9	(0.5)	5.6	(0.9)	<0.001	7.9	(0.9)	7.0	(0.6)
Ectopic	0.4	(0.3)	0.2	(0.2)	0.69	1.1	(0.4)	0.7	(0.3)
Expulsions	12.5	(1.4)	12.8	(1.3)	0.87	11.1	(1.1)	11.8	(0.8)
Perforations	0.0	(0.0)	0.2	(0.2)	0.18	0.1	(0.1)	0.1	(0.1)
Total medical removals	40.2	(2.1)	39.0	(2.2)	0.69	36.8	(1.7)	37.3	(1.3)
Total pain or bleeding	35.5	(2.1)	34.3	(2.2)	0.67	30.2	(1.7)	31.6	(1.3)
Pain	13.0	(1.3)	11.3	(1.4)	0.37	10.5	(1.2)	10.7	(0.9)
Bleeding	22.0	(2.0)	22.6	(2.1)	0.85	17.2	(1.5)	19.1	(1.2)
Pain and bleeding	4.9	(1.0)	4.3	(1.0)	0.66	5.9	(0.8)	5.3	(0.7)
Pelvic inflammatory disease	1.1	(0.5)	0.9	(0.4)	0.70	0.3	(0.2)	0.6	(0.2)
Other medical removals	6.1	(1.1)	6.3	(1.2)	0.91	9.1	(1.2)	7.9	(0.9)
Total use-related discontinuations	48.8	(2.0)	50.0	(2.0)	0.67	48.8	(1.6)	49.0	(1.2)
Total nonmedical removals	53.9	(2.0)	54.0	(2.0)	0.99	43.6	(1.6)	47.8	(1.3)
Wish to become pregnant	27.0	(1.7)	24.3	(1.7)	0.26	22.4	(1.3)	23.2	(1.0)
No further need	24.4	(2.1)	29.1	(2.3)	0.14	18.2	(1.6)	22.5	(1.3)
Other nonmedical removals	16.5	(1.9)	14.3	(1.8)	0.38	11.0	(1.2)	12.3	(1.0)
Loss to follow-up	38.4	(2.3)	38.8	(2.2)	0.91	33.2	(1.7)	35.4	(1.4)
Other discontinuations (devices not removed)	15.2	(1.8)	15.2	(1.7)	0.99	2.5	(0.5)	7.9	(0.8)
Continuation rate	12.3	(0.9)	12.0	(0.9)	0.77	18.8	(0.9)	15.9	(0.7)
Number of insertions	1,396		1,396			1,881		3,277	
Number of women completing the interval	172		167			174		341	
Woman-years experience	7,159		7,018			10,080		17,098	

Note: Data are for 12 years (4,380 days).

(Reprinted by permission of the publisher from Rowe PJ, for United Nations Development Programme/United Nations Population Fund/World Health Organization/World Bank, Special Programme of Research, Development, and Research Training in Human Reproduction: Long-term reversible contraception: Twelve years of experience with the TCu380A and TCu220C. *Contraception* 56:341–352, copyright 1997 by Elsevier Science Inc.)

Results.—There were 3 insertion failures in the TCu220C group and no insertion failures in the TCu380A group. The TCu380A had a significantly lower pregnancy rate than the TCu220C group. Between the eighth and twelfth years of use, there were 7 pregnancies in the TCu220C group, and none in the TCu380A group. There were 14 TCu220C expulsions and 5 TCu380A expulsions (Table 4). Most of the removals for medical reasons were for pain and bleeding. The annual removal rates were about 3% for each device, but the TCu380A had a consistently higher removal rate. The 12-year combined study removal rate for the TCu220C was 0.6/100 women. There were 8 histologically confirmed ectopic pregnancies with the TCu220C and 2 with the TCu380A.

Conclusion.—The results of the largest international multicenter, long-term clinical trial of 2 IUDs, the TCu380A and the TCu220C, confirm that these devices are safe and effective for at least 12 years of use. The TCu380A is significantly more effective than the TCu220C and is a potentially reversible, nonsurgical alternative to sterilization or depot hormonal methods for long-term female contraception.

► The copper TCu380A intrauterine device is an extremely effective reversible form of contraception. The data in this large, long-term multicenter study of nearly 1,400 parous women inserted with this contraceptive device indicate that it has a similar effectiveness as tubal sterilization, with a failure rate after 12 years of only 2.2%. No pregnancies occurred after the eighth year of use. Only 2 ectopic pregnancies occurred with use of this intrauterine device, both in the first few years after insertion, and there were only 5 removals for pelvic inflammatory disease.

The intrauterine device is the most widely used method of contraception worldwide because of its high prevalence of use in China. However, less than 1 million women in the United States use this effective method of contraception because of a lack of understanding about its long-term safety. The results of this study should reduce concerns about problems associated with this excellent form of long-acting contraception.

D.R. Mishell, Jr., M.D.

Randomised Controlled Trial of Prophylactic Antibiotics Before Insertion of Intrauterine Devices

Walsh T, for the IUD Study Group (California Family Health Council, Los Angeles; Univ of California, San Francisco; Harbor-Univ of California, Los Angeles Med Ctr, Torrance; et al)

Lancet 351:1005–1008, 1998 15–9

Introduction.—Many countries have limited the use of intrauterine devices because of concern about infection of the upper genital tract. However, the risk of infection lasts only a few weeks after insertion. The bacteria are usually introduced during the insertion process, and it is unknown whether the antibiotic prophylaxis before intrauterine device

TABLE 2.—Status of Intrauterine Devices 90 Days After Insertion

Outcome	Placebo Group (n=915)	Antibiotic Group (n=918)
Removed		
Heavy bleeding	10	11
Cramping/abdominal pain	6	8
Adnexal or uterine pain*	5	1
Personal reason	1	3
Infection of lower genital tract	1	2
Perforation	1	1
Salpingitis	0	1
Pregnancy	0	1
Other medical reason	7	7
All removals	31 (3·4%)	35 (3·8%)
Expelled		
Partly	27	30
Fully	4	2
All expulsions	31 (3·4%)	32 (3·5%)
Retained	853 (93·2%)	851 (92·7%)

*Did not meet diagnostic criteria for salpingitis.

(Courtesy of Walsh T, for the IUD Study Group: Randomized controlled trial of prophylactic antibiotics before insertion of intrauterine devices. *Lancet* 351:1005–1008, copyright 1998 by The Lancet Ltd.)

insertion would reduce upper genital tract infection. The effect of prophylaxis in a population of intrauterine device users was examined.

Methods.—There were 1,985 women who requested intrauterine device insertion and were at low risk of sexually transmitted infection, according to self-reported medical history. They were randomly assigned to receive placebo capsules or 500 mg azithromycin, taken about 1 hour before insertion of a Copper T 380A intrauterine device. An intrauterine device was not inserted in 118 women. For at least 90 days after insertion, the remaining 18,933 women were studied. The rate of removal of the intrauterine device, within the 90 days after insertion, for reasons other than partial expulsion was used as an indicator of acute or subacute pelvic infection.

Results.—In the antibiotic group, the rate of intrauterine device removal for any reason other than partial expulsion was 3.8% (38 of 918), and in the placebo group, it was 3.4% (31 of 915) (Table 2). The 2 treatment groups sought medical attention with equal frequency, with a mean of 38 visits per 100 women. Only 1 woman from each group had salpingitis, as defined by established criteria, during the 90 days after intrauterine device insertion.

Conclusion.—The likelihood that a woman would retain her intrauterine device at 90 days and the frequency of postinsertion medical attention were not affected by prophylaxis with azithromycin. With or without the administration of prophylactic antibiotics, the risk of upper-genital-tract infection after intrauterine device insertion, in appropriately screened women, is negligible.

► Worldwide, the intrauterine device (IUD) is the most commonly used method of contraception, mainly because of its frequent use in China. In several European countries, about one fourth of women using contraception elect to use the IUD. Nevertheless, in the United States the IUD is used by less than 1% of women of reproductive age. One of the major reasons for the infrequent use of this extremely effective and completely reversible method of contraception is the fear of both providers and consumers that the IUD increases the risk of pelvic infection. Although the shield IUD, with its multifilament tail string, did facilitate the ascent of bacteria from the vagina to the upper genital tract, all IUDs in current use have a monofilament tail string that does not permit bacteria to ascend to the upper genital tract. Thus, the only way that the IUD can cause salpingitis is by transporting pathogens to the upper genital tract at the time of insertion. If pathogens are not present in the endocervical canal, the other organisms that are transported to the endometrial cavity at the time of IUD insertion are nearly always eliminated by the body's host defense. The results of this study indicate that in a large number of women who had no clinical or bacteriologic evidence of pathogenic organisms in the cervix, the risk of developing salpingitis within 3 months of IUD insertion was extremely low, about 1 per 1,000 insertions. With this low incidence of infection, prophylactic use of antibiotics just prior to insertion of the IUD was not found to be beneficial or cost-effective.

D.R. Mishell, Jr., M.D.

New Estimates of the Effectiveness of the Yuzpe Regimen of Emergency Contraception

Trussell J, Rodríguez G, Ellertson C (Princeton Univ, NJ; The Population Council, New York)

Contraception 57:363–369, 1998 15–10

Background.—The Yuzpe method of emergency contraception consists of 2 doses of combined estrogen and progestin pills, each dose containing 100 μg of ethinyl estradiol and 1 mg of norgestrel. The first dose is taken within 72 hours after intercourse, and the second is taken 12 hours later. New estimates of the efficacy of this regimen are presented.

Methods.—Seven studies identified in a review of the literature were analyzed. All included treatment outcomes by cycle day of unprotected intercourse relative to expected day of ovulation. The probabilities of conception by cycle day of intercourse among women not using contraception and the associated variance-covariance matrix from 5 other data sets were also estimated. These estimates were used to evaluate treatment efficacy.

Findings.—On the basis of analyses of the 7 studies separately and combined, as well as 5 sets of conception probabilities by cycle day, the 40 estimates of efficacy ranged from 44.2% to 88.7%. According to preferred point estimation, emergency contraceptive pills decreased the risk of pregnancy by 75.4%, with a 95% confidence interval of 65.6% to 82.4%. The true efficacy is likely to be greater than 75%, as the treatment failures included women who were already pregnant when treated and women who became pregnant after treatment.

Conclusions.—The efficacy of the Yuzpe regimen of emergency contraception is at least 75%. These new estimates indicate that this regimen is as effective as previously reported, or more so.

▶ The results of this analysis indicate that when emergency contraceptive pills (ECPs) are used correctly after a single incident of unprotected intercourse, about 3 of 4 pregnancies that would have occurred will be prevented. However, because in the great majority of cycles in which ECPs are used, pregnancy would not normally occur; the actual pregnancy rate in 7 studies of ECP varied between 1% and 2%. Greater use of ECPs should markedly reduce the number of unwanted pregnancies in the United States.

D.R. Mishell, Jr., M.D.

The Effects of Self-administrating Emergency Contraception

Glasier A, Baird D (Edinburgh Healthcare Natl Health Service Trust Family Planning and Well Woman Services, Scotland; Univ of Edinburgh, Scotland)

N Engl J Med 339:1–4, 1998 15–11

Background.—Postcoital contraception could prevent 1.7 million unintended pregnancies each year in the United States. Currently, such contraception requires a doctor's prescription, although it must be taken within 72 hours of intercourse. This study examined the effect of readily available emergency contraceptives on the behavior of healthy, sexually active women.

Methods.—The study group consisted of 1,083 women, aged 16–44, who were recruited following consultation for emergency contraception or therapeutic abortion from 1994 through 1996. Of these women, 553 were assigned a replaceable supply of emergency contraceptive pills (treatment group) and 530 women were assigned to require a doctor's prescription (control group). The incidence of unwanted pregnancy, the use of other contraceptives, and the use of emergency contraceptives were assessed.

Results.—Follow-up information was available for 69% of the treatment group and 62% of the control group. Emergency contraception was employed at least once by 47% of the women in the treatment group and 27% of those in the control group. Emergency contraception was used correctly 98% of the time, and there were no adverse effects. The women in the treatment group were not more likely to use emergency contraception repeatedly and continued to use other methods of contraception. There were 18 unintended pregnancies in the treatment group and 25 in the control group.

Conclusions.—The results of this large study on the effects of making emergency contraception readily available to sexually active women indicated that emergency contraception is used correctly, does no harm, and may reduce the risk of unwanted pregnancy.

▶ The use of 2 doses of 2 tablets of levonorgestrel containing oral contraceptives taken 12 hours apart within 72 hours of unprotected intercourse has been estimated to prevent about 75% of the pregnancies that would occur without their use. The resulting pregnancy rate with this method of emergency contraception is 3%, because most episodes of midcycle coitus do not result in pregnancy. Although the subjects in this study were highly selected, either having previously used emergency contraception or having an elective abortion, the results indicate that women would be more likely to use this method of pregnancy prevention if the pills are readily available than if they need to visit a clinic to obtain the medication. Clinicians should offer to prescribe emergency contraception when young women have their routine health maintenance visit. If the necessity for use occurs, women would not have to undergo the difficulties of obtaining a prescription for emergency contraception at an inconvenient time.

D.R. Mishell, Jr., M.D.

16 Abortion

Exposure to Video Display Terminals and Risk of Spontaneous Abortion
Grasso P, Parazzini F, Chatenoud L, et al (Istituto di Ricerche Farmacologiche "Mario Negri," Milan, Italy; Università di Milano, Italy)
Am J Ind Med 32:403–407, 1997 16–1

Background.—Some research has shown that exposure to low-frequency electromagnetic fields results in reproductive failure. The association between video display terminal (VDT) exposure and risk of miscarriage was further explored in a case-control study.

Methods.—Five hundred eight women hospitalized for spontaneous abortion composed the case group. The control group consisted of 1,148 women delivering healthy infants at term at the same hospitals.

Findings.—Spontaneous abortion was associated with previous spontaneous abortion, with an odds ratio (OR) of 1.9, and with the consumption of alcohol, coffee, and tobacco, with ORs of 1.6, 1.8, and 1.6, respectively. However, spontaneous abortion was not associated with VDT exposure, even at greater lengths of exposure. The multivariate OR of spontaneous abortion for VDT exposure during word processing, which was the main work done with the VDT, was 1.3, of borderline significance (Table 2).

TABLE 2.—Distribution of Cases and Controls According to VDT Exposure, Milan, Italy, 1992–95

	Spontaneous abortions No. (%)	Controls No. (%)	OR (95% CI) MH*	MLV**
Use of VDT				
Never	332 (65.4)	740 (64.5)	1+	1+
Ever	176 (34.6)	408 (35.5)	1.0 (0.8–1.2)	1.1 (0.8–1.4)
How often do you use it (hours/week)?				
< 11	51 (34.4)	115 (32.8)	1.0 (0.7–1.4)	1.0 (0.7–1.5)
11–20	29 (19.6)	81 (23.1)	0.9 (0.5–1.4)	1.0 (0.6–1.6)
≥ 20	68 (46.0)	155 (44.1)	1.0 (0.7–1.4)	1.1 (0.8–1.6)
Main use of VDT				
Word Processing	137 (81.1)	269 (69.5)	1.2 (0.9–1.5)	1.3 (1.0–1.7)
Others	32 (18.9)	118 (30.5)	0.6 (0.4–1.0)	0.7 (0.4–1.1)

Conclusions.—Video display terminal exposure did not increase the risk of spontaneous abortion in this study. Strengths of the current methodology include an adequate sample size and a small number of missing data.

▶ The use of VDTs in the workplace is becoming common. Therefore, a large number of women in early pregnancy are being exposed to low-frequency electromagnetic fields. Although a few studies in the late 1970s suggested that users of VDTs may have an increased rate of spontaneous abortion, the results of this case-control study and several other epidemiologic studies performed between 1989 and 1992 found no significant association between VDT exposure and the risk of miscarriage. Clinicians can inform women about these conclusions to alleviate their possible concerns. It is of interest that this study confirmed findings of other studies, which have shown that alcohol and tobacco consumption is associated with significantly increased risk of miscarriage. In this study, use of either agent increased the risk of spontaneous abortion by 60%. It was also found that coffee consumption increased the risk of spontaneous abortion. Both caffeine and tobacco have been shown to increase the risk of infertility. Thus, these agents should not be used by women trying to conceive or after conception has occurred.

D.R. Mishell, Jr., M.D.

Factor V Leiden Mutation as a Risk Factor for Recurrent Pregnancy Loss

Ridker PM, Miletich JP, Buring JE, et al (Harvard Med School, Boston; Washington Univ Med Ctr, St Louis)

Ann Intern Med 128:1000–1003, 1998 16–2

Background.—Although the cause of recurrent pregnancy loss is often not understood, hypercoagulability has been proposed as a contributing factor. The factor V Leiden mutation is the most common inherited predisposition to thrombosis. A case–control study examined whether hypercoagulability from the factor V Leiden mutation is associated with an increased risk for spontaneous abortion.

Study Design.—The study group consisted of 113 consecutive Caucasian women referred to the Recurrent Miscarriage Clinic at Brigham and Women's Hospital from July 1995 to June 1996 with a history of at least 3 spontaneous abortions and no chromosomal abnormality. Controls were 437 Caucasian women who participated in the Women's Health Study and had a history of successful pregnancy without pregnancy loss. None of the study participants had a history of venous thromboembolism. All women were tested for the factor V Leiden mutation. Mutation status was also determined for 387 Caucasian participants in the Women's Health Study who reported at least 1 pregnancy loss.

Findings.—The prevalence of factor V Leiden mutation was significantly higher among cases than among controls. In the sub–group of cases with at least 3 pregnancy losses and no successful pregnancies, the prevalence of this mutation was 9%. Among the women in the Women's Health Study with at least 3 pregnancy losses, the prevalence of this mutation was similar to that of the case-patients.

Conclusions.—The results of this study are compatible with the idea that hypercoagulability from factor V Leiden mutation, the most common inherited predisposition to thrombosis, plays a role in some cases of recurrent pregnancy loss. Large scale studies are needed to confirm these observations.

▶ This study confirms the finding of several other recent reports that women with a history of recurrent abortion without a demonstrated etiology show a significantly increased incidence of activated protein C resistance compared with a control population. It remains to be determined whether treatment of these women with heparin and aspirin will increase the likelihood of a viable birth, as apparently occurs among women with recurrent miscarriage and the presence of lupus anticoagulant or anticardiolipin antibodies.

D.R. Mishell, Jr., M.D.

Are Serum Progesterone Levels Predictive of Recurrent Miscarriage in Future Pregnancies?

Ogasawara M, Aoyama T, Kajiura S, et al (Nagoya City Univ, Japan)

Fertil Steril 68:806–809, 1997 16–3

Background.—Various investigators have reported a possible luteal phase defect (LPD) in women who have recurrent miscarriage and infertility. This concept has been questioned by other investigators because there is no accurate means of diagnosing LPD; diagnosis is made by a single determination of the midluteal phase serum progesterone (P) level. In normal pregnancies, studies have reported significantly higher single serum P levels than in pregnancies that result in spontaneous abortion, though such levels were measured early in the pregnancies. Studies have also reported lowered luteal P/E_2 ratios after ovulation induction at the time of implantation in cycles that result in abortion.

Methods.—Prepregnancy hormones and the degree of association with abortion were investigated in 197 untreated women who had 2 consecutive unexplained abortions in the first trimester. All women conceived naturally within 12 months of the day of P evaluation. Assays were conducted for P, E_2, and prolactin in blood samples obtained at least 3 months after the second abortion and before the next conception. In at least 2 cycles, blood samples were collected 5–9 days after ovulation. The criterion for LPD was a midluteal phase single serum P level of less than 10 ng/mL.

Results.—Of the 197 subjects, 46 had an LPD. Also of the 197 subjects, 38 had another abortion; 20.5% were LPD-negative; and 15.2% were LPD-positive. This difference was not significant. In women who had another successful pregnancy, the mean value of E_2 was 129 pg/mL and the mean value of the P/E_2 ratio was 121. In women who had another abortion, the mean value of E_2 was 137 pg/mL and the mean value of the P/E_2 ratio was 128. These differences between groups were not significant. When excluding miscarriages caused by these abnormal chromosomes, 16.1% of women who were LPD-negative had a miscarriage and 11.4% of women who were LPD-positive had a miscarriage.

Discussion.—These results indicate that in women who have recurrent miscarriage, preconceptional P and P/E_2 ratio do not predict miscarriage in a later pregnancy, in spite of reports of such an association on a case-by-case basis in the literature. Preconceptional diagnosis of an LPD appears to have little value for women who have recurrent miscarriage.

▶ It is generally believed that LPD is a cause of recurrent abortion as well as infertility. Various criteria have been utilized for the diagnosis of LPD and none are universally accepted. There are data indicating that LPD is a fairly common sporadic event in normal fertile women. Luteal phase defect needs to be shown in at least 2 cycles to establish the diagnosis, whether the diagnosis is determined by low midluteal serum P levels or by retarded endometrial histology.

Data indicating that LPD is a cause of recurrent abortion are limited to a few case series. The results of this study in which women with an unexplained cause of recurrent abortion had LPD diagnosed on the basis of a single serum P suggest that LPD is not a cause of recurrent abortion. More studies utilizing stricter criteria for the diagnosis of LPD need to be done to determine whether this entity is really a cause of recurrent abortion. If LPD is found to cause abortion, then randomized clinical trials need to be performed to determine whether P supplementation will increase the rate of viable births.

D.R. Mishell, Jr., M.D.

Low-dose Aspirin in Prevention of Miscarriage in Women With Unexplained or Autoimmune-related Recurrent Miscarriage: Effect on Prostacyclin and Thromboxane A2 Production

Tulppala M, Marttunen M, Söderström-Anttila V, et al (Univ Central Hosp of Helsinki; The Family Federation of Finland, Helsinki; Natl Public Heath Inst, Helsinki)

Hum Reprod 12:1567–1572, 1997 16–4

Background.—Although the cause of recurrent spontaneous abortion (RSA) is unknown in most cases, the histories of these women indicate a deficiency in prostacyclin (PGI_2), detectable levels of anticardiolipin antibodies (ACA), and/or an overproduction of thromboxane A_2 (TXA_2). Data are available indicating that low-dose aspirin (LDA) may improve pregnancy outcome in RSA women. In this article, results of a randomized, placebo-controlled study on the effect of LDA on PGI_2 and TXA_2 produc-

TABLE 1.—Outcome of Pregnancy in Women Using Low-dose Aspirin (LDA, n = 33) or Placebo (PLA, n = 33)

	LDA (*n* = 33)	PLA (*n* = 33)
Miscarriage	9/33 (27.3)	7/33 (21.2)
gestation at miscarriage (weeks)	10.9 (8.0–16.0)	11.6 (8.0–19.0)
Ectopic pregnancy	1/33 (3.0)	3/33 (9.1)
Failed pregnancy (total)	10/33 (30.3)	10/33 (30.3)
Late pregnancy complications		
pre-eclampsia	1/23 (4.3)	3/23 (13.0)
IUGR	3/23 (13.0)	3/23 (13.0)
gestational diabetes	1/23 (4.3)	4/23 (17.4)
Delivery	23	23
vaginal	19/23 (82.6)	20/23 (87.0)
abdominal	4/23 (17.4)	3/23 (13.0)
Blood loss during delivery (ml)	695.7 ± 157.9	500.0 ± 60.3
Length of gestation at delivery (weeks) (range)	39.9 (38.0–42.0)*	39.3 (37.0–42.0)*
Birthweight (g)	3604.1 ± 101.4	3498.2 ± 112.1

Note: Values are given as mean ± SEM with percentages shown in parentheses.
Abbreviation: IUGR, intrauterine growth retardation.
(From Tulppala M, Marttunen M, Söderström-Anttila V, et al: Low-dose aspirin in prevention of miscarriage in women with unexplained or autoimmune-related recurrent miscarriage: Effect on prostacyclin and thromboxane A_2 production. *Hum Reprod* 12:1567–1572, 1997. By permission of Oxford University Press, copyright European Society for Human Reproduction and Embryology.)

tion and on the rate of abortion in RSA women with or without detectable levels of ACA were assessed.

Methods.—Of 82 RSA (3 to 8 miscarriages) women, average age 32.7 years, 66 (80.5%) who became pregnant were given either LDA (50 mg/d) (n = 33) or placebo (n = 33) as soon as home pregnancy tests were positive. The level of ACA in venous blood was measured.

Results.—Sixteen (19.5%) of 82 women had elevated IgG ACA levels. Twelve (75%) became pregnant, 6 taking LDA and 6 taking placebo. Ultrasound demonstrated viable pregnancies in 30 LDA patients (5 with elevated ACA levels and 25 with normal ACA levels) and in 28 placebo patients (3 with elevated ACA levels and 25 with normal ACA concentrations). Four (80%) LDA patients with elevated ACA levels and 3 (12%) with normal ACA levels miscarried. Two (61.7%) placebo patients with elevated ACA concentrations and 3 (12%) with normal ACA concentrations miscarried. Women who miscarried had higher levels of ACA than women who did not miscarry (Table 1). The remaining pregnancies resulted in the birth of a healthy term infant. LDA significantly inhibited platelet TXB_2 production in women with and without ACA, in women who carried to term (7.0 ng/mL in the LDA group versus 254.5 ng/mL in the placebo group), and in women who miscarried (13.8 ng/mL versus 233.6 ng/mL). LDA also significantly reduced urine output in successful pregnancies and in miscarried pregnancies. LDA did not affect output of 2, 3-dinor-6-keto-$PGF_{1\alpha}$. Growth retardation was 13.0% in both the treatment and placebo groups. Pre-eclampsia developed in 1 LDA-treated woman and 3 placebo-treated women.

Conclusion.—LDA did not improve pregnancy outcome in RSA women with or without detectable levels of ACA.

▶ The results of this well-designed randomized clinical trial indicate that the ingestion of 50 mg of aspirin daily in early pregnancy to women with a history of unexplained recurrent spontaneous abortion does not improve the rate of live births as compared with placebo ingestion. It is of interest that of the 58 pregnancies in which a live embryo was found to be present during sonographic imaging in early pregnancy 46 (79%) ended in term birth of a viable healthy infant. This study group had a prior history of 3–8 consecutive abortions. The high rate of viable births in both arms of the study demonstrates the necessity of performing randomized clinical trials with a placebo in all studies investigating the effectiveness of possible therapies for recurrent spontaneous abortion.

D.R. Mishell, Jr., M.D.

A Woman With Five Consecutive Fetal Deaths: Case Report and Retrospective Analysis of Hyperhomocysteinemia Prevalence in 100 Consecutive Women With Recurrent Miscarriages

Quere I, Bellet H, Hoffet M, et al (Centre Hospitalier Universitaire, Nîmes, France)

Fertil Steril 69:152–154, 1998 16–5

Background.—Mild to moderate hyperhomocysteinemia has been found to be a cause of recurrent miscarriages. Homocysteine plasma levels are controlled by the C677T gene mutation and folates. The C677T methylene tetrahydrofolate reductase variant, occurring with a frequency of 12% for the homozygous mutant genotype, is a genetic risk for hypercysteinemia.

Case Report.—Woman, 35, had a history of 5 consecutive fetal deaths, 2 stillbirths, and 3 early abortions. Antiphospholipid antibodies were negative. Plasma antithrombin, protein C, and protein S activities were normal. Fibrinolytic response was essentially absent in 3 10-minute venous occlusion tests. Her homocysteine levels were 46 μmol/L (normal, less than 10 μmol/L). She carried the C677T homozygous genotype. After daily treatment for 1 month with 15 mg folic acid, and 500 mg vitamin B6, her homocysteine returned to a normal level, her fibrinolytic response was restored, and she conceived. The folic acid plus vitamin B6 treatment was continued throughout the pregnancy, and she delivered a healthy boy at 32 weeks by cesarean section.

Discussion.—In a retrospective analysis of 100 women with multiple miscarriages, 12 were found to have total plasma homocysteine levels greater than the 95th percentile of a control group. Twenty percent of the patients had the C677T homozygous genotype and 28% had the wild-type genotype versus 14% and 32% of controls (NS). Low levels of folic acid were found in 15% of patients. The highest homocysteine levels were found in patients with folic acid deficiency and the C677T homozygous genotype.

Conclusion.—Recurrent miscarriages are apparently related to hypercysteinemia. The folate deficiency potentiated by the C677T homozygous genotype results in decreased remethylation of homocysteine to methionine, an effect that allows the buildup of homocysteine.

► An earlier study from the Netherlands reported that hyperhomocysteinemia might be a cause of recurrent spontaneous abortion (RSA). The findings in this case report and review of 100 women with RSA of unknown cause provide additional evidence of a causal relation between these 2 conditions. Clinicians may wish to measure serum homocystein levels in women with RSA and, if they are elevated, treat them with folic acid and pyridoxine. To determine whether such therapy is truly beneficial, a randomized clinical trial must be performed. Until such a trial is performed, administration of the 2 agents to women with hyperhomocysteinemia is innocuous and may be beneficial.

D.R. Mishell, Jr., M.D.

Short-term Therapy for Recurrent Abortion Using Intravenous Immunoglobulins: Results of a Double-blind Placebo-controlled Italian Study
Perino A, Vassiliadis A, Vucetich A, et al (Univ of Palermo, Italy; Univ of Milan, Italy; Univ of Naples, Italy; et al)
Hum Reprod 12:2388–2392, 1997 16–6

Background.—In a multicenter, randomized trial, the effect of IV immunoglobulins on pregnancy outcome in women who had had more than 3 spontaneous abortions, no live birth, and no apparent cause (chromosomal, anatomical, infective, or autoimmune) of their reproductive problems was investigated.

Methods.—In a double-blind, placebo-controlled study, 46 women younger than 42 years were confirmed to be negative for antinuclear antibodies, have normal concentrations of IgG and IgM anticardiolipin antibodies, and be negative for lupus anticoagulant. Of the 46 women, 22 were given immunoglobulins in 2 initial doses of 25 g/day on 2 consecutive days in 5 100-mL phials, and a third dose of 25 g 3 weeks later after US confirmation of an ongoing pregnancy; 24 women received placebo. Therapy was administered immediately after a positive result on a pregnancy test to avoid any bias from the identification of a viable pregnancy by US scanning.

Results.—Among the 22 study subjects, 16 pregnancies (1 twin gestation) progressed beyond week 12. The success rate was 72.7%, with 5 pregnancies ending between week 5 and 10. Among the 24 control subjects, 19 pregnancies progressed to term and 4 abortions occurred between week 6 and 8.

Discussion.—These results suggest that treatment with immunoglobulins based on an assumption that an undefined immune problem causes reproductive problems does not benefit women who have recurrent abortion. Pregnancy progressed beyond week 12 in 73% of women given immunoglobulins and 83% of women given placebo. Women who have recurrent abortion may benefit from a thorough medical screening and emotional support during the first few weeks of gestation.

► It has been postulated that an abnormality in the immune system may be a cause for recurrent spontaneous abortion (RSA) when another cause is not found to be present. Therefore, women with recurrent spontaneous abortion have been treated with infusions of paternal white blood cells to overcome a deficiency in the normal immune response to the foreign protein in the gestational tissue. Several randomized clinical trials have failed to confirm a benefit of such therapy for the treatment of RSA. In the past few years, several groups have reported that IV administration of immunoglobulins (IVIG) may increase the viable birth rate in women with no diagnosed cause of RSA. The results of this small randomized clinical trial indicate that the administration of a high dose of IVIG early in gestation does not improve the viable birth rate. The 80% viable birth rate found in the women receiving placebo is similar to the high rate others have reported with the use of intensive psychologic support during pregnancies of women with a history of RSA of no known cause.

D.R. Mishell, Jr., M.D.

Intravenous Immunoglobulin Therapy for Recurrent Spontaneous Abortion: A Meta-Analysis

Daya S, Gunby J, Clark DA (McMaster Univ, Hamilton, Ont, Canada)
Am J Reprod Immunol 39:69–76, 1998 16–7

Background.—The results of randomized studies of IV immunoglobulins (IVIG) in the treatment of recurrent spontaneous abortion (RSA) are conflicting. The current evidence was systematically reviewed to further explore the efficacy of IVIG for RSA.

Methods.—Four randomized, double-blind comparisons of IVIG with placebo in patients with RSA were identified in a thorough literature search. Live birth rates were extracted for the meta-analysis, and the overall odds ratios and absolute treatment effect were calculated.

Findings.—Two trials showed an increase in successful pregnancy outcomes with IVIG treatment. The other 2 did not. The overall odds ratio was 1.48 favoring IVIG. The absolute treatment effect was 10.1%. When pregnancy failures with an obvious cause were excluded, treatment results were significant; however, this approach may be subject to bias (Fig 1).

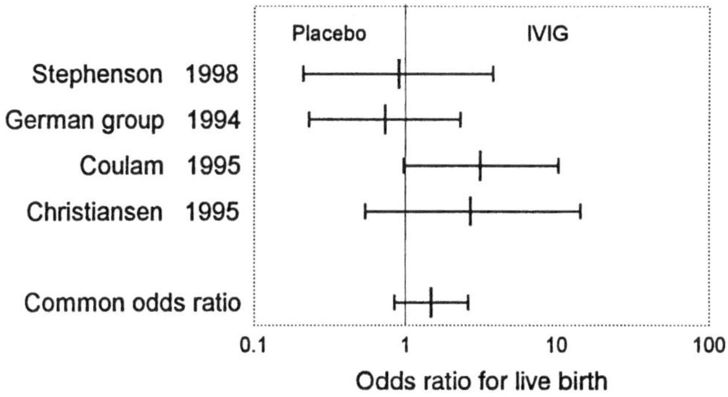

FIGURE 1.—Odds ratios and proportions for live birth (Breslow and Day test for homogeneity of treatment effect = 5.11, $P = 0.16$). *Abbreviation*: *IVIG*, IV immunoglobulin. (Courtesy of Daya S, Gunby J, Clark DA: Intravenous immunoglobulin therapy for recurrent spontaneous abortion: A meta-analysis. *Am J Reprod Immunol* 39:69–76, 1998.)

Conclusion.—The meta-analysis suggests that IVIG may be beneficial in the treatment of RSA. However, the evidence is still not conclusive.

▶ In 30% to 40% of women with RSA, no cause for the problem can be determined after a complete diagnostic evaluation. It is believed by some investigators that the cause of the recurrent pregnancy loss is an immunologic mechanism. There have been about 23 case series in which IVIG has been given to women with unexplained RSA and 4 randomized clinical trials in which IVIG was compared with placebo. The time of initiation of IVIG therapy, the dose, and the frequency of administration varied in the 4 trials. In none of the trials was IVIG therapy found to be sufficiently more effective than placebo.

In this report, when the data were combined by a meta-analytic technique, the summary risk of a viable pregnancy with IVIG therapy was about 1.5. However, this increase in live birth rate was not statistically significant. Therapy with IVIG is expensive and not risk free. At the present time, its use as therapy for RSA should be limited to investigational protocols, as its benefit for unexplained RSA has not been proven.

D.R. Mishell, Jr., M.D.

Randomised Trial of Expectant Versus Surgical Management of Spontaneous Miscarriage

Chipchase J, James D (Univ Hosp, Nottingham, England)

Br J Obstet Gynaecol 104:840–841, 1997 16–8

Background.—The potential complications of retained products after spontaneous abortion are thought to justify curettage. However, the natural course of spontaneous abortion and its complications in the current population are unknown. Short- and medium-term outcomes associated with expectant management and surgical treatment of first-trimester spontaneous abortion were compared.

Methods.—Thirty-five women with retained products of conception after spontaneous abortion were randomly assigned to expectant or surgical treatment. The women were evaluated at 1 and 2 weeks and at 6 months.

Findings.—The number of days of pain, bleeding, sick leave, or return-to-normal periods did not differ significantly between groups. Three fourths of the women receiving expectant management, and two thirds of those undergoing surgery were able to conceive within 6 months of spontaneous abortion.

Conclusions.—The short- and medium-term effects of expectant management are comparable to those of surgical treatment for retained products of conception after spontaneous abortion. These data provide additional reassurance for women and clinicians considering expectant management for first-trimester miscarriages.

▶ The standard of care for women who have an incomplete abortion in the first trimester is to surgically evacuate the remaining intrauterine conceptional tissue by curettage. The results of this randomized comparative trial indicates that if the sonographic diameter of the tissue retained in the intrauterine cavity is less than 50 mm a curettage is probably unnecessary. When women with this amount of tissue were treated expectantly, the conceptional tissue was passed spontaneously and resulted in no significant difference in the duration of bleeding, pain, or time to return of regular menses than when a curettage was performed. Clinicians with access to transvaginal sonography may elect to treat some women with incomplete abortions expectantly instead of surgically.

D.R. Mishell, Jr., M.D.

Medical Abortion or Vacuum Aspiration? Two Year Follow Up of a Patient Preference Trial

Howie FL, Henshaw RC, Naji SA, et al (Univ of Aberdeen, Foresterhill; Univ of Adelaide, Woodville, South Australia; Univ of York, Heslington; et al)

Br J Obstet Gynaecol 104:829–833, 1997 16–9

Introduction.—A satisfactory alternative to surgical vacuum aspiration is medical abortion of a first trimester pregnancy using mifepristone (RU486). Up to 60% of women prefer to have medical abortion. Women who are allowed a choice of method say that both procedures are equally acceptable. However, after more than 50 days of amenorrhea, medical abortion is more painful and less effective. At higher gestations, women who are unsure which method they would prefer are usually advised to consider vacuum aspiration. Between the 2 procedures, there is little economic difference. No comparisons have been made with surgical vacuum aspiration and medical abortion to determine longer term sequelae.

Health outcomes of women who had either medical abortion or vacuum aspiration were compared.

Methods.—During a 2-year period, there were 363 women who had either vacuum aspiration or medical abortion using mifepristone and gemeprost during the first trimester. Women having medical abortion swallowed 600 mg of mifepristone and were admitted to the hospital 36–48 hours later when they received a gemeprost 1-mg vaginal pessary. Women having vacuum aspiration were given general anesthesia. Women having medical abortion experienced significantly more pain and unpleasant symptoms during the procedure but not after discharge from the hospital.

Results.—No significant differences were seen in the reproductive, general, or psychological health of women who had vacuum aspiration or medical abortion. The provision of choice of termination was valued highly by almost all the women. Among women who had been randomized to a method of termination, there was a significant difference in perception of long-term procedure of acceptability.

Conclusion.—The method of termination should be chosen by women. Higher levels of acceptability, particularly at gestations of less than 50 days of amenorrhea, will result when women have the opportunity to choose the method.

▶ In many areas of the world, women who elect to terminate their pregnancy in early gestation now have the choice of utilizing medical or surgical methods. The results of this long-term follow-up indicate that when mifepristone plus a prostaglandin is used as the medical method, the effects upon general, reproductive, and psychological health outcomes are similar to those after vacuum aspiration. More than 80% of women in each group had regular menses and less than 20% sought medical care for psychiatric morbidity. The results of this study indicate that women can be counseled that the use of medical abortion has not been shown to cause long-term adverse reproductive effects.

D.R. Mishell, Jr., M.D.

Early Pregnancy Termination With Mifepristone and Misoprostol in the United States

Spitz IM, Bardin CW, Benton L, et al (Ctr for Biomedical Research, New York)

N Engl J Med 338:1241–1247, 1998 16–10

Introduction.—The antiprogestin mifepristone (RU 486) causes abortion by competitively blocking progesterone receptors. Whether mifepristone is used with gemeprost or misoprostol, both prostaglandin E1 compounds, the rates of termination of pregnancies 49 days old or less are similar, ranging from 96% to 99%. Up to 200,000 women die annually of complications after illegal abortions in developing countries. Greater access to safer abortion services could result with the availability of medical

TABLE 1.—Results of Mifepristone and Misoprostol in Women Seeking Termination of Pregnancy

Outcome	Pregnant ≤49 Days (N=827)	Pregnant 50 to 56 Days (N=678)	Pregnant 57 to 63 Days (N=510)
	number (percent [95% confidence interval])		
Success	762 (92 [90–94])	563 (83 [80–86])*	395 (77 [74–81])*†
After mifepristone alone	40 (5)	12 (2)‡	4 (0.8)*
Failure (need for surgical intervention)			
Medical indication for intervention	13 (2)	26 (4)‡	21 (4)‡
Patient's request for intervention	5 (0.6)	13 (2)	
Incomplete abortion	39 (5)	51 (8)‡	12 (2)*
Ongoing pregnancy	8 (1)	25 (4)*	36 (7)
			46 (9)*§
Total	65 (8)	115 (17)*	115 (23)*†

*P less than 0.001 for the comparison with the 49-days or less group.
†P=0.02 for the comparison with the 50- to 56-days group.
‡0.001 less than 0.03 for the comparison with the 49-days or less group.
§P less than 0.001 for the comparison with the 50- to 56-days group.
(Courtesy of Spitz IM, Bardin W, Benton L, et al: Early pregnancy termination with mifepristone and misoprostol in the United States. *N Engl J Med* 338:1241–1247, 1998. Reprinted by permission of the New England Journal of Medicine, copyright Massachusetts Medical Society. All rights reserved.)

abortion in the United States and elsewhere. To determine whether the combination of mifepristone and misoprostol could be used to terminate pregnancies of up to 63 days' duration, a multicenter trial was conducted.

Methods.—There were 2,121 women seeking termination of their pregnancies who received 600 mg of mifepristone, and 400 μg of misoprostol 2 days later. After the administration of misoprostol, the women were observed for 4 hours, and they returned on day 15 for final assessment. The final assessment was completed by 2,015 women.

Results.—In 762 of 827 women pregnant for 49 days or less (92%), pregnancy was terminated. In 563 of 678 women pregnant for 50–56 days (83%), pregnancy was terminated. In 395 of the 510 women pregnant for 56–63 days (77%), pregnancy was terminated. In 49% of all women, termination occurred within 4 hours after the administration of misoprostol, and in 75% of the women, termination occurred within 24 hours. Failure, defined as women requiring surgical intervention for medical reasons or because the patient requested it, the abortion was incomplete, or the pregnancy was ongoing, increased with increasing duration of pregnancy (Table 1). The largest increase was in failures representing ongoing pregnancy, which increased from 1% in the 49-days-or-less group to 9% in the 56–63 days group. Abdominal pain, nausea, vomiting, diarrhea, and vaginal bleeding increased with advancing gestational age. Hospitalization, surgical intervention, and intravenous fluids were given to 2% of women in the 49-days-or-less group, as compared with 4% in each of the other 2 groups. In the 49-days-or-less group, the median duration of bleeding or spotting was 13 days, and in the other 2 groups, it was 15 days (Fig 3).

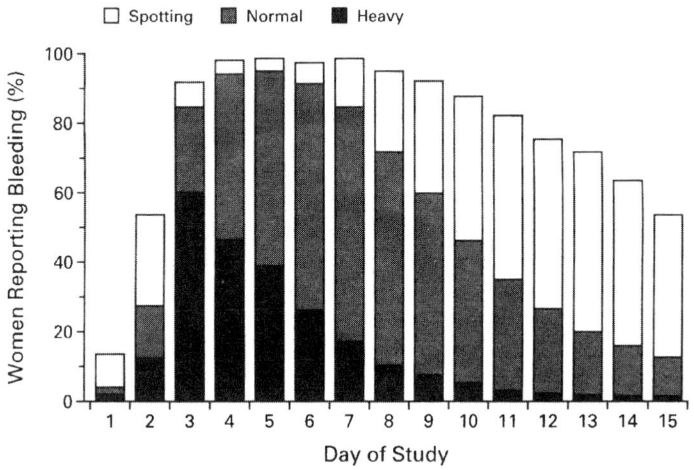

FIGURE 3.—Types of vaginal bleeding as recorded by the women from day 1 (administration of mifepristone) to day 15. The data are from 1,606 women who did not undergo surgical termination of pregnancy and who recorded the types of bleeding they had from the study day 1 to day 15 on menstrual-diary cards. Bleeding was characterized as *spotting*, as similar to normal menstrual bleeding (*normal*), or as heavier than normal menstrual bleeding (*heavy*). (Courtesy of Spitz IM, Bardin W, Benton L, et al: Early pregnancy termination with mifepristone and misoprostol in the United States. *N Engl J Med* 338:1241–1247, 1998. Reprinted by permission of the *New England Journal of Medicine*, copyright Massachusetts Medical Society. All rights reserved.)

Conclusion.—The mifepristone-misoprostol regimen is effective in terminating pregnancies, especially in women with pregnancies of 49 days' duration or less.

▶ Each year in the United States, slightly more than 6 million women become pregnant. About half of these pregnancies are unintended and half of these (one fourth of all pregnancies) or 1.4 million are terminated by elective surgical abortion. Many women in this country who wish to terminate their pregnancies are unable to do so because of a lack of providers of surgical abortion in many areas. If a safe effective medical method of abortion, such as the combination of mifepristone and misoprostol used in this study, were available and approved by the U.S. Food and Drug Administration, many additional women who wished to terminate their pregnancies could do so. Although the results of this trial confirm the safety and efficacy of this medical regimen, mifepristone is not currently being manufactured in facilities that are approved by the Food and Drug Administration for production of pharmaceutical agents. Thus, it is unlikely that mifepristone will become available for U.S. women in the next few years, until the drug is manufactured in a Food and Drug Administration-approved facility.

D.R. Mishell, Jr., M.D.

Medical Abortion With Oral Methotrexate and Vaginal Misoprostol

Creinin MD, Vittinghoff E, Schaff E, et al (Univ of Pittsburgh, Pa; Univ of California, San Francisco; Univ of Rochester, NY; et al)

Obstet Gynecol 90:611–616, 1997 16–11

Background.—For medical abortion, methotrexate given orally would offer advantages over parenteral administration. The efficacy of oral methotrexate followed by vaginal misoprostol for abortion at up to 49 days' gestation was determined.

Methods.—Three hundred women seeking elective abortion were enrolled in a prospective multicenter study. The women were given methotrexate, 50 mg orally, followed 5–6 days later by misoprostol, 800 μg vaginally. If abortion did not occur, the dose was repeated.

Findings.—Complete abortion occurred in 91.3% of the women. In 77.9%, abortion occurred within 8 days of methotrexate administration. In the remaining 13.4%, abortion occurred at a mean of 23.5 days. Vaginal bleeding lasted means of 15 and 11 days in immediate and delayed abortions, respectively. The rates of complete abortion declined linearly as body surface area increased. The adverse effects of methotrexate and misoprostol were nausea, in 37% and 33%, respectively; vomiting, in 11% and 18%; diarrhea, in 12% and 18%, and subjective fever or chills, in 15% and 31%.

Conclusion.—Oral methotrexate followed by vaginal misoprostol is an effective method for medical abortion. Thus, oral administration is an acceptable alternative to IM administration.

► Intramuscular methotrexate followed by vaginal insertion of misoprostol is currently the most common method of performing medical elective abortion in the United States. The results of this large study show that in pregnancies of less than 7 weeks' gestation, 50 mg of methotrexate given orally instead of by injection and followed 6–7 days later by vaginal insertion of misoprostol results in an abortion rate of 91%, similar to that obtained with methotrexate given by injection. Side effects after administration of both drugs was common, and about one fourth of the subjects did not abort until a mean of 3 weeks after receiving misoprostol. Despite these problems, some women may elect to have their early pregnancies terminated medically by this technique instead of by suction aspiration.

D.R. Mishell, Jr., M.D.

17 Ectopic Pregnancy

Epidemiology of Repeat Ectopic Pregnancy: A Population-based Prospective Cohort Study

Skjeldestad FE, Hadgu A, Eriksson N (Norwegian Univ, Trondheim, Norway; Natl Ctrs for Disease Control and Prevention, Atlanta, Ga; Orkdal Hosp, Orkanger, Norway)

Obstet Gynecol 91:129–135, 1998 17–1

Background.—Studies of the effect of ectopic pregnancy on subsequent fertility have been problematic. Pregnancy outcomes after the first (index) ectopic pregnancy were further investigated, with a focus on risks during the index pregnancy associated with a repeat event.

Methods.—Six hundred ninety-seven women aged 37 years or younger at the time of their first ectopic pregnancy were studied. None had had tubal surgery before the index pregnancy. The women were followed up for 1–17 years. Three hundred fifty-three women had a total of 555 pregnancies.

Findings.—Pregnancy order was the stronger correlate of the subsequent occurrence of ectopic pregnancy. The frequency of repeat ectopic pregnancy declined by one third for each pregnancy from the first to the third. Women diagnosed as having infectious pathologic conditions had a risk of another ectopic pregnancy almost 3 times greater than that among women without such conditions. Other variables associated with repeat ectopic pregnancy were age of 24 years or less at the index pregnancy, history of repeat ectopic pregnancy, initiation of infertility work-up, and conception with an intrauterine device at the index pregnancy. Surgical procedure was not related to repeat ectopic pregnancy (Table 4).

Conclusions.—Assisted reproduction should be considered for women who have had 2 ectopic pregnancies. After 2 ectopic pregnancies, the chances of a completed intrauterine pregnancy was only about 4%.

▶ This study provides much useful data for the practitioner to use when counseling a woman with an ectopic pregnancy about the outcome of a subsequent conception. The entry criteria included only women who had a spontaneous subsequent conception, excluding those who had a subsequent pregnancy after treatment for infertility or those with a history of prior tubal surgery. Among this group of women who were less than 38 years of age at the time of their ectopic pregnancy and were not using an intrauterine

TABLE 4.—Odds of Repeat Ectopic Pregnancy in Subsequent Pregnancies

	Adjusted OR	95% CI
Pregnancy order		
1st subsequent	11.8	2.0, 68.0
2nd subsequent	3.0	0.5, 21.1
3rd or more subsequent	1.0	Reference
Repeat ectopic pregnancy		
1 repeat (2nd) ectopic pregnancy	9.5	2.5, 36.6
No repeat (1st) ectopic pregnancy	1.0	Reference
Status at index ectopic pregnancy		
Age (y)		
≤24	3.1	1.1, 8.9
≥25	1.0	Reference
Infectious pathology*		
Yes	2.7	1.5, 5.0
No	1.0	Reference
Have started infertility work-up		
Yes	2.3	1.0, 5.1
No	1.0	Reference
Conceived with intrauterine device in situ at index pregnancy		
Yes	0.4	0.1, 0.9
No	1.0	Reference

*Defined as either adhesions or macroscopic damage to the contralateral tube or both.
Abbreviation: OR, odds ratio; *CI*, confidence interval.
(Reprinted with permission from American College of Obstetricians and Gynecologists [*Obstetrics and Gynecology*, 1997, 91(1) 129–135].)

device (IUD) for contraception, if they conceived again, their overall rate of repeat ectopic pregnancy was 21%. About one fourth of the pregnancies ended in spontaneous or induced abortions and slightly more than half were viable gestations. The risk of repeat ectopic pregnancy was increased three fold in women whose first ectopic pregnancy occurred when they were less than 25, as well as those who had gross or histologic evidence of prior tubal infection compared to women with normal oviducts. Women with a history of infertility evaluation prior to their ectopic pregnancy had about a 2-fold increased risk of their subsequent pregnancy being ectopic compared to women without such a history. Those who had an ectopic pregnancy while wearing an IUD had about a 60% reduction in risk of the subsequent pregnancy being ectopic compared with non–IUD users. If a woman's first pregnancy after her ectopic was also ectopic, her chances of having a subsequent intrauterine gestation was only 4%. However, if her first subsequent pregnancy was intrauterine, her chances of having an ectopic pregnancy in a subsequent gestation was reduced to 5%. The type of surgical procedure performed on the oviductal site of ectopic pregnancy did not affect the risk of ectopic pregnancy in a subsequent gestation.

D.R. Mishell, Jr., M.D.

Treatment, Failures and Complications of Ectopic Pregnancy: Changes Over a 20–year Period

Landström G, Thorburn J, Bryman I (Göteborg Univ, Sweden)
Hum Reprod 13:203–207, 1998 17–2

Introduction.—The changes in treatment of ectopic pregnancy and their effects on complication rates from 1975–1994 were retrospectively examined in a cohort of Swedish patients.

Study Design.—The study group consisted of 225 patients who were operated on for ectopic pregnancy between 1992 and 1994 at Sahlgrenska University Hospital in Göteborg, Sweden. Their treatment was compared to that from the same hospital from 1975–1979, 1981–1982, and 1986–1987.

Findings.—Trend analysis demonstrated a significant decrease in the proportion of radical procedures during the 20–year period. There was a decrease in laparotomy procedures and an increase in laparoscopic surgery. There were no laparoscopic procedures in 1975–1979. By 1992–1994, the percentage of laparoscopic procedures rose to 84.5%. The incidence of pre–shock/shock, bleeding, and tubal rupture deceased throughout the study period. The complication rate was 1.2% in 1975 to 1979, and complications were only observed after conservative procedures. The complication rate increased to 7.3% in 1986–1987 after the introduction of laparoscopic procedures but continued to increase to 14.2% in 1992–1994 after this procedure became well established. Complication rates were significantly higher after laparoscopy rather than laparotomy and after conservative rather than radical procedures.

Conclusions.—This study examined changes in treatment and complication rates for ectopic pregnancy from 1975–1994. The introduction of laparoscopic surgery was accompanied by an increase in the overall complication rate, which increased further after this technique was well established. The failure and complication rate of laparoscopic conservative surgery remains too high. More attention must be paid to patient selection and surgical skills in the use of these difficult procedures.

▶ With the use of sensitive rapid assays for human chorionic gonadotropin and transvaginal sonography, the diagnosis of ectopic pregnancy is much more frequent before tubal rupture than in the past. Nearly all unruptured ectopic pregnancies are now treated by laparoscopic salpingostomy. The postpartum complication rate is greater after salpingostomy than salpingectomy. For women without a history of infertility and a grossly appearing normal contralateral oviduct, subsequent pregnancy rates do not appear greater when salpingostomy is performed instead of salpingectomy. Knowledge of this information, as well as the 25% complication rate when laparoscopic salpingostomy was performed during the years 1992–1994, may have accounted for the trend of increasing incidence of radical surgical procedures in this institution between 1986 and 1992. If no future fertility is desired, the treatment of choice of unruptured ectopic pregnancy is salpingectomy. But for those women desiring future fertility, salpingostomy is still the treatment of choice.

D.R. Mishell, Jr., M.D.

Medical Treatment of Ectopic Pregnancy With Methotrexate

Theon LD, Creinin MD (Univ of Pittsburgh, Pa)

Fertil Steril 68:727–730, 1997 17–3

Background.—Outpatient medical management is now an accepted approach for the treatment of ectopic pregnancy (EP). One experience with low-dose intramuscular methotrexate was reviewed.

Methods.—Fifty women with EP were treated with 50 mg/m^2 of methotrexate intramuscularly. This dose was repeated if the β-hCG concentration did not decline by 15% or more between 4 and 7 days or if a plateau or increase occurred during weekly follow-up assessment. Surgery was indicated by significant abdominal pain in the presence of hemodynamic instability or signs of peritoneal irritation on physical examination.

Findings.—Methotrexate treatment was successful in 91.5% of the women. Seven women needed a second dose. Four women underwent surgery after the failure of medical treatment. Mean time from treatment initiation to resolution in successfully treated women was 25 days. Increased abdominal pain prompted 27.7% of the women to make additional visits to the emergency department.

Conclusions.—A greater awareness of the side effects associated with medical therapy for EP may improve success rates. The decision to perform surgery should be based on defined guidelines, such as the development of peritoneal signs, declining hemoglobin concentrations, or hemodynamic instability.

▶ Medical management of unruptured ectopic pregnancy with intramuscularly administered methotrexate is being used with increasing frequency because the success rate is high and an expensive surgical procedure is avoided. The results of only a few series of more than 20 women with ectopic pregnancy treated with methotrexate have been published. The reported success rates in these studies vary from 75%–94%. Since most women treated with methotrexate develop some pain afterwards due to abortion of the tubal pregnancy, a surgical procedure should not be performed for pain alone. A surgical procedure should be performed only if the pain is accompanied by evidence of hemodynamic instability, decreasing serial hemoglobin level, or signs of peritoneal irritation. With the use of the strict criteria required before medical treatment, as reported in this study, and the avoidance of performing a post-methotrexate surgical procedure for pain alone, a success rate for medical therapy of more than 90% should be obtained.

D.R. Mishell, Jr., M.D.

A 6-year Clinical Trial of Methotrexate Therapy in the Treatment of Ectopic Pregnancy

Jiménez-Caraballo A, Rodríguez-Donoso G (Hospital Universitario 'Virgen Macarena,' Seville, Spain)

Eur J Obstet Gynecol Reprod Biol 79:167–171, 1998 17–4

Background.—Methotrexate therapy has been used in the treatment of ectopic pregnancy. A 6-year experience with intrasacular and intramuscular methotrexate in women with unruptured ectopic pregnancy was reported.

Methods.—Sixty patients were treated between November 1990 and December 1996. Fourteen received an intrasacular injection of 15 mg, 45 received an intramuscular dose of 50 mg/m², and 1 received methotrexate by both routes.

Findings.—Forty-six patients (76.7%) responded to treatment, including 10 who received the drug intrasacularly and 36 who received it intramuscularly. Minor adverse effects occurred in 33.3% of the patients. The most common was mild abdominal pain. Declining leukocyte concentrations on the third day after initiation of treatment may be a fairly accurate criterion for predicting a patient's response.

Conclusions.—Methotrexate therapy is a reliable alternative to surgery in the treatment of unruptured ectopic pregnancy. Intramuscular administration with laparoscopy seems to be the most convenient route and is associated with relatively few complications.

► This is another study showing that where a small (less than 3.5 cm) unruptured ectopic pregnancy is present, treatment with intramuscular methotrexate may be used as an alternative to surgical excision. The success rate of 76% reported in this study is lower than the 98.6% reported by Stovall but is similar to the 78% to 80% success rate reported by other authors. Many women treated with methotrexate experience abdominal pain soon after the injection, without the occurrence of tubal rupture. If there is no ancillary evidence of tubal rupture, such as a falling hematocrit, the pain usually resolves within a few days and laparoscopy, which lowers the success rate, is unnecessary.

D.R. Mishell, Jr., M.D.

Single-dose Methotrexate for Unruptured Ectopic Pregnancy

Lecuru F, Robin F, Bernard J-P, et al (Hôpital Boucicau, Paris; Necker-Enfants Malades, Paris)

Int J Gynaecol Obstet 61:253–259, 1998 17–5

Background.—Minimally invasive approaches for the treatment of unruptured ectopic pregnancies (UEP), such as methotrexate (MTX) therapy, have been developed. In the current study, the efficacy of single-dose MTX was compared with that of laparoscopic salpingostomy.

Methods.—Seventy-five patients were included in this prospective, nonrandomized study. Thirty-seven received single-dose MTX (group 1), and 38 had laparoscopic salpingostomy (group 2). Methotrexate, 1 mg/kg, was given intramuscularly on an outpatient basis when β-human chorionic gonadotropin (hCG) levels were less than 5,000 IU/L, the hematosalpinx diameter was less than 3 cm, and the peritoneal fluid was less than 300 cm^3 on transvaginal sonography.

Findings.—Ninety-two percent of group 1 patients were cured with 1 to 3 doses of MTX. The remainder required laparoscopy. Seventy-three percent of this latter group were treated as outpatients. Mean time to hCG resolution was 26.7 days. The initial β-hCG level was significantly associated with the need for surgery and time to β-hCG resolution. All patients with β-hCG levels less than 3,600 IU/L were cured with 1 injection, with no need for hospitalization. Eighty-two percent of group 2 patients were cured with laparoscopy. Sixteen percent were given an MTX injection for persistent UEP. Mean hospitalization was significantly longer for patients needing MTX injection, but follow-up was shorter, requiring significantly fewer clinical examinations, sonograms, and biologic tests. The efficacy of single-dose MTX and laparoscopic salpingostomy was comparable.

Conclusions.—A single dose of MTX is as effective as laparoscopy in the treatment of UEP. Patients should be rigorously selected to maximize the success rates of outpatient treatment with a short follow-up.

► This nonrandomized prospective study provides additional data indicating that the use of intramuscular MTX is an effective means of treating small UEPs. In this study, the success rate with MTX was 92%. An interesting finding of this study is that the pretreatment serum hCG level was a good prognostic indicator of success with MTX. All women with a small (less than 3 cm) UEP were cured with a single dose of MTX if their hCG level was less than 3,600 IU/L. The authors suggest that all women with hCG levels above 3,600 IU/L be treated by laparoscopy.

D.R. Mishell, Jr., M.D.

Randomised Trial of Systemic Methotrexate Versus Laparoscopic Salpingostomy in Tubal Pregnancy

Hajenius PJ, Engelsbel S, Mol BWJ, et al (Univ of Amsterdam; Onze Lieve Vrouwe Gasthuis, Amsterdam)

Lancet 350:774–779, 1997 17–6

Objective.—Laparoscopic salpingostomy for tubal pregnancy preserves fertility. Methotrexate offers a nonsurgical option. Results of a randomized study comparing treatment success, tubal preservation, and homolateral tubal patency of systemic methotrexate versus laparoscopic salpingostomy for treatment of tubal pregnancy are presented.

Methods.—Between January 1, 1994, and September 1, 1996, 100 patients in 6 Dutch hospitals were randomly allocated to receive systemic methotrexate (n = 51) or laparoscopic salpingostomy (n = 49) for treatment of tubal pregnancy diagnosed noninvasively by sonography and measurement of human chorionic gonadotropin (hCG). One course of methotrexate involved 4 1-mg/kg doses IM of methotrexate on days 0, 2, 4, and 6 and 4 0.1-mg/kg doses PO of folinic acid on days 1, 3, 5, and 7. Side effects and any methotrexate toxicity were recorded. Hysterosalpingography was performed 3 months after treatment to assess tubal patency. Serum hCG was monitored to assure treatment success.

Results.—One course of methotrexate was successful in 42 (82%) patients; 2 (4%) patients required a second course because of persistent trophoblast, and 7 (14%) patients required surgery. Two patients needing surgery underwent laparoscopic salpingostomy because of bleeding, and 1 underwent laparoscopic nettoyage because of tubal rupture. Laparoscopic salpingostomy was successful in 35 (72%) patients; conservative surgery failed in 4; and 10 (20%) required additional methotrexate treatment because of persistent trophoblast. Twenty (39%) patients in the methotrexate group and 38 (78%) in the salpingostomy group had no complications or side effects, 37% and 4% experienced abdominal pain, and 25% and 8% had nausea/vomiting. Eighteen (35%) methotrexate patients had conjunctivitis. Median serum hCG clearance time was 19 days in the methotrexate group, and 14 days in the salpingostomy group. Homolateral tubal patency was 62% in the methotrexate group and 66% in the salpingostomy group.

Conclusion.—Although both treatments were equally successful, more patients who underwent salpingostomy had persistent trophoblasts and more patients who received methotrexate required surgical intervention. The treatment of choice will be determined by subsequent fertility outcomes, patient quality of life, patient preference, and cost.

► This study is the first published randomized clinical trial comparing the effects of systemic methotrexate with laparoscopic salpingostomy for the treatment of unruptured tubal pregnancy. The study had the advantage that prior to randomization the diagnosis of unruptured tubal pregnancy was confirmed by diagnostic laparoscopy. A similar degree of success was achieved with each treatment methodology. In the group treated medically, 14% required surgical intervention, while in the group treated surgically, 20% required methotrexate treatment for persistent ectopic pregnancy (PEP). This incidence of PEP is higher than the usually reported rate of 5%. Since the location of most PEP is proximal to the laparoscopic incision used to perform salpingostomy, we now extend the original incision 1 to 2 cm proximally to the grossly visualized ectopic gestation. Since performing this modification, the incidence of PEP in our institution is only 1% to 2%.

D.R. Mishell, Jr., M.D.

18 Sexuality and Premenstrual Syndrome

A Double-blind Provocative Study of Chocolate as a Trigger of Headache

Marcus DA, Scharff L, Turk D, et al (Univ of Pittsburgh, Pa; Univ of Washington, Seattle)

Cephalalgia 17:855–862, 1997 18–1

Background.—Chocolate is often cited as a trigger of headache. Chocolate contains various vasoactive amines, which some investigators believe are precipitants of headache. The evidence of this, however, is mixed. In a large sample of patients with migraine, tension-type, or combined migraine and tension-type headache, the ability of chocolate to provoke headache was determined.

Methods.—There were 63 female patients with recurrent headache who completed the double-blind study, mean age 28.3. During a 2-week washout period, the patients ate a diet that restricted vasoactive amine–rich foods and recorded headache activity 4 times a day. They then underwent a series of 4 provocative trials with chocolate or carob placebo.

Results.—Overall, the most common triggers of headache were stress, changes in sleep pattern, menstruation, and hunger; 17.5% of patients reported that chocolate triggered their headache. No significant differences were found in reports of headache after eating chocolate or carob. No differences in incidence of headache after eating chocolate were seen among the headache diagnostic groups.

Discussion.—In this general sample of individuals with recurrent headache, chocolate did not provoke headache. Future prospective trials should study additional dietary factors to determine the true role of diet in headache in the general headache population and in selected subpopulations.

▶ It is widely believed that chocolate as well as other foods containing a high level of vasoactive amines, such as certain cheeses, meats, peanuts, and alcohol, can trigger the onset of headaches, particularly those of the migraine type. The majority of people with headaches are women, and women are more likely than men to report that ingestion of certain foods can trigger the onset of headaches. The results of this fairly large, well-done double-blind, clinical trial suggest that ingestion of chocolate does not act as a trigger to induce headaches of the migraine or tension type. It is possible that a craving for ingestion of sweets is a prodromal symptom for the onset of headaches. Therefore, chocolate may alleviate this sweet craving, but its ingestion is not a true cause of the headaches.

D.R. Mishell, Jr., M.D.

Comparison of Fluoxetine, Bupropion, and Placebo in the Treatment of Premenstrual Dysphoric Disorder

Pearlstein TB, Stone AB, Lund SA, et al (Brown Univ, Providence, RI; Univ of Massachusetts, Worcester; Deaconess Waltham Hosp, Mass)

J Clin Psychopharmacol 17:261–266, 1997 18–2

Background.—Many clinicians now use serotonergic antidepressants as first-line therapy for premenstrual dysphoric disorder (PMDD). The efficacy of nonserotonergic antidepressants has not been studied as thoroughly. Fluoxetine, bupropion, and placebo were compared in the treatment of women with PMDD.

Methods.—Thirty-four women with PMDD were enrolled in the 2-center, parallel design, placebo-controlled, randomized study. The patients completed 1 month of single-blind placebo and 2 months of fluoxetine, 20 mg/day; bupropion, 100 mg 3 times a day; or placebo. In each of 3 treatment cycles, Clinical Global Impressions Scale (CGIS), an expanded form of the Hamilton Rating Scale for Depression (HAM-D), and Global Assessment Scale (GAS) ratings were obtained before menstruation.

Findings.—The CGIS ratings differed significantly among the 3 groups, with fluoxetine being superior to bupropion and placebo. Comparison of HAM-D and GAS scores before and after treatment also showed that fluoxetine was superior to placebo. Bupropion scores were intermediate between the 2 and did not differ significantly from either (Table 1).

TABLE 1.—Number of Subjects With Good Improvement at Completion of Trial

	N	%
Fluoxetine	10/10	100*†
Bupropion	4/12	33.3
Placebo	2/12	16.7

Note: "Good improvement" is represented by a Clinical Global Impressions Scale score of 1 or 2.
*$\chi^2 = 12.1$, $df = 1$, $P < 0.001$, fluoxetine vs. placebo.
†$\chi^2 = 7.8$, $df = 1$, $P < 0.005$, fluoxetine vs. bupropion.
(Courtesy of Pearlstein TB, Stone AB, Lund SA, et al: Comparison of fluoxetine, bupropion, and placebo in the treatment of premenstrual dysphoric disorder. *J Clin Psychopharmacol* 17(4):261–266, 1997.)

Conclusion.—Fluoxetine is significantly better than bupropion or placebo in the treatment of PMDD. Some improvements occurred with bupropion, and both agents were tolerated well. However, patient satisfaction was greatest with fluoxetine.

Fluoxetine in the Treatment of Premenstrual Syndrome

Özeren S, Çorakçi A, Yücesoy I, et al (Univ of Kocaeli, Turkey)

Eur J Obstet Gynecol Reprod Biol 73:167–170, 1997 18–3

Background.—Although the etiology of premenstrual syndrome (PMS) is not known, some authors have speculated that it may be associated with a deficiency in central serotonergic activity. The efficacy of fluoxetine in the treatment of PMS was investigated.

Methods.—Thirty-five women meeting criteria for PMS, including psychiatric interviews, were included in the double-blind, placebo-controlled trial. By random assignment, placebo or fluoxetine, 20 mg/day, was given for 3 menstrual cycles. PROZAC

Findings.—Fluoxetine was significantly better than placebo in alleviating PMS symptoms. Twelve of the 15 fluoxetine recipients responded to therapy (Fig 1). After treatment, total luteal Calendar of Premenstrual Experiences scores were 58% lower, compared with a 23% decrease in the placebo group. Fluoxetine improved both behavioral, affective, and physical symptoms (Fig 2). The most common adverse effects were gastrointestinal irritability, occurring in 15%; insomnia, occurring in 11%; and sexual dysfunction, occurring in 8.5%.

Conclusion.—Fluoxetine, 20 mg/day, is significantly better than placebo in relieving the symptoms of PMS. It is also well tolerated.

► In 1994, premenstrual syndrome was renamed premenstrual dysphoric disorder (PMDD) in the Diagnostic and Statistical Manual of Mental Disor-

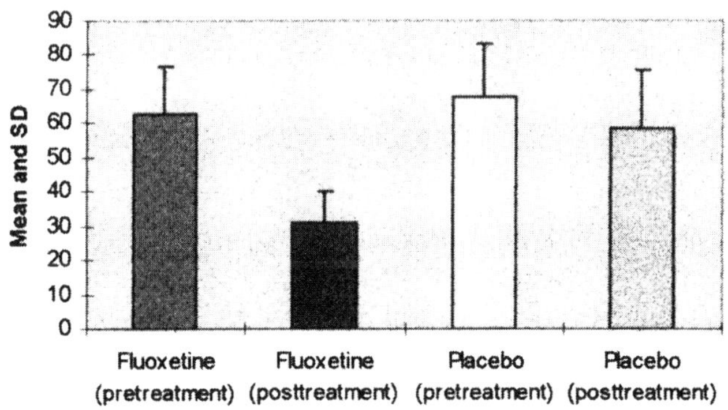

FIGURE 1.—Luteal phase Calendar of Premenstrual Experiences scores before and after 3 menstrual cycles of treatment. (Courtesy of Özeren S, Çorakçi A, Yücesoy I, et al: Fluoxetine in the treatment of premenstrual syndrome. *Eur J Obstet Gynecol Reprod Biol* 73:167–170, copyright 1997, with kind permission from Elsevier Science Ireland Ltd., Bay 15K, Shannon Industrial Estate, Co. Clare, Ireland.)

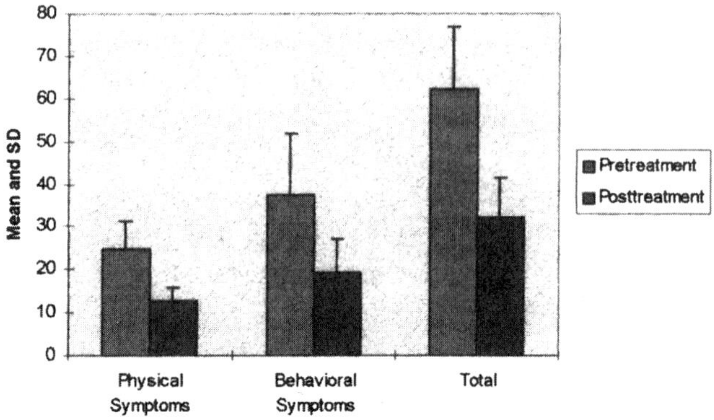

FIGURE 2.—Physical and behavioral luteal symptom scores before and after fluoxetine treatment. (Courtesy of Özeren S, Çorakçi A, Yücesoy I, et al: Fluoxetine in the treatment of premenstrual syndrome. *Eur J Obstet Gynecol Reprod Biol* 73:167–170, copyright 1997, with kind permission from Elsevier Science Ireland Ltd., Bay 15K, Shannon Industrial Estate, Co. Clare, Ireland.)

ders published by the American Psychiatric Association. The etiology of this common disorder is not completely known, but recent data suggest that women with PMDD have abnormalities in the regulation of the neurotransmitter serotonin.

Several studies, including the 2 clinical trials summarized in these abstracts (Abstracts 18–2 and 18–3), have shown that when the selective serotonin reuptake inhibitor fluoxetine (Prozac) was given to women with this disorder, there was a significantly greater improvement in objectively measured symptom scores when compared with both a placebo and a nonserotoninergic antidepressant. The antidepressant effect of fluoxetine is believed to be the result of increased availability of serotonin, as this agent blocks reuptake of serotonin. In both studies, a single oral dose of 20 mg of fluoxetine was used. Side effects with this dosage included nausea, insomnia, and fatigue, but they occurred in a minority of subjects. Clinicians should consider using this agent to treat women with disabling symptoms of PMDD.

D.R. Mishell, Jr., M.D.

19 Diagnostic Gynecology

Plasma Organochlorine Levels and the Risk of Breast Cancer

Hunter DJ, Hankinson SE, Laden F, et al (Harvard Med School; Harvard School of Public Health, Boston; Mount Sinai Hosp, New York)

N Engl J Med 337:1253–1258, 1997 19–1

Objective.—There is growing evidence that environmental and lifestyle factors are major causes of breast cancer, with suspicion falling on environmental pollutants such as 1,1-dichloro-2,2-bis(*p*-chlorophenyl)ethylene (DDE) and polychlorinated biphenyls (PCBs) as causative agents. Levels of PCBs and DDE were measured in blood samples prospectively collected in 1989 and 1990 from 240 women with a diagnosis of breast cancer before June 1, 1992, and 240 control women in the Nurses' Health Study.

Methods.—In the breast cancer group, there were 200 women with invasive cancer, 39 with carcinoma in situ, and 1 with cancer of uncertain histology. Levels of PCBs (in 230 pairs) and DDE (in 236 pairs) for women with cancer and controls were compared statistically.

Results.—The age range of women in the study was 43–69 years and 68% of both groups were menopausal. Both DDE and PCB plasma levels significantly increased with age. Plasma DDE levels were significantly correlated with body mass index. Plasma DDE levels were lower in women with breast cancer than in controls, and plasma PCB levels were similar in the 2 groups (Table 2).

Conclusion.—There was no association between high plasma levels of DDE and PCBs and risk of breast cancer.

► I include this article on the risk of breast cancer and environmental weak estrogens because of great current interest. In this case, plasma levels of environmental carcinogens of pesticides were evaluated as its metabolite DDE and the much-studied PCBs. The results showed no difference in plasma levels between women with breast cancer and controls. The study failed to substantiate any link between these agents and breast cancer.

In the accompanying thoughtful editorial, Dr. Safe[1] notes the conflicting evidence in this area, and he further notes the great publicity in the public

TABLE 2.—Plasma Levels of DDE and PCBs Among Case Patients With Breast Cancer and Controls in the Nurses' Health Study

	Case Patients and Controls*	Mean (±SD) Value	Median Value	P Value†
	no.	parts per billion		
DDE				
Case patients	236	6.01 ± 4.56	4.71	
Controls	236	6.97 ± 5.99	5.35	0.14
PCBs				
Case patients	230	5.08 ± 2.51	4.49	
Controls	230	5.16 ± 2.26	4.68	0.72

Note: The plasma levels of DDE and PCBs were measured after adjustment for plasma cholesterol concentrations.

*Values of DDE were missing for 1 member of 4 case-control pairs, and PCB values were missing for an additional 6 pairs because of lost samples or evidence of contamination.

†The Wilcoxon signed-rank test was used.

Abbreviations: DDE, 1,1-dichloro-2,2-bis (*p*-chlorophenyl) ethylene; *PCBs*, polychlorinated biphenyls.

(Courtesy of Hunter DJ, Hankinson SE, Laden F, et al: Plasma organochlorine levels and the risk of breast cancer. *N Engl J Med* 337:1253–1258, Reprinted by permission of the *New England Journal of Medicine*, copyright 1997, Massachusetts Medical Society.)

press on the problem of environmental carcinogens and weak estrogens in the causation of breast cancer. He made the important point that one should not assume a so-called "paparazzi science" relationship in the absence of credible scientific evidence. Both the article and the editorial have a useful message.

A.L. Herbst, M.D.

Reference

1. Safe SH: Xenoestrogens and breast cancer (editorial). *N Engl J Med* 337:1303–1305, 1997.

Survival of *BRCA1* Breast and Ovarian Cancer Patients: A Population-based Study From Southern Sweden

Jóhansson OT, Ranstam J, Borg A, et al (Univ Hosp, Lund, Sweden)

J Clin Oncol 16:397–404, 1998 19–2

Introduction.—Positive family history of breast cancer is a well-known risk factor for breast cancer, but how family history influences survival of patients with breast cancer is still not clear. Mutations in the gene *BRCA1* confers a high risk of developing breast and ovarian cancer, but whether carriers of *BRCA1* have a better or worse survival than other patients with breast or ovarian cancer is not known. Survival of patients with breast and ovarian cancer belonging to families carrying *BRCA1* germline mutations was compared with the survival of a population-based comparison group.

Methods.—A population-based group that consisted of 28,281 invasive breast cancers and 7,011 ovarian cancers diagnosed in a 37-year period was compared with 71 *BRCA1*-associated cancer patients (33 breast cancer, 7 breast and ovarian cancer, and 31 ovarian cancer patients from 21 families with *BRCA1* germline mutations).

Results.—Upon direct comparison, no apparent survival advantage was found for *BRCA1*-associated breast cancers. Survival was equal to or worse than that of the comparison group after adjustment for age and calendar year of diagnosis. Survival appeared equal or worse in comparison with an age- and stage-matched control group. An initial survival advantage was noted that disappeared with time for *BRCA1*-associated ovarian cancers. Multivariate analyses cannot adequately be analyzed because of this time dependency. Survival again appeared equal or worse when compared with the age- and stage-matched control group.

Conclusions.—For carriers of a *BRCA1* mutation, survival may be similar or worse than that for ovarian or breast cancer in general. This finding is consistent with the adverse histopathologic features found in *BRCA1* tumors. Families that carry a *BRCA1* mutation must be under surveillance.

► There is great interest in inherited ovarian cancer and the *BRCA1* gene. As noted by the authors and in the accompanying editorial by Lynch and Watson,[1] there are conflicting reports about the prognosis in these patients. It is reported by Rubin et al.[2] that patients with ovarian cancer and *BRCA1* have a better prognosis. In their study, the patients were matched for age and stage, but treatments were at different times and at different hospitals for the controls. The current study encompasses patients treated at the same time at 1 hospital in southern Sweden—which helps to eliminate some bias—and this study shows no survival advantage. The number of patients with ovarian cancer in any of these series is small, but it does appear that those with *BRCA1* may not have a survival advantage when compared with appropriate controls.

A.L. Herbst, M.D.

References

1. Lynch HT, Watson P: BRCA 1, pathology and survival (editorial). *J Clin Oncol* 16:395–396, 1998.
2. Rubin S, Benjamin I, Behbakht K, et al: Clinical and pathological features of ovarian cancer in women with germ-line mutations of *BRCA1*. *N Engl J Med* 335:1413–1416, 1996.

The Effect of Intrauterine Diethylstilbestrol Exposure on Ovarian Reserve Screening

Sangvai M, Thie J, Hofmann GE (Bethesda Hosp, Cincinnati, Ohio)
Am J Obstet Gynecol 177:568–572, 1997 19–3

Introduction.—Diethylstilbestrol, a nonsteroidal synthetic estrogen, was initially thought to be safe and effective for preventing threatened abortion and stillbirth. Up to 2 million women were exposed to diethylstilbestrol between 1940 and 1970. In 1971, it was demonstrated that this estrogen was associated with clear-cell adenocarcinoma of the vagina in women who were exposed in utero, and was subsequently banned by the Food and Drug Administration. Little is known about ovarian function in diethylstilbestrol-exposed women. The potential role of diethylstilbestrol in accelerating the process of oocyte loss as a possible cause of reduced reproductive potential in women exposed to this synthetic estrogen was investigated.

Methods.—Ovarian reserve screening was conducted in 402 women, 20 of whom had intrauterine diethylstilbestrol exposure and 382 who did not. The 2 groups were compared with respect to their age, incidence of diminished ovarian reserve, and cycle length. Comparison of the total human menopausal gonadotropin dose, the day of human chorionic gonadotropin administration, the peak estradiol level, and the number of mature follicles was conducted on 9 women with and 204 women without diethylstilbestrol exposure.

Results.—The non–diethylstilbestrol-exposed women were similar in average age (35 years) to the diethylstilbestrol-exposed women (37 years). Diminished ovarian reserve was seen in 3 of 20 exposed women (15.8%) and in 57 of 382 nonexposed women (15.3%). There were also similarities between the exposed and nonexposed women in the amounts of human menopausal gonadotropin (30 vs. 33.7 ampules) required to achieve peak estradiol levels (633 vs. 817 pg/mL) with comparable numbers of follicles (5.7 vs. 5.4) on the day of human chorionic gonadotropin administration.

Conclusions.—A similar incidence of diminished ovarian reserve and a similar follicular response to gonadotropin was observed in the diethylstilbestrol-exposed and nonexposed women. The ovarian follicular apparatus is not affected by intrauterine exposure to diethylstilbestrol.

► This is a nonrandomized study from an infertility clinic of 20 patients exposed in vitro to diethylstilbestrol (DES) and 388 unexposed. It was found that the DES-exposed women were slightly but not significantly older (37 ± 3.4 years vs. 36 ± 4.4 years in controls). Although higher estradiol levels were seen in controls, the number of follicles and mean number of human menopausal gonadotropin (HMG) ampules (33.7 vs. 30) were slightly higher but not significantly higher in the DES-exposed women. As noted by the authors, these data do not demonstrate decreased ovarian reserve in the DES population.

A.L. Herbst, M.D.

Serum CA 125 Concentrations in Women of Different Ages, Hormonal Statuses, or Clinical Conditions

Koper NP, Thomas CMG, Massuger LFAG, et al (Univ of Nijmegen, The Netherlands)

Int J Gynecol Cancer 7:405–411, 1997 19–4

Objective.—Serum cancer antigen (CA) 25 can be used to make a differential diagnosis, monitor a patient's response to therapy, detect disease before second-look surgery, and make a prognostic assessment during follow up of ovarian cancer patients. The magnitude of changes in serum CA 125 levels during the normal menstrual cycle, the suppressed or stimulated cycle, pregnancy, and hormone replacement therapy after menopause were retrospectively evaluated to gain a better understanding of factors that influence the serum CA 125 concentration.

Methods.—Serum CA 125 concentrations were studied in 300 women aged 16 to 61 years. Between-group and within-group comparisons were analyzed statistically.

Results.—In women with a healthy normal-cycle and in women using oral contraceptives, serum CA levels were an average of 14% and 11% higher, respectively, in the early follicular period than in the luteal phase. Concentrations of CA 125 were essentially unchanged in women undergoing ovarian stimulation. Normal pregnant women had the highest CA 125 concentrations during the first trimester, whereas concentrations in the second and third trimester were similar to those in normal-cycle women. In postmenopausal women taking hormone replacement therapy, mean serum CA 125 concentrations increased from a pretreatment level of 9.9 U/mL to 11.5 U/mL in nonhysterectomy patients but declined by 1.5 U/mL in patients who had had a hysterectomy.

Conclusion.—Variations in levels of sex hormones have little effect on serum CA 125 levels. Changes in endometrial tissue appear to have a larger influence on serum CA 125 levels.

► In view of the widespread interest in CA 125, I thought it worthwhile to reproduce this article on 300 women in various clinical circumstances whose CA 125 had been measured. The main messages are that increases in CA 125 are particularly notable in the first trimester of pregnancy and also occurred during the follicular phase of the cycle. However, an increase was not seen during ovulation induction. In addition, postmenopausal women were found to have markedly lower values—usually less than 10 U/mL—and the authors suggest that it may be wise to use a value lower than the usual 35 U/mL in the postmenopausal group. This seems to me to be a wise clinical guideline.

A.L. Herbst, M.D.

20 Human Papillomavirus

Natural History of Cervicovaginal Papillomavirus Infection in Young Women

Ho GYF, Bierman R, Beardsley L, et al (Albert Einstein College of Medicine, Bronx, NY; Rutgers Univ, New Brunswick, NJ)

N Engl J Med 338:423–428, 1998 20–1

Introduction.—One of the most common sexually transmitted diseases is genital infection with human papillomavirus (HPV), with a prevalence ranging up to 46%. Cervical dysplasia and cervical cancer have been associated with genital HPV, but information about its natural history is limited, including whether genital HPV is transient, whether specific types

TABLE 3.—Risk Factors for Persistence of Human Papilloma Virus Infection for ≥ 6 Months in College Women*

Risk Factor	Adjusted Odds Ratio (95% CI)	P Value
Age (per additional yr)	1.1 (1.1–1.2)	0.05
No. of cigarettes smoked/day since previous visit		
None	1.0	0.003†
≤5	0.8 (0.5–1.3)	
>5	0.3 (0.2–0.7)	
Status of HPV infection at previous visit‡		
New infection	1.0	
Already persistent for 6 mo	2.3 (1.4–3.8)	0.001
Already persistent for >6 mo	3.1 (1.8–5.6)	<0.001
Infection of unknown duration	1.4 (0.9–2.2)	0.19
Multiple types detected at previous visit	4.1 (2.7–6.3)	<0.001
High-risk types detected at previous visit	1.5 (1.1–2.2)	0.03

*Results were obtained from a time-dependent generalized linear regression model with a generalized estimating-equation approach. CI denotes confidence interval.

†P value is for linear trend.

‡Human papilloma virus results of 2 consecutive visits were grouped as a pair. An infection at the previous visit was classified as a new infection if the HPV types had not been detected at previous visits, as a continual type-specific persistent infection if at least one of the types had been detected 6 or more months before, or as an infection of unknown duration if the most recent visit was the baseline visit or if no information from previous visits was available. (Courtesy of Ho GYF, Bierman RK, Beardsley L, et al: Natural history of cervicovaginal papillomavirus infection in young women. *N Engl J Med* 338:423–428, 1998. Reprinted by permission of *The New England Journal of Medicine*.

TABLE 4.—Relative Risk for the Association Between Continual Human Papilloma Virus Infection and the Development of Squamous Intraepithelial Lesions*

HPV Status	Relative Risk (95% CI)	P Value
HPV-negative at the previous or current visit	1.0	
HPV-positive at both visits†	20.9 (8.6-51.0(	<0.001
With different HPV types	14.7 (4.5–48.3)	<0.001
Non-high risk types at current visit	9.6 (1.9–47.6)	0.006
High-risk types at current visit	22.2 (5.5–89.5)	<0.001
With the same HPV types	25.5 (10.2–63.7)	<0.001
Non-high risk types	6.9 (1.4–34.1)	0.02
High-risk types	37.2 (14.6–94.8)	<0.001

*Results were obtained from univariate time-dependent proportional-hazards regression analysis. Continual HPV infection was determined by the HPV results at 2 consecutive visits—the current visit when a Pap smear was taken and the previous 6-month visit. CI denotes confidence interval.

†Women who were positive for HPV at both visits were subclassified according to whether they had continual infection of different types or of the same type and whether high-risk types were involved. The relative-risk estimates were obtained from separate univariate analyses for each classification, with the women who were negative for HPV at one or both visits as the reference group.

(Courtesy of Ho GYF, Bierman RK, Beardsley L, et al: Natural history of cervicovaginal papillomavirus infection in young women. *N Engl J Med* 338:423–428, 1998. Reprinted by permission of *The New England Journal of Medicine*. Copyright Massachusetts Medical Society.)

are associated with cervical cancer, and whether these high-risk types have natural histories that are different from those of other types. Risk factors for HPV infection, its incidence, and duration were examined.

Methods.—For 3 years, 608 college women were studied at 6-month intervals. Information about lifestyle and sexual behavior was collected at each visit. For the detection of HPV DNA by polymerase chain reaction and Southern blot hybridization, cervicovaginal lavage samples were obtained. Annual Papanicolaou smears were taken.

Results.—There was a 43% cumulative 36-month incidence of HPV infection. Younger age, Hispanic ethnicity, black race, an increased number of vaginal-sex partners, high frequencies of vaginal sex and alcohol consumption, anal sex and certain characteristics of partners, (such as regular partners with an increased number of lifetime partners), and not being in school were significantly associated with an increased risk of HPV infection (Table 3). The median duration of new infections was 8 months. Older age, types of HPV associated with cervical cancer, and infection with multiple types of HPV, but not smoking were related to the persistence of HPV for 6 months or more. Persistent HPV infection, particularly with high-risk types, increased the risk of abnormal Papanicolaou smears (Table 4).

Conclusion.—There is a high incidence of HPV infection in sexually active young college women. The associated cervical dysplasia should be managed conservatively because of the short duration of most HPV infections in these women.

▶ This is an interesting study of the natural history of HPV infection. A couple of important points are worth emphasizing. First, in sexually active young women, the frequency of HPV infection is high, and in most individuals the duration is short (i.e., a median of about 8 months in this study). Although an abnormal Papanicolaou smear was more likely in those with persistent HPV infection, Table 3 indicates that multiple types detected at a previous visit are actually greater risk factors than the high-risk types. Table 4 shows that if high-risk types were detected at both a previous visit and the current visit, the relative risk is the greatest, but there is still a significant increase in elevated risk, even if non-high-risk types are detected. The ongoing National Cancer Institute trial to evaluate management of low-risk Papanicolaou smears low grade squamous intraepithelial lesion and atypical squamous cells of undetermined significance has recently closed the LGSIL arm for HPV testing. Part of the reason is that so many subjects in the trials are positive for the virus and HPV testing did not yield useful results. All of this information adds to the evidence that HPV testing for clinical management of abnormal smears is not yet ready to be implemented in clinical practice.

A.L. Herbst, M.D.

Prospective Seroepidemiologic Study of Human Papillomavirus Infection as a Risk Factor for Invasive Cervical Cancer

Dillner J, Lehtinen M, Björge T, et al (Karolinska Inst, Stockholm; Natl Public Health Inst at Helsinki; Inst for Epidemiological Cancer Research, Oslo, Norway; et al)

J Natl Cancer Inst 89:1293–1299, 1997 20–2

Objective.—Human papillomavirus (HPV) infection and other sexually transmitted diseases such as *Chlamydia trachomatis* and cigarette smoking are risk factors for invasive cervical cancer. The individual contributions of each of these risks has not been established. The HPV-associated risk for invasive cervical cancer was assessed in a prospective study.

Methods.—Blood samples were obtained from 700,000 residents of Finland, Norway, and Sweden. Women were studied for 5 years, and the 182 women who had diagnoses of invasive cervical cancer were age-matched with 538 controls in a nested-case control study. Human papillomavirus, *Chlamydia*, and serum serology were determined at enrollment. Relative risks for cervical cancer were estimated using conditional regression analysis.

Results.—Infection with HPV was associated with an increased risk of cervical cancer (relative risk [RR] = 2.4). Neither smoking nor *C. trachomatis* infection increased the risk significantly. An HPV16 infection increased the relative risk of squamous cell carcinoma in the low sexually transmitted disease prevalence cohort (RR = 11.8). An HPV18 infection increased the relative risk of adenocarcinoma in all cohorts (RR = 3.4).

Conclusion.—An HPV16 infection increased the relative risk of squamous cell carcinoma in the low sexually transmitted disease prevalence cohort (RR = 11.8), and HPV18 infection increased the relative risk of adenocarcinoma in all cohorts (RR = 3.4). Smoking and *C. trachomatis* infection did not increase those risks.

▶ I have included this Scandinavian study because of the interesting finding that HPV seropositivity was most predictive of invasive cervical cancer in patients with a low prevalence of antibodies against other sexually transmitted parasites (e.g., in this case, *C. trachomatis*). It is of interest that in patients with evidence of high prevalence of other infections, the association did not hold. This suggests that HPV clinical testing may prove to be the most useful in populations without a high prevalence of sexually transmitted diseases.

A.L. Herbst, M.D.

Stringent Criteria for Histological Diagnosis of Koilocytosis Fail to Eliminate Overdiagnosis of Human Papillomavirus Infection and Cervical Intraepithelial Neoplasia Grade 1 CIN 1

Abadi MA, Ho GYF, Burk RD, et al (Albert Einstein College of Medicine, Bronx, NY)

Hum Pathol 29:54–59, 1998 20–3

Introduction.—The causative agent of cervical intraepithelial neoplasia and cervical cancer is human papillomavirus (HPV). The diagnosis of cervical intraepithelial neoplasia has been associated with infection with HPV types 16, 18, 31, 33, 35 and other oncogenic types. There may be an overdiagnosis of cervical intraepithelial neoplasia 1 that would affect clinical management and related health care costs. The validity of the histopathologic diagnosis of koilocytosis in detecting genital HPV infection in low-grade lesions using molecular detection of HPV DNA as the gold standard was evaluated. The extent of false positivity or overdiagnosis of HPV infection was estimated.

Methods.—Strict criteria for histologic diagnosis of koilocytosis were determined by using polymerase chain reaction and Southern blot hybridization as the gold standard for diagnosis of koilocytosis. There were 511 patients with colposcopic biopsy specimens, including 76 with referral diagnoses of negative cervix and 241 with cervical intraepithelial neoplasia 1 or koilocytosis.

Results.—Human papillomavirus-infected and uninfected patients were not distinguished with referral diagnoses for low-grade lesions. There was a 74.8% false-positive rate for prediction of HPV infection. There was an increase in the prevalence of HPV infection among patients with biopsy specimens showing negative (43.7%), minimal (52.4%), or definite (69.5%) features of koilocytosis after stringent diagnostic criteria were applied (Table 3). There was a greater likelihood of infection among patients infected with high viral load or oncogenic HPV infection. A significant number of women with a diagnosis of cervical intraepithelial

TABLE 3.—Revised Diagnoses and Prevalence of Human Papillomavirus (*HPV*) Infection

	Negative (*N* = 71)	Minimal (*N* = 36)	Definite (*N* = 118)	*P*
HPV positive*	31 (43.7)	33 (52.4)	82 (69.5)	.001
High viral load	20 (28.2)	16 (25.4)	56 (47.5)	.004
High-risk type	20 (28.2)	20 (31.8)	50 (42.4)	.040

NOTE: All biopsy specimens were reviewed and classified as having no evidence of koilocytosis (group A), minimal features of koilocytosis (group B), or definite features of koilocytosis.

*Subjects with HPV detected in each diagnostic group; numbers in parentheses are the proportion with HPV infection.

(Courtesy of Abadi MA, Ho GYF, Burk RD, et al: Stringent criteria for histological diagnosis of koilocytosis fail to eliminate overdiagnosis of human papillomavirus infection and cervical intraepithelial neoplasia grade 1. *Hum Pathol* 29:54–59, 1998.)

neoplasia grade 1/koilocytosis (34%) did not have HPV infection, despite the increased predictive value of stringent diagnostic criteria.

Conclusions.—Patients with histologic diagnosis of cervical intraepithelial neoplasia grade 1 or HPV infection should be observed for several months before definite ablative treatment is begun because most low-grade lesions spontaneously regress. The primary predictor of outcome of cervical intraepithelial neoplasia continues to be histologic grading until cost-effective and sensitive modalities for molecular detection of high viral load or oncogenic HPV infections become available.

▶ It is frequently stated that stringently diagnosed koilocytosis is usually accompanied by HPV infection and that high viral load increases the likelihood of a positive morphological reaction. This study appears to provide different data using the very sensitive polymerase chain reaction (PCR) and less sensitive Southern blot testing for multiple HPV types. Active infection was found in only 69.5% of those with significant criteria for koilocytosis/HPV. The authors did not test the tissue directly by in situ hybridization, which may have altered the results, but the authors suggest their results indicate that aggressive therapy of low-grade lesions based on their data is not warranted, because many of these patients have lesions that will regress. I think that their concern that these lesions may frequently be overly diagnosed is correct.

A.L. Herbst, M.D.

Human Papillomavirus Testing as Triage for Atypical Squamous Cells of Undetermined Significance and Low-grade Squamous Intraepithelial Lesions: Sensitivity, Specificity, and Cost-effectiveness

Kaufman RH, Adam E, Icenogle J, et al (Baylor College of Medicine, Houston; Ctrs for Disease Control and Prevention, Atlanta, Ga)

Am J Obstet Gynecol 177:930–936, 1997 20–4

Introduction.—In the development of intraepithelial and invasive carcinoma of the cervix, the role of infection with human papillomavirus is well established. No study has previously evaluated the cost-effectiveness, sen-

TABLE 2.—Colposcopically Directed Biopsy Results from 462 Women With Atypical Squamous Cells of Undetermined Significance or Low-grade Squamous Intraepithelial Lesions on Referral Papanicolaou Smear According to Cytology and High-risk HPV Triage Algorithms

	Cytology triage				*High-risk HPV triage*				*Combined triage*			
Colposcopically indicated	*No.*	*No CIN*	*Grade 1 CIN*	*Grade 2 or 3 CIN*	*No.*	*No CIN*	*Grade 1 CIN*	*Grade 2 or 3 CIN*	*No.*	*No CIN*	*Grade 1 CIN*	*Grade 2 or 3 CIN*
Yes	194	36	116	42 (21.6*)	140	39	96	45 (25.0)	257	57	145	55 (21.4)
No	268	101	142	25 (8.6)	282	98	162	22 (7.8)	205	80	113	12 (5.9)
Sensitivity				62.7				67.2				82.1
Specificity				61.5				65.8				48.9
Positive predictive value				21.6				25.0				21.4
Negative predictive value				90.7				92.2				94.1

Percentage of all in each row.

(Courtesy of Kaufman RH, Adam E, Icenogle J, et al: Human papillomavirus testing as triage for atypical squamous cells of undetermined significance and low-grade squamous intraepithelial lesions: Sensitivity, specificity, and cost-effectiveness. *Am J Obstet Gynecol* 177:930–936, 1997.)

TABLE 3.—Follow-up of 462 Women—Cost-effectiveness (colposcopy $150, HPV testing $65)

Method	Follow-up without HPV No.	Follow-up without HPV Cost	Follow-up with HPV No.	Follow-up with HPV Cost	Both methods No.	Both methods Cost
Colposcopy	194	$29,100	180	$27,000	257	$38,550
HPV testing	0	—	462	$30,030	462	$30,030
TOTAL		$29,100		$57,030		$68,580
Grade 2 or 3 CIN identified by biopsy	42/67 (62.7%)*,†		45/67 (67.2%)*,‡		55/67 (82.1%)†,‡	

*$p = 0.71$.
†$p = 0.02$.
‡$p = 0.07$.
(Courtesy of Kaufman RH, Adam E, Icenogle J, et al: Human papillomavirus testing as triage for atypical squamous cells of undetermined significance and low-grade squamous intraepithelial lesions: Sensitivity, specificity, and cost-effectiveness. *Am J Obstet Gynecol* 177:930–936, 1997.)

sitivity, and specificity of Papanicolaou (PAP) smear alone with Pap smear with human papillomavirus (HPV) deoxyribonucleic acid testing for women with low-grade squamous intraepithelial lesions (LGSIL) or with women showing atypical squamous cells of undetermined significance (ASCUS).

Methods.—Repeat Pap smear, cervical colposcopy, directed cervical biopsy, and endocervical curettage were performed on 462 women who had Papanicolaou smear reports of ASCUS or (LGSIL). The Food and Drug Administration's approved HPV Profile test was also conducted on the women. A comparison was made of sensitivity, specificity, and cost-effectiveness of colposcopy on the basis of repeat cytologic testing vs. incorporating repeat cytologic testing and human papillomavirus screening.

Results.—In relation to increasing severity of cervical intraepithelial neoplasia, high-risk human papillomavirus deoxyribonucleic acid was detected with greater frequency, as expected. The follow-up smear was negative in 268 women. In 23.5% of these women, high-risk human papillomavirus types were found. Cervical biopsy confirmed grade 2 or 3 cervical intraepithelial neoplasia in 5.9% of women who were human papillomavirus-negative. Of those who had a positive result, 20% had confirmation on cervical biopsy. There was only a 52% sensitivity of a positive result predicting the presence of grade 2 or 3 cervical intraepithelial neoplasia. There was no difference in the frequency of biopsy-provided grade 2 or 3 cervical intraepithelial neoplasia among the women who showed ASCUS undetermined significance or LGSIL in a follow-up clinical Pap smear or between those women who had a positive test result and those with a negative test result. Because of a repeat clinic smear revealing ASCUS, LGSIL, or a high-grade squamous intraepithelial lesion, colposcopy would have been recommended for 194 women (Table 2). Biopsy showed grade 2 or 3 cervical intraepithelial neoplasia on 21.6% of these women. Because of high-risk human papillomavirus results or a high-grade squamous intraepithelial lesions being detected at the clinic visit, colposcopy would have been recommended for 180 women. Biopsy showed grade 2 or 3 cervical intraepithelial neoplasia in 25% of this group. The cost of human papillomavirus tests was nearly double that of triage based on repeat cytologic testing alone, although sensitivity and specificity were virtually identical for the 2 algorithms.

Conclusion.—For patients referred with Pap smears reported as showing ASCUS or LGSIL, the Food and Drug Administration-approved HPV Profile test is not a cost-effective triage (Table 3).

▶ The debate on HPV testing in clinical practice continues. A recent article by Cox et al.[1] suggested a cocktail of high-risk HPV types measured by hybrid capture had promise as a tool to triage low-grade or ASCUS smears.

This article by Kaufman et al. reaches a markedly different conclusion using the current FDA-approved multiple HPV typing kit. The authors appropriately note in the discussion they are probably dealing with a different population than Cox et al did. They also make the important point that they have tested the sensitivity of both the HPV kit and hybrid capture technique used by Cox et al and found them similarly sensitive.

Newer, more sensitive hybrid capture techniques may improve the result, but as shown in Tables 2 and 3 above, the technique may not be sufficiently sensitive or specific (Table 2) and is certainly more expensive (Table 3).

A.L. Herbst, M.D.

Reference

1. Cox TJ, Lorincz AT, Schiffman MH: Human papillomavirus testing by Hybrid Capture appears to be useful in triaging women with a cytologic diagnosis of atypical squamous cells of undetermined significance. *Am J Obstet Gynecol* 1996; 171:946–954.

21 Cervical Cytology

The Value of Repeat Pap Smear at the Time of Initial Colposcopy

Spitzer M, Ryskin M, Chernys AE, et al (Queens Hosp Ctr, Jamaica, NY)

Gynecol Oncol 67:3–7, 1997 21–1

Background.—It is standard practice in the United States to perform a repeat Papanicolaou (Pap) smear at the time of initial colposcopy. Whether the clinical benefits of this repeat Pap smear justify its cost was determined.

Study Design.—A record review was performed for all patients who had an initial colposcopy at Queens Hospital Center between 1984 and 1995. A repeat Pap smear was defined as clinically valuable if it would have changed patient management.

Findings.—The study group consisted of 2,969 women who underwent initial colposcopy at this institution during the study period. Of these women, only 139 had no repeat Pap smear. Based on the triage protocols of this institution, the repeat Pap smear at the time of initial colposcopy would have indicated a need for cone biopsy in 1.1% and a more careful follow-up in 1.6% of these patients. No cancers would have been missed in the absence of repeat Pap smears. The cost savings of skipping the repeat Pap smear would have been $24.23 per patient or $68,580 for the entire study group. At the national level, skipping the repeat Pap smear would save more than $24 million per year.

Conclusions.—Repeating the Pap smear at initial colposcopy provided little additional information. A Pap smear just before colposcopy may interfere with the colposcopic examination. Considering its cost and the limited clinical benefit provided, the practice of routine repeat Pap smear before initial colposcopy does not appear to be justified.

▶ This article and its accompanying editorial by Noller[1] call for a change in current practice. It has long been the usual practice to repeat an abnormal Pap smear at the time of colposcopy, but as Spitzer et al. and Noller indicate, this is probably more costly than worthwhile. The issue is, of course, cost.

I believe the argument not to repeat the Pap smear at the time of colposcopy is compelling. However, if the smear has been done and analyzed at an outside institution, I would repeat the Pap before colposcopy, using the endocyte brush or similar device to check the endocervix. But I would not send it to the cytology laboratory unless the colposcopy were unsatisfactory or the colposcopy findings were negative (just to be sure the first smear was not erroneous), particularly if dealing with a previously reported HGSIL. If one is dealing with a low-grade lesion, it is probably adequate to repeat the smear in 6 months.

A.L. Herbst, M.D.

Reference

1. Noller KL: When one more Pap smear is one too many (editorial). *Gynecol Oncol* 67:1–2, 1997.

Clinical Evaluation of Atypical Glandular Cells of Undetermined Significance on Cervical Cytology

Duska LR, Flynn CF, Chen A, et al (Massachusetts Gen Hosp, Boston)
Obstet Gynecol 91:278–282, 1998 21–2

Background.—In 1988, the Bethesda system for categorizing the results of Papanicolaou tests was introduced. One of the categories introduced was "atypical glandular cells of undetermined significance" (AGCUS). This category is not as well defined as its squamous counterpart. The risk factors and incidence for a clinically significant AGCUS diagnosis were determined.

Methods.—Three years of patients with AGCUS were identified through a computer search. The cytologic diagnosis was reviewed for 73 patients who had been examined in the colposcopy clinic. Only high-grade squamous intraepithelial lesions (SIL), endocervical glandular atypia, carcinomas, and lesions worse than the aforementioned were considered clinically significant.

Results.—The AGCUS diagnosis rate was 0.167%. Colposcopy was performed on all patients, and endocervical curettage was performed on 88%. Approximately one third of patients had clinically significant diagnoses, including 8.2% who had cancer. Researchers determined a risk of

TABLE 3.—Final Diagnosis by Menopausal Status

Diagnosis	Premenopausal $n = 46$	Postmenopausal $n = 27$	Total
Benign/low-grade SIL	28	20	48
Endocervical atypia	2	1	3
High-grade SIL	14	2*	16
Endocervical carcinoma	1	0	1
Endometrial carcinoma	0	3	3
Ovarian carcinoma	1	1	2
Clinically significant lesions	18 (39%)	7 (27%)*	

*$P = 0.04$.
†$P = 0.31$.
Abbreviation: SIL, squamous intraepithelial lesion.
(Courtesy of Duska LR, Flynn CF, Chen A, et al: Clinical evaluation of atypical glandular cells of undetermined significance on cervical cytology. *Obstetrics and Gynecology* 91:278–282, 1998. Reprinted with permission from The American College of Obstetricians and Gynecologists.)

25.5% for an AGCUS diagnosis. A 50% risk was determined for a concurrent squamous diagnosis. High-grade SIL was found to be much more prevalent in premenopausal (30.4%) than in postmenopausal (7.4%) patients (P = 01.04) (Table 3). The category "suggestive of reactive" predicted nonsignificant lesions with 95% confidence.

Conclusion.—With further studies, the most cost-effective and appropriate method for clinical evaluation of AGCUS will be determined, and triage algorithms can be established.

▶ The diagnosis of AGCUS, as mentioned elsewhere in this section, causes particular difficulty for clinicians. The category is still not clearly defined, and the meaning of the diagnosis may vary from laboratory to laboratory. This study evaluates a small group of 73 patients (81 smears). About one third had biopsy evidence of a significant lesion, and, perhaps surprisingly, invasive cancer was found in 8.2%. As has been reported in many other series, the cytologic category of AGCUS frequently is accompanied by a squamous lesion. I was surprised at the high rate of abnormality among the premenopausal patients. Our cytology laboratory provides us with the modifiers of "favor reactive" or "favor neoplasia," which I find quite useful. I have followed up the reactive group with a smear in 6 months, but I have a workup done for those that are in the "favor neoplasia" category. I do an endometrial biopsy on postmenopausal patients who are in the "favor neoplasia" category, even though it was not found to be a useful maneuver in this study. I particularly would perform a biopsy on a postmenopausal patient for whom no explanation of the AGCUS smear is available.

A.L. Herbst, M.D.

Biopsy Findings in Five Hundred Thirty-One Patients With Atypical Glandular Cells of Uncertain Significance as Defined by the Bethesda System

Eddy GL, Strumpf KB, Wojtowycz MA, et al (State Univ of New York, Syracuse; Croose Hosp, Syracuse, NY; Pathology Associates of Syracuse, NY)

Am J Obstet Gynecol 177:1188–1195, 1997 21–3

Background.—The histologic findings of previous biopsy specimens from patients with "atypical glandular cells of uncertain significance" (AGCUS) were examined to determine the limitations and utility of this category of the Bethesda system.

Methods.—Researchers examined 3 years of computerized records and discovered 1,117 patients given a diagnosis of AGCUS, of which 531 had undergone biopsies within 1 year of the AGCUS-detecting Papanicolaou smear. These 531 biopsy patient records were examined to determine the validity of the AGCUS categorization.

Results.—Table 4 shows a portion of the histologic findings listed by AGCUS subcategory. Of the 531 patients originally classified as having

TABLE 4.—Biopsy Specimen Results in 27 Patients With Atypical Glandular Cells of Uncertain Significance and Squamous Intraepithelial Lesions

AGCUS subcategory	*Total*	*Neg./react.*	*SIL*
Favor reactive	11	3	8
Unable to further classify	15	5	10
Favor premalignant/malignant	1	0	1
Favor endocervical adenocarcinoma in situ	0	0	0
Suspicious for endometrial carcinoma	0	0	0
All subcategories	27	8	19

Abbreviations: AGCUS, atypical glandular cells of uncertain significance; *Neg./react.*, normal tissue/reactive changes; *SIL*, squamous intraepithelial lesions.

(Courtesy of Eddy GL, Strumpf KB, Wojtowycz MA, et al: Biopsy findings in five hundred thirty-one patients with atypical glandular cells of uncertain significance as defined by the Bethesda system. *Am J Obstet Gynecol* 177:1188–1195, 1997.)

AGCUS, 36% had preinvasive (83%) or invasive (17%) lesions as determined by biopsy. Of the preinvasive lesions, 89% were squamous. Of the invasive lesions, 97% were glandular. Twenty-eight (88%) patients with invasive and preinvasive lesions were found to have endometrial carcinomas (Table 7).

Conclusion.—Nearly 75% of all patients that were categorized as having AGCUS had squamous rather than glandular lesions. Thus, the name AGCUS does not differentiate between the significant risk of the usually glandular malignant lesions that arise from the endometrium and the less threatening presence of atypical squamous cells of uncertain significance.

▶ This is a large series of smears with a diagnosis of AGCUS. The series is much larger and with slightly different results than the Duska article (see Abstract 21–2). This series is somewhat biased because the review was only of cases that had biopsies. There were 1,117 patients with AGCUS diagnoses, but this report deals only with the 531 for whom biopsy or hysterectomy information was available. Slightly more than one third (36%) had neoplasia, and, interestingly, 89% of the preinvasive diagnoses were squamous, whereas 97% of the invasive tumors were glandular.

Tables 4 and 7 show the yield of premalignant and invasive lesions by AGCUS category. Although the "favor reactive" category had a surprising 25% SIL rate, the results were twice as high for SILs in the "favor neoplasia" category. The positive predictive value for the latter reached 95%.

As noted by the authors, in this report as well as in numerous others referred to in the article, a diagnosis of AGCUS on cytologic examination is accompanied by a preinvasive SIL in about one third of cases. The risk is highest among those cases with a "favor neoplasia" designation. We still need more experience with this perplexing category; however, I do triage (colposcopy and biopsy) those cases categorized as favoring neoplasia, and I repeat the smear in half a year for those reliable patients who fit in the "favor reactive" category.

A.L. Herbst, M.D.

TABLE 7.—Invasive Lesion Detected by Biopsy in Patients With Atypical Glandular Cells of Uncertain Significance With or Without Atypical Squamous Cells of Uncertain Significance or Squamous Intraepithelial Lesion Listed by Subcategory

AGCUS subcategory	*Patients*	*Endometrial*	*Vulvar*	*Cervical*	*Other*	*Total*
Favor reactive	289	1 (0.3%)	0	0	0	1 (0.3%)
Unable to further classify	198	9 (4.5%)	1 (0.5%)	1 (0.5%)	0	11 (5.6%)
Favor premalignant/malignant	22	2 (9.1%)	0	0	2 (9.1%)*	4 (18%)
Favor endocervical adenocarcinoma in situ	4	0	0	0	0	0
Suspicious for endometrial carcinoma	18	16 (89%)	0	0	0	16 (89%)
TOTAL	531	28 (5.3%)	1 (0.2%)	1 (0.2%)	2 (0.4%)	32 (6.0%)

*One case of metastic breast carcinoma and 1 case of metastatic ovarian carcinoma.

Abbreviations: AGCUS, Atypical glandular cells of uncertain significance.

(Courtesy of Eddy GL, Strumpf KB, Wojtowycz MA, et al: Biopsy findings in five hundred thirty-one patients with atypical glandular cells of uncertain significance as defined by the Bethesda system. *Am J Obstet Gynecol* 177:1188–1195, 1997.)

22 Cervical Intraepithelial Neoplasia

Outcomes After Cervical Cold Knife Conization With Complete and Incomplete Excision of Abnormal Epithelium: A Review of 699 Cases
Mohamed-Noor K, Quinn MA, Tan J (Royal Women's Hosp, Melbourne, Victoria, Australia)
Gynecol Oncol 67:34–38, 1997 22–1

Objective.—Ablative techniques and cervical conization have replaced hysterectomy as the treatment of choice for carcinoma in situ. Studies have shown that even incomplete removal of neoplastic epithelium during conization can result in cure of cervical intraepithelial neoplasia (CIN). A retrospective analysis of outcome after complete and incomplete conization as treatment for CIN was conducted.

Methods.—A total of 699 cone biopsy specimens, obtained at the Royal Women's Hospital in Melbourne between 1966 and 1992, were examined histologically. Patients were followed up for 2 months to 21 years.

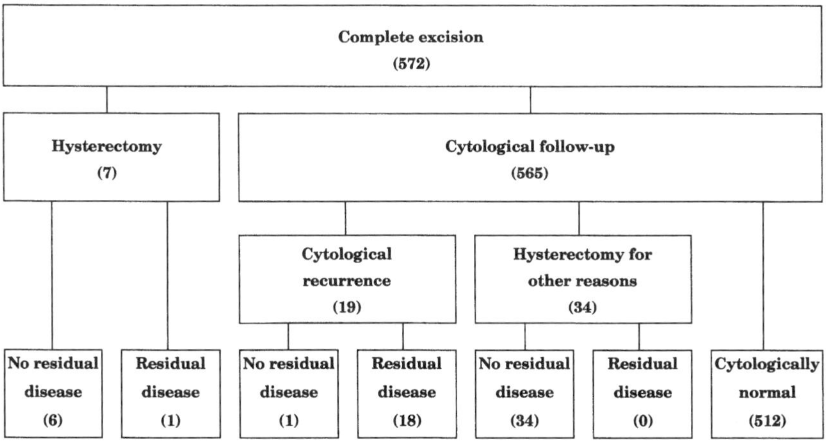

FIGURE 1.—Follow-up and outcomes after complete conization. (Courtesy of Mohamed-Noor K, Quinn MA, Tan J: Outcomes after cervical cold knife conization with complete and incomplete excision of abnormal epithelium: A review of 699 cases. *Gynecol Oncol* 67:34–38, 1997.)

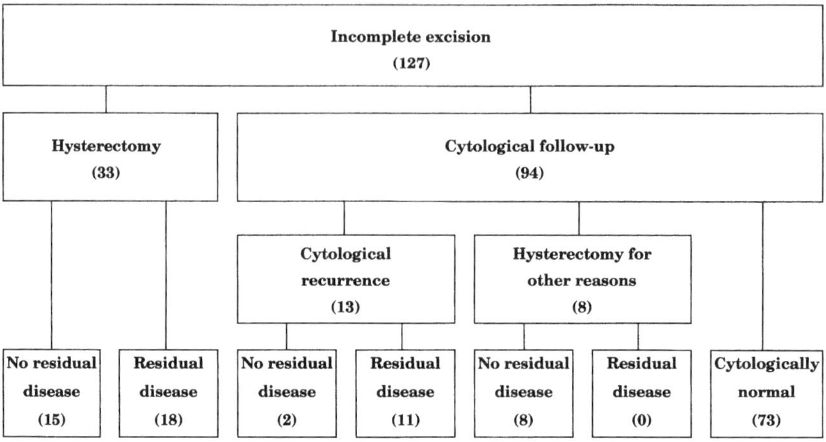

FIGURE 2.—Follow-up and outcomes after incomplete conization. (Courtesy of Mohamed-Noor K, Quinn MA, Tan J: Outcomes after cervical cold knife conization with complete and incomplete excision of abnormal epithelium: A review of 699 cases. *Gynecol Oncol* 67:34–38, 1997.)

Results.—Abnormal epithelium was completely excised in 572 patients (Fig 1). Abnormal epithelium was incompletely excised in 127 patients (Fig 2). The cure rate for complete excision was 96.7%. The cure rate for incomplete excision was 77% but varied depending on the site of the disease. In this study, cone biopsy carried an overall cure rate of 93%, which is comparable to the results of Bjerre et al. of 87% and Ahlgren et al. of 93%. Incomplete excision was detected in 18% of cone biopsies. Possible recurrences after complete excision are the result of multifocal disease, inadequate examination of the biopsy specimen, or recurrence relating to ongoing exposure to human papillomavirus infection.

Conclusion.—Cone biopsy results in a cure of CIN in 96.7% of patients when the excision is complete. Because recurrent disease is always a possibility, these patients should be followed up closely. Most patients (77%) with incomplete excision are also cured of their disease.

▶ This large study from Australia reconfirms that cold knife conization is excellent therapy for CIN. Figures 1 and 2 nicely summarize the data from this study of 699 conizations. A few points are worth explaining. First, a cone with complete excision (i.e., negative margins,) yields an excellent cure rate of almost 97%. However, long-term follow up is mandatory because 3.3% of the lesions do recur, presumably as a result of multifocal disease recurrence. For those with positive margins in this series, the cure rate was obviously lower, but still an impressive 77%, emphasizing that, even with positive margins, a conization can be curative, particularly if the involved margin is ectocervical.

A.L. Herbst, M.D.

Residual and Recurrent Disease After Laser Conization for Cervical Intraepithelial Neoplasia

Skjeldestad FE, Hagen B, Lie AK, et al (Norwegian Univ, Trondheim, Norway)
Obstet Gynecol 90:428–433, 1997 22–2

Introduction.—The incidence of cervical cancer can be reduced by up to 90% with organized screening with Papanicolaou (Pap) smears, but guidelines for the screening interval differ as well as the follow-up interval after treatment of precancerous lesions of the cervix uteri. The risks for residual and recurrent disease were assessed by studying women treated by laser conization for high-grade lesions of the cervix uteri. Data were provided to refine the Pap smear follow-up interval after treatment.

Methods.—A total of 1,081 women were treated for cervical intraepithelial neoplasia grade II to III during a 10-year period. They were followed up for residual or recurrent disease, which was verified histologically. Survival analyses were used to assess the cumulative incidence of recurrent disease. Clinical features at initial treatment that were associated with the risk of residual or recurrent disease were predicted using logistic regression analysis.

Results.—In 20 study participants (1.9%), residual disease was diagnosed. There was an extremely low cumulative incidence of recurrent disease, increasing nearly linearly with an annual incidence of 3 per 1,000 woman-years. Residual disease and recurrent disease were significantly associated with involved resection margins when compared with disease-free resection margins as reference (Fig 1).

Conclusions.—Depending upon the histologic evaluation of cone margins, a differential follow-up interval is recommended. Women with free resection margins should return at a 3-year interval for follow-up, if there is no residual disease. Pap smears are recommended at annual intervals for

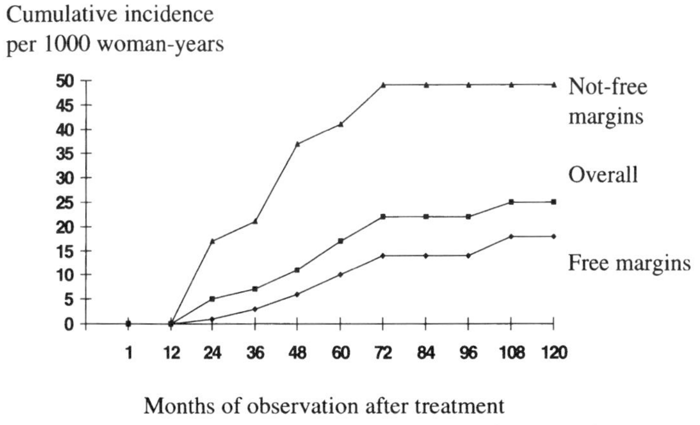

FIGURE 1.—Cumulative incidence of recurrence by histologic findings in the resection margin. (Courtesy of Skjeldestad FE, Hagen B, Lie AK, et al: Residual and recurrent disease after laser conization for cervical intraepithelial neoplasia. *Obstet Gynecol* 90:428–433. Copyright 1997, reprinted with permission of The American College of Obstetricians and Gynecologists.)

women who have disease extended to the cone margins through the fourth postoperative year, before returning at a 3-year interval as practiced in the general screening program.

▶ Although this article deals with laser cone, the results probably apply to other excisional procedures. It is worth noting the "accepted" protocol in Norway was 4 visits for a repeat Pap in year 1, 2 in year 2, and then annually thereafter. This changed in 1993 to only 2 visits the first year, then annually.

In their study the authors did defocus the laser beam to vaporize the entire cone bed. As shown in Figure 1, there was a low rate of recurrence even in patients with positive margins. The authors appropriately note that other studies have shown higher recurrence rates, which are likely related to the size of the cone. Based on this study the authors recommend a 1-year smear with negative margins and 4 annual smears if the margins are positive, to be followed by a smear at 3-year intervals because the risk of recurring disease was so low. I would like to see more studies before adopting these guidelines, but 2 smears the first year followed by annual follow up seems reasonable.

A.L. Herbst, M.D.

Duration of Pregnancy After Carbon Dioxide Laser Conization of the Cervix: Influence of Cone Height

Raio L, Ghezzi F, Di Naro E, et al (Kantonssiptal, Münsterlingen, Switzerland; Univ of Pavia, Varese, Italy; Univ of Bari, Italy; et al)

Obstet Gynecol 90:978–982, 1997 22–3

Introduction.—Patients with a history of cervical conization have a higher incidence of preterm labor and delivery. The outcome of women undergoing laser conization is still controversial. This article determines whether carbon dioxide laser conization of the cervix is a risk factor for preterm delivery in subsequent gestation, and evaluates whether there is any relationship between duration of pregnancy and cone measurements.

Methods.—The study included 64 women with singleton pregnancies after carbon dioxide laser conization and 64 controls. They were followed for reproductive events. Recordings were taken of pregnancy duration, rate of preterm birth, and mode of delivery to investigate the relationship between cone height and subsequent preterm delivery. Logistic regression analysis and Cox proportional hazard modeling were used.

Results.—In the rate of preterm delivery or in the duration of pregnancy, there was no difference found in the 2 groups. There was a higher rate of preterm delivery for women with cone height of at least 10 mm than for women with a cone height of less than 10 mm or the controls (Fig 2). In predicting the occurrence of preterm delivery and the duration of pregnancy after adjusting for known risk factors, cone height of at least 10 mm remained significant.

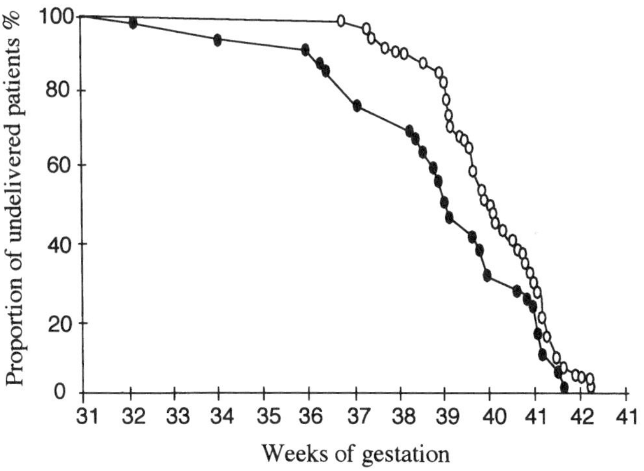

FIGURE 2.—Survival curve analysis of patients with cone height of at least 10 mm (*closed circles*) and those with cone height less than 10 mm (*open circles*). (Courtesy of Raio L, Ghezzi F, Di Naro E, et al: Duration of pregnancy after carbon dioxide laser conization of the cervix: Influence of cone height. *Obstet Gynecol* 90:978–982, 1997. Reprinted with permission from The American College of Obstetricians and Gynecologists.)

Conclusion.—For the occurrence of preterm delivery in the subsequent gestation and for the duration of pregnancy, cone height of at least 10 mm is an independent risk factor.

► This is a case control study of 64 women who underwent laser cone compared to 64 matched controls. The numbers are small, but the results are important. For those with a cone height greater than 10 mm, there was a significantly greater risk of preterm delivery when compared to controls or to those whose cone heights were less than 10 mm. These analyses were limited to subsequent singleton pregnancies. It is of interest that, overall, the difference between the cone and no-cone cases was insignificant. The authors, however, note that the study was small and had limited power to demonstrate an increase in preterm delivery in between cases and controls overall or between pregnancies before and after conization.

This study adds to the body of literature that conization adds to the risk of preterm delivery and that this risk is related to the size of the tissue removed. I believe this observation is valid regardless of the technique used, i.e., laser, cold knife cone or large loop electrical excision procedure, and this is a concern the gynecologist should remember when doing these procedures on reproductive-age females.

A.L. Herbst, M.D.

Endocervical Curettage, Cone Margins, and Residual Adenocarcinoma In Situ of the Cervix

Denehy TR, Gregori CA, Breen JL (Saint Barnabas Med Ctr, Livingston, NJ)
Obstet Gynecol 90:1–6, 1997 22–4

Objective.—Adenocarcinoma in situ of the cervix is a rare cancer that usually affects women in their 30s. Whether conservative management is the treatment of choice is controversial because of the unclear natural history of the lesion. The roles of endocervical curettage (ECC) and the margin status of cervical cones in the treatment of adenocarcinoma in situ and their ability to predict residual disease reliably were evaluated in a retrospective descriptive study.

Methods.—A total of 49 cone specimens from 42 women, aged 18–65 years (average age 37 years), were evaluated for the presence or absence of cervical adenocarcinoma in situ and endocervical glandular dysplasia at the surgical margins.

Results.—All patients had abnormal cervicovaginal cytology diagnoses. In 27 patients (64%), results showed mixed lesions of adenocarcinoma in situ and squamous dysplasia. Fifteen patients had adenocarcinoma in situ. There were 40 ECCs performed at colposcopy or after conization in 32 patients. These results were compared with the pathologic findings of 28 conizations and 12 hysterectomies performed shortly thereafter in the same patients (Table 2). The rate of positive cone margins was 43%.

TABLE 2.—Residual Adenocarcinoma In Situ in Subsequent Surgical Specimen According to Endocervical Curettage (ECC) Status and Type of Surgery

	Negative ECC		Positive ECC	
	Cone (n = 18)	Hysterectomy (n = 9)	Cone (n = 10)	Hysterectomy (n = 3)
Adenocarcinoma in situ	9	2	3	0
Adenocarcinoma in situ with squamous dysplasia	6	1	3	0
Adenocarcinoma in situ with endocervical glandular dysplasia	0	0	0	3
Adenocarcinoma in situ with squamous dysplasia and adenocarcinoma	0	0	1	0
Subtotal	15/18	3/9	7/10	3/3
Total	18/27		10/13	

(Courtesy of Denehy TR, Gregori CA, Breen JL: Endocervical curettage, cone margins, and residual adenocarcinoma in situ of the cervix. *Obstet Gynecol* 90:1–6, 1997. Reprinted with permission from the American College of Obstetricians and Gynecologists.)

Conclusions.—Negative ECCs and negative cone margins do not necessarily confirm the absence of adenocarcinoma in situ. Any cytologic abnormality should be thoroughly evaluated. Patients with negative cone margins and ECC managed conservatively should be followed carefully and frequently.

► Adenocarcinoma in situ is a perplexing disease, and sufficiently rare that it is difficult to obtain adequate data to provide useful guidelines for the clinician.

This study by Denehy et al. indicates that there is a risk of residual disease in the cervix if there is a negative ECC done at colposcopy. For ECCs done before conization, 18 of 27 patients with negative ECCs were found to have adenocarcinoma in situ either in the subsequent cone or hysterectomy specimens. Follow-up information was available on 19 of the patients who were followed conservatively. One of these eventually developed disease, and invasive adenocarcinoma. All 19 patients had regular follow-up.

Clearly this is a difficult disease to treat, and it would appear wise to advocate hysterectomy for patients beyond their childbearing years. For those in their childbearing years with negative cone margins and a negative ECC done *after* the conization, I would favor follow-up every 4 months for the first year, every 6 months for up to 2 years, and then at least annually. Unfortunately I do not have any data to support this recommendation other than the fact that in this, and other series, recurrent disease is rare for patients who have close follow-up—in this small series approximately 6% of the patients developed recurrence. For those with positive cone margins desiring fertility preservation, I would try to do a repeat conization before attempting conservative follow-up.

A.L. Herbst, M.D.

The Case for Cytologic Follow-up After LEEP

Hanau CA, Bibbo M (Thomas Jefferson Univ Hosp, Philadelphia)
Acta Cytol 41:731–736, 1997 22–5

Objective.—The loop electrocautery excision procedure (LEEP) for squamous intraepithelial lesions (SILs) can be performed in a physician's office using local anesthesia. The technique takes less time, results in less bleeding than the cold knife cone, and yields histologic specimens for microscopic examination. The incidence of abnormal post-LEEP follow-up and its relationship to marginal status of LEEP specimens were evaluated.

Methods.—Diagnosis, margin readability, and margin positivity or negativity were evaluated by reviewing records and slides of 162 LEEP procedures performed between January 1992 and April 1994.

Results.—Length of follow-up averaged 10.9 months. In 67 patients, results at follow-up were normal; in 54 patients, abnormal results (atypical squamous cells of undetermined significance [ASCUS or SIL]) were noted;

and 41 patients had no follow-up. The 54 abnormal results were diagnosed as high-grade SIL in 16 patients (13.2% of follow-up cases), low-grade SIL in 27 patients (22.3% of follow-up cases), and ASCUS in 11 patients. Of the 54 specimens with abnormal results, 37 had readable margins, and 17 had unreadable margins. Of the 67 specimens with normal results, 50 had readable margins, and 17 had unreadable margins.

Conclusion.—The marginal status of LEEP specimens is unreliable in predicting recurrence of SIL. All these patients should be followed up carefully and regularly.

▶ This article correctly concludes that one needs cytologic follow-up after the LEEP procedure. With only a short follow-up of approximately 11 months, about one third of the cases have a positive result regardless of the status of the LEEP margins histologically. Some of the unreliability is probably the result of thermal artifact. Most disturbingly, one quarter of the cases failed to have follow-up. All patients treated for intraepithelial neoplasia need follow-up, usually at 6 months after the procedure. Assuming the results of the first few Papanicolaou smears are negative, annual follow-up with cytology is appropriate. I usually desire at least 3 negative smears before returning to annual follow-up.

A.L. Herbst, M.D.

Invasive Cervical Cancer After Conservative Therapy for Cervical Intraepithelial Neoplasia

Soutter WP, de Barros Lopes A, Fletcher A, et al (Hammersmith Hosp, London; Gateshead Hosps NHS Trust, England; London School of Hygiene and Tropical Medicine; et al)

Lancet 349:978–980, 1997 22–6

Background.—Ablative methods for treating cervical intraepithelial neoplasia (CIN) have been replaced by more conservative methods such as diathermy, laser vaporization, cold coagulation, and cryotherapy. These treatments are used to prevent invasive cervical cancer. However, there have not been many long-term studies on the efficacy of conservative CIN treatments. Using the life-table method, this study combines unpublished information with data from five other studies to determine the long-term results of conservative CIN treatments.

Methods.—Researchers collected data from the time that test-subjects were treated with diathermy, laser vaporization, cold coagulation, or cryotherapy to the time that invasive cervical cancer developed. Follow-up data beyond the scope of the original studies were collected through phone interviews with family physicians, through cytology, and through colposcopy. Researchers examined patient records to determine further cases of invasive cancer. Life-table methods were used to analyze follow-up data. The data were used to determine the duration of risk and the rate of invasive disease after conservative treatment.

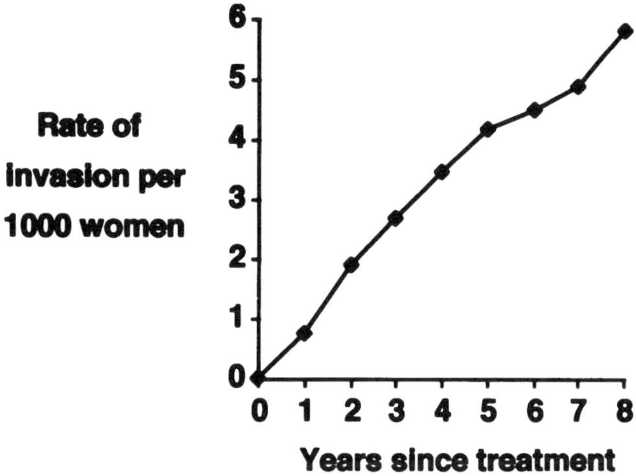

FIGURE 1.—Cumulative rate of invasion calculated from pooled data on individual patients for first 8 years after treatment. (Courtesy of Soutter WP, de Barros Lopes A, Fletcher A, et al: Invasive cervical cancer after conservative therapy for cervical intraepithelial neoplasia. *Lancet* 349:978–980, copyright by The Lancet Ltd. 1997.)

Results.—Of 2,116 test-subjects, 33 developed invasive cancer. (Fig 1) Microinvasion occurred in 14 of these 33 women. Eight years after the completion of treatment, the cumulative invasion rate was 58 in 1,000 women. Risk for developing cancer remained constant during the eight-year study period.

Conclusion.—During the first 8 years after conservative CIN treatment, the risk of invasive cervix cancer was reduced by 95%. Nonetheless, women treated for CIN are 5 times more likely to develop invasive cervical cancer than the general female population. Thus, annual cytological follow up is necessary every year for at least 10 years after treatment.

▶ This article has useful follow-up information on the conservative management of cervical intraepithelial neoplasia (CIN). Soutter et al. nicely show that the conservative treatment of 2,116 women followed up for 8 years was 95% effective in eliminating cervical cancer. The cumulative risk rate for cervical cancer was 6 per 1,000 women at 8 years of follow-up. Of the 33 women who had invasive disease, 14 had cases of microinvasion. The authors note that conservative therapy for CIN is effective, but long-term follow-up is mandatory.

A similar message is conveyed in a previous article on conization by Mohamed-Noor et al., (Abstract 22–1), which demonstrates a 96.7% cure rate with conization and negative margins. If the margins of the cone are involved with CIN, the cure rate obviously drops; however, even in this latter case, more than three fourths appear to be cured. These authors also note that conservative treatment is effective, but the need for long-term follow-up is the pertinent message.

A.L. Herbst, M.D.

23 Cervical Cancer

Early Invasive Carcinoma of the Cervix (3 to 5 mm Invasion): Risk Factors and Prognosis: A Gynecologic Oncology Group Study

Creasman WT, Zaino RJ, Major FJ, et al (Med Univ of South Carolina, Charleston; Pennsylvania State Univ, Hershey; Univ of Colorado, Denver)

Am J Obstet Gynecol 178:62–65, 1998 23–1

Introduction.—The histologic definition of stage IA carcinoma of the cervix was quantified for the first time in 1985 and was defined as the earliest form of invasion in which minute foci of invasion are visible only microscopically. Stage IA_2 was a macroscopically measurable microcarcinoma that should not exceed 5 mm in depth and 7 mm in width. There are considerable data on histopathologic parameters, treatment, and results of stage IA_2, but those patients with 3–5 mm of invasion have not been fully studied. The risk factors and prognosis in patients with stage IA squamous cell carcinoma of the cervix and 3–5 mm of invasion were evaluated.

Methods.—Patients with stage I carcinoma of the cervix were prospectively reviewed during a 3-year period. Patients with squamous cell carcinoma of the cervix who were treated with radical hysterectomy and pelvic lymphadenectomy and who had disease confined to the uterus, with or without microscopically positive lymph nodes, were part of a selective study group.

Results.—Central pathology review determined 188 patients had invasion of 3, 4, or 5 mm. This report focused on patients who satisfied the 3- to 5-mm invasion definition of the current stage IA_2 classification of the International Federation of Gynecology and Obstetrics (1995).

Conclusions.—There is a very low risk for lymph node metastases, recurrences, or death caused by cancer in patients with stage IA_2 carcinoma of the cervix who have 3–5 mm of invasion present on conization without invasion in the hysterectomy specimen. It is still unknown whether the recurrences and cancer deaths would remain constant with more conservative therapy. It may be time to reconsider whether radical therapy is indicated in all patients with 3–5 mm of invasion because the main concern about these patients has been the rate of lymph node metastases.

▶ This collaborative Gynecologic Oncology Group (GOG) study provides important data on a small group of patients who had microinvasive carcinoma of the cervix with 3–5 mm of invasion diagnosed at conization. The 51 patients who satisfied these criteria and had no residual disease at radical hysterectomy are the subject of this report (stage IA_2). Of interest, about one fourth of these patients were noted to have vascular space involvement microscopically. Among the 51 patients, there were no lymph node metastases discovered at subsequent operation, and the 5-year survival was an impressive 100%. As noted by the authors, there are reports in the literature of lymph node metastases in a small proportion of patients (perhaps 2%) who are stage IA_2. They advise considering a simple hysterectomy in those found to have negative nodes. Even a conization in someone who desires to preserve fertility could be considered, if the margins of the cones are negative. Obviously it would be useful to have reassuring lymph node information in such a patient, but that is a topic of debate. I believe that it is reasonable to consider conization in the early microinvasive group for those wanting to preserve fertility.

A.L. Herbst, M.D.

Neoadjuvant Chemotherapy in the Treatment of Locally Advanced Cervical Carcinoma in Pregnancy: A Report of Two Cases and Review of Issues Specific to the Management of Cervical Carcinoma in Pregnancy Including Planned Delay of Therapy

Tewari K, Cappuccini F, Gambino A, et al (Univ of California, Orange; Univ of Brescia, Italy)

Cancer 82:1529–1534, 1998 23–2

Objective.—Invasive cervical carcinoma during pregnancy is rare but confronts patients with a difficult decision. Two cases are reported of pregnant patients with locally advanced cervical cancer who received neoadjuvant chemotherapy so that they could continue their pregnancies.

Case 1.—Woman, 34, with scleroderma, had invasive, poorly differentiated, nonkeratinizing, papillary, squamous cell carcinoma of the cervix, diagnosed at 5 weeks' gestation. Her disease was classified as International Federation of Gynecology & Obstetrics stage IIA. After 3 cycles of vincristine and cisplatin followed by 3 cycles of cisplatin, her tumor had shrunk to 3 cm^2 from 4.5 cm^2 with diminished involvement of the anterior wall. A healthy female infant was delivered by cesarean section. However, despite a radical hysterectomy with pelvic lymphadenectomy and lateral ovarian transposition and external beam irradiation, the disease recurred 5 months later. The patient received salvage chemotherapy.

Case 2.—Woman, 36, had International Federation of Gynecology & Obstetrics stage IB_2, moderately differentiated, squamous cell carcinoma of the cervix diagnosed at 21 weeks' gestation. Four courses of vincristine and cisplatin reduced the tumor to 3 cm from 7 cm. A healthy male infant was delivered by cesarian section, which was followed by a radical hysterectomy and pelvic lymphadenectomy. After 2 years she is free of disease.

Discussion.—Before 20 weeks gestation, a short treatment delay for pregnant patients with FIGO stage I squamous cell lesions, can be acceptable. Use of antineoplastic agents during the second and third trimesters can result in low birth weight, intrauterine growth restriction, impaired mental development, infertility, carcinogenesis, and second-generation teratogenesis.

▶ Fortunately, invasive cancer during pregnancy is rare. Tewari et al. report 2 cases treated with vincristine and cisplatin, both after the twentieth week of gestation when organogenesis is complete. Patient 2 had a stage IB tumor that responded to chemotherapy, and she had no evidence of disease 2 years after a radical hysterectomy at 32 weeks of gestation; the results in her case were excellent. The authors reviewed the literature as shown in Table 2 which involved a mixture of varying types of patients, most of whom had low-stage tumors. As noted by the authors, most of the patients did well in spite of delays of a number of months. Although there was one reported death and one progression of disease during pregnancy, the good results are similar to what my colleagues and I noted for clear-cell adenocarcinoma,[1] with no demonstrable effects from treatment delay during pregnancy. In their discussion, the authors note the potential adverse effects of chemotherapy during the second and third trimesters of pregnancy, including intrauterine growth retardation, hematopoietic suppression, potential carcinogenesis, etc.

My conclusion is somewhat different from the authors'. For the patient who wishes to maintain the pregnancy, I would wait for fetal viability and then treat after delivery, but I am not comfortable giving chemotherapy during pregnancy.

A.L. Herbst, M.D.

Reference

1. Senekjian EK, Hubby M, Bell D, et al: Clear cell adenocarcinoma (CCA) of the vagina and cervix in association with pregnancy. *Gynecol Oncol* 24:207, 1986.

Radiotherapeutic Management of Cervical Carcinoma That Complicates Pregnancy

Sood AK, Sorosky JI, Mayr N, et al (Univ of Iowa, Iowa City)

Cancer 80:1073–1078, 1997 23–3

Objective.—Whereas surgical management of cervical cancer during pregnancy has been shown to be safe and effective, little information is available about the effects of radiation treatment. Outcomes of pregnant patients with cervical cancer after treatment with radiation were analyzed retrospectively to assess the effects of pregnancy on tumor control, survival, and morbidity associated with radiation therapy.

Methods.—Of 86 pregnant women with cervical cancer diagnosed at the University of Iowa Hospitals and Clinics between 1960 and 1994, 26 received external beam radiation (average dose 46.7 Gy) and intracavity radiation (average dose 56.5 Gy) treatment. These patients were age-, histology- disease stage-, treatment modality-, and year of treatment-matched with nonpregnant women with cervical cancer.

Results.—Eighteen infants were born healthy, and 8 infants died. Two patients had radiation treatments interrupted, 1 because of an infected pelvic hematoma after a cesarean section and 1 because of drug-related granulocytopenia. Most cancer patients and controls experienced diarrhea and weight loss. Long-term complications included 3 fistulas in cancer patients and 3 in controls, 2 bowel obstructions in controls, and 2 cases of bowel necrosis in controls. At follow-up, 11 cancer patients and 12 controls had no evidence of disease, 11 cancer patients and 6 controls had died of their disease, and 4 cancer patients and 8 controls had died with no evidence of disease.

Conclusion.—Radiation for pregnant women with advanced cervical cancer is safe and effective, but may need to be delayed or interrupted depending on stage. Short-term toxicity was similar between groups. Long-term complications were more common in the control group.

► This is a small, but useful series on the radiation treatment of cervical carcinoma during pregnancy. None of us has extensive experience with this and there is a temptation to "treat the cancer" as soon as possible. The authors satisfactorily used radiation to treat these tumors with no clear difference between case-patients and controls. They advocate delay in therapy for those in the latter part of the second or in the third trimester with improved neonatal ICU results and pregnancy after delay to older ages. I believe we may be obviously faced with the problem of carcinoma of the cervix in an older primipara. I favor delaying therapy until fetal viability in the third trimester, assuming this is consistent with the patient's wishes. For those in the first trimester and with stage 1B lesions, especially for lesions less than 4 cm, I prefer to try to carry out treatment by radical hysterectomy. As noted by the authors, however, radiation can be used effectively in the pregnant patient, especially in early pregnancy.

A.L. Herbst, M.D.

Extended Field Radiation and Cisplatin for Stage IIB and IIIB Cervical Carcinoma

Malfetano JH, Keys H, Cunningham MJ, et al (Albany Med Ctr, NY)
Gynecol Oncol 67:203–207, 1997 23–4

Background.—Even though radiotherapy has been used since the beginning of this century in treating cervical carcinomas, the 5-year survival rate

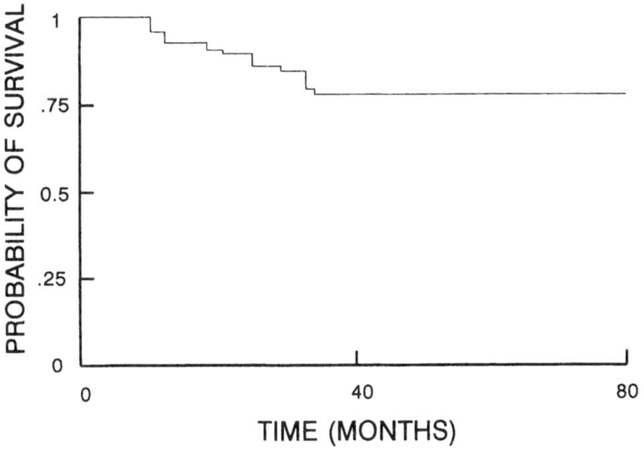

FIGURE 2.—Kaplan-Meier survival curve for FIGO stages IIB and IIIB (67 patients) squamous cell carcinomas. *Abbreviation: FIGO*, International Federation of Gynecology and Obstetrics. (Courtesy of Malfetano JH, Keys H, Cunningham MJ, et. al: Extended field radiation and cisplatin for stage IIB and IIIB cervical carcinoma. *Gynecol Oncol* 67:203–207, 1997.)

after treatment is still between 30% and 65%, and almost 60% of patients experience disease relapse. Most of the progress made in the treatment of cancer has resulted from early detection rather than improved treatment methods. Patients with FIGO IIB and IIIB cervical squamous cell carcinomas were studied. Patients were treated with prophylactic para-aoratic radiation and a radiation sensitizer (cisplatin) to determine survival, control, and morbidity.

Methods.—Forty-four patients with IIB and 23 patients with IIIB cervical carcinomas served as test research subjects receiving up to 60 mg (1 mg/kg) of cisplatin weekly. All patients also underwent extended field radiotherapy, both external and intracavitary. Survival rates were determined using the Kaplan-Meier survival curve method (Fig 2).

Results.—Ninety-four percent of patients given treatment responded completely. After an average 47.5 months of follow-up, 75% of patients had no evidence of disease and were living.

Conclusion.—Concomitant weekly cisplatin used in combination with extended field radiation deserves further investigation as a treatment for cervical carcinomas considering the 75% survival rate determined in this study.

▶ As noted by the authors, convincing proof that chemoradiation confers a survival advantage to patients undergoing therapy for advanced cervical carcinomas is certainly debated. Nonetheless, I continue to be impressed by the results of many selected series, including this one.

The authors used weekly cisplatin (1 mg/kg) up to 60 mg and extended field radiotherapy that included the para-aortic nodes. That approach also is debatable in these advanced-stage tumors. Brachytherapy was also used to complete treatment. I believe that the results are impressive; an excellent overall 5-year survival rate is calculated, as shown in Figure 2. There were only 2 major complications requiring operative intervention. I look forward to further reports of this combined approach for advanced cervical cancer.

A.L. Herbst, M.D.

Carcinoma of the Cervical Stump: Retrospective Analysis of 77 Cases
Hannoun-Lévi J-M, Peiffert D, Hoffstetter S, et al (Centre Alexis Vautrin, France)
Radiother Oncol 43:147–153, 1997 23–5

Introduction.—Up to 9% of cervical carcinomas are carcinomas of the cervical stump. It would be beneficial to assess therapeutic results in patients with carcinoma of the cervical stump. A clinical series of patients with carcinoma of the cervical stump who were mainly treated with radical radiation therapy is reviewed.

Methods.—Treatment for an infiltrating carcinoma of the cervical stump was provided for 77 patients in a 16-year period. There were 9% adenocarcinomas and 91% squamous cell carcinomas. Stage I tumors accounted for 35%, stage II accounted for 45%, stage III accounted for 18%, and stage IV accounted for 2% of the patients. Plesiobrachytherapy and external-beam radiation therapy were performed as treatment with some patients and some had surgery or interstitial brachytherapy. External beam radiation therapy was first delivered to patients with bulky tumor or advanced stage and/or lymphatic node involvement. Treatment with plesiobrachytherapy was initiated in most of the stage I and II patients. Exclusive radiation therapy was performed on 95% of the patients. Complications were recorded.

Results.—In 56 of the 66 patients (76.5%), 3-year pelvic control was achieved. In Stage I tumors, 3-year pelvic control probabilities were 89%; in stage II tumors, they were 73.7%; and in Stage III tumors, they were 56%. For the entire series, the 3-year pelvic control probability was 77%. The 5-year overall survival probability was 66.4%, and the 10-year overall survival probability was 61.2%. Seventeen late complications occurred in 10 patients at 12.8%. Nine patients had gastrointestinal complications.

Conclusion.—Patients with carcinoma of the cervical stump and those with carcinoma of the intact uterus have similar treatment results. Because of the pelvic anatomic modifications induced by the subtotal hysterectomy and its consequences on the new organization of critical organs into the treated volume, it is sometimes difficult to perform a correct plesiobrachytherapy.

▶ This article from France summarizes the authors' experience of treating cervical stump carcinoma with radiation. The total numbers are small—77 patients in 16 years—but the results are quite respectable with 5-year survival of Stages I and II at about 70%. Excellent pelvic control was obtained. An important point is their success at pelvic control, and survival is dependent on having a sufficiently long cervical canal to allow effective brachytherapy with an endocervical source.

The authors believe this is a declining disease, but with more supracervical hysterectomies being done with laparoscopic surgery, we may see an increase in this problem.

A.L. Herbst, M.D.

24 Endometrial Cancer

Uterine Side Effects of Tamoxifen: A Need for Systematic Pretreatment Screening

Berlière M, Charles A, Galant C, et al (Catholic Univ of Louvain, Brussels, Belgium)

Obstet Gynecol 91:40–44, 1998 24–1

Introduction.—The risk of endometrial cancer appears to increase with tamoxifen, perhaps 2–3 times greater than in women with breast cancer not treated with tamoxifen. In women at high risk of breast cancer, tamoxifen is being studied as a preventive agent, but its side effects should be evaluated carefully before it is extensively used as preventive treatment. The effect of tamoxifen on the endometrium was studied in postmenopausal women with breast cancer. Women at higher risk of developing endometrial cancer on the basis of gynecologic pretreatment were identified.

Methods.—Participants were 264 postmenopausal women with breast cancer who had pelvic US in a 3-year period. If US abnormalities were detected, outpatient hysteroscopy and endometrial biopsy were done. Before treatment with tamoxifen was started (20 mg daily), and annually thereafter, initial endometrial evaluation was done. Endometrial lesions and endometrial hyperplasia were focused on. There were 2 categories of endometrial hyperplasia—hyperplasia without cytologic atypia and hyperplasia with cytologic atypia. A well-differentiated endometrial carcinoma confined to the endometrial mucosa without myometrial invasion was the definition of adenocarcinoma in situ.

Results.—Asymptomatic endometrial lesions were diagnosed in 46 women (17.4%) before starting tamoxifen, and 2 were atypical lesions. Patients with initial lesions and those without initial lesions were followed up separately. In women with lesions initially, the incidence of atypical lesions was significantly higher at 3 years of follow-up in comparison with those without (Table 2). There were 3 atypical lesions among 9 women with lesions initially, compared with 1 atypical lesion among 51 women who did not have lesions initially.

Conclusions.—On the basis of endometrial evaluation before tamoxifen therapy, a group of high-risk women can be defined. Because of the high

TABLE 2.—Patient Follow-up

Treatment		Without initial lesions			Initial lesions (treated)		
(year)	*n*	*n*	Benign	Atypical	*n*	Benign	Atypical
0	264	218	—	—	46	44	2
1	220	185	7 (3.8%)	0	35	3	0
2	140	120	11 (9.2%)	0	20	3	1
3	60	51	5 (9.8%)	1	9	1	3
Total			23	1		51	6

(Courtesy of Berlière M, Charles A, Galant C, et al: Uterine side effects of tamoxifen: A need for systematic pretreatment screening. *Obstet Gynecol* 91:40–44, Copyright 1998. Reprinted with permission from the American College of Obstetricians and Gynecologists.)

incidence of severe atypical lesions, these women should be followed up carefully.

▶ This study deals with a topic of great concern; namely, endometrial neoplasia in patients taking tamoxifen for breast cancer. The authors note that the frequency of atypical lesions were significantly higher in women who had lesions noted before tamoxifen was started. The results are summarized in Table 2. It shows 3 of 9 cases of atypical lesions in those who initially were found to have lesions before therapy vs. 1 of 51 in the group who were negative before therapy. While the difference is statistically significant, and there is no doubt that tamoxifen increases the risk of endometrial neoplasia in these patients, it is worth noting that the total effect is really quite low. For example, of 220 women followed up for 1 year, there were no atypical lesions; among 140 followed up for 2 years, there was 1; and among 60 followed up for 3 years, there were 4. Put in different terms, the risk for atypical lesions in the entire group without an endometrial lesion before treatment was 0.2 per 100 women-years, and rose to 4 per 100 women-years in the group with pretreatment benign endometrial abnormalities.

A.L. Herbst, M.D.

Iatrogenic Risks of Endometrial Carcinoma After Treatment for Breast Cancer in a Large French Case-Control Study

Mignotte H, for the Fédération Nationale des Centres de Lutte Contre le Cancer (Centre Léon Bérard, Lyon, France; Centre Alexis Vautrin, Nancy, France; Centre Paul Strauss, Strasbourg, France; et al)

Int J Cancer 76:325–330, 1998 24–2

Background.—Tamoxifen is widely used to treat breast cancer and has been proposed to prevent it. Thus, the endometrial effects of this agent must be studied thoroughly. The association between endometrial cancer and tamoxifen use in women with breast cancer was evaluated in a case-control study.

Methods.—One hundred thirty-five women with diagnosed endometrial cancer after breast cancer treatment were compared with 467 women with an intact uterus matched for age, year of breast cancer diagnosis, and hospital and survival times.

Findings.—Women given tamoxifen were significantly more likely to have endometrial cancer diagnosed than those not given tamoxifen. In univariate and adjusted analyses, the risk of endometrial cancer increased with length of treatment or cumulative tamoxifen dose, regardless of the daily dose. The risk of endometrial cancer was also higher in women who had had pelvic radiotherapy. After adjustment for confounding variables, an increased risk was associated with tamoxifen use, treatment exceeding 3 years, and pelvic radiotherapy. Women with endometrial cancer who had received tamoxifen had more advanced disease and a poorer prognosis than women with endometrial cancer who had not received tamoxifen.

Conclusions.—Tamoxifen appears to play a causal role in endometrial cancer. Pelvic radiotherapy in women with breast cancer may also be a contributing factor. Women treated with tamoxifen for breast cancer should be offered gynecologic surveillance during and after therapy. Further research is needed to establish the long-term risk-benefit ratio of tamoxifen as a preventive treatment for breast cancer.

► This retrospective study associates the rare development of endometrial carcinoma with tamoxifen therapy in breast cancer patients. The crude relative risk was 4.9, with longer duration (more than 3 years) and higher cumulative dose increasing the risk. Interestingly, the endometrial carcinomas in this cohort had a poorer prognosis, suggesting these are less well differentiated tumors low in estrogen and progesterone receptors.

Parenthetically, the authors also noted that the benefit-risk relationship for tamoxifen in the prevention of breast cancer is not established. Recently, U.S. investigators halted the trial of breast cancer prevention with tamoxifen because of fewer cancers developing in the tamoxifen-treated group. Our European colleagues have continued the trial on the basis that mortality is the proper end point and therefore the U.S. trial has not proven efficacy for that end point, nor have all the potential long-term adverse consequences necessarily occurred. I believe the Europeans are correct on this issue.

A.L. Herbst, M.D.

Value of Preoperative CA 125 Level in the Management of Uterine Cancer and Prediction of Clinical Outcome

Sood AK, Buller RE, Burger RA, et al (Univ of Iowa, Iowa City; Univ of California, Irvine)

Obstet Gynecol 90:441–447, 1997 24–3

Introduction.—Uterine cancer is the fourth most common malignancy in American women. It would make economic and medical sense to better identify selected candidates with uterine cancer who might be treated as

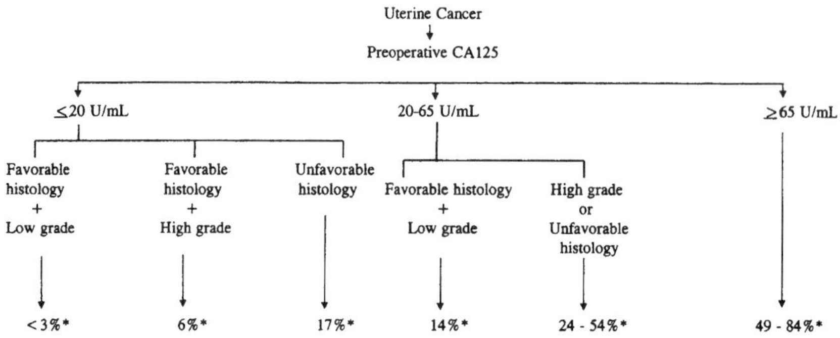

FIGURE 2.—Algorithm for management of uterine cancer based on preoperative CA 125 values. *Unfavorable histology*, papillary serous, clear cell, or sarcoma; *high grade*, grade II or III. *Asterisk*, percentages represent likelihood of extrauterine disease. Under categories for which a range is given, the exact risk depends on various combinations of histology and grade. (Courtesy of Sood AK, Buller RE, Burger RA, et al: Value of preoperative CA 125 level in the management of uterine cancer and prediction of clinical outcome. *Obstet Gynecol* 90:441–447. Copyright 1997, reprinted with permission of The American College of Obstetricians and Gynecologists.)

effectively by vaginal hysterectomy as by the abdominal route. CA 125 is a circulating antigen in patients with epithelial ovarian cancer and is elevated in a variety of gynecologic malignancies including ovarian, endometrial, fallopian tube, and endocervical cancers. It was determined whether a preoperative CA 125 level would prognosticate the likelihood of metastatic disease and determine overall survival.

Methods.—There were 210 women with endometrial carcinoma who were retrospectively reviewed for their preoperative CA 125 levels. The relationship between various preoperative and postoperative histopathologic factors and preoperative CA 125 levels was investigated.

Results.—Higher stage, higher grade, increased depth or myometrial invasion, positive cytology, pelvic or para-aortic lymph node metastases, and reduced actuarial survival correlated with elevated CA 125 of more than 35 U/mL. The most important predictor for poor survival was an elevated CA 125 level, according to multivariate analysis. The most significant predictor of extrauterine disease was a preoperative CA 125 level of more than 65 U/mL, carrying a 6.5-fold higher risk. The logistic model to predict extrauterine disease had a sensitivity of 62%, specificity of 91%, positive predictive value of 69%, and negative predictive value of 88%. The likelihood of finding extrauterine disease would be less than 3% with a preoperative CA 125 value of 20 U/mL or less when favorable histology and low grade are present (Fig 2).

Conclusions.—For all women with uterine cancer, a CA 125 level should be included as part of the preoperative workup. Candidates for vaginal hysterectomy are women with a preoperative CA 125 level of 20 U/mL or less, unless unfavorable histology or a high-grade (grade II or III) tumor is present. Up to 24% of the abdominal staging procedures would have been eliminated with this approach, resulting in a risk of less than 3% for extrauterine disease. Treatment-related morbidity would have been lowered, and costs in the treatment of this common female cancer would have been reduced.

▶ This interesting study demonstrates the usefulness of preoperative CA 125 in the management of endometrial carcinoma. It is well known that the test is useful for prognosis and particularly follow up of ovarian carcinoma. Sood et al. have demonstrated that in good prognosis disease—grade I, stage I, and a CA 125 level of 20 U/mL or less—the risk of extrauterine disease is about 3%, rising to about 6% for grade II and III (non-clear clear and nonpapillary serous). As the authors note, this is useful information for managing the patient who is at high risk for abdominal surgery who could be considered for vaginal hysterectomy, particularly when the patient has a CA 125 level of 20 U/mL or less and a grade I adenocarcinoma.

A.L. Herbst, M.D.

Risk of Endometrial Cancer in Relation to Use of Low-dose, Unopposed Estrogens

Cushing KL, Weiss NS, Voight LF, et al (Univ of Washington, Seattle)

Obstet Gynecol 91:35–39, 1998 24–4

Introduction.—Menopausal symptoms such as hot flashes have been alleviated with unopposed estrogen, which also reduces the risk of osteoporosis and cardiovascular disease, but the risk of endometrial cancer is increased. A lower dose of unopposed estrogens could conceivably have a lesser impact on the endometrium. The impact of exclusive use of 0.3 mg/day of unopposed estrogens has not been assessed in a large study. Whether a low dosage (0.3 mg/day) of unopposed conjugated estrogens can be used without incurring an elevated risk of endometrial cancer was evaluated.

Methods.—A total of 484 women with diagnosed endometrial cancer in a 6-year period were compared with 780 controls to obtain basic demographic and medical history information and specific information about hormone use.

Results.—There were 18 patients and 8 controls who took 0.3 mg/day of unopposed conjugated estrogens with no other dose or preparation estrogens. In women whose use of this dosage was both current and of more than 8 years' duration, the risk was particularly high. The daily unopposed use of 0.625 mg of conjugated estrogens had a similar elevation in risk as users of 0.3 mg/day.

Conclusions.—An increased risk of endometrial cancer is associated with a dosage of 0.3 mg per day of unopposed conjugated estrogens, but the association could be biased by unmeasured confounders. Even though this was considered to be a large study, the number of women who used

0.3 mg/day of unopposed estrogen was modest and the estimate of altered risk may be somewhat imprecise.

▶ Most of us prescribe 0.625 mg of conjugated estrogens with a progestin. Rarely, I have encountered a patient who is taking a low dose of 0.3 mg for a variety of reasons, and this article indicates that these patients do have an increased risk of endometrial cancer if they do not have accompanying progestin therapy. Specifically for those taking low-dose hormone replacement therapy for more than 8 years, the relative risk was particularly high (RR = 9.2; 95% confidence interval, 2.9–29.0). I was surprised to learn that this magnitude was similar to those ingesting the higher dose of 0.625 mg, which means even those patients on low-dose unopposed estrogen require monitoring for endometrial changes. In the asymptomatic patient, a vaginal ultrasound demonstrating an endometrial stripe less than 4 mm would indicate that the patient needs only to be followed up.

A.L. Herbst, M.D.

Progestin Treatment of Atypical Hyperplasia and Well-differentiated Carcinoma of the Endometrium in Women Under Age 40

Randall TC, Kurman RJ (Johns Hopkins Med Institutions, Baltimore, Md)
Obstet Gynecol 90:434–440, 1997 24–5

Introduction.—The most frequent malignant tumor in the female genital tract is endometrial cancer. The immediate precursor of endometrial carcinoma is atypical hyperplasia; untreated, it has a 25% risk of progressing to carcinoma. Hysterectomy is the standard treatment of atypical hyperplasia. Medical treatment, such as treatment with progestin, is desirable for young women who desire to preserve their fertility. A retrospective study of women younger than 40 with atypical hyperplasia or well-differentiated carcinoma on endometrial biopsy or curettage was conducted to determine whether conservative hormonal treatment was effective in eradicating atypical hyperplasia and well-differentiated carcinoma, and whether they could bear children afterward. Another aim of the study was to estimate the baseline extent of disease in women managed conservatively.

Methods.—Atypical hyperplasia or well-differentiated carcinoma of the endometrium was diagnosed in 67 women younger than 40 over a 6-year period. Available biopsy, curettage, and hysterectomy specimens were reviewed. Follow-up was conducted with the women's gynecologists.

Results.—Well-differentiated carcinoma was found in 35 women, and atypical hyperplasia was found in 32 women. Eight of 27 patients with atypical hyperplasia had hysterectomy, 2 had ovulation induction, and 17 were given progestin; of the women treated with progestin, 16 had regression of their lesions, and 1 had a persistent lesion. Seventeen of 19 women were managed conservatively for atypical hyperplasia, and 16 (94%) had regression to benign endometrial findings (Table 3). Nineteen of 33 women

TABLE 3.—Follow-up of 19 Patients With Atypical Hyperplasia Treated With Hormones

Case	Initial diagnosis	Treatment	Final diagnosis	Follow-up
Regression				
1	AH	Megestrol acetate 160 mg/day × 3 months	Proliferative endometrium	A + W, 9 months
2	AH in multiple polyps	Megestrol acetate 40 mg/day × 3 months	Inactive endometrium with marked decidual change	A + W, 10 months
3	Focal AH in proliferative endometrium	Medroxyprogesterone 10 mg/day × 4 months	Secretory endometrium	A + W, 10 months
4	AH	Medroxyprogesterone 10 mg/day × 3 months	Secretory endometrium	A + W, 17 months
5	AH	Megestrol acetate 80 mg/day continuous	Complex hyperplasia with no atypia	A + W, 61 months
6	Focal AH in simple hyperplasia	Medroxyprogesterone 10/mg day continuous	Complex hyperplasia with no atypia	A + W, 41 months
7	AH in a polyp	Megestrol acetate 40 mg/day × 4 months, then Medroxyprogesterone × 12 months	Proliferative endometrium	A + W, 27 months
8	AH	Medroxyprogesterone 10 mg/day × 24 months, then ovulation induction	Complex hyperplasia with no atypia	A + W, 48 months
9	AH	Megestrol acetate 80 mg/day × 3 months, then oral contraceptives continuous	Secretory endometrium	A + W, 37 months
10	AH	Megestrol acetate × 6 months	Proliferative endometrium	A + W, 36 months
11	AH in a polyp	Megestrol acetate 80 mg/day continuous	Secretory endometrium and benign polyps	A + W, 38 months
12	AH in a polyp	Medroxyprogesterone 10 mg/day × 6 months, then 30 mg/day × 6 months	Scant inactive endometrium	A + W, 45 months

(*Continued*)

TABLE 3 (cont.)

Case	Initial diagnosis	Treatment	Final diagnosis	Follow-up
13	AH	Megestrol acetate 120 mg/day continuous	Inactive endometrium with marked decidual change	A + W, 59 months
14	AH	Megestrol acetate 160 mg/day × 12 months, then ovulation induction	Inactive endometrium with marked decidual change	A + W, 54 months
15	AH in a polyp	Megestrol acetate 40 mg/day × 4 months, then ovulation induction	Inactive endometrium with marked decidual change	A + W, 64 months
16	AH	Medroxyprogesterone 10 mg/day × 12 months, then Medroxyprogesterone + tamoxifen × 6 months	Scant inactive endometrium	A + W, 79 months, full-term pregnancy
17	AH in a polyp	Ovulation induction × 11 cycles, then in vitro fertilization × 4 cycles	Proliferative endometrium	A + W, 40 months full-term pregnancy
Persistence				
18	AH	Megestrol acetate 120 mg/day × 4 months	Focal AH in inactive endometrium with marked progestin effect	A + W, 63 months*
Progression				
19	AH	Ovulation induction × 11 cycles	WDC confined to the endometrium on hysterectomy	A + W, 41 months

*Moderately differentiated carcinoma confined to the endometrium found at hysterectomy 3 years after discontinuing progestin. This patient has no evidence of disease 19 months after hysterectomy.

AH = atypical hyperplasia; A + W = alive and well; WDC = well-differentiated endometrioid adenocarcinoma. (Courtesy of Randall TC, Kurman RJ: Progestin treatment of atypical hyperplasia and well-differentiated carcinoma of the endometrium in women under age 40. *Obstet Gynecol* 90:434–440, 1997. Reprinted with permission from The American College of Obstetricians and Gynecologists.)

TABLE 4.—Follow-up of 14 Patients With Well-Differentiated Carcinoma Treated With Hormones

Case	Initial diagnosis	Treatment	Final diagnosis	Follow-up
Regression				
20	Focal WDC	Megestrol acetate 160 mg/day × 3 months	Inactive endometrium with marked progestin effect	A + W, 9 months
21	WDC	Megestrol acetate 160 mg/day + bromocriptine for increased prolactin × 6 months	Atrophic endometrium with marked decidual change	A + W, 10 months
22	Focal WDC in AH	Megestrol acetate 80 mg/day × 6 months	Simple hyperplasia, no atypia	A + W, 32 months, full-term pregnancy
23	WDC	Megestrol acetate 40 mg/day continuous, + tamoxifen × 1 month	Complex hyperplasia, no atypia	A + W, 21 months
24	Focal WDC in AH	Megestrol acetate 80 mg/day × 12 months	Proliferative endometrium	A + W, 38 months
25	WDC	Megestrol acetate 80 mg/day × 2 months, then oral contraceptives continuous	Proliferative endometrium	A + W, 43 months
26	WDC*	Megestrol acetate 160 mg/day × 9 months	Proliferative endometrium	A + W, 42 months full-term pregnancy × 2
27	WDC	Megestrol acetate 160 mg/day × 6 months, then Medroxyprogesterone 10 mg/day continuous	Proliferative endometrium	A + W, 42 months
28	Focal WDC	Megestrol acetate 120 mg/day × 18 months, then Medroxyprogesterone 10 mg/day, 10 days/month	Proliferative endometrium	A + W, 78 months, full-term pregnancy × 2
29	Focal WDC	Bromocriptine 10 mg/day × 6 months	Secretory endometrium	A + W, 24 months

(*Continued*)

TABLE 4 (cont.)

Case	Initial diagnosis	Treatment	Final diagnosis	Follow-up
Persistence				
30	WDC	Megestrol acetate 400 mg/day × 6 months, then self-discontinued	AH	A + W, 14 months
31	WDC	Megestrol acetate 240 mg/day × 3 months	WDC confined to the endometrium on hysterectomy	A + W, 61 months
32	WDC in secretory endometrium	Oral contraceptives × 12 months	AH in hysterectomy specimen	A + W, 72 months
33	WDC with extensive squamous differentiation	Megestrol acetate 80 mg/day × 4 months, + platinum × 4 cycles	WDC confined to the endometrium in hysterectomy specimen	A + W, 62 months

WDC = well-differentiated endometrioid adenocarcinoma; A + W = alive and well; AH = atypical hyperplasia.
*Diagnosis made in curettage performed because of an incomplete abortion.
(Courtesy of Randall TC, Kurman RJ: Progestin treatment of atypical hyperplasia and well-differentiated carcinoma of the endometrium in women under age 40 *Obstet Gynecol* 90:434–440, 1997. Reprinted with permission from The American College of Obstetricians and Gynecologists.)

with well-differentiated carcinoma had hysterectomy, one received bromocriptine, one was given oral contraceptives, and 12 were given progestin; of these, 9 had regression of their lesions and 3 had persistent lesions (Table 4). The median length of treatment required for a regression was 9 months. All women were alive and well, without evidence of progressive disease, at a mean follow-up of 40 months. Pregnancy was attempted by 25 women, of whom 5 were delivered of healthy infants at term.

Conclusion.—A safe alternative to hysterectomy in women under age 40 appears to be treatment of atypical hyperplasia and well-differentiated carcinoma of endometrium with progestin.

▶ Progestin has been used effectively in the treatment of premalignant endometrial hyperplasia for decades. The use of this agent for treatment of well-differentiated carcinoma has also been reported to have some success.

The current article describes a comparatively large series of cases successfully treated, as shown in Tables 3 and 4. The patients were treated for a mean duration of 9 months with median follow-up of 40 months. All patients were under age 40, and 5 were delivered of healthy infants; one of the latter patients was treated with ovulation induction. It is worth noting that 2 patients with hyperplasia and 4 with well-differentiated carcinoma underwent hysterectomy for persistent disease (1 case of hyperplasia progressed to carcinoma). All patients were well and free of disease, with follow-up as long as 6½ years in some. This treatment is both feasible and successful, but these patients require lifetime monitoring because the risk of carcinoma in the future in this high-risk group remains.

A.L. Herbst, M.D.

Total Abdominal Hysterectomy and Bilateral Salpingo-Oophorectomy: A Sufficient Treatment for Patients With Low Risk Endometrial Carcinoma

Leijon T, Rosenberg P, Boeryd B (Univ Hosp of Linkoping, Sweden)

Int J Gynecol Cancer 7:376–380, 1997 24–6

Objective.—Simple hysterectomy with bilateral salpingo-oophorectomy is usually advocated as the primary treatment for endometrial carcinoma. Whether adjuvant radiation therapy is important is debated. The clinical outcome and value of post-treatment follow-up were evaluated in patients with stage I endometrial carcinoma with favorable prognostic features who had undergone a simple hysterectomy and bilateral salpingo-oophorectomy only.

Methods.—Of 757 patients with uterine cancer diagnosed between January 1988 and December 1994, 248 women, aged 34–88, with low-risk endometrial carcinoma underwent a total abdominal hysterectomy and bilateral salpingo-oophorectomy without additional adjuvant therapy. Patients were followed up for a median of 42 months. They were examined at 3, 6, and 12 months and twice yearly thereafter for up to 5 years. Clinical outcome and relapse rate were were the end points.

Results.—At 5 years, 242 patients were still alive, 2 with evidence of disease, for disease-free and total survival rates of 96.7% and 97.5%, respectively. There were 9 relapses (3.6%), 5 local to the vagina, 1 to the pelvis, and 3 to multiple sites. Seven relapses occurred within 24 months of surgery, and 3 patients died of their disease within the 5-year period.

Conclusion.—Total abdominal hysterectomy and bilateral salpingo-oophorectomy as treatment for patients with low-risk endometrial carcinoma resulted in disease-free and total survival rates of 96.7% and 97.5% during a median observation period of 42 months.

▶ The authors report on 248 patients with low-risk endometrial carcinoma. They define this as stage Ia or Ib and grades 1 or 2. In addition, they did a DNA analysis and restricted low grade to a diploid tumor. However, the determination of ploidy is not used on a widespread clinical basis, so perhaps it is worth noting that of the 181 patients with grade 1 tumors, stage Ia or Ib, 152 tumors were identified as diploid, 14 as nondiploid, and 15 as undetermined. Among the grade 2 cases of similar stage, there were 122 tumors, 96 of which were diploid, 22 of which were not diploid, and 4 of which were not determined. It is perhaps not surprising that among the grade 2 cases, there was a higher rate of tumors that were not diploid.

Overall, the results were excellent: a 3% recurrent rate with a median observation time of 42 months. The authors emphasized the importance of regular follow-up insofar as they detected recurrences in 7 of 9 cases. The authors believe that this justifies routine follow-up, which I certainly continue to do for my patients. For those with local recurrence (usually in the vagina), radiation can be given. In many cases, this is successful, but in this series it salvaged only 2 of 9 patients.

The issue for debate is the treatment of the stage Ib, grade 2 tumors. As noted above, in this series, these tumors had a higher rate of nondiploid DNA index. I think it is still not clear what the best treatment is for stage Ib, grade 2 disease, particularly if the tumor penetrates close to halfway through the myometrium.

A.L. Herbst, M.D.

Advanced Endometrial Adenocarcinoma Following Endometrial Ablation: A Case Report and Review of the Literature

Klein Z, Markovitch O, Altaras M, et al (Sapir Med Ctr, Kfar Saba, Israel)

Int J Gynecol Cancer 7:163–165, 1997 24–7

Objective.—Patients undergoing endometrial ablation must be selected carefully to rule out malignancy or hyperplasia and thus to avoid the potential for malignancy developing in unablated areas. A case of advanced stage endometrial adenocarcinoma diagnosed after endometrial ablation is discussed.

Case.—Postmenopausal woman, 52, with well-differentiated, papillary, endometrial adenocarcinoma, had a prior history of bleeding that began 2 years after menopause. She was not taking hormone replacement therapy and had an unremarkable physical examination. An ultrasound showed a fibroid uterus and normal endometrium and ovaries. She was treated with hormone therapy with progesterone, but bleeding recurred after 3 months. A hysterectomy was offered, but because of her cardiac history she requested endometrial ablation. During the procedure a biopsy revealed well-differentiated papillary adenocarcinoma. Ultrasound showed a fibroid uterus and no abnormality, and a left ovarian cyst. The patient underwent total abdominal hysterectomy, bilateral salpingo-oophorectomy, and pelvic lymph node sampling. At histopathology, moderately differentiated adenocarcinoma of the endometrium was found, with more than 50% invasion of the myometrium and a metastatic lesion of the left ovary. She was treated with adjuvant radiation therapy.

Conclusion.—Whereas development of endometrial carcinoma under these conditions is extremely uncommon and may have resulted from a missed small lesion in 2 hysteroscopies, the retrograde spread of malignant cells after ablation cannot be ruled out. Careful patient selection and meticulous evaluation before endometrial ablation are imperative.

▶ This case report describes an endometrial carcinoma discovered at the time of endometrial ablation after prior negative hysteroscopies. The authors note that isolated case reports in the literature[1-3] demonstrate the development of endometrial carcinoma after endometrial ablation.

Although these reports are rare, it reminds us that endometrial ablation does not destroy all endometrial tissue and that malignancy can arise subsequently, which will be difficult to diagnose due to the lack of symptoms and bleeding. Obviously, there should not be evidence of endometrial hyperplasia in patients undergoing this procedure.

A.L. Herbst, M.D.

References

1. Horowitz IR, Copas PR, Aaronoff M, et al: Endometrial adenocarcinoma following endometrial ablation for postmenopausal bleeding. *Gynecol Oncol* 56:460–463, 1995.
2. Ramey JW, Koonings P, Given FT, et al: The process of carcinogenesis for endometrial adenocarcinoma could be short: Development of a malignancy after endometrial ablation. *Am J Obstet Gynecol* 170:1370–1371, 1994.
3. Copperman A, DeCherney A, Olive D: A case of endometrial cancer following endometrial ablation for dysfunctional uterine bleeding. *Obstet Gynecol* 82:640–642 1993.

Stage IA Uterine Serous Carcinoma: A Study of 13 Cases

Carcangiu ML, Tan LK, Chambers JT (Yale Univ, New Haven, Conn; Mem Sloan-Kettering Cancer Ctr, New York)

Am J Surg Pathol 21:1507–1514, 1997 24–8

Background.—The myometrial invasion depth associated with endometrioid carcinomas is a gauge for predicting survival. However, the accuracy of this predictor has not been determined in cases of serous carcinomas (SCs). Thirteen patients with endometrial polyps or endometria exhibiting SCs which were completely staged as IA, were tracked.

Methods.—The follow-up, including an extensive histologic examination, ranged from 10–93 months. Only patients without myometrial invasion were studied. In 6 cases, endometrial polyps were present. In 4, both endometrial polyps and the endometrium were recorded as sites of SCs. In 3 cases, only the endometrium was affected. Twelve patients had multifocal serous intraepithelial carcinomas.

Results.—The overall survival rate for the course of the study was 83%. Two patients died—1 at 10 months, the other at 14.

Conclusion.—This study shows that the most reliable way to predict SC is to use careful histologic examinations to determine an accurately assessed stage.

▶ This useful series describes the outcome of 13 cases of early (stage Ia) SC of the endometrium. All of us associate this histologic diagnosis with a poor prognosis. Indeed, in spite of the very early presentation (no myometrial invasion), 2 of the patients eventually had disseminated disease and died (median follow-up, 38 months).

As emphasized by the authors, complete staging laparotomy is indicated because disseminated disease can exist in spite of a stage IA presentation with SC in an endometrial polyp. The authors also note that this lesion has been described in endometrial polyps in patients who have been receiving long-term tamoxifen treatment for breast cancer. A major take-home message is that these patients deserve a full staging laparotomy.

A.L. Herbst, M.D.

Uterine Papillary Serous Carcinoma: Evaluation of Long-term Survival in Surgically Staged Patients

Grice J, Ek M, Greer B, et al (Virginia Mason Med Ctr, Seattle; Milton S Hershey Med Ctr, Hershey, Pa)

Gynecol Oncol 69:69–73, 1998 24–9

Background.—Previous research has shown that the uterine papillary serous carcinoma (UPSC) variant of endometrial carcinoma has a high rate of recurrence, even when disease appears to be limited to the uterus. Survival among patients with surgically staged UPSC was determined.

TABLE 1.—Survival Status and Treatment for Stage I and II UPSC

Patient	Status	Survival	Treatment	ADD XRT	Chemo
MH IA	NED	19 months	None	None	
CD IA	NED	54 months	None	None	
HG IA	NED	78 months	None	None	
VW IA	NED	28 months	WART	None	
ME IB	DOC	28 months	None	None	
IR IB	NED	54 months	None	None	
AT IB	NED	32 months	WPXRT	Preop T & O	
EC IB	NED	64 months	WPXRT	None	
EK IC	DOD	30 months	WPXRT	None	After REC
NR IC	NED	41 months	WPXRT/VB	None	
CR IC	DOD	57 months	WPXRT/VB	None	After REC
EP IC	DOC	94 months	WPXRT	None	
BA IIB	NED	45 months	None	Preop T & O	
GH IIB	NED	68 months	WART/PB/VB	None	

Abbreviations: ADD, additional; *NED*, no evidence of disease; *DOD*, died of disease; DOC, died of other causes without evidence of disease; *AWD*, alive with disease; *WART*, whole abdominal radiation therapy; *WPXRT*, whole pelvis radiation therapy; *VB*, vaginal boost; *PB*, pelvic boost; *REC*, recurrence; *T&O*, tandem and ovoid.

(Courtesy of Grice J, Ek M, Greer B, et al: Uterine papillary serous carcinoma: Evaluation of long-term survival in surgically staged patients. *Gynecol Oncol* 69:68–73, 1998.)

Methods.—Thirty-six patients with UPSC were identified retrospectively, and their records were reviewed. All patients had had a total abdominal hysterectomy and bilateral salpingo-oophorectomy, lymph node dissection, and peritoneal cytology.

Findings.—The International Federation of Gynecology and Obstetrics stages of these patients were stage I in 12, stage IIB in 2, stage III in 13, and stage IV in 9. Six of the 14 patients with stage I or II disease were not given adjuvant therapy, 5 underwent whole pelvic radiation, and 3 were given whole abdominal radiation therapy (WART). After a median follow-up of 50 months, only 14% of this group had a recurrence. Both of these 2 recurrences were in patients with stage IC disease who were given radiation. One patient had a recurrence in the radiation field. Of the 5 patients with stage IIIA disease, 3 patients declined treatment and 2 received WART. The latter 2 patients and 1 declining treatment are currently alive without disease. Of the 8 patients with stage IIIC disease, 2 declined postoperative treatment, 2 underwent WART, and 4 underwent whole pelvic radiation with an extended field that included para-aortic nodes. After a median 48 months of follow-up, 4 of the 6 patients with stage IIIC disease treated with curative intent had no disease, and another had died from unrelated causes. Both the patients with stage IIIC disease who declined treatment had a recurrence. Eight of the 9 patients with stage IV disease died from their disease (Table 1).

Conclusions.—The prognosis of UPSC is good when surgical staging shows that disease is limited to the uterus. Surgical findings can be used to tailor individual adjuvant radiation therapy. The optimal treatment for women with metastatic UPSC remains unclear.

▶ Uterine papillary serous carcinoma is recognized as an aggressive malignancy.

This retrospective study of 36 patients provides some useful data. Complete surgical staging offers prognostic and therapeutic information. As shown in Table 1 (reproduced above), a variety of therapies were used for stages I and II, but some patients were NED without any postoperative treatment. Only 2 of the 14 patients with stage I and II had recurrences.

For advanced-stage disease, the results, as expected, were worse, with survivals in only those patients who had post-operative therapy, usually with radiation treatment. For stage III patients, 7 of 13 were NED at 29–93 months, while 8 of 9 with stage IV were dead of disease at the time of the report.

The authors recommend aggressive initial operative staging for these tumors, and I agree. These authors are studying a regimen of chemotherapy and whole abdominal for postoperative treatment, but at this point the optimal approach is not known. Certainly this article provides some evidence that postoperative treatment (radiation or chemotherapy or both) is worthwhile.

A.L. Herbst, M.D.

Effective Treatment of Stage I Uterine Papillary Serous Carcinoma With High Dose-Rate Vaginal Apex Radiation (^{192}Ir) and Chemotherapy

Turner BC, Knisely JPS, Kacinski BM, et al (Yale Univ, New Haven, Conn; Glens Falls Hosp, NY)

Int J Radiat Oncol Biol Phys 40:77–84, 1998 24–10

Objective.—Uterine papillary serous carcinoma (UPSC) is a high-grade, highly invasive form of endometrial cancer. There is no general agreement on the treatment of choice, and the type of treatment appears to depend on the stage of the disease. The condition has a poor overall survival rate, a high recurrence rate, is frequently understaged, and has a poor response to salvage treatment. The presentation, pathology, local and distant control, survival, salvage rate, and complications of UPSC for patients undergoing whole-pelvis radiation therapy (WPRT), whole-abdomen radiation therapy (WART), low-dose–rate (LDR) intracavitary brachytherapy, or high-dose–rate (HDR) vaginal apex brachytherapy and chemotherapy were retrospectively reviewed.

Methods.—Between 1975 and 1993, 38 patients with Federation International of Gynecology and Obstetrics (FIGO) stage I UPSC were treated with combinations of total abdominal hysterectomy, bilateral salpingo-oophorectomy, radiation therapy, and chemotherapy. Fifteen patients underwent surgical staging. Twenty patients underwent LDR, WART, or WPRT. In this group, 2 also had cisplatin chemotherapy, 18 had vaginal brachytherapy (5 of these also had chemotherapy), and 6 had both brachytherapy and external beam radiotherapy.

Results.—The FIGO stage I patients who were completely surgically staged and treated with postoperative HDR vaginal apex brachytherapy and chemotherapy had a 5-year actuarial overall survival rate of 100%.

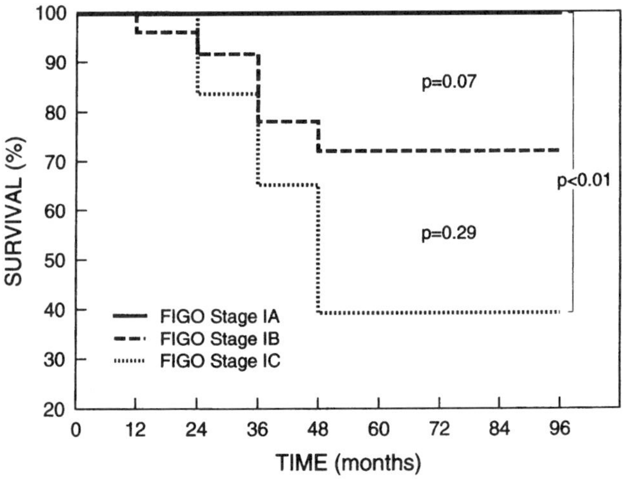

FIGURE 3.—Actuarial disease-free survival by depth of myometrial invasion was determined for Federation International of Gynecology and Obstetrics (*FIGO*) stage I patients with uterine papillary serous carcinoma (UPSC) who had undergone complete surgical staging. Survival for stage IA (*solid line*), IB (*dashed line*), and IC (*dotted line*) UPSC patients was determined by the Kaplan-Meier method. (Reprinted by permission of the publisher from Turner BC, Knisely JPS, Kacinski BM, et al: Effective treatment of stage I uterine papillary serous carcinoma with high dose-rate vaginal apex radiation (^{192}Ir) and chemotherapy. *Int J Radiat Oncol Biol Phys* 40:77–84, copyright 1998 by Elsevier Science Inc.)

Stage I patients treated with preoperative and postoperative LDR brachytherapy, WPRT, and/or WART had a 5-year actuarial overall survival rate of 65%. These findings are in agreement with results of previous studies. None of the 6 stage I patients who underwent complete surgical staging, LDR therapy, and WART/WPRT had a recurrence. Five-year actuarial disease-free survival rate for stage IA, IB, and IC patients who underwent complete staging were 100%, 71%, and 40% (Fig 3). The salvage rate for distant and local recurrence was 0%. Sixteen percent of patients undergoing HDR vaginal apex brachytherapy had Radiation Therapy Oncology Group (RTOG) grades 1 and 2 toxicity, whereas 15% of patients undergoing WART/WPRT and/or LDR had RTOG grades 3 and 4 toxicity.

Conclusion.—Patients with UPSC can be effectively treated with complete surgical staging and HDR vaginal apex brachytherapy and chemotherapy. Overall survival and disease-free survival depend on the depth of myometrial invasion. Salvage rates for distant and local recurrence are very low. A minority of patients undergoing HDR vaginal apex brachytherapy experienced RTOG grades 1 and 2 toxicity.

▶ This article demonstrates that UPSC can be effectively treated, particularly in stage IA. I think an important point made by the authors is that patients with these tumors deserve a full-staging laparotomy consistent with the approach we use for ovarian carcinoma. The therapies used in this small series of 38 patients varied widely, and, for that reason, it is difficult to draw any definitive therapeutic conclusions.

The authors did demonstrate that HDR vaginal apical radiation therapy can be effectively given, but I am not certain that this therapy has been shown to make a difference in survival for these patients. I am very much in favor of using chemo-radiation for patients with this disease, but, as noted by the authors, this, too, is controversial.

A.L. Herbst, M.D.

Conservative Management of Endometrial Stromal Sarcoma in Young Women

Lissoni A, Cormio G, Perego P, et al (Univ of Milan, Italy)

Int J Gynecol Cancer 7:364–367, 1997 24–11

Objective.—Total abdominal hysterectomy and bilateral salpingo-oophorectomy are standard therapy for endometrial stromal sarcoma (ESS), a rare tumor with a poor prognosis. Fertility-sparing therapy in younger women has not been well studied. Pathologic characteristics, clinical outcome, and subsequent pregnancies of 6 patients conservatively managed for ESS of the uterus were presented.

Methods.—The number of mitotic figures per 10 high power fields (HPF), cytologic atypia, presence of necrosis, and margin status were determined in 6 nulliparous women, aged 18 to 36 years with ESS of the uterus. Patients were informed of the risk of recurrence after conservative surgery. No patient had postoperative adjuvant therapy. Examinations, ultrasonography, and hysteroscopy were performed every 3 months for 2 years, and chest X-ray studies and abdominal MRI or CT were performed every 6 months for 2 years and then annually thereafter. Patients were followed for a median of 51 months.

Results.—One patient had high-grade ESS (12 mitoses/10 HPF), and 5 had low-grade ESS. In 5 patients, the tumor was completely resected with a margin of at least 2 mm. Two patients had a second surgical procedure. At follow-up, all patients were alive and well and had no recurrences. Two patients had 2 successful pregnancies and a third had a miscarriage at week 8.

Conclusion.—Conservative management of ESS can be used in selected patients who wish to become pregnant. Rigorous follow-up is necessary.

▶ This is an interesting report on conservative fertility-sparing therapy for a rare disease that is usually treated by hysterectomy. The number of patients treated was quite small, but among the 6 patients with a median age 27 years, myoma resection was the treatment modality. Five patients had a low mitotic rate averaging 4/10 HPF. However, 1 patient had a markedly higher grade lesion with an average of 12 mitoses/10 HPF, and she, too, was treated conservatively. All of the patients had a tumor-free resection margin of at least 2 mm and, most impressively, all were recurrence free, with a median survival of 51 months.

This is an impressive record, especially for the patient with the higher-grade lesion. None of the patients received any postoperative chemotherapy and it is certainly questionable, if adjuvant chemotherapy prolongs survival even for high-grade endometrial stromal sarcomas. In spite of the small number in this study, it appears that this is an approach worth considering for young patients with this disease—particularly those with a low mitotic rate—who desire to preserve fertility.

A.L. Herbst, M.D.

25 Gynecologic Oncology

Ovarian

The Malignant Potential of Small Cystic Ovarian Tumors in Women Over 50 Years of Age

Bailey CL, Ueland FR, Land GL, et al (Univ of Kentucky Med Ctr, Lexington)

Gynecol Oncol 69:3–7, 1998 25–1

Background.—The risk of malignancy is believed to be high for large complex tumors with wall abnormalities and lower for unilocular cystic tumors. The malignant potential of ovarian tumors less than 10 cm in diameter, detected by transvaginal sonography in asymptomatic postmenopausal women, was investigated.

Methods.—The size and morphology of all cystic ovarian tumors detected by transvaginal sonography screening in asymptomatic women who were postmenopausal or age 50 or older were recorded. Histologic findings of all tumors removed at surgery were documented.

Findings.—Unilocular cystic tumors were found in 256 (3.3%) of 7,705 women. All tumors were less than 10 cm in diameter, and 90% were less than 5 cm. Forty-nine percent of the cysts resolved spontaneously within 60 days. Tumors were removed surgically in 45 patients with persisting ovarian cysts. Thirty-two patients had ovarian serous cystadenomas, and the rest had benign lesions. No ovarian carcinoma was found in this group, nor in the 86 patients studied every 3–6 months without surgery. Three percent of the patients had complex cystic ovarian tumors, all less than 10 cm in diameter, and 89% had tumors less than 5 cm. Fifty-five percent of these tumors resolved spontaneously within 60 days. One hundred fourteen of the 115 patients with persisting lesions underwent surgery. Ovarian

TABLE 1.—Spontaneous Resolution of Unilocular Cystic Ovarian Tumors Related to Patient Age

Age (years)	Number	Spontaneous tumor resolution	Significance
50–60	210	114 (54.3%)	$P<0.03$
>60	46	11 (23.9%)	

(Courtesy of Bailey CL, Ueland FR, Land GL, et al: The malignant potential of small cystic ovarian tumors in women over 50 years of age. *Gynecol Oncol* 69:3–7, 1998.)

TABLE 2.—Pathology of Patients With Unilocular Cystic Ovarian Tumors (n = 45)

Pathology	Number
Serous cystadenoma	32
Paratubal cyst	4
Paraovarian cyst	3
Endometriotic cyst	2
Mucinous cystadenoma	2
Hydrosalpinx	1
Peritoneal cyst	1
Total	45

(Courtesy of Bailey CL, Ueland FR, Land GL, et al: The malignant potential of small cystic ovarian tumors in women over 50 years of age. *Gynecol Oncol* 69:3–7, 1998.)

carcinoma was found in 7 patients, peritoneal cancer in 1, and metastatic breast cancer of the ovary in 1 (Tables 1 and 2).

Conclusions.—The risk for ovarian cancer associated with unilocular ovarian cysts less than 10 cm in diameter appears to be minimal in asymptomatic, postmenopausal women. By contrast, the risk for malignancy associated with complex ovarian cysts with wall abnormalities or solid areas is significant.

▶ There has been a great deal of interest in vaginal US screening to detect ovarian cancer. The technique has, thus far, not proved to be cost-effective, but this article does provide some useful data.

A unilocular ovarian cyst in menopausal women can regress, as shown in Table 1. Spontaneous regression is less frequent in older women, but even those over age 60 have a regression rate of about 25%.

The article also shows that unilocular masses less than 10 cm (usually less than 5 cm) are not malignant. The results are different for complex masses, as shown in Table 2, also reproduced above.

As noted by the authors, approximately 3% of asymptomatic postmenopausal women will be found to have ovarian cysts less than 5 cm. Most of these cysts resolve spontaneously, but those which are complex or grow under observation require operative intervention.

A.L. Herbst, M.D.

Ovarian Tumors of Low Malignant Potential: A Retrospective Study of 234 Patients

Sykes PH, Quinn MA, Rome RM (Royal Womens Hosp, Melbourne, Australia)

Int J Gynecol Cancer 7:218–226, 1997 25–2

Objective.—Most patients with low malignant potential (LMP) ovarian tumors have a good prognosis. Prognostic factors include surgical stage, histologic type, presence of pseudomyxoma, DNA-ploidy, histology of

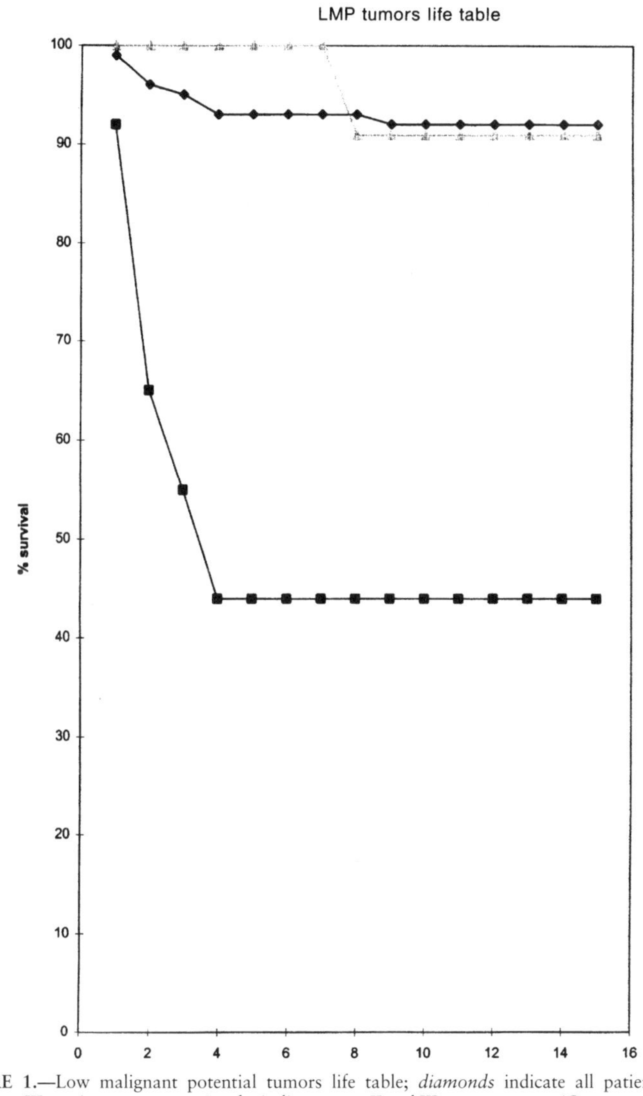

FIGURE 1.—Low malignant potential tumors life table; *diamonds* indicate all patients; *squares* indicate stage III mucinous tumors; *triangles* indicate stage II and III serous tumors. (Courtesy of Sykes PH, Quinn MA, Rome RM: Ovarian tumors of low malignant potential: A retrospective study of 234 patients. *Int J Gynecol Cancer* 7:218–226, 1997).

implants, and pathologic grading. In this study, the malignant potential of pseudomyxoma was established, high-risk patients were identified, and recommendations for surgical staging and postoperative management were reviewed.

Methods.—An epithelial ovarian tumor with low malignant potential was diagnosed in 234 consecutive patients, aged 16–93 years, seen at the Royal Womens Hospital in Melbourne between 1972 and 1994. Six patients with synchronous intra-abdominal malignancy and 6 with early stromal invasion were considered separately.

Results.—Histologically, tumors were mucinous in 53%, serous in 37%, mixed in 7%, endometrioid in 3%, and clear cell in 0.4%. Twenty-four percent of tumors were bilateral including 39% serous, 15% mucinous, and 24% mixed. Significantly more serous than mucinous tumors were bilateral. Fourteen patients had pseudomyxoma peritonei associated with mucinous tumors. Extra ovarian implants were found in 34% of patients with serous tumors, 13% with mucinous tumors, and 24% with mixed tumors. Four patients had positive lymph nodes and 5 patients with serous tumors had invasive implants. There were 175 patients with clinical stage I disease, 19 with stage II, and 28 with stage III. A total of 173 patients were followed for an average of 54 months. Six of 13 patients who died had pseudomyxoma peritonei. Seven of 12 patients with invasive malignancies died. No patients with stage Ia of Ib disease had a recurrence (Fig 1).

Conclusion.—Adjuvant therapy is not necessary for patients with early-stage ovarian tumors. In this study, no patients with stage Ia or Ib disease had a recurrence. The prognosis is good, except for those patients with synchronous intra-abdominal malignancy or pseudomyxoma peritonei, and fertility can be maintained.

▶ It is well established that low malignant potential tumors have an indolent course and, in general, do not respond to adjuvant therapy. Operation is the mainstay of treatment. However, as noted in this study, a few of these patients do die and, as shown in Fig 1, the results in the mucinous group can be particularly discouraging. This is partially because of the occurrences of pseudomyxoma peritonei among these patients.

Eliminating those with pseudomyxoma pertitonei, the overall 5-year survival rate for all patients was a respectable 93%. Patients with stage II and III serous disease had a 10-year survival rate of 90%, as determined by life table analysis. Interestingly, but not surprisingly, no patient with surgical stage Ia or Ib tumors had a recurrence. As emphasized by the authors, extra ovariandisease worsens the prognosis, but there is little evidence that chemotherapy helps with survival in this group. It is still debated which group, if any, should receive chemotherapy, and—although the evidence is, at best, fragmentary—I usually restrict it to those rare patients who have extraovarian disease with invasive "implants."

A.L. Herbst, M.D.

Ovarian Serous Borderline Tumors With Invasive Peritoneal Implants

Gershenson DM, Silva EG, Levy L, et al (Univ of Texas, Houston)

Cancer 82:1096–1103, 1998 25–3

Background.—There is no accepted standard postoperative treatment for women with serous borderline tumors with peritoneal implants. A

TABLE 6.—Disease Recurrence and Death From Tumor in Patients with Stage II–IV Serous Borderline Tumors With Invasive Peritoneal Implants

Study	No. with recurrence	No. dead of tumor
Kliman et al.	0/2	0/2
Manchul et al.	1/5	0/5
Russell	3/6	3/6
Michael and Roth	1/8*	1/8*
McCaughey et al.	5/11†	4/11†
Bell et al.	5/6	4/6
De Nictolis et al.	4/9	4/9
Seidman and Kurman	8/13‡	6/13‡
Total	27/60 (45%)	22/60 (37%)

*4 patients had been followed for 2 years or less.
†6 patients who did not have a recurrence had been followed for 1 year or less.
‡11 patients' primary tumors were classified as "micropapillary serous carcinoma."
(Courtesy of Gershenson DM, Silva EG, Levy L, et al: Ovarian serous borderline tumors with invasive peritoneal implants. *Cancer* 82:1096–1103, ©1998, American Cancer Society. Reprinted by permission of Wiley-Liss, Inc., a subsidiary of John Wiley & Sons, Inc.)

large retrospective series of these patients, studied to understand prognostic factors and the effects of postoperative treatment, was described.

Study Design.—The study group consisted of 39 women, aged 17 to 60 years, diagnosed with primary ovarian serous borderline tumor with invasive peritoneal implants, who were seen at the M.D. Anderson Cancer Center of the University of Texas from 1956 through 1966. Invasive implants were subdivided into early and frankly invasive types. All patients had surgery as the initial treatment. For those who had second-look surgery, surgicopathologic response was evaluated. There was a median follow-up of 111 months. The Cox proportional hazards model was used for identification of prognostic factors.

Findings.—Of these 39 patients, 30 had both noninvasive and invasive peritoneal implants. Early invasive implants were detected in 35 patients and frankly invasive implants were detected in 9, with 5 patients having both types. Postoperative chemotherapy was used in 31 patients, of whom 22 received platinum-based and 9 received melphalan chemotherapy. At second-look surgery in 18 patients, 11 had no macroscopic disease and findings were either negative (9 patients) or demonstrated involvement of only the residual ovary (2 patients). Of the remaining 7 patients, 1 had a complete surgicopathologic response to chemotherapy, 3 had a partial response, and 3 had no response. During follow-up, 12 patients experienced progression or recurrence, with a median time from diagnosis of 24 months. Time to progression was significantly longer for those patients with no macroscopic residual disease after initial surgery and for those with early invasive peritoneal implants. Platinum-based chemotherapy was associated with significantly shorter progression-free survival.

Conclusion.—This largest retrospective study of women with ovarian serous borderline tumors with invasive peritoneal implants revealed that more than 30% of these women will have progressive or recurrent tumor (Table 6). The most important prognostic factor was the presence of macroscopic residual tumor after initial surgery. In this study, the role of postoperative therapy could not be defined. Further study is necessary to determine appropriate postoperative treatment for women with ovarian serous borderline tumors with invasive peritoneal implants.

► The therapy of serous borderline ovarian tumors of advanced stage remains controversial, primarily because there is a lack of data on tumor behavior and response to therapy. This report from the M.D. Anderson Cancer Center of the University of Texas of a comparatively large series of these tumors with invasive implants illustrates the difficulty. The authors usefully restricted their analyses of 39 patients to those with invasive implants, and for those patients, the primary factor affecting survival was the eradication of all tumor at initial operation. I have included Table 6 from the paper, which summarizes a number of articles regarding patients with invasive implants. Overall, 37% of patients died of disease.

Interestingly, in this series the use of platinum therapy was associated with a *shorter* progression-free interval. As noted by the authors, this may be the result of selection bias. I would avoid postoperative therapy in those who are disease free after initial surgery. For those with residual disease, the issue is unclear. Of those evaluable, only 1 of 7 in this series had a complete response to therapy. As noted by the authors, a prospective Gynecologic Oncology Group trial will, hopefully, provide some answers.

A.L. Herbst, M.D.

Tumor Recurrence in Stage I Ovarian Serous Neoplasms of Low Malignant Potential

Silva EG, Tornos C, Zhuang Z, et al (Univ of Texas, Houston; NIH, Bethesda, Md)

Int J Gynecol Pathol 17:1–6, 1998 25–4

Objective.—Rare recurrences of serous neoplasm of low malignant potential (SNLMP) in patients with stage I disease are retrospectively reviewed.

Methods.—Eleven patients, aged 26–43 years at diagnosis, with SNLMP, had a clinical recurrence after a disease-free interval of 1 year or more after bilateral salpingo-oophorectomy and a total abdominal hysterectomy.

Results.—The clinicopathologic characteristics of the patients were analyzed (Table 1). Nine patients had radiotherapy, and 2 had chemotherapy. Time to recurrence ranged from 7–39 years. Recurrences were treated with surgical resection in 9 patients and with chemotherapy in 10 patients. Recurrence rates were independent of age, gravidity, size of the ovarian tumor, degree of epithelial proliferation, or number of mitoses. There was a significant relationship between papillary excrescences on the external surface and extraovarian endosalpingiosis (7 of 13 lesions) suggesting a relationship between exophytic SNLMPs, peritoneal implants, and endo-

TABLE 1.—Ovarian Serous Neoplasm of Low Malignant Potential, Cases That Recurred

		Primary ovarian tumor			Recurrence			
Patient no.	Age (yrs)	Size (cm)	External surface	Endosalpingiosis	Time to recurrence (yr)	Site	Type of tumor	Follow-up after recurrence (yr)
1	31	4 × 4 × 3	Smooth	Fallopian tube	22	Omentum	Serous ca	DOD, 2
2	43	9 × 9 × 8	Unknown	Uterine serosa	20	Neck	Serous ca	DOD, 2
3	39	15 × 15 × 15 19 × 6 × 5	Papillary	Uterine serosa	8	Pelvis	Serous ca	DOD, 4
4	26	8 × 6 × 5	Smooth	—	10	Pelvis	Serous ca	DOD, 4
5	26	14 × 11 × 8 6 × 4 × 3	Papillary	Uterine serosa and fallopian tube	17	Pelvis	Serous LMP	NED, 9
6	42	8 × 8 × 8 5 × 5 × 5	Smooth	—	24	Abdomen	Serous ca	Died[a], 10
7	27	6 × 6 × 6 5 × 5 × 5	Smooth	Omentum, appendix, and uterine serosa	12	Abdomen	Serous ca	DOD, 4
8	32	10 × 7 × 7 4 × 4 × 3	Papillary	—	16	Abdomen	Serous ca	DOD, 5
9	33	7 × 5 × 3 4.5 × 3.5 × 2.5	Papillary	Fallopian tube	18	Pleura	Serous ca	DOD, 3
10	41	13 × 13 × 13 8 × 6 × 6	Papillary	Uterine serosa	7	Neck	Serous ca	AWPD, 7
11	27	6 × 5 × 5	Papillary	Uterine serosa	39	Abdomen	Serous ca	AWPD, 1

Abbreviations: ca, carcinoma; *DOD*, died of disease; *LMP*, low malignant potential; *NED*, no evidence of disease; *AWPD* alive with progressive disease.
[a]This patient died of leukemia with recurrent ovarian tumor. (Courtesy of Silva EG, Tornos C, Zhuang Z, et al: Tumor recurrence in stage I ovarian serous neoplasms of low malignant potential. *Int J Gynecol Pathol* 17:1–6, 1998.)

salpingiosis. A correct diagnosis of recurrent disease is important, because patients whose disease recurred as serous carcinoma died or are alive with recurrent disease. Patients whose disease recurred as SNLMP are alive with no evidence of disease 9 and 26 years after resection of the original tumor.

Conclusion.—No features that predicted recurrence of stage I ovarian SNLMP were identified. Patients who died or were alive with recurrent disease had serous carcinoma, whereas those with recurrent SNLMP were alive with no evidence of disease at last follow-up. Those with recurrent disease also had extraovarian endosalpingiosis.

► This article provides long-term follow-up on recurrence of serous ovarian tumors with low malignant potential. As noted by the authors, recurrences are rare and, unfortunately, this study does not help predict which features of these tumors in stage I are more likely to recur. However, those recurrences were in patients with an increased frequency of extraovarian endosalpingiosis. Of interest is that 10 of the 11 tumors that recurred were low-grade invasive serous carcinoma and the one patient whose recurrence was borderline is alive with no evidence of disease. As can be seen from Table 1, the recurrences were truly late (7–39 years), and we have little evidence that therapies other than operation have any beneficial effect.

A.L. Herbst, M.D.

Fertility After Conservative Treatment of Ovarian Immature Teratomas

Edraki B, Schwartz PE (Univ of Texas, Houston; Yale Univ, New Haven, Conn)

Int J Gynecol Cancer 7:227–232, 1997 25–5

Objective.—The majority of rare immature teratomas occur in children and young adults. For patients who have not yet had children, preservation of fertility is important. The survival and reproductive experience of patients treated conservatively for immature teratomas of the ovary were reported.

Methods.—Charts of 35 consecutive patients, aged 7–47 years, with pure immature teratomas of the ovary were retrospectively reviewed. These patients were followed for an average of 110 months. All patients had primary surgery. Two had no other treatment, 25 were treated with vincristine, dactinomycin, and cyclophosphamide (VAC), and 8 were treated with a cisplatin regimen. Reproductive potential was preserved in 26 patients (74.3%), aged 7 to 32 years. All patients had primary surgery. Two patients had surgery alone, 20 were treated with VAC in addition to surgery, and 4 were given a cisplatin regimen. These patients were followed for an average of 125.5 months.

Results.—One surgery-only patient had a recurrence. Two VAC-treated patients failed treatment but were salvaged, and 1 had her fertility preserved. Three patients treated with a cisplatin regimen had a recurrence. Two died and 1 was salvaged. Of the 26 whose fertility was initially spared, 2 had primary treatment failure but were salvaged, 3 had secon-

TABLE 3.—Characteristics of Patients Achieving Pregnancy

Stage	Grade	Therapy	Wedge biopsy	Second look surgery	Gravida	Para	Abortion
IA	1	Ovarian cystectomy	N	N	5	3	2
IA	2	USO + VAC × 12	N	Y	2	2	—
IA	2	USO + PVB × 1 + BEP × 3	Y	N	3	1	2
IA	2	USO + VAC × 8	?	N	3	2	1
IA	3	USO + VAC × 6	N	N	2	2	—
IC	1	USO + VAC × 18	Y	Y	2	1	1*
IC	3	USO + VAC × 6	Y	N	1	1	—
IC	3	USO + VAC × 12	N	Y	2	1	1
III A	1	USO + VAC × 6	N	N	2	2	—
III A	2	USO + BEP × 3 + VAC × 3	Y	N	2	2	—
III B	2	USO + VAC × 6 + BADV × 16	Y	N	2	2	—

*Delivery followed by a hysterectomy.

Abbreviations: USO, unilateral salpingo-oophorectomy; *VAC*, vincristine, dactinomycin, cyclophosphamide; *PVB*, cisplatin, vinblastine, bleomycin; *BEP*, bleomycin, etoposide, cisplatin; *BADV*, bleomycin, dactinomycin, imidazole carboximide, vinblastine.

(Courtesy of Edraki B, Schwartz PE: Fertility after conservative treatment of ovarian immature teratomas. *Int J Gynecol Cancer* 7:227–232, 1997.)

dary loss of fertility, 1 had a total abdominal hysterectomy and contralateral salpingo-oophorectomy for what was found to be a benign ovarian cyst, 2 were incompletely developed sexually, and 1 had an unwanted pregnancy and subsequent bilateral tubal ligation. The remaining 20 were able to conceive. Seven did not attempt pregnancy, but the remaining 13 achieved 26 pregnancies (Table 3).

Conclusion.—Primary or salvage treatment of patients with ovarian immature teratomas can preserve reproductive function, and the majority of patients who desire to become pregnant can do so.

▶ This study reports on 35 consecutive patients with ovarian immature teratoma who were treated conservatively to preserve fertility. Twenty-three of the patients in this series had fertility-preserving treatment and 13 of them attempted pregnancy, with 11 successes. The characteristics of these 11 patients are shown in Table 3. It is of interest that 10 of 20 patients also had a wedge resection of the contralateral ovary. I believe that this is probably not necessary if the contralateral ovary appears normal, particularly with the current availability of vaginal US follow-up. However, it is worth remembering that these patients were treated over a 20-year period.

As shown in the table, many of the patients had a grade 2 or grade 3 immature teratoma, and 6 were higher than stage Ia. This report successfully emphasizes the effectiveness of chemotherapy in this disease and shows the wisdom of the conservative approach used by the Yale group to treat these young patients.

A.L. Herbst, M.D.

Prognostic Factors in Adult Granulosa Cell Tumor of the Ovary

Miller BE, Barron BA, Wan JY, et al (Univ of Tennessee, Memphis; Univ of Kansas, Wichita; Univ of Texas, Houston)

Cancer 79:1951–1955, 1997 25–6

Background.—Adult granulosa cell tumor of the ovary is characterized by indolent growth usually leading to large tumor size at diagnosis. Recurrent disease is not uncommon, although frequently after a long interval. To identify prognostic factors in this slowly progressing disease, the clinical and pathologic features of recurrent and nonrecurrent granulosa cell tumors were retrospectively compared over a 35-year period in a multisite study.

Study Design.—Tumor registries from 4 sites were reviewed for all patients treated between 1958 and 1993 for primary or recurrent adult granulosa cell tumors of the ovary. For comparison, these 70 cases were subdivided into 51 patients without recurrence (NED group) and 19 with recurrent disease (REC group).

Findings.—Logistic regression analysis indicated that only tumor stage was significantly different between these 2 groups. Pathologic examination demonstrated that Call-Exner bodies occurred more commonly in tumors from NED patients. Atypia was significantly more common in tumors from the REC group. Early-recurring tumors had fewer Call-Exner bodies, higher mitotic rates, and more atypia than late-recurring tumors, which were more similar to tumors of NED patients.

Conclusion.—Tumor stage is the only clinical parameter with prognostic significance in patients with adult granulosa cell tumor of the ovary. Cellular atypia and, to some extent, mitotic rate and the absence of Call-Exner bodies are the only significant pathologic prognostic factors in these patients. These pathologic parameters can be used to identify tumors with higher proliferation rates but cannot be used to predict late recurrences of these slow-growing tumors.

► This report on 70 patients with granulosa cell tumor, treated at M.D. Anderson Hospital of the University of Texas, is a large experience for 1 institution. Unfortunately, the authors were unable to uncover any features—except initial tumor stage and tumor size—that were prognostic. Most of these tumors are indolent, with large recurrences when they occur. Those with recurrence tended to have cellular atypia, a high mitotic rate, and fewer Call-Exner bodies, but these were not sufficient to make useful predictions.

I agree with the authors, these tumors can show different biological behaviors, i.e., some are indolent and others more aggressive. Unfortunately, we cannot yet predict the future in an individual case, and I have not been impressed with the use of adjuvant chemotherapy for these patients.

A.L. Herbst, M.D.

Primary Ovarian Sarcoma: Analysis of Prognostic Variables and the Role of Surgical Cytoreduction

Sood AK, Sorosky JI, Gelder MS, et al (Univ of Iowa, Iowa City; Presbyterian Hosp, Charlotte, NC; Univ of Florida, Gainesville)

Cancer 82:1731–1737, 1998 25–7

Background.—The value of cytoreduction and cell histology in women with ovarian sarcomas has not been thoroughly investigated. The role of surgical cytoreduction, preoperative CA 125 levels, stage, histology, and platinum-based chemotherapy in the primary treatment of ovarian sarcomas was studied.

Methods and Findings.—Forty-seven women with primary ovarian sarcomas were studied retrospectively. Eighty-seven percent had advanced-stage disease. Optimal surgical cytoreduction was achieved in 53%. Eighty-five percent had a malignant mixed mullerian tumor, and 15% had pure sarcoma. Mixed mullerian tumors were homologous in 18 and heterologous in 22. Treatment response was significantly more likely with platinum-based chemotherapy than with other regimens. There was also a survival advantage with platinum-based chemotherapy. In 93% of the patients, preoperative CA 125 levels exceeded 35 U/mL. A preoperative

CA 125 level of less than 75 U/mL was correlated with improved survival. In a multivariate analysis, the most significant prognostic factor was optimal surgical cytoreduction, followed by histologic subtype.

Conclusions.—Preoperative CA 125 levels should be obtained in all women with suspected ovarian carcinoma or sarcoma. Surgical cytoreduction to a residual tumor burden of 1 cm or less improves outcomes. Although the optimal consolidation chemotherapy regimen has yet to be established, platinum should be included.

▶ Primary ovarian sarcoma is extraordinarily rare, so I believe that including this report of 41 patients is useful. The prognosis is poor, in part because the patients had advanced-stage disease when initially seen.

The authors recommend surgical cytoreduction to the greatest extent possible, and (presumably) this will improve the outcome. Not surprisingly, there is no clear-cut recommendation for chemotherapy, but I agree with the authors' suggestion that platinum should be included.

A.L. Herbst, M.D.

Secondary Cytoreductive Surgery at Second-look Laparotomy in Advanced Ovarian Cancer: A Gynecologic Oncology Group Study

Williams L, Brunetto VL, Yordan E, et al (Vanderbilt Univ, Nashville, Tenn; Roswell Park Cancer Inst, Buffalo, NY; Rush–Presbyterian St. Luke's Med Ctr, Chicago, et al)

Gynecol Oncol 66:171–178, 1997 25–8

Objective.—One of the potential advantages of second-look laparotomy (SLL) for patients with advanced ovarian cancer is to provide an opportunity for debulking a macroscopic tumor if found. The effect on survival of this procedure has not been studied. The technical feasibility of secondary cytoreduction and the effect of this surgery on survival were assessed.

Methods.—Second-look laparotomy was performed on 153 women aged 20–79 years, with stage III or IV epithelial ovarian cancer. Cytoreduction was performed on 36 patients. Tumor size before and remaining after cytoreduction was estimated. Survival estimates were determined using the Kaplan-Meier method, and risk factors for survival were evaluated using Cox's proportional hazards model.

Results.—There were 66 patients 60 years of age or older and 36 with stage IV disease. There were 127 women with no clinically measurable disease at the time of SLL. At SLL, 69 patients had a tumor greater than 1 cm, which was cytoreduced to leave a microscopic residual in 15 patients and to macroscopic small tumor in 18 patients. At SLL, 55 patients had a tumor of 1 cm or less, which was cytoreduced to macroscopic small tumor in 21 patients. At SLL, 29 patients had microscopic disease. Cytoreduction to microscopic disease was accomplished in 36 (29%) of 124 patients with macroscopic tumor. Survival depended on tumor size found at SLL and on residual tumor size after debulking (Fig 2). Patients whose debulked tumor

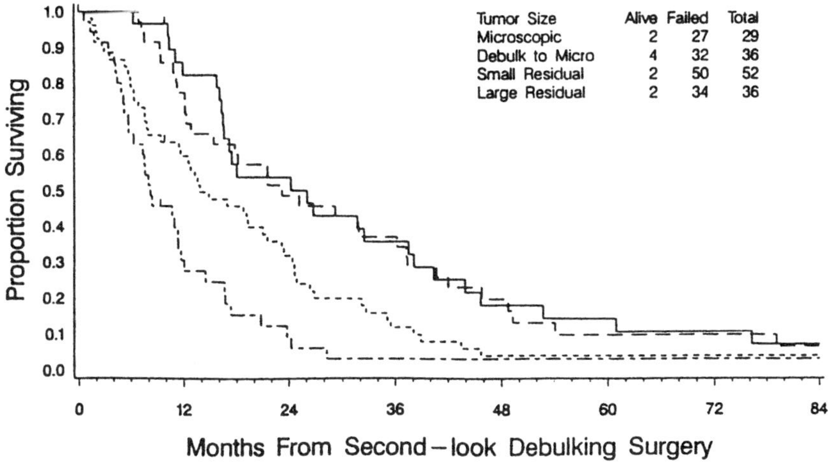

FIGURE 2.—Survival by residual tumor size. (Courtesy of Williams L, Brunetto VL, Yordan E, et al: Secondary cytoreductive surgery at second-look laparotomy in advanced ovarian cancer: A Gynecologic Oncology Group study. *Gynecol Oncol* 66:171–178, 1997).

was greater than 1 cm had significantly shorter survival times than patients in other categories. Survival was unaffected in patients with microscopic disease and those whose tumors were cytoreduced to microscopic disease. Risk of death was decreased in patients whose tumors were cytoreduced to a lower category. There were few intraoperative complications. Postoperative complications were not evaluated.

Conclusion.—Whether cytoreductive surgery is beneficial and improves outcomes cannot be determined. A randomized prospective trial is necessary to answer these questions.

▶ These data add controversy to the debate concerning the value of SLL and further cytoreduction. The results appear to suggest benefit insofar as those whose tumors were debulked to a lower category, i.e., 1 cm or less, to microscopic disease, greater than 1 cm to 1 cm or less, and greater than 1 cm to microscopic disease, all experienced a survival advantage. As noted by the authors selection bias may be at work here, because the more biologically favorable tumors may have been those that were most readily cytoreduced. I agree with the authors' suggestions of a randomized clinical trial. It is discouraging that long-term survivors between the 4 groups are similar at 4–5 years (see Figure 2). Only a few patients appear to have benefited from the 153 operations performed. The median survival for those following SLL with microscopic disease was 13 months, for those with microscopic disease it was 26 months, and for those with small macroscopic disease, 21 months. Although all this is significant on a statistical basis, we still are faced with the problem of effective therapy for patients who have failed primary chemotherapy.

A.L. Herbst, M.D.

Analysis of Failures After Negative Second-Look in Patients With Advanced Ovarian Cancer: An Italian Multicenter Study

Gadducci A, Sartori E, Maggino T, et al (Univ of Pisa, Italy; Univ of Brescia, Italy; Univ of Padova, Italy; et al)

Gynecol Oncol 68:150–155, 1998 25–9

Objective.—Whereas the 5-year survival rate in patients with ovarian cancer is 40.9%, a negative second look is associated with improved survival. A multicenter Italian retrospective study examined the patterns of failures and the prognostic factors for recurrences in patients with advanced ovarian cancer after a negative second look.

Methods.—Between 1980 and 1994 second-look surgery was performed in 192 ovarian cancer patients, aged 30 to 74 at diagnosis. Patients were in pathologic complete response at second look.

Results.—After a second look, 39.7% had no more treatments, 1.5% had external abdomen-pelvic irradiation, 0.5% received intraperitoneal chronic phosphorus, and 57.2% had consolidation chemotherapy. At 4 to 150 months after second-look surgery, 87 patients were still alive. Recurrent disease developed in 94 patients at a median of 18 months—47.9% in the pelvis, 44.7% in the abdomen, 13.8% in the retroperitoneal lymph nodes, and 21.1% at distant sites. Five-year and 7-year disease-free survival rates after second-look surgery were 47.4% and 44.5%, respectively. According to the log rank test, disease-free survival was associated with FIGO stage, tumor grade, size of residual disease, and type of second-look surgery (laparoscopy vs. laparotomy). Survival rates for patients without further treatment and for those having consolidation chemotherapy were similar. According to the Cox proportional hazard model, tumor grade, size of residual disease, and type of second-look surgery were independent and significant predictors of disease-free survival. The risk ratio for relapse was 1.877 in patients with residual disease of 1-2 cm, 2.156 in patients with residual disease greater than 2 cm, 2.386 in patients with G2 disease, 3.118 in patients with G3 disease, and 1.826 in patients with laparoscopy vs. laparotomy.

Conclusion.—Approximately half of these patients had a recurrence. A high tumor grade and large residual disease after surgery were strong predictors of recurrence.

► This is a large and important study of negative second-look procedures after primary chemotherapy. First, the 6- and 7-year survival rates are 47.4% and 44.5%; that is, even after a negative second look, more than half of the patients succumbed to their disease within 5 years. Not surprisingly, initial FIGO stage, tumor grade, and size of residual disease after initial operation were all prognostic. It is of interest that the patients who had laparotomy did better than those who had laparoscopy, perhaps because the former procedure was more comprehensive. As noted by the authors, consolidation chemotherapy did not appear to improve survival in those with a negative second look, nor do other studies support the addition of P32.

Thus, we can conclude that patients with stage III and IV disease will do well if all or most of their disease can be removed, and the outlook is clearly better for low-grade tumors.

The series suggests that if one is to do a second-look procedure, laparotomy may be superior to laparoscopy, but part of these results may be confounded by the extent of the laparoscopic procedure. The problem remains that we do not have established effective treatment for those patients who relapse after a second-look operation.

A.L. Herbst, M.D.

Five-year Survival After Second-line Cisplatin-based Intraperitoneal Chemotherapy for Advanced Ovarian Cancer

Recio FO, Piver MS, Hempling RE, et al (Roswell Park Cancer Inst, Buffalo, NY)

Gynecol Oncol 68:267–273, 1998 25–10

Background.—The efficacy of intraperitoneal chemotherapy (IPC) as salvage treatment in patients with epithelial ovarian cancer should be judged by meaningful long-term survival as well as tumor response rates. The 5-year survival rates of second-line IPC in advanced stage ovarian cancer were determined.

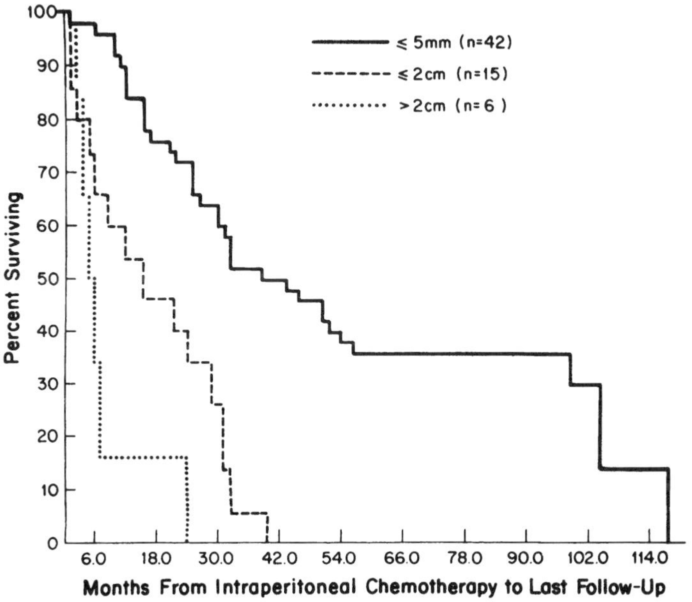

FIGURE 3.—Percentage of survival from time of intraperitoneal chemotherapy according to size of residual disease at second-look laparotomy. (Courtesy of Recio FO, Piver MS, Hempling RE, et al: Five-year survival after second-line cisplatin-based intraperitoneal chemotherapy for advanced ovarian cancer. *Gynecol Oncol* 68:267–273, 1998.)

Methods and Findings.—Sixty-three patients with advanced epithelial ovarian cancer were given intraperitoneal cisplatin and cytarabine chemotherapy as second-line therapy between 1985 and 1991. Median survival from the start of IPC was 29.1 months. Twenty-one patients had a response to first- and second-line treatment. These patients had a significantly better 5-year survival rate (40%) and 5-year progression-free survival rate (37%) than patients who only responded to first-line therapy (with respective rates of 6% and 0). Thirteen patients failed to respond to both first- and second-line treatment. None of these patients survived for 5 years. Forty-two patients had residual disease of 5 mm or less at the time of IPC initiation. This group had a 5-year survival of 36% and a 5-year progression-free survival of 31%. By contrast, none of the 21 patients with residual disease greater than 5 mm at IPC initiation survived for 5 years (Fig 3).

Conclusions.—Although this study was not randomized, it suggests that salvage platinum-based IPC results in significant 5-year survival and 5-year progression-free survival in selected patients whose tumor burden is 5 mm or less at the time of IPC initiation. Such patients have survival rates after second-line therapy that approach those attained by first-line platinum-based IV chemotherapy in patients with advanced stage ovarian cancer with comparable tumor burden at the start of treatment.

► The group at Roswell Park has had a long interest in intraperitoneal therapy. After the initial enthusiasm, disappointing results have tempered the use of this modality for ovarian cancer treatment. This nonrandomized study of 63 patients over a 6-year period indicates that patients who have residual disease of less than 5mm at second-look laparotomy can do well, as shown in the survival curve (Fig 3). As noted by the authors, these results compare favorably with first-line treatment, and it appears that this modality can be useful in patients who responded initially to platinum-based treatment. A larger national randomized study is needed to evaluate this further.

A.L. Herbst, M.D.

A Phase II Trial of Intraperitoneal Cisplatin and Etoposide as Consolidation Therapy in Patients With Stage II–IV Epithelial Ovarian Cancer Following Negative Surgical Assessment

Barakat RR, Almadrones L, Venkatraman ES, et al (Mem Sloan-Kettering Cancer Ctr, New York)

Gynecol Oncol 69:17–22, 1998 25–11

Background.—Combined intraperitoneal cisplatin and etoposide is effective in patients with recurrent ovarian cancer previously responding to systemic platinum. Forty percent of patients with residual disease of less than 0.5 cm before intraperitoneal therapy reportedly have complete responses. The efficacy of 3 courses of intraperitoneal cisplatin (CDDP) and etoposide (VP-16) as consolidation therapy after pathologically negative second-look surgical reassessment for stage IIC to IV epithelial ovarian cancer (EOC) was determined.

Methods.—Forty patients were given consolidation therapy consisting of 3 cycles of intraperitoneal CDDP, 100 mg/m^2, and VP-16, 200 mg/m^2, between 1988 and 1996. Thirty-six patients, mean age 52 years, were evaluable. Forty-six contemporaneous patients undergoing observation only comprised the comparison group. The median age of this group was 52 years. Both groups were followed up for 36 months.

Findings.—Thirty-nine percent of the patients in the treatment group and 54% in the control group had recurrences. Median disease-free survival, not yet reached in the treatment group, was 28.5 months in the control group. Disease-free survival distribution between the 2 groups was significant. In a multivariate analysis, the protocol treatment was the only significant predictor of improved disease-free survival.

Conclusions.—Intraperitoneal consolidation with CDDP/VP-16 after negative second-look reassessment in patients with advanced epithelial ovarian cancer significantly increased disease-free survival compared with observation alone. The role of intraperitoneal consolidation should be further investigated.

▶ This is another article on intraperitoneal therapy of ovarian cancer. The authors have addressed the important point of trying to improve survival of patients who are free of the disease at second-look operation. They have a survival of less than 50% without further therapy. With a 3-year follow-up at the time of the report, 39% of the treated group had recurrence of disease vs. 54% of the untreated group. Statistical analyses indicated that the use of consolidation intraperitoneal treatment did significantly improve the outlook for these patients. Further evaluation by a randomized trial is currently ongoing, and the results will be extremely important as we try to improve treatment of this difficult disease.

A.L. Herbst, M.D.

Cost-Utility Analysis of Paclitaxel in Combination With Cisplatin for Patients With Advanced Ovarian Cancer

Ortega A, Dranitsaris G, Sturgeon J, et al (Ontario Cancer Inst/Princess Margaret Hosp, Toronto)

Gynecol Oncol 66:454–463, 1997 25–12

Objective.—Most patients with ovarian cancer are diagnosed with stage III or IV disease. These patients usually receive chemotherapy with cyclophosphamide and cisplatin after surgical debulking. Whereas progression-free survival is approximately 13 months in these patients, encouraging results have been observed with taxane paclitaxel. Total treatment costs, progression-free survival benefit, and patients' and societal preferences were incorporated into a cost-utility analysis to estimate the incremental cost of the taxane paclitaxel combination to the Canadian health care system.

Methods.—Data from a randomized comparative trial of first-line paclitaxel vs. cisplatin were fitted into a decision model. Treatment costs were estimated based on costs incurred by 12 patients with stage III or IV epithelial ovarian cancer who received first-line paclitaxel compared with costs incurred by 12 age- and disease-stage–matched (on a 1:2 basis) control patients who received primary cisplatin chemotherapy. Patient preferences for alternate health states were determined using a cohort of 20 patients and 40 healthy volunteers. A cost-utility analysis compared first-line therapies for advanced ovarian cancer.

Results.—Taxane paclitaxel treatment costs were 4 times larger than cisplatin treatment costs (Canadian $1,911 vs. Canadian $459). When preference values and overall health care utilization costs per patient were combined, the incremental cost of paclitaxel per quality-adjusted progression-free year ranged from Canadian $11,600 with second-line tamoxifen to Canadian $24,200 with ifosfamide.

Conclusion.—The cost-utility analysis shows that first-line therapy with paclitaxel confers a considerable quality-adjusted progression-free survival benefit for advanced ovarian cancer for a reasonable health care cost.

▶ We will presumably be seeing more cost-utility studies as efforts are made to control spending on medical care. This interesting study notes that paclitaxel (Taxol) is much more expensive, but that its providing a disease-free incremental survival of 5 months may be sufficient to justify its use. The difference in cost between paclitaxel-platinum and cisplatin-cyclophosphamide was greater (Canadian $1,911 vs. Canadian $459) per cycle and Canadian $12,000 vs. Canadian $24,000 per quality-adjusted progression-free year. The latter is a complicated calculation, but the point is made that paclitaxel is most useful both therapeutically and probably financially as first-line therapy. It is probably not so useful as salvage therapy after failure of first-line treatment.

A.L. Herbst, M.D.

Second-line Therapy With Paclitaxel and Carboplatin for Recurrent Disease Following First-line Therapy With Paclitaxel and Platinum in Ovarian or Peritoneal Carcinoma

Rose PG, Fusco N, Fluellen L, et al (Univ MacDonald Womens Hosp/Univ Hosps of Cleveland, Ohio; Case Western Reserve Univ, Cleveland, Ohio)
J Clin Oncol 16:1494–1497, 1998 25–13

Background.—The most active first-line treatment for advanced ovarian carcinoma is combined paclitaxel and a platinum compound. The efficacy of repeating this combination in patients with recurrent ovarian or peritoneal carcinoma was assessed.

Methods.—Twenty-five patients, with disease recurring 6 months or more after complete response with first-line paclitaxel and platinum chemotherapy, were retreated with 135 mg/m^2 paclitaxel in a 24-hour infusion and with carboplatin at an area under the concentration-time curve of 5–6 every 21 days. Treatment response was classified as measurable or evaluable.

Findings.—Median time to recurrence after initial treatment was 10 months. Twenty patients had measurable or evaluable disease. Seventy percent had a complete clinical response, and 20% a partial clinical response. Response rate with measurable disease was 91%, and with evaluable disease 89%. For all patients, the median progression-free interval was 9 or more months. For nonevaluable disease, it was 7 or more months. Sixty percent of the patients had a recurrence after repeat treatment at a median of 9 months. Only 2 patients died, between 2 and 21 months after repeat therapy.

Conclusions.—Retreatment with paclitaxel and platinum chemotherapy produces a high response rate and long progression-free interval in patients with recurrent ovarian or peritonal cancer. When platinum resistance develops in such patients, alternative agents need to be considered.

▶ Most oncologists are aware that patients with recurrent ovarian cancer will do better if the recurrence develops late. I was surprised, however, that these authors obtained such good results in their 25 patients who had recurrent disease, with a lower limit of more than 6 months after initial therapy. The authors repeated the paclitaxel and carboplatin combination and achieved a 70% complete response rate. This certainly is not "the answer," because patients will have recurrences again, but the approach does appear to offer useful palliation, particularly in the absence of truly effective therapy for recurrent disease.

A.L. Herbst, M.D.

Prolonged Oral Etoposide as Second-line Therapy for Platinum-resistant and Platinum-sensitive Ovarian Carcinoma: A Gynecologic Oncology Group Study

Rose PG, Blessing JA, Mayer AR, et al (Case Western Reserve Univ, Cleveland, Ohio; Roswell Park Cancer Inst, Buffalo, NY; Walter Reed Army Med Ctr, Washington, DC; et al)

J Clin Oncol 16:405–410, 1998 25–14

Introduction.—In ovarian carcinoma, intravenous etoposide has had response rates of 0% to 25%. The availability of etoposide orally has allowed prolonged administration. Previous studies showed that oral etoposide had an effect on tumors that were not affected by intravenous etoposide. The effectiveness of prolonged oral etoposide as second-line therapy for ovarian carcinoma was investigated. After initial demonstration of activity of this regimen, the study was reopened to investigate the activity in platinum-resistant and platinum-sensitive patients.

Methods.—Progression on platinum-based chemotherapy or recurrence within 6 months of completing therapy was the definition for platinum-resistant disease. The initial dosage was 50 mg/m^2 per day for 21 days, every 28 days. An escalation of dosage to a maximum dosage of 60 mg/m^2 per day was prescribed.

Results.—There was a 26.8% response rate among the 41 platinum-resistant patients. The median progression-free interval was 5.7 months, the median response duration was 4.3 months, and the median survival time was 10.8 months. Paclitaxel was previously given to 25 of 41 platinum-resistant patients, of whom 8 (32%) responded. There was a 34.1% response rate among 41 platinum-sensitive patients; they had a median progression-free interval of 6.3+ months, a median response duration of 7.5 months, and a median survival time of 16.5+ months. Grade 3 or grade 4 hematologic toxicity was common in 97 patients assessable for toxicity, with 41.2% having leukopenia, 45.5% having neutropenia, 9% having thrombocytopenia, and 13.4% having anemia. Treatment-related deaths occurred in 3 patients, 1 from thrombocytopenic bleeding after an overdose and 2 from neutropenic sepsis. Leukemia developed in 1 patient.

Conclusions.—In platinum-resistant and platinum-sensitive ovarian carcinoma, and in paclitaxel-resistant ovarian carcinoma, this regimen is active.

► We are still searching for better therapies for patients with ovarian cancer who fail first-line chemotherapy. This study looked at platinum-resistant and platinum-sensitive patients, and I believe that it is reasonable to assume, as the authors suggest, that the same type of results would be obtained with patients sensitive or resistant to paclitaxel platinum protocols. For the resistant patients in this study, oral etoposide accomplished a complete response rate of only 7.3% with a 5.7-month median progression-free survival. For the chemotherapy-sensitive group, the comparable results were 14.6% complete response and median progression-free survival of only 6.3 months. Even though this is considered to be an active second-line agent in the treatment of ovarian carcinoma, it is worth noting that few patients have a complete response and that the positive effect lasts for approximately one half year. The treatment of this disease with second-line chemotherapy remains a difficult problem for gynecologic oncology.

A.L. Herbst, M.D.

Phase II Study of "Dose-Dense" High-Dose Chemotherapy Treatment With Peripheral-Blood Progenitor-Cell Support as Primary Treatment for Patients With Advanced Ovarian Cancer

Aghajanian C, Fennelly D, Shapiro F, et al (Mem Sloan-Kettering Cancer Ctr, New York; St Vincents Hosp, Dublin, Ireland)

J Clin Oncol 16:1852–1860, 1998 25–15

Background.—The standard therapy for patients with advanced epithelial ovarian cancer is a combination of a platinum agent, up to 25 mg/m^2/week of cisplatin, plus paclitaxel. Beyond this dosage, toxicity appears to outweigh benefit. Peripheral blood progenitor (PBP) cells can be used to reduce toxicity and increase the dose of chemotherapy that can be tolerated by cancer patients. A phase II pilot study was performed to examine rapidly sequenced high-dose chemotherapy rescued with autologous peripheral-blood progenitor cells for patients with previously untreated advanced ovarian cancer.

Methods.—The phase II pilot study group consisted of 21 patients with stage IIC to IV ovarian cancer. A single cycle of mobilization was used, primed with cyclophosphamide, paclitaxel, and filgrastim (granulocyte colony stimulating factor) followed by 3 cycles of high-dose carboplatin/paclitaxel and 1 cycle of high-dose melphalan. Each cycle was rescued with peripheral-blood progenitor cells (PBPs). All 56 consecutive patients with advanced ovarian cancer treated with high-dose chemotherapy containing paclitaxel were reviewed to assess outcome.

Results.—Although there were no treatment-related deaths in the phase II pilot study group, 34 of 98 treatment cycles were complicated by hospitalization, usually for neutropenic fever. Grades 3 to 4 gastrointestinal toxicity occurred in 76% of patients and grades 2 to 3 neuropathy occurred in 62%. Of the 15 patients in the pilot study group who underwent second-look surgery, 5 attained a complete response. Of the 56 patients reviewed overall, 44 had second-look surgery and 15 achieved a complete response. The pathologic complete response rate in patients with optimal-disease was 55%, but it was only 13% in suboptimal patients.

Conclusion.—This phase II pilot study has demonstrated that high-dose chemotherapy with PBP support is feasible as a primary treatment for patients with advanced ovarian cancer, although it is frequently complicated by severe toxicity. In patients with optimally debulked stage III ovarian cancer, a pathologic complete response rate of 55% was obtained, whereas in suboptimal stage III and IV patients, there was no benefit of this high-dose regimen. Based on these findings, the Gynecologic Oncology Group has begun a pilot phase II trial of high-dose chemotherapy with PBP rescue for patients with optimally debulked advanced ovarian cancer. There is currently insufficient evidence to support the use of this aggressive treatment protocol outside of a clinical trial.

► I have included this Gynecologic Oncology Group study on high-dose chemotherapy and peripheral stem cell support to illustrate the limited efficacy of this toxic treatment. Fortunately, there were no treatment-related deaths. However, most of the patients required subsequent hospitalization for complications, primarily neutropenic fever, and 1 patient died of sepsis.

For suboptimally debulked patients, the results, as noted by the authors, are dismal, i.e., a 13% pathologic complete response. For optimally debulked patients, there was a 50% complete response rate.

It seems that there is a great deal of toxicity with lack of a clearly demonstrable increase in efficacy, except possibly for the optimally debulked group. This type of therapy will need further evaluation, but only in a study setting with established protocols as is being undertaken by the Gynecologic Oncology Group.

A.L. Herbst, M.D.

A Retrospective Review of Paclitaxel-associated Gastrointestinal Necrosis in Patients With Epithelial Ovarian Cancer

Seewaldt VL, Cain JM, Goff BA, et al (Univ of Washington, Seattle; Pennsylvania State Univ, Hershey; Univ of Washington, Seattle)

Gynecol Oncol 67:137–140, 1997 25–16

Introduction.—The leading cause of gynecologic cancer deaths in the United States is epithelial ovarian cancer. Treatment involves aggressive surgical resection and combination chemotherapy, and patients are put at high risk for bowel complications. Studies have shown an association between gastrointestinal necrosis and paclitaxel administration. It is still not understood how gastrointestinal necrosis developed after paclitaxel chemotherapy. A literature review and a retrospective review of gastrointestinal necrosis in patients treated with paclitaxel for epithelial ovarian cancer was conducted.

Methods.—A retrospective review was conducted of 7 patients with gastrointestinal necrosis after paclitaxel chemotherapy. An analysis was conducted of any history of abdominal pain, bowel perforation, typhlitis, fistulae formation, neutropenic sepsis, and ischemic colitis. Platinum refractory disease was seen in 4 patients, and 3 had primary paclitaxel therapy.

Results.—Fever was the most common clinical presentation, followed by neutropenia and abdominal pain. After the first cycle of paclitaxel chemotherapy, all 7 patients developed gastrointestinal necrosis. A direct drug effect on the gastrointestinal epithelium may be the cause of gastrointestinal necrosis, which may involve a synergistic interaction between paclitaxel-induced mitotic arrest and compromised bowel.

Conclusion.—In patients with platinum refractory disease, the incidence of gastrointestinal necrosis is 4 of 108 patients, or 3.7%. For patients with neutropenic fever and abdominal pain after paclitaxel chemotherapy, gastrointestinal necrosis should be strongly suspected.

▶ Paclitaxel (Taxol) is a popular drug widely used by all gynecological oncologists particularly against ovarian cancer. I was surprised by the frequency the authors have seen serious gastrointestinal complications in the form of necrosis, i.e., 3.7% of 108 patients that were previously treated with platinum and 2.3% of 128 patients who had received paclitaxel as primary treatment. The authors' conclusion is worth remembering; i.e., a high index of suspicion of gastrointestinal necrosis should exist for patients receiving paclitaxel who present with neutropenic fever and abdominal pain. The complications here occurred within 5–16 days after paclitaxel administration.

A.L. Herbst, M.D.

Vulvar

Cofactors With Human Papillomavirus in a Population-based Study of Vulvar Cancer

Madeleine MM, Daling JR, Carter JJ, et al (Fred Hutchinson Cancer Ctr, Seattle; Univ of Washington, Seattle; The Johns Hopkins Univ, Baltimore, Md)

J Natl Cancer Inst 89:1516–1523, 1997 25–17

Objective.—Vulvar cancer has been linked to human papillomavirus (HPV) infection. Other factors such as smoking and infection with herpes simplex virus type 2 (HSV2) have also been suggested as possibly being involved in the pathogenesis of HPV-related genital cancers. Whether exposure to HPV, cigarette smoking, or HSV2 independently or together increases the risk of vulvar cancer was examined in a population-based study.

Methods.—Between January 1980 and July 1994, serum samples from 400 women with squamous cell vulvar cancer in situ and 110 women with invasive squamous cell vulvar cancer were analyzed for antibodies against HPV and HSV2 and compared with samples from 1,403 controls. Human papillomavirus DNA was detected using the polymerase chain reaction. The relative risk of cancer was estimated.

Results.—Polymerase chain reaction analysis of tumor samples from 308 of 510 patients showed the presence of HPV DNA in almost 70% of in situ cancers and 28 (50.9%) of 55 invasive cancers. The odds ratio (OR) of vulvar cancer associated with the presence of HPV16 was 3.6 for in situ disease and 2.8 for invasive disease. The ORs (odds ratios) associated with smoking and in situ and invasive disease were 6.4 and 3.0, and with HSV2 seropositivity were 1.9 and 1.5, respectively. The OR associated with HPV16 seropositive- and HPV16 DNA-positive results and risk of squamous cell vulvar cancer was 4.5. The OR associated with current smoking history and HPV16 seropositivity was 18.8.

Conclusion.—Smoking, HPV infection, and HSV infection are risk factors for vulvar cancer. The risk increases for women who both smoke and are HPV16 seropositive.

► The findings of this population-based study relied upon interview of control subjects and those with vulvar neoplasia as well as serologic testing for HPV16. Herpes simplex virus type 2 was also tested and found to be a factor, but the major emphasis is on smoking and HPV16, both of which attained statistical significance. The association became particularly striking in those who were seropositive for HPV16 and also smoke, and their data provide further evidence linking these risk factors to disease development.

A.L. Herbst, M.D.

Intraepithelial and Invasive Squamous Cell Neoplasia of the Vulva: Trends in Incidence, Recurrence, and Survival Rate in Norway

Iversen T, Tretli S (Univ of Bergen, Norway)

Obstet Gynecol 91:969–972, 1998 25–18

Background.—The number of patients diagnosed with vulvar intraepithelial neoplasia has been increasing, which may be genuine or the result of better diagnostic procedures. No major changes have occurred in the incidence rate of invasive cancer. Time trends in the incidence of intraepithelial and invasive vulvar neoplasia, transition of intraepithelial vulvar neoplasia to invasive cancer, and survival rate based on a total population were reported.

Methods.—Cases were identified using the Cancer Registry of Norway. Data were obtained on all residents with squamous cell carcinoma of the vulva diagnosed between 1956 and 1990 and all those with intraepithelial vulvar neoplasia diagnosed between 1973 and 1992.

Findings.—From 1973–1977 to 1988–1992, the incidence rate of intraepithelial neoplasia increased threefold, with 3.4% changing to invasive disease. In a multivariate analysis, age was a significant variable. The age-adjusted incidence rate for squamous cell carcinoma remained constant during the period. The ratio of recurrence to total number of invasive cancers ranged from 21% to 31%. Five-year survival rates did not change significantly. Age was a powerful prognostic indicator, with an excess death rate associated with increasing age (Tables 1 and 2).

Conclusions.—The incidence of vulvar intraepithelial neoplasia has risen markedly in the past 40 years. However, the incidence of invasive vulvar cancer has not changed markedly.

► This population-based study from Norway confirms the general impression that we all are seeing an increased frequency of cases of vulvar intraepithelial neoplasia (VIN). During the 20 years of the study, the incidence of VIN tripled, while the age-adjusted incidence rate for invasive vulvar cancer remained relatively constant (Tables 1 and 2). Although the

TABLE 1.—New Cases per Year and Relative Risk of Intraepithelial Squamous Cell Neoplasia*

Age (y)	1973–77	1978–82	1983–87	1988–92	RR adjusted for period of diagnosis (95% CI)
0–29	6 (1)	2	11	23	1.00 (reference group)
30–34	3 (1)	4	16	20	6.04 (3.95, 9.24)
35–39	9	10	11 (1)	18	7.23 (4.78, 10.94)
40–44	4	13	10	17	7.29 (4.77, 11.13)
45–49	5	7	10	23 (1)	8.49 (5.58, 12.93)
50–54	12	11	9 (2)	10	8.54 (5.57, 13.10)
55–59	3	16	12	14	8.89 (5.84, 13.54)
60–64	5	18 (1)	12 (1)	10 (1)	8.55 (5.61, 13.02)
65–69	3	8 (1)	4	21	6.92 (4.44, 10.81)
70–74	3	11 (1)	9 (1)	13	7.76 (4.97, 12.11)
75–79	0	4	7	8 (1)	5.13 (2.98, 8.82)
80+	1 (1)	7	4 (2)	11	5.32 (3.20, 8.85)
Total	54 (3)	111 (3)	115 (7)	188 (3)	
Age-adjusted incidence rate†	0.5	0.8	0.9	1.4	
RR adjusted for age (95% CI)	1.00 (reference group)	1.98 (1.43, 2.75)	1.99 (1.44, 2.75)	3.15 (2.32, 4.26)	

*In parenthesis, 16 patients who progressed to cancer.
†Incidence rate per 100,000 women per year. (The world standard population is used.)
Abbreviations: RR, relative risk; *CI*, confidence interval.
(Courtesy of Iversen T, Tretli S: Intraepithelial and invasive squamous cell neoplasia of the vulva: Trends in incidence, recurrence, and survival rate in Norway. *Obstet Gynecol* 91:969–972, 1998. Reprinted with permission of the American College of Obstetricians and Gynecologists.)

TABLE 2.—New Cases per Year of Squamous Cell Carcinoma of the Vulva

Age (y)	1956–60	1961–65	1966–70	1971–75	1976–80	1981–85	1986–90
0–49	12	9	15	11	12	18	22
50–59	15	19	18	19	23	24	14
60–69	45	30	39	59	46	43	40
70–79	55	72	59	78	62	68	72
80+	19	18	35	33	49	48	67
Total	146	148	166	200	192	201	215
Age-adjusted incidence rate	1.1	0.9	1.0	1.1	1.0	1.0	0.9

(Courtesy of Iversen T, Tretli S: Intraepithelial and invasive squamous cell neoplasia of the vulva: Trends in incidence, recurrence, and survival rate in Norway. *Obstet Gynecol* 91:969–972, 1998. Reprinted with permission of the American College of Obstetricians and Gynecologists.)

survival rates for the cancer patients were also constant during the 20-year period, older patients did demonstrate a worse prognosis.

As the authors note, precise conclusions are difficult but it would appear that VIN is related to human papillomavirus (HPV) infection, and that these cases either have a low rate of conversion to invasive cancer, with only 3.4% of VIN III cases progressing to invasive cancer, or there is a very long latency period. Interestingly, the status of resection margins in operatively treated VIN cases did not appear to be prognostic for the development of invasive cancer.

A.L. Herbst, M.D.

Trends in Squamous Cell Carcinoma of the Vulva: The Influence of Vulvar Intraepithelial Neoplasia

Jones RW, Baranyai J, Stables S (Natl Women's Hosp, Auckland, New Zealand)

Obstet Gynecol 90:448–452, 1997 25–19

Introduction.—Squamous cell carcinoma of the vulva usually originates in a background of abnormal skin in women who are older. Squamous cell cancer of the vulva seems to be representative of 2 distinct entities: the common keratinizing squamous cell cancer, and the less common human papilloma virus (HPV)-related warty or basaloid carcinoma. A striking increase in the frequency of vulvar intraepithelial neoplasia has been observed in the past 2 decades in younger women, which may be associated with changing sexual mores, human papillomavirus (HPV) infection, and smoking. The clinical features and histopathology of squamous cell carcinoma of the vulva and the adjacent skin in 2 cohorts of women separated by 20–30 years were examined to determine trends in vulvar carcinoma and whether there is an increasing frequency of vulvar intraepithelial neoplasia in young women.

Methods.—Fifty-six women with squamous cell carcinoma who were seen initially during 1965–1974, and 57 women with squamous cell carcinoma who were seen initially during 1990–1994 were retrospectively studied. Concurrent analysis was conducted of pathologic specimens.

Results.—Only 1 of 56 women (1.8%) was younger than 50 years in the 1965–1974 cohort, whereas 12 of 57 women (21%) were younger than 50 years in the 1990–1994 cohort. Warty or basaloid vulvar intraepithelial neoplasia was associated with their invasive carcinoma in 10 of 13 women younger than 50 years, compared with 13 of 100 women older than 50 years. In women younger than 50 years, cigarette smoking and multiple lower genital tract neoplasia were both significantly more common.

Conclusions.—A subset of women younger than 50 years with squamous cell carcinoma of the vulva has emerged in the last 2 decades. The increasing incidence of vulvar intraepithelial neoplasia seen in young women during the past 2 decades seems to be presently reflected in vulvar intraepithelial neoplasia–associated squamous cell carcinoma of the vulva in younger women.

▶ This hospital-based study from New Zealand of vulvar carcinoma compares the clinicopathologic aspects of vulvar carcinoma from a group of patients treated in 1965–1974 with 1 treated in 1990–1994. The results are not surprising and confirm that the disease is occurring with greater frequency in younger women (defined in this article as younger than 50), and most of these tumors are associated with vulvar intraepithelial neoplasia (VIN). All of this is consistent with an increase in frequency of VIN in younger women, usually associated with HPV infection. The resulting tumors appear to have a warty basiloid appearance. Fortunately these tumors appear to have a somewhat improved prognosis compared with the common keratinizing squamous cell cancer not usually associated with HPV. Vulvar cancers continue to be comparatively rare, but unfortunately they do occur in young women even in their late 20s and early 30s.

A.L. Herbst, M.D.

Prophylactic Chemoradiation of Inguinofemoral Lymph Nodes in Patients with Locally Extensive Vulvar Cancer

Leiserowitz GS, Russell AH, Kinney WK, et al (Univ of California, Davis Med Ctr, Sacramento; Radiological Associates of Sacramento Med Group, Calif; Mercy San Juan Hosp, Carmichael, Calif)

Gynecol Oncol 66:509–514, 1997 25–20

Objective.—Approximately one third of vulvar cancer cases are advanced (International Federation of Gynecology and Obstetrics clinical stages III and IV). Surgery may compromise function of midline structures, and radical inguinofemoral node dissection may result in significant morbidity and permanent and disabling complications. Chemoradiation has achieved complete clinical and pathologic response. The outcome of elective inclusion of groin nodes with the irradiated volume in a group of women undergoing initial chemoradiation for $T_{2,3,4}$ squamous cancers of the vulva was reviewed to test the efficacy of prophylactic groin irradiation in a population at higher risk of nodal metastases.

Methods.—A group of 23 previously untreated patients aged 13–90 years, with primary invasive squamous cancer of the vulva (2 T_2, 20 T_3, and 1 T_4) were treated with radiation administered for 26–61 days twice daily with a 6-hr minimum interval between treatments. The inguinal node dose was delivered at the depth of the femoral artery, ranging from 4 to 8 cm, as determined by CT scans or estimated with a lateral simulation radiograph. Chemotherapy, usually 4 days of continuous IV 5-fluorouracil at 1,000 mg/m^2/24 hr, was administered concurrently.

Results.—After chemoradiation, 9 patients had local excision, and only 2 showed persistent cancer. Fourteen patients had a complete clinical response (Table 1). No patient failed in the groin. Future patients will be

TABLE 1.—Summary of Patient Characteristics and Outcomes

Patient	Age	Indication	Initial tumor (TNM)	Groins (TNM)	Postradiation excision	Residual disease	Complete clinical response	Status	Time to recurrence (months)	Length of follow-up (months)	Comments
1	66	Midline structures	T3	N2	Yes	No	Yes	DID	7	17.5	Exenteration for local recurrence, died with persistent bowel obstruction, NED at death
2	83	Midline structures	T3	N1	No		Yes	DOD	47	58	Local recurrence, no failure in groins
3	71	Exenteration needed	T4	N1	No		Yes	DOD	66	73.5	Local recurrence, no failure in groins
4	13	Midline structures	T3	N2	No		Yes	DID	94	98.5	Local recurrence (possible new primary) Undefined immune defect Died of pneumonia
5	67	Midline structures	T3	N0	No		Yes	NED		24	
6	40	Midline structures	T3	N2	Yes	No	No	NED		7.5	Groin node biopsy prior to radiation negative, persistent vulvar thickening at end of radiation
7	53	Midline structures	T3	N1	Yes	No	No	NED		9	
8	64	Midline structures	T3	N0	No		Yes	NED		6	
9	50	Midline structures	T3	N0	No		Yes	NED		6	
10	66	Midline structures	T3	N0	No		Yes	NED		32	

11	75	Midline structures	T3	N0	No		Yes	DID	8	Biopsy postradiation negative, died of gangrene of leg
12	41	Midline structures	T2	N2	Yes	No	No	NED	33	FNA of groin node prior to radiation negative
13	90	Midline structures	T3	N0	Yes	No	Yes	DID	51.5	Died of heart failure
14	87	Midline structures	T3	N0	Yes	No	Yes	NED	31.5	
15	71	Midline structures	T3	N1	Yes	No	Yes	DID	42	Died of primary squamous cancer of lung, heavy smoker
16	62	Exenteration needed	T3	N0	Yes	Yes	No	DID	18	Died of pyoderma, osteomyelitis; NED at death
17	53	Unresectable disease	T3	N2	Yes	Yes	No	NED	57	FNA of groin node prior to radiation negative
18	72	Midline structures	T3	N0	No		Yes	NED	86.5	
19	84	Midline structures	T3	N0	No		Yes	NED	63.5	
20	58	Midline structures	T3	N0	No		Yes	NED	85.5	
21	65	Medical contraindications	T2	N0	No		Yes	DID	60	Severe emphysema, died of emphysema
22	49	Midline structures	T3	N0	No		Yes	NED	75	
23	75	Midline structures	T3	N0	No		Yes	NED	97	

Note: TNM tumor, node, metastasis. The TNM staging of the inguinofemoral lymph nodes used the 1969 International Federation of Gynecology and Obstetrics system (as described in the text.)

Abbreviations: DID, died of intercurrent disease; *DOD*, died of disease; *NED*, no evidence of disease; *FNA*, fine-needle aspiration.

(Courtesy of Leiserowitz GS, Russell AH, Kinney WK, et al: Prophylactic chemoradiation of inguinofemoral lymph nodes in patients with locally extensive vulvar cancer. *Gynecol Oncol* 66:509–514, 1997.)

enrolled in the larger Radiation Therapy Oncology Group (RTOG) study, which uses radiation doses of 45 Gy in 25 daily fractions of 1.8 Gy for 5 weeks and 2 cycles of concurrent 5-fluorouracil infusion with mitomycin C at 10 mg/m^2.

Conclusion.—Chemoradiation of the inguinofemoral lymph nodes for locally advanced vulvar cancer is effective and has acceptable toxicity and few complications. It is preferable to groin dissection in these patients.

▶ Table 1 gives the pertinent details of this small series, and it shows that results really reflect a mixed bag of chemoradiation and operative treatment. I have personally seen recurrence of vulvar cancer in patients treated for positive nodes by radiation so I found this article that reports no recurrences, albeit for only 23 patients, of interest. I think 1 of the most important messages is buried in the methods section, which is that the authors have increased the depth of groin therapy to include the femoral artery. They hypothesize that previously recorded[1] failures may result from the depth of treatment being more superficial. In addition, they give radiation in twice-daily fractions only while the patient receives chemotherapy. The approach is being tested in a radiation therapy oncology group (RTOG) study, which it is hoped will provide a definitive answer.

A.L. Herbst, M.D.

Reference

1. Stehman FB, Bundy BN, Thomas G. et al: Groin dissection versus groin radiation in carcinoma of the vulva: A Gynecologic Oncology Group study. *Int J Radiat Oncol Biol Phys* 24:389–396, 1992.

Fallopian Tube

Adenocarcinoma of the Fallopian Tube: Results of a Multi-institutional Retrospective Analysis of 72 Patients

Wolfson AH, Tralins KS, Greven KM, et al (Univ of Miami, Fla; Bowman Gray School of Medicine, Winston-Salem, NC; Univ of Alabama, Birmingham; et al)

Int J Radiat Oncol Biol Phys 40:71–76, 1998 25–21

Introduction.—Primary carcinoma of the fallopian tube is one of the rarest gynecologic malignancies and has an incidence of less than 2% of all female genital cancers. Determining the role of adjuvant therapy after initial surgery would require a multicentric, prospective trial because of the limited patient numbers. Prognostic factors that affect survival and patterns of failure were identified by a retrospective analysis of 72 patients obtained from the tumor registries of 6 major medical centers.

Methods.—A total of 72 patients with primary adenocarcinoma of the fallopian tube were identified in a 35-year period. The Dodson modification of the International Federation of Gynecology and Obstetrics surgical staging for carcinoma of the fallopian tube was used. Overall and disease-free survival were the end points for outcome. Prognostic significance and patterns of failure were determined by univariate analysis of host, tumor, and treatment factors.

Results.—The women had a median age of 61 years, and 33% had stage I disease, 28% had stage II, 33% had stage III, and 6% had stage IV. Seventy-five percent of patients received adjuvant chemotherapy, and 31% received postoperative radiotherapy. In the latter treatment group, whole pelvic external beam irradiation was administered to 64%, of patients, whole abdominal radiotherapy was administered to 23% of patients, P-32 instillation was used in 9% of patients, and vaginal brachytherapy alone was used in 4% of patients. In 67% of stage I disease and in 79% of stages II/III/IV disease, chemotherapy was used. In stage I disease, radiotherapy was more commonly used than in the other stages. The 5-year overall survival was 44.7%, and the 5-year disease-free survival was 27.3%. The 8-year overall survival was 23.8%, and the 8-year disease-free survival was 17%. Fifteen-year overall and disease-free survival were 18.8% and 14%, respectively. Stage I and age of 60 years or less at diagnosis were significant prognostic factors of overall survival. Disease-free survival could be predicted by only stage I disease. Patterns of failure were 18% pelvic, 36% upper abdominal, and 19% distant. The more frequently found failures found in stages II, III, and IV were upper abdominal failures. For only 15% of patients with failures, relapses solely outside of what would be included in standard whole abdominal radiotherapy portals occurred. Those most likely to die were patients having any recurrence (including the upper abdomen), compared with those without any type of relapse.

Conclusions.—In predicting the overall and disease-free survival of patients with carcinoma of the fallopian tube, the importance of the International Federation of Gynecology and Obstetrics staging was demonstrated.

▶ As noted by the authors, primary fallopian tube carcinoma is an extraordinarily rare disease. A new finding in this series is that younger patients (60 years or younger) appear to do better than older patients. Not surprisingly, those with stage I disease do the best.

Combination chemotherapy with drugs active against ovarian carcinoma have been reported to be effective in this disease. The authors hypothesize that whole abdominal radiation may also be effective for stage II or III disease (30 Gy at 150 centigray fraction with a pelvic boost). They advise that intraperitoneal disease should be small (less than 1 cm), and such an approach might be worthwhile for posthysterectomy patients with small-volume intraperitoneal disease.

A.L. Herbst, M.D.

General

Management of Placental Site Trophoblastic Tumors

Newlands ES, Bower M, Fisher RA, et al (Charing Cross Hosp, London)
J Reprod Med 43:53–59, 1998 25–22

Introduction.—A rare variant of gestational trophoblastic tumor is placental site trophoblastic tumor (PSTT), which consists of a monomorphic population of nonvillous trophoblasts that is derived from the intermediate trophoblasts of the placental bed. Surgery plays a major role in the management of PSTT. The genetic background of tumors in women with PSTTs was analyzed, and the clinical outcome was examined in women treated for this rare variant of trophoblastic disease.

Methods.—Seventeen women with PSTTs were seen over a 20-year period. Polymerase chain reaction allelotyping and GeneScan software were used to study the molecular genetics of a group of PSTTs. To test the significance of differences in survival distributions, the log rank method was used.

Results.—Of 7 women who had detailed molecular analysis, 4 had PSTTs from diploid, biparental pregnancies and 3 had androgenetic tumors that followed monospermic complete hytadiform moles. The treatment of choice is hysterectomy for women with PSTT localized to the uterus. PSTT show variable sensitivity to current cytotoxic chemotherapy. Several women using the etoposide, methotrexate, actinomycin D-cyclophosphamide, vincristine schedule were cured, but clinical impressions suggest that cisplatin probably should be introduced into the chemotherapy schedule from the outset. The schedule should include etoposide, cisplatin/etoposide, methotrexate, and actinomycin D.

Conclusion.—A major adverse prognostic variable is a long interval from the antecedent pregnancy to clinical presentation, and there is a poor outcome in women whose last known pregnancy was more than 2 years before the appearance of PSTTs. For women whose disease is limited to the uterus, the treatment of choice is hysterectomy. Chemotherapy is indicated for women with more extensive or metastatic disease, but the clinical outcome is variable.

► Placental site trophoblastic tumor is extraordinarily rare. The group at Charing Cross Hospital has extensive experience with trophoblastic disease, and this review of seven cases confirms that, if the tumor is confined to the uterus, hysterectomy is the treatment of choice. This tumor is much less sensitive to chemotherapy than most cases of trophoblastic disease, but the authors report that multiple-agent chemotherapy can induce remission. They note that etoposide and platinum are useful, with one complete remission reported in a patient treated with etoposide, methotrexate, and actinomycin D. These patients should be optimally treated in centers used to handling this rare disease.

A.L. Herbst, M.D.

A Randomized Study Comparing Retroperitoneal Drainage With No Drainage After Lymphadenectomy in Gynecologic Malignancies

Benedetti-Panici P, Maneschi F, Cutillo G, et al (Catholic Univ of the Sacred Heart, Rome; 'S Carlo di Nancy' Hosp, Rome)

Gynecol Oncol 65:478–482, 1997 25–23

Introduction.—Prophylactic drainage of the retroperitoneum following lymphadenectomy in gynecologic oncologic surgery is advocated to promptly identify postoperative hemorrhage and decrease postoperative morbidity. This technique has been brought into question because careful hemostasis makes postoperative hemorrhage extremely rare, lymphocyst formation does not seem to be prevented by closed suction drainage, the prevention of ureteral fistula is related to surgical technique, and febrile morbidity can be reduced by intraoperative antibiotic prophylaxis. The clinical effectiveness of retroperitoneal prophylactic drainage after systematic lymphadenectomy was compared with no drainage.

Methods.—There were 137 patients who had systematic lymphadenectomy performed for gynecologic malignancies. Sixty patients received retroperitoneal drainage, and 69 did not. After node dissection, the pelvic peritoneum and the paracolic gutters were not sutured. Recordings were taken of perioperative data and complications.

Results.—In the 2 groups, clinical and surgical parameters were comparable. In the group that did not receive retroperitoneal drainage, postoperative hospital stay was significantly shorter; and the complication rate was significantly higher in the group that had retroperitoneal drainage (Table 3). A significant increase in lymphocyst and lymphocyst-related

TABLE 3.—Postoperative Complications Occurring in Drained and Not-Drained Patients Within 30 Days

	Drains			
	Yes (%)	No (%)	RR	CI
No. of patients	68	69		
Pts with complications[a]	29 (43%)	15 (22%)*	1.96	1.16–2.23
Symptomatic lymphocyst	16 (23%)	5 (7%)†	3.2	1.7–8.4
Pelvic abscess	—	2 (3%)	—	—
Sepsis	—	1 (1%)	—	—
Febrile morbidity	7 (10%)	3 (4%)	2.4	0.6–8.8
Deep venous thrombosis	3 (4%)	1 (1%)	3.04	0.3–28.5
Leg edema	8 (12%)	3 (4%)§	2.7	0.7–9.8
Hemoperitoneum	—	1 (1%)	—	—
Symptomatic ascites	2 (3%)	3 (5%)	0.6	0.1–3.9
Subocclusion	5 (7%)	1 (1%)	5.07	0.6–42.3
Wound dehiscence	1 (1%)	1 (1%)	1.01	0.06–15.8
Ureteral fistula	1 (1%)	1 (1%)	1.01	0.06–15.8
Nerve injury	—	1 (1%)	—	—

[a]Some patients had one complication or more.
$*P = 0.01$
$†P = 0.007$
$‡P = 0.006$
$§P = 0.02$

(Courtesy of Benedetti-Panici P, Maneschi F, Cutillo G, et al: A randomized study comparing retroperitoneal drainage with no drainage after lymphadenectomy in gynecologic malignancies. *Gynecol Oncol* 65:478–482, 1997.)

morbidity accounted for these differences. In 18% of drained and in 36% of non-drained patients, sonographic monitoring for lymphocyst showed free abdominal fluid. In 2 drained patients (3%) and in 3 nondrained patients (4%), symptomatic ascites developed.

Conclusion.—Lymphadenectomy-related morbidity and postoperative stay seems to increase with prophylactic drainage of the retroperitoneum. When the retroperitoneum is left open, routine drainage following lymphadenectomy seems no longer to be indicated.

▶ I was trained to drain the closed retroperitoneum after pelvic lymphadenectomy. The authors have done a randomized trial on 137 patients which, according to their calculations, should have been adequate to detect a 50% decrease in their prior published complications rate. It turns out that leaving the retroperitoneal open, which has become increasingly popular, does not seem to have an adverse effect; and in fact, in this study, those who were drained did worse, as shown in Table 3. I know of no evidence, at present, that long-term complications (adhesions, bowel obstruction) are more frequent in the open retroperitoneal group. Absent such evidence, leaving the peritoneum open seems like a reasonable technique.

A.L. Herbst, M.D.

A Prospective Controlled Trial of Early Postoperative Oral Intake Following Major Abdominal Gynecologic Surgery

Schilder JM, Hurteau JA, Look KY, et al (Indiana Univ, Indianapolis)

Gynecol Oncol 67:235–240, 1997 25–24

Introduction.—Oral intake has traditionally been delayed until evidence of bowel function is present postoperatively, because of concern about postoperative ileus. However, recent studies suggest that early oral intake may actually be beneficial and is well tolerated with few side effects. There is little information on early postoperative feeding in gynecologic literature. A study was conducted to determine whether early oral intake after major gynecologic surgery led to a shorter hospitalization than delayed feeding.

Methods.—Ninety-six patients undergoing major abdominal gynecologic surgery were randomized into 1 of 2 groups. The control group was treated traditionally; oral intake began only after documentation of bowel function, which was defined by bowel sounds, flatus or bowel movement, and subjective hunger. The early oral intake group was given a clear liquid diet on the first day after surgery. A regular diet was given once 500 mL was tolerated. The women were evaluated daily for flatus, bowel sounds, bowel movement, vomiting, hunger, nausea, and need for nasogastric tube decompression. Recordings and comparisons were made on length of hospital stay, length of postoperative ileus, and incidence of adverse effects, such as vomiting, nausea, and postoperative complications.

Results.—In the number of patients who required postoperative antiemetics or postoperative biscodyl suppositories, the groups did not vary statistically. For patients on the early-feeding regimen, there was a statis-

TABLE 5.—Postoperative Outcome

	Group 1	Group 2	*P* value
LOS (days)	4.02 ± 0.30	3.12 ± 0.16	0.008
Tolerated solid (POD)	2.72 ± 0.14	1.88 ± 0.14	<0.0001
Episodes of emesis	0.32 ± 0.10	0.39 ± 0.13	0.04

(Courtesy of Schilder JM, Hurteau JA, Look KY, et al: A prospective controlled trial of early postoperative oral intake following major abdominal gynecologic surgery. *Gynecol Oncol* 67:235–240, 1997.)

tically significant reduction in the length of hospitalization. The control group had an average length of stay of 4.02 days, whereas the experimental group had an average length of stay of 3.12 days (Table 5). A higher incidence of emesis was seen in the study group but was not associated with any untoward outcome, and these patients could tolerate a solid diet almost 1 full day earlier than the control group (2.72 days vs. 1.88 days).

Conclusion.—When compared with traditional dietary management in patients having abdominal surgery, early postoperative oral intake results in a decreased length of hospitalization.

▶ Most of us have been trained to be cautious in postoperative feeding of gynecology patients to avoid ileus, emesis, and postoperative bowel dysfunction. This study appears to show a different approach that is effective and allows earlier discharge. The protocol is worth noting; i.e., solid food was started once 500 mL clear liquids were tolerated; as shown in the table, this led to shorter length of stay and earlier ingestion of solid food. However, these aggressively treated patients did have significantly more emesis. All in all, this appears to be a well-done study that can reduce length of hospital stay.

A.L. Herbst, M.D.

Size of the Urogenital Hiatus in the Levator Ani Muscles in Normal Women and Women With Pelvic Organ Prolapse

Delancey JOL, Hurd WW (Univ of Michigan, Ann Arbor)

Obstet Gynecol 91:364–368, 1998 25–25

Introduction.—Pelvic organ prolapse has been associated with damage to the levator ani muscles. It may be possible that loss of the levator ani muscles' ability to close the hiatus is a factor contributing to prolapse, because pelvic organ prolapse occurs through the urogenital hiatus in the levator ani muscles. The size of the urogenital hiatus was determined in women with normal support, and the degree of its enlargement in women with prolapse was quantified.

Methods.—In 300 women whose support was scored according to a modified Baden system, the sagittal and transverse urogenital hiatus diameters were measured and hiatus area was calculated.

Results.—Hiatus area was 5.4 cm^2 in women with normal support who had not had prior surgery. The area of the hiatus was enlarged to 9.6 cm in women with uncorrected clinical prolapse at grade 2-3; with progressive prolapse, the area became larger. Patients with prolapse had a larger hiatus than normal women when matched for age and parity. A larger hiatus was seen in women with recurrent prolapse (13.3 cm^2) than in cured women (8.1 cm^2) or women with recurrence after one operation (8.9 cm^2). In women who were surgically cured, the hiatus size did not return to normal. An increase in anteroposterior diameter correlated with increasing area of the hiatus, was less attributable to increased transverse diameter, and was not related to thickness of the perineal body.

Conclusion.—Increasing urogenital hiatus size is associated with increasing pelvic organ prolapse. After several unsuccessful operations, the hiatus is larger than after successful surgery or a single failure. The hiatus is progressively larger in women with increasingly severe prolapse, and it is largest in those who had several unsuccessful surgical repairs. It is still not known what factor is responsible for enlargement of the urogenital hiatus.

▶ This article by Delancey and Hurd is an interesting study of pelvic support. Many years ago, the late Howard Ulfelder studied the biomechanics of pelvic support and noted that the levator was an extremely important part of the support process. Many of us who were trained years ago were taught always to perform a posterior repair if anything was done to the anterior vagina or the bladder neck. I have become aware that in recent years some individuals do not follow this practice. I believe that is a mistake, and I believe that the current article provides some impressive evidence of why it is important to reconstitute the levators in the midline when operating for pelvic relaxation, even though it may appear that the relaxation is predominantly confined to the anterior wall.

A.L. Herbst, M.D.

Long-term Complications Associated With Prosthetic Repair of Incisional Hernias

Leber GE, Garb JL, Alexander AI, et al (Tufts Univ, Springfield, Mass)
Arch Surg 133:378–382, 1998 25–26

Background.—Incisional hernia complicates 2% to 11% of abdominal procedures. After primary repair of the hernia, recurrent herniation develops in 30% to 50%. Using prosthetic material to create a tension-free repair has reportedly decreased the rate of recurrent hernias to 0 to 10%. Whether the type of prosthetic material and technique of placement affect long-term complications after repair of incisional hernias was determined.

Methods.—Two hundred patients undergoing open repair of abdominal incisional hernias with prosthetic material between 1985 and 1994 were included in the retrospective cohort study. Four types of prosthetic material were used: monofilamented polypropylene mesh (Marlex), doublefilamented mesh (Prolene), expanded polytetrafluroethylene patch (Gore-Tex), and multifilamented polyester mesh (Mersilene). The materials were placed by an onlay, underlay, sandwich, or finger interdigitation technique.

Findings.—In a univariate analysis, the Mersilene was associated with a significantly greater mean number of complications per patient, a higher incidence of fistula formation, more infections, and more recurrent hernias than the other materials. Also, the additional mean length of stay to treat complications was significantly longer when Mersilene was used. Multiple logistic regression confirmed the deleterious effect of this material on long-term complications. Placement method did not affect outcome.

Conclusions.—The incidence of complications associated with Mersilene is substantially greater than for Marlex, Gore-Tex, and Prolene. Thus, multifilamented polyester mesh should no longer be used for repairing incisional hernias.

► This is a study of 300 incisional abdominal hernia repairs. While most obstetrician gynecologists are not concerned with this procedure, it is encountered especially by gynecologist oncologists. The results of the study seem clear-cut. Of the various materials that are available, the highest complication rate was noted with polyester mesh (Mersilene) and the results suggest that polyester mesh should no longer be used; Marlex, Prolene, or Gore-Tex are preferable.

A.L. Herbst, M.D.

26 Breast Disease

Coronary Heart Disease Mortality and Adjuvant Tamoxifen Therapy
Costantino JP, Kuller LH, Ives DG, et al (Univ of Pittsburgh, Pa)
J Natl Cancer Inst 89:776–782, 1997 26–1

Introduction.—The results of randomized clinical trials suggest that giving tamoxifen to women with breast cancer may not only improve survival but also reduce the risk of coronary heart disease (CHD). Data from the National Surgical Adjuvant Breast and Bowel Project (NSABP) were analyzed to determine mortality from CHD among tamoxifen-treated patients with early breast cancer.

Methods.—The analysis included 2,885 patients from the NSABP B-14 trial of tamoxifen therapy. In the first phase of the trial, all patients were randomly assigned to receive 5 years of either tamoxifen or placebo. Records were received to classify causes of heart disease-related death: deaths from definite fatal myocardial infarction, death from definite fatal CHD possible myocardial infarction, and death from possible fatal CHD. The findings were compared by treatment group according to the average annual hazard rates and the corresponding relative hazard of death.

Results.—Patients receiving tamoxifen had a lower average annual rate of death from coronary heart disease, but not significantly so (Table 3). Eight patients receiving tamoxifen died of definite heart-related causes, for an average annual rate of 0.62/1,000 patients. Twelve patients in the placebo group died of definite heart-related causes, for an average annual rate of 0.94/1,000 patients. Relative hazard of death from definite fatal heart disease was thus 0.66. Another 11 deaths in the tamoxifen group and

TABLE 3.—Rates of Coronary Heart Disease-related Deaths Among Patients Included in Phase 1 of the National Surgical Adjuvant Breast and Bowel Project Protocol B-14

	Placebo		Tamoxifen			
Type of coronary heart disease-related death	No. of patients	Rate per 1000	No. of patients	Rate per 1000	Relative hazard	95% confidence interval
All definite coronary heart disease*	12	0.94	8	0.62	0.66	0.27–1.61
Definite and possible coronary heart disease	22	1.73	19	1.48	0.85	0.46–1.58

*Includes cases of definite fatal myocardial infarctions and definite fatal coronary heart disease.

(Courtesy of Costantino JP, Kuller LH, Ives DG, et al: Coronary heart disease mortality and adjuvant tamoxifen therapy. *J Natl Cancer Inst* 89:776–782, 1997.)

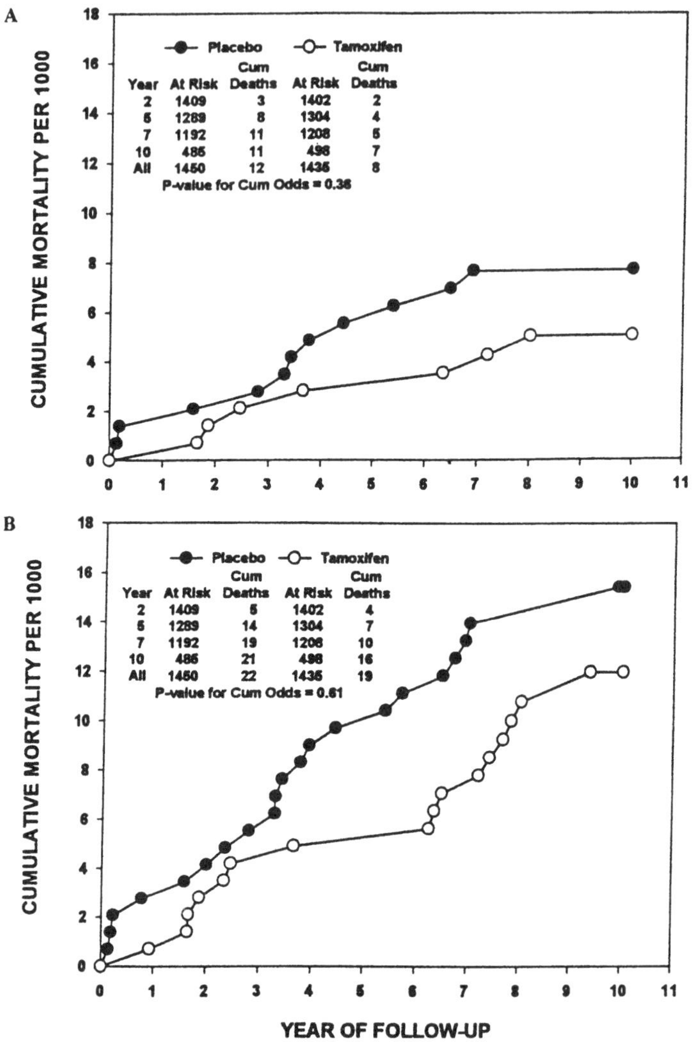

FIGURE 2.—Ten-year cumulative (*Cum*) mortality from coronary heart disease among patients included in the National Surgical Adjuvant Breast and Bowel Project protocol B-14. A, definite coronary heart disease-related deaths. B, definite and possible coronary heart disease-related deaths. At risk = number of patients at risk. The P values are 2-sided. (Courtesy of Costantino JP, Kuller LH, Ives DG, et al: Cornary heart disease mortality and adjuvant tamoxifen therapy. *J Natl Cancer Inst* 89:776–782, 1997, by permission of Oxford University Press.)

10 deaths in the placebo group were regarded as possibly caused by fatal CHD. On combined analysis of the possible and definite cases, the average annual rate of heart disease-related deaths was 1.48/1,000 in the tamoxifen group and 1.73/1,000 in the placebo group (Fig 2). Relative hazard of death was 0.85.

Conclusions.—Analysis of randomized trial data supports the notion that tamoxifen therapy for early breast cancer may reduce the rate of death from CHD. Final conclusions will require longer follow-up of patients from the NSABP trials of preventive tamoxifen therapy. One key question will be whether stopping tamoxifen after 5 years affects the subsequent risk for coronary artery disease.

► Longer term follow-up data, such as in this analysis, continue to accumulate showing that tamoxifen (despite early concerns that it might have antiestrogenic effects on the cardiovascular system) actually has "positive" estrogenic effects on the coronary arteries and results in decreased coronary artery-related mortality. Analogues of tamoxifen with altered site-specific estrogenic and antiestrogenic effects are being developed and tested in clinical trials. In addition, prospective clinical trials need to be done comparing the effects of tamoxifen and of estrogen replacement therapy (physiologic dosages of conjugated equine estrogen or equivalents) on the coronary artery and cardiovascular illness.

W.H. Hindle, M.D.

Standards for Diagnosis and Management of Invasive Breast Carcinoma

Winchester DP, Cox JD (American College of Surgeons; American College of Radiology; College of American Pathologists)

CA Cancer J Clin 48:83–107, 1998 26–2

Background.—This article discusses the various diagnostic strategies and treatments used to identify and treat invasive breast carcinoma.

TABLE 1.—Prospective Randomized Trials Comparing Conservative Surgery and Radiation With Mastectomy for Early-Stage Breast Cancer

Trial	Treatment Period	Total No. of Patients	Stage	Surgery for Primary	Adjuvant Therapy
Milan Cancer Institute Trial I	1973–1980	701	I	Quandrantectomy, radical mastectomy	CMF
Institut Gustave-Roussy	1972–1980	179	I	Wide excision, modified radical mastectomy	None
NSABP B-06	1976–1984	1,219	I–II	Wide excision, modified radical mastectomy	Melphalan, 5-FU
National Cancer Institute	1979–1987	237	I–II	Local excision, modified radical mastectomy	AC
EORTC	1980–1986	874	I–II	Local excision, modified radical mastectomy	CMF
Danish Breast Cancer Group	1983–1989	904	I–III	Quandrantectomy, wide excision, modified radical mastectomy	CMF, T

Abbreviations: A, doxorubicin; *C*, cyclophosphamide; *CMF*, cyclophosphamide, methotrexate, fluorouracil (5-FU); *EORTC*, European Organization for Research and Treatment of Cancer; *NSABP*, National Surgical Adjuvant Breast and Bowel Project; *T*, tamoxifen.

(Courtesy of Winchester DP, Cox JD: Standards for diagnosis and management of invasive breast carcinoma. *CA Cancer J Clin* 48:83–107, 1998.)

TABLE 2.—Comparison of Survival After Conservative Surgery and Radiation With That After Mastectomy in Prospective Randomized Trials

Trial	Endpoint (years)	Overall Survival (%) CS & R (P value)	Overall Survival (%) Mastectomy	Disease-Free Survival (%) CS & R (P value)	Disease-Free Survival (%) Mastectomy
Milan Cancer Institute Trial I	18	65 (NS)	65	N/A	N/A
Institut Gustave-Roussy	15	73 (.19)	65	N/A	N/A
NSABP B-06	12	63 (.12)	59	50 (.21)	49
National Cancer Institute	10	77 (.89)	75	72 (.93)	69
EORTC	8	54 (NS)	61	N/A	N/A
Danish Breast Cancer Group	6	79 (NS)	82	70 (NS)	66

Abbreviations: CS & R, conservative therapy and radiation; *EORTC,* European Organization for Research and Treatment of Cancer; *N/A,* data not available; *NS,* not significant; *NSABP,* National Surgical Adjuvant Breast and Bowel Project.

(Courtesy of Winchester DP, Cox JD: Standards for diagnosis and management of invasive breast carcinoma. *CA Cancer J Clin* 48:83–107, 1998.)

Mastectomy vs. Conservative Treatment.—Six large randomized prospective trials have compared mastectomy and breast conservation plus radiation therapy (Table 1). Neither shows a clear advantage in overall survival (Table 2) or disease-free survival (Table 3). Six large randomized prospective trials have compared conservative surgery alone with conservative surgery plus radiotherapy (Table 4). Overall and disease-free survival was improved with radiation therapy (Table 5). Numerous nonrandomized trials also support this improvement (Tables 6 and 7).

Diagnostic Methods.—The history and physical examination can reveal the patient's general health and thus her suitability for a conservative approach. Bilateral mammography is used to determine the extent of disease, to investigate multicentricity, and to evaluate the contralateral breast. Vascular or lymphatic invasion, necrosis, inflammatory infiltrate, and extensive ductal component increase the risk of disease recurrence. The degree of tubule formation, nuclear grade, mitotic rate, and estrogen and progesterone receptor status should also be noted. Frozen-section slices should not be used. The patient's expectations should also be evaluated.

TABLE 3.—Comparison of Local Recurrence After Conservative Surgery and Radiation With That After Mastectomy in Prospective Randomized Trials

Trial	Endpoint	Local Recurrence (%) CS & R	(P value)	Mastectomy
Milan Cancer Institute Trial I	Cumulative incidence at 18 years	7	(NS)	4
Institut Gustave-Roussy	Cumulative incidence at 15 years	9	(NS)	14
NSABP B-06	Cumulative incidence at 8 years	10	(NS)	8
National Cancer Institute	Crude incidence, median follow-up 10.1 years	19	(.01)	6
EORTC	Crude incidence at 14 years	17	(NS)	14
Danish Breast Cancer Group	Crude incidence, median follow-up 3.3 years	3	(NS)	4

Abbreviations: CS & R, conservative therapy and radiation; *EORTC,* European Organization for Research and Treatment of Cancer; *NS,* not significant; *NSABP* National Surgical Adjuvant Breast and Bowel Project.

(Courtesy of Winchester DP, Cox JD: Standards for diagnosis and management of invasive breast carcinoma. *CA Cancer J Clin* 48:83–107, 1998.)

TABLE 4.—Prospective Randomized Trials Comparing Conservative Surgery Alone With Conservative Surgery and Radiation Therapy

Trial	No. of Patients	Tumor Size (cm)	Nodal Status	Surgery	Systemic Therapy
Uppsala-Orebro Breast Cancer Study Group	381	<2.0	Negative	Quadrantectomy	None
Milan Cancer Institute Trial III	601	<2.5	Negative or positive	Quadrantectomy	CMF or tamoxifen for positive nodes
NSABP B-06	1,265	<4.0	Negative or positive	Local excision	L-PAM; 5-FU for positive nodes
Ontario Clinical Oncology Group	837	<4.0	Negative	Local excision	None
Scottish Cancer Trials Breast Group	556	<4.0	Negative or positive	Wide excision	CMF or tamoxifen for positive nodes
British Trial	399	≤5.0	Negative or positive	Wide excision	CMF or tamoxifen for positive nodes

Abbreviations: CMF, cyclophosphamide, methotrexate, fluorouracil (5-FU); *L-PAM*, L-phenylalanine mustard; *NSABP*, National Surgical Adjuvant Breast and Bowel Project.

(Courtesy of Winchester DP, Cox JD: Standards for diagnosis and management of invasive breast carcinoma. *CA Cancer J Clin* 48:83–107, 1998.)

Patients in whom radiation after lumpectomy is contraindicated include those with 2 or more primary tumors in different quadrants, those with previous radiation therapy, pregnant patients, those in whom microcalcifications appear diffuse and malignant, and those in whom margins remain positive despite repeated attempts. Relative contraindications are collagen vascular disease, 2 or more tumors in the same quadrant, tumor size, and breast size.

TABLE 5.—Local Recurrence and Survival in Prospective Randomized Trials Comparing Conservative Surgery Alone and Conservative Surgery and Radiation Therapy

Trial	Breast Recurrence (%)		Overall Survival (%)		Interval Results
	CS	CS + RT	CS	CS + RT	Reported (years)
Uppsala-Orebro Breast Cancer Study Group	18	2	90	91	5*
Milan Cancer Institute Trial III	18	2	92	92	5*
NSABP B-06	35	10	58	62	12*
Ontario Clinical Oncology Group	40	18	72	74	10*
Scottish Cancer Trials Breast Group	28	6	85	88	5*
ER-positive	25	3	N/A	N/A	N/A
ER-negative	4	14	N/A	N/A	N/A
British Trial	35	13	N/A	N/A	5

Abbreviations: CS, conservative surgery; *CS + RT*, conservative surgery and radiation therapy; *ER*, estrogen receptor; *N/A*, data not available; *NSABP*, National Surgical Adjuvant Breast and Bowel Project.

*Calculated as actuarial years.

(Courtesy of Winchester DP, Cox JD: Standards for diagnosis and management of invasive breast carcinoma. *CA Cancer J Clin* 48:83–107, 1998.)

TABLE 6.—Survival After Conservative Surgery and Radiation Therapy for Early-Stage Breast Cancer in Nonrandomized Studies

Study	No. of Patients	10-Year Survival (%)
	Stages I and II	
Fowble et al	697	83
Haffty et al	278	67
Leung et al	493	68
Mansfield et al	1,070	80*
Spitaller et al	1,133	80
Stotter et al	490	74
	Stage I	
Dewar et al†	757	79
Veronesi et al	1,232	78
Perez et al	520	85*
Zafrani et al.†	434	86

*Cause-specific.
†Includes small T2.
(Courtesy of Winchester DP, Cox JD: Standards for diagnosis and management of invasive breast carcinoma. *CA Cancer J Clin* 48:83–107, 1998.)

Surgical Approaches.—Curvilinear skin incisions provide a more cosmetic result, although a radial incision is preferred in the mid-inner aspect of the breast and in the lower part of the breast. Cosmetic results are best if the incision is placed close to the tip of the biopsy wire, if the subcutaneous tissue is preserved, and if the breast is not reapproximated. The biopsy site should be reexcised to check margins. When invasive tumors are 1 cm or less and histologic type is favorable, it is sufficient to remove level I axillary nodes. The thoracodorsal and long thoracic nerves, the medial pectoral nerve, and, when possible, the intercostal brachial nerve should be preserved. The preferred drainage method is closed suction.

TABLE 7.—Recurrence in the Breast After Conservative Surgery and Radiation Therapy for Early-Stage Breast Cancer in Nonrandomized Studies

Study	No. of Patients	Maximum Primary Tumor Size (cm)	Breast Recurrence at 10 Years (%)
Clark et al	1,130	5	14
Dewar et al	757	3	8
Fourquet et al	518	5	11
Fowble et al	697	5	18
Gage et al	1,628	5	13
Haffty et al	433	5	19
Halverson et al	511	5	14
Kurtz et al	1,593	5	14
Leung et al	493	5	10
Mansfield et al	1,070	5	14
Stotter et al	490	5	19
Veronesi et al	1,232	2	8

(Courtesy of Winchester DP, Cox JD: Standards for diagnosis and management of invasive breast carcinoma. *CA Cancer J Clin* 48:83–107, 1998.)

Radiation Therapy.—Irradiation can usually be started 2 to 4 weeks after conservative surgery. Each field (rather than a bolus) should be treated each day.

Follow-up Care.—Physical examinations should be performed every 3 to 6 months for the first 3 years, every 6 months in years 4 and 5, and yearly thereafter. Mammography should be performed 3 to 9 months after surgery and thereafter at least annually; this should include the ipsilateral breast.

▶ This authoritative review and clinical guidelines are recommended for all clinicians involved in women's health care and are available online at http://www.ca.journal.org. In easily readable language, it reviews the current clinically applicable knowledge concerning the diagnosis and treatment of invasive breast cancer. Here are keenly useful data and pertinent facts that you can use in counseling your patients and answering their questions about breast cancer. The tables represent a summation of the clinical trials reported in the English-language medical literature. The references and selected bibliography are extensive. It is well worth your time to read the original article in its entirety (20 pages). I urge you to keep a copy handy in your office for quick reference and to make it available to those women with intense concerns or family affliction with invasive breast cancer. The authors and the American Cancer Society have done health care providers for women a profound service by creating this timely, lucid, and precise overview of the current clinical status of invasive breast cancer.

W.H. Hindle, M.D.

Suggested Readings

Hann LE, Giess CS, Bach AM: Endometrial Thickness in Tamoxifen-Treated Patients: Correlation with Clinical and Pathologic Findings. *AJR Am J Roentgenol* 168:657–661, 1997.

▶ This observational review of the Memorial Sloan-Kettering Cancer Center experience of endometrial abnormalities in women receiving tamoxifen therapy can serve as a guide to clinicians in formulating a plan of evaluation and management for their patients receiving tamoxifen. Multiple endometrial abnormalities can occur in women on tamoxifen therapy. The incidence of these abnormalities increases with the duration of tamoxifen therapy. Ultrasound measurement of endometrial thickness alone is not a reliable predictor of malignancy or a valid surgical call to action. Sonohysterography is effective in demonstrating endometrial thickness accurately and often allows identification of other endometrial abnormalities, e.g. endometrial polyps. Women receiving tamoxifen who experience vaginal (uterine) bleeding should be expeditiously evaluated by sonohysterography or hysteroscopy. Of course all suspicious endometrial lesions should be biopsied for definite histology diagnosis.

Bonnier P, Romain S, Dilhuydy JM, et al: Influence of Pregnancy on the Outcome of Breast Cancer: A Case-Control Study. *Int J Cancer* 72:720–727, 1997.

▶ This retrospective nationwide study from 23 French institutions collected 154 pregnancy-associated (defined as diagnosed during pregnancy or in the first six months postpartum) breast cancer patients during 1960–1993. The case-control group consisted of 308 patients. The observational findings are recorded and analyzed in detail. The authors conclude "that pregnancy was an independent and significant prognostic factor" with an adverse effect on outcome and an associated poor response to chemotherapy. However, the multifactorial nature of breast cancer incidence, histologic type, and biologic behavior, and the confounding variables such as selection, diagnosis, and treatment require caution in drawing conclusions that are meaningful in clinical practice.

Stuver SO, Chung-Cheng H, Bertone E, et al: The association between lactation and breast cancer in an international case-control study: A re-analysis by menopausal status. *Int J Cancer* 71:166–169, 1997.

▶ This is a reanalysis of a previously published hospital-based international case-control study of breast cancer.[1] The data cover 4,671 parous premenopausal and 7,200 parous postmenopausal women. The critical findings are (1) "examination of cumulative duration of lactation did not support an inverse association between breast cancer and increased length of total breast-feeding;" and (2) that after adjusting for known covariables, data "did not reveal a protective effect of lactation or duration of lactation against breast-cancer occurrence among the premenopausal, parous women." Although conflicting published data exist, there seems to be no significant effect of breast-feeding upon the incidence of breast cancer.

Reference

1. MacMahon B, Lin TM, Lowe CR, Mirra AP, et al: Lactation and cancer of the breast: A summary of an international study. *Bull WHO* 42:185–194, 1970.

Surbone A, Petrek JA: Childbearing Issues in Breast Carcinoma Survivors. *Cancer* 79:1271–1278, 1997.

▶ This review of the pertinent literature on pregnancy and breast cancer from the Memorial Sloan-Kettering Cancer Center summarizes the clinical data and could serve as an overview for interested patients. Noting that no prospective studies exist, the authors state that "The survival of women with breast carcinoma is not decreased by subsequent pregnancy in any of the published series." The authors are initiating a multicenter prospective study.

W.H. Hindle, M.D.

Twelve Years of Experience of Breast Cancer at the Institut Curie: Improvement of Survival and Value of Screening Mammographics

Salmon RJ, Asselain B, Le Gal M, et al (Institut Curie, Paris)

Breast J 6:202–205, 1997 26–3

Introduction.—The role of mammography in screening requires classification because some authors suggest a harmful effect in women younger than age 50, even though the value of mammography in diagnosing breast cancer is clearly established. The detection of smaller tumors should result with early detection of breast cancers by a mass screening programming. One of the major prognostic factors is the size of the tumor at the time of

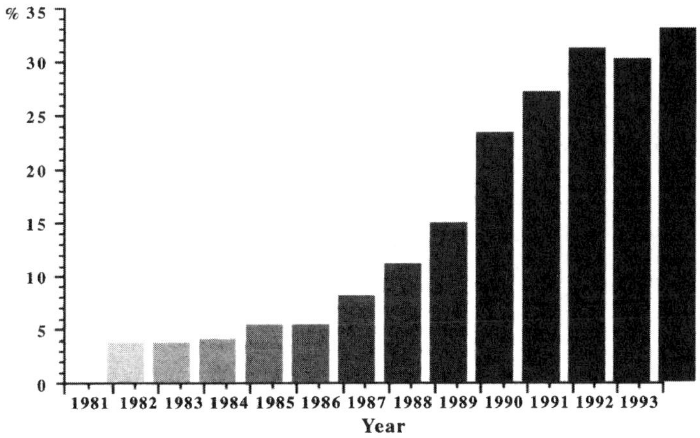

FIGURE 1.—Breast cancer, Institut Curie: Evolution of breast cancer diagnosed by screening mammography, 1981–1993. (Courtesy of Salmon RJ, Asselain B, Le Gal M, et al: Twelve years of experience of breast cancer at the Institut Curie: Improvement of survival and value of screening mammographics. *Breast J* 6:202–205, 1997.)

the initial diagnosis. The results of systematic prospective registrations of all patients treated for breast cancer in an institute were reported.

Methods.—There were 13,248 epithelial breast cancers registered in a 12-year period for women who were untreated at the time of the first visit. All patients had a similar protocol. Patients were reviewed 2–4 times a year after treatment, depending on protocols applied for a period of 10 years with no age limit. Patients had laboratory, clinical, and mammographic monitoring. They were sent follow-up reminders. There was no organized screening program.

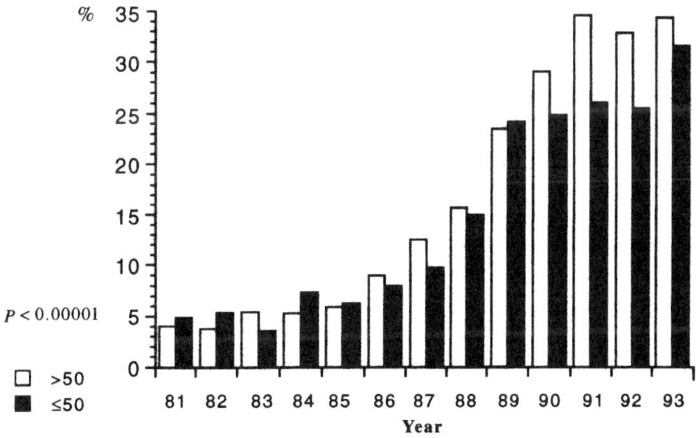

FIGURE 2.—Breast cancer, Institut Curie: Evolution of breast cancer diagnosed by screening mammography, 1981–1993. (Courtesy of Salmon RJ, Asselain B, Le Gal M, et al: Twelve years of experience of breast cancer at the Institut Curie: Improvement of survival and value of Screening Mammographics. *Breast J* 6:202–205, 1997.)

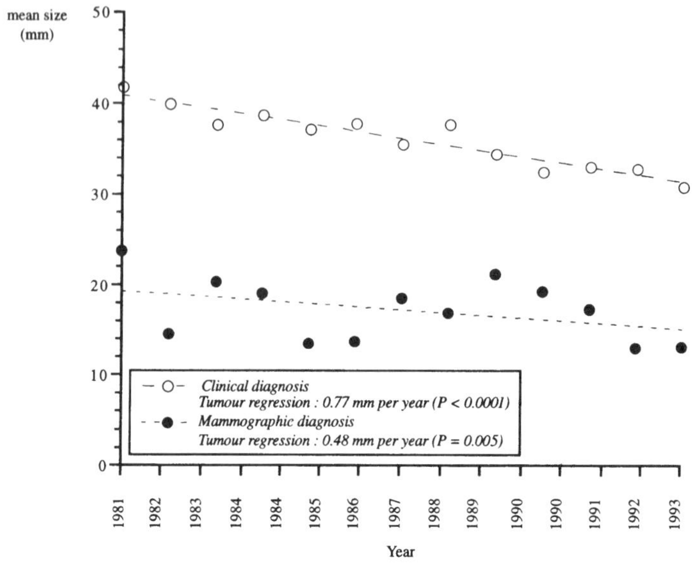

FIGURE 3.—Clinical size. (Courtesy of Salmon RJ, Asselain B, Le Gal M, et al: Twelve years of experience of breast cancer at the Institut Curie: Improvement of survival of screening mammographics. *Breast J* 6:202–205, 1997.)

Results.—T0–T1 increased from 22.9% to 53.1% in the number of cancers detected, T2 decreased from 44% to 34% in the number of cancers detected, and T3 decreased from 20.5% to 7.3%. Over the same 12-year period the rate of detection by screening mammography rose from 4% to 34% in the absence of any organized campaign (Fig 1) and was not related to age (Fig 2). In cancers detected by screening mammography, the decrease in size was very evident (Fig 3). Conservation therapy as a first choice of treatment increased from 20% to 63% of patients during the same period. The 5-year survival rose from 77% to 85%, regardless of stage.

Conclusion.—In the last 10 years, there has been an improvement in the detection rate, which is most likely related to information programs directed to the public and to doctors. Development of specific therapeutic trials of small tumors and in situ carcinomas are justified by the increasing number of these tumors and carcinomas being demonstrated by mammographic screening.

▶ The number of women with diagnosed breast cancer registered at the Curie Institute in Paris (13,248) during this 12-year interval is impressive. This single institution's experience gives a clear picture of the impact and utilization of screening mammography. The graph (Figure 2) shows that at the Curie Institute women younger than 50 with breast cancer are being diagnosed by screening mammography at approximately the same frequency as are women 50 and older with breast cancer. These data reflect the practice patterns of the physicians referring patients to the Curie Institute because during this time the Institute did not have an organized or publicized screening mammography campaign. As a result of the fractionated, geographically diverse medical care in the United States, it is difficult to obtain comparable data here. The fact that 63% of women at the Curie Institute received breast conserving therapy as a first treatment in 1993 (the last year covered in this report) is outstanding.

W.H. Hindle, M.D.

Survival of Women Ages 40–49 Years With Breast Carcinoma According to Method of Detection

McPherson CP, Swenson KK, Jolitz G, et al (HealthSystem Minnesota, Minneapolis; TUMORS, St Paul, Minn; Univ of Minn, Minneapolis)
Cancer 79:1923–1932, 1997 26–4

Background.—The impact of mammographic screening on breast cancer mortality in women younger than the age of 50 is still unclear. Previous randomized trials were flawed by inadequate sample sizes, prolonged screening intervals, questionable randomization, and/or cross-contamination between intervention groups. In the current study, a historical prospective cohort design was used to assess differences in prognostic factors at the time of breast carcinoma diagnosis and in overall survival among women 40 to 49 years old according to the method of detecting breast carcinoma.

Methods.—Nine hundred seventy-one women, aged 40 to 49 diagnosed as having invasive breast carcinoma between 1986 and 1992 were included in the analysis. Tumor size, lymph node status, and overall survival were compared among groups whose tumors were detected by self-examination, by clinical examination, incidentally by the patient, and by mammography.

Findings.—The mean size of tumors found by mammography was significantly smaller than that of tumors detected by the other methods. Mammographically detected tumors were also significantly more likely to

TABLE 4.—Relative Risk of Death for Women in Each Breast Carcinoma Detection Method Group After Deleting First Year of Follow-Up for Patients in the Mammogram Group

Method of detection	Relative risk of death	95% Confidence interval	*P* value
Mammogram[a]	1.0		
Breast self-exam	1.9	1.05–3.23	0.03
Clinical breast exam	2.0	1.09–3.73	0.03
Patient incidental	2.1	1.25–3.39	0.005

Note: Results of Cox Proportional Hazards Regression (n = 966).

(Courtesy of McPherson CP, Swenson KK, Jolitz G, et al: Survival of women ages 40–49 years with breast carcinoma according to method of detection. *Cancer* 79:1923–1932, 1997. Reprinted by permission of Wiley-Liss, Inc., a subsidiary of John Wiley & Sons, Inc.)

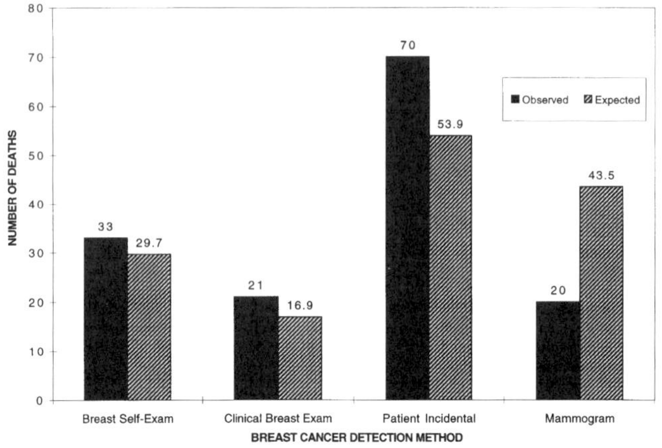

FIGURE 3.—Observed vs. expected deaths by breast carcinoma detection method among women ages 40–49 years are shown. The number of deaths expected was based on the total number of deaths in the cohort and the distribution of patients among the detection method group. Overall chi-square test =22.048, $P < 0.0001$. (Courtesy of McPherson CP, Swenson KK, Jolitz G, et al: Survival of women ages 40–49 years with breast carcinoma according to method of detection. *Cancer* 79:1923–1932, 1997. Reprinted by permission of Wiley-Liss, Inc., a subsidiary of John Wiley & Sons, Inc.)

be localized than those found by other methods. Survival was significantly better in the mammography group than in the other groups, especially among women with smaller tumors, even after adjustment for lead time bias (Table 4; Figs 3 and 4).

Conclusion.—Women aged 40–49 whose invasive breast carcinoma is detected mammographically have significantly smaller tumors and more

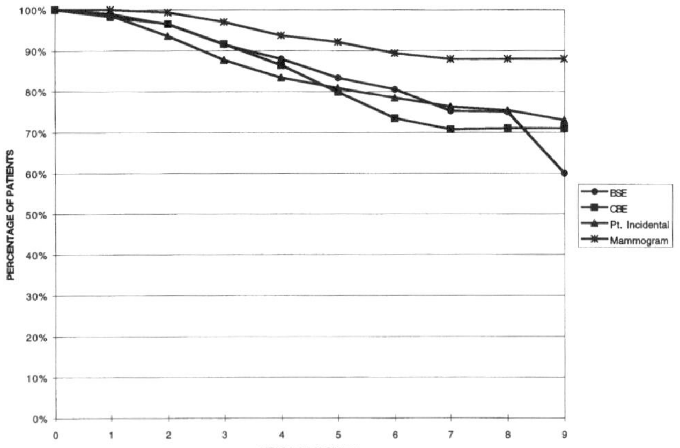

FIGURE 4.—Survival curves by breast carcinoma detection method are shown for women ages 40–49 years (n = 971). Women in the mammogram group had better survival than women in the breast self-examination group ($P = 0.0008$), the clinical breast examination group ($P = 0.0008$), or the patient incidental detection group (P 0.0001) (log rank test). (Courtesy of McPherson CP, Swenson KK, Jolitz G, et al: Survival of women ages 40–49 years with breast carcinoma according to method of detection. *Cancer* 79:1923–1932, 1997. Reprinted by permission of Wiley-Liss, Inc., a subsidiary of John Wiley & Sons, Inc.)

localized disease. The risk of mortality in these women may also be lower than in women whose tumors are detected by other methods.

▶ This historical, prospective, cohort-designed analysis from the University of Minnesota of 971 women aged 40–49 diagnosed with invasive breast cancer documents that those diagnosed by mammography had smaller cancers with more localized disease and a lower risk of mortality. Thus, the overall breast cancer survival was significantly greater for women whose cancers were detected by mammography than by other methods of detection. This result seems logical because the mammography-detected lesions are almost all nonpalpable with associated favorable prognosis compared to palpable cancers. It is of interest that cancers detected by breast self-examination (BSE) yielded about the same prognosis as those found at clinical breast examination (CBE) or accidentally by the patient. This data should provide clinicians with strong incentives to make it their goal to diagnose all breast cancers by mammography before the cancers have grown to a size large enough to be palpated. Based upon review of all the currently available published data, my recommendation remains that annual screening mammography should begin at age 40 and continue throughout a woman's life.

W.H. Hindle, M.D.

Early-onset Breast Cancer: Histopathological and Prognostic Considerations

Kollias J, Elston CW, Ellis IO, et al (Nottingham City Hosp, England)

Br J Cancer 75:1318–1323, 1997 26–5

Background.—It is generally believed that young patients with breast cancer have a poor prognosis. Some studies have indicated that the prognosis of younger and older patients is similar, and that management of young patients with breast cancer should be dictated by clinical and histopathologic criteria. Prognostic factors and survival were compared in young and older patients with breast cancer.

Methods.—Between 1973 and 1993, 2,879 patients aged 70 years or younger were treated surgically for primary operable breast cancer. Patients were categorized according to age: younger than 35 years, 35–50 years, and 51–70 years. The predictive value of age, invasive tumor size, histologic tumor grade, and lymph node stage was analyzed. Patients were evaluated every 3–6 months for 5 years, and once a year thereafter.

Results.—There were 120 patients younger than 35 years, 1,003 patients aged 35–50 years, and 1,756 patients aged 51–70 years. Significantly lower metastasis disease-free survival and actuarial survival were seen in patients younger than 35 years compared to the other 2 groups (Fig 1 and Fig 2). More high-grade cancers and vascular invasion were seen in patients younger than 35 years at diagnosis. There were no differences in tumor size or lymph nodes among groups. The Nottingham Prognostic

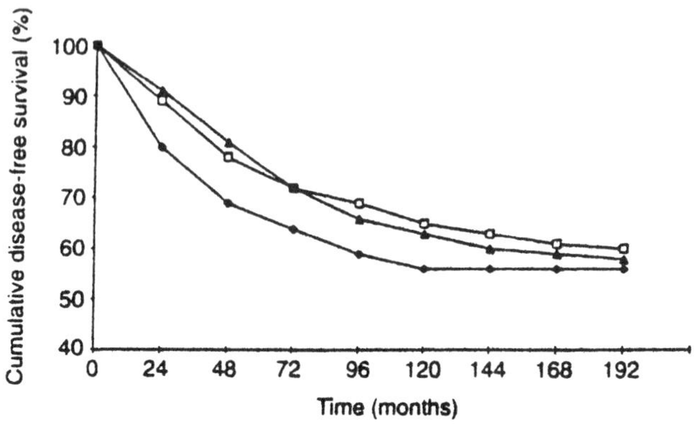

No at risk

Group I	120	107	70	49	32	22	15	11	8
Group II	1003	920	646	459	322	218	157	96	59
Group III	1756	1622	1138	762	479	320	205	116	65

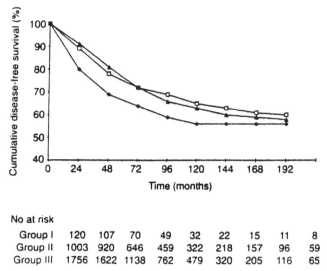

FIGURE 1.—Metastases disease-free survival curves for age group 1 (*diamonds*, age younger than 35), group II (*squares*, age 35–50), and group III (*triangles*, age 51–70 years. χ^2 = 9.32. P = 0.01 (2 df). (Courtesy of Kollias J, Elston CW, Ellis IO, et al: Early-onset breast cancer: Histopathological and prognostic considerations. *Br J Cancer* 75:1318–1323, 1997.)

Index was used to classify cancers in each age group. Patients younger than 35 years were more likely to be in the group with poor prognosis because of their higher prevalence of high-grade tumors. Within each prognostic group, there was no difference in actuarial survival among age groups (Fig 3).

Discussion.—The difference in survival between patients younger than 35 years and older patients with breast cancer is explained by the higher

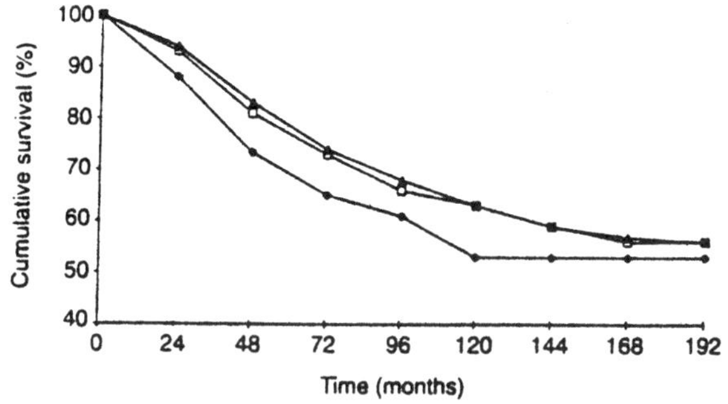

No at risk

Group I	120	107	70	49	32	22	15	11	8
Group II	1003	920	646	459	322	218	157	96	59
Group III	1756	1622	1138	762	479	320	205	116	65

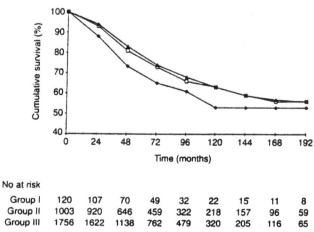

FIGURE 2.—Actuarial survival curves for age group I (*diamonds*, age younger than 35), group II (*squares*, age 35–50), and group III (age 51–70). χ^2 = 6.6 P = 0.03 (2 df). (Courtesy of Kollias J, Elston CW, Ellis IO, et al: Early-onset breast cancer: Histopathological and prognostic considerations. *Br J Cancer* 75:1318–1323, 1997.)

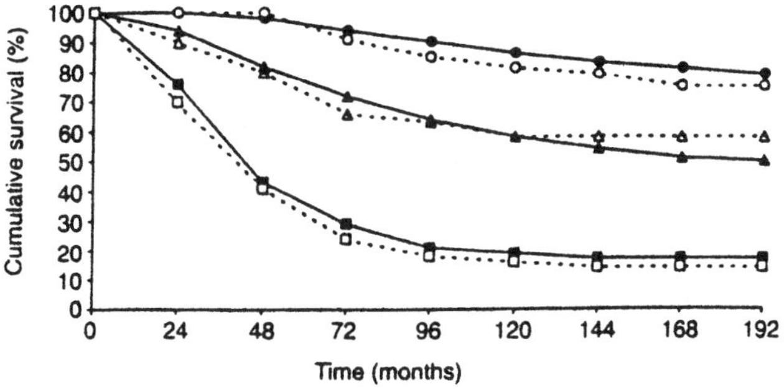

FIGURE 3.—Actuarial survival of patients according to Nottingham Prognostic Index and age; (*filled circles*). Good prognostic group for all ages, n = 891; (*open circles*), good prognostic group for patients younger than 35 years, n = 16; (*filled triangles*) medium prognostic group for all ages, n = 1,369; (*open triangles*) medium prognostic group for patients younger than 35 years, n = 61; (*filled squares*) poor prognostic group for all ages, n = 415; (*open squares*) poor prognostic group for patients younger than 35 years, n = 34. Within any one Nottingham Prognostic Index group, no difference was seen according to age. (Courtesy of Kollias J, Elston CW, Ellis IO, et al: Early-onset breast cancer: Histopathological and prognostic considerations. *Br J Cancer* 75:1318–1323, 1997.)

rate of high-grade tumors and vascular invasion in the younger patients. Young age alone is not an independent predictive factor of outcome in patients with primary breast cancer. Young women, however, tend to have more adverse intrinsic biological factors.

► Contrary to a commonly held misconception, the authors conclude that "age itself had no influence on the prognosis of the individual" woman younger than 35 with a diagnosis of invasive breast cancer, compared to other age groups. However, the cancers of these women were generally of high-grade (poorly differentiated, anaplastic) and they commonly exhibited vascular invasion when compared to cancers in the older age groups. It does seem logical that "aggressive" breast cancer would be more common in the younger age group and that those cancers with a slow indolent growth pattern would tend to be diagnosed in the older age groups, thus giving the "bad reputation" (e.g., poor prognosis) for breast cancer diagnosed in young women. Because obstetrician-gynecologists commonly see patients of reproductive age, they often have an opportunity to screen for and diagnose breast cancer in women such as those younger than 35 years in this study.

W.H. Hindle, M.D.

Alcohol and Breast Cancer in Women: A Pooled Analysis of Cohort Studies

Smith-Warner SA, Spiegelman D, Yaun S-S, et al (Harvard School of Public Health, Boston; Harvard Med School, Boston; Univ of Maastricht, The Netherlands; et al)

JAMA 279:535–540, 1998 26–6

Introduction.—Numerous studies have examined the association between alcohol consumption and breast cancer risk, but findings have been inconsistent. A pooled analysis of 6 prospective studies, each with at least 200 incident breast cancer cases, assessed the risk of invasive breast cancer associated with total and beverage-specific alcohol consumption. Also examined were the effects of dietary and nondietary factors on the association between alcohol and breast cancer.

Methods.—The 6 studies were conducted in Canada, The Netherlands, Sweden, and the United States. All included an assessment of long-term intake of foods and nutrients and a validation study of the diet assessment method. Food frequency questionnaires were used in each study to estimate alcohol intake.

Results.—The studies included 322,647 women who were evaluated for up to 11 years; 4,335 participants had a diagnosis of incident invasive breast cancer. Nondrinkers accounted for 22.5% to 55.3% of controls in the cohorts. Among controls who were drinkers, mean alcohol intakes ranged from 3.22 to 12.58 g/day across the studies. There was a positive association between alcohol consumption and the risk of invasive breast cancer, and the risk increased linearly with increasing intake among women with alcohol intakes of less than 60 g/day (an intake reported by more than 99% of participants). Compared with nondrinkers, women with total alcohol intakes between 30 and 60 g/day (about 2 to 5 drinks) had a multivariate-adjusted relative risk of 1.41. Other factors, such as body mass index and hormone replacement therapy, did not modify the association between alcohol intake and breast cancer, and the specific type of alcoholic beverage consumed did not strongly influence risk estimates.

Conclusion.—This pooled analysis of cohort studies indicates that alcohol consumption increases the risk of breast cancer in women. Compared with nondrinkers, women consuming approximately 2.3 to 4.5 bottles of beer, 2.8 to 5.6 glasses of wine, or 2.0 to 4.0 shots of liquor had a 41% higher risk of invasive breast cancer. Reduction of regular alcohol consumption is likely to reduce the risk of breast cancer in women.

► Alcohol consumption is 1 of the confounding variables of breast cancer risk that continues to be debated. Conflicting studies persist, and the clinical implications of most of them are not clear. Although this pooled analysis does reach statistical significance because of the large numbers involved, the resultant relative risk is low (less than 2.0), which qualifies as an epidemiologic "weak association" and still may be the result of chance. The analysis demonstrates some dose effect but no duration effect. This is consistent with other recent reports, such as Bowlin et al.,[1] that suggest that intensity of drinking is a risk factor. After covariate adjustment there was no difference between premenopausal and postmenopausal women. Again, the odds ratios were all less than 1.50.

Alcohol consumption seems to fit with other factors—such as smoking, overweight, lack of regular exercise, fatty diet, and stress—that may play some role in increasing the incidence of breast cancer, although their impact upon breast cancer is modest at most. Furthermore, modifications of these factors have yet to be documented as being effective or practical for breast cancer prevention.

W.H. Hindle, M.D.

Reference

1. Bowlin SJ, Leske MC, Varma A, et al: Breast cancer risk and alcohol consumption: Results from a large case-control study. *Int J Epidemiol* 26:915–923, 1997.

Breast Cancer Risk Assessment and Counseling: A Clinician's Guide

Kelly PT (John Muir Med Ctr, Walnut Creek, Calif)
Breast J 3:311–316, 1997 26–7

Objective.—More and more patients are asking about their risk of breast cancer, and whether they should undergo genetic testing. However, at present, most of these patients will not benefit from genetic testing. This article presents an overview of the Cancer Risk Assessment and Counseling process.

Breast Cancer Risk Assessment and Counseling.—Initial assessment should include ordering medical records on the patient's affected relatives. In an example case described by the author, a reported case of "stomach cancer" in the patient's grandmother turned out to have been ovarian cancer. Patients with a family history of breast cancer who are diagnosed with atypia should understand there is no additive or multiplicative increase in risk from these findings. Patients also need to know about the effects of hormone replacement therapy (HRT) on breast cancer risk. Most studies suggest that breast cancer risk does not decrease when HRT stops, making HRT an unlikely causative agent. Studies suggesting an increased risk of breast cancer in women taking HRT likely reflect chance fluctuations. There are no large studies showing a clinically significant increase in risk, i.e., 2– to 3–fold or greater. Smaller risks could be attributable to confounding variables. Women should understand they are far more likely to die of cardiac or cerebrovascular disease than of breast cancer.

Patients who carry a BRCA–1 or BRCA–2 mutation may be at increased risk of various cancers, including colon, pancreatic, endometrial, or thyroid cancer; lymphoma; multiple myeloma; or Hodgkin's disease. Patients should understand that current genetic testing approaches cannot detect all BRCA–1 or BRCA–2 mutations, and that some genes relevant to hereditary cancer risk may not have been identified yet. All of this information can help patients reach a rational decision about handling their increased cancer risk, and living with their anxiety about cancer.

Discussion.—Although most patients with a family history of breast cancer are not at increased hereditary risk, many can benefit from risk analysis. This analysis should include not only a family history, but also an assessment of nonhereditary risks. Patients should understand that genetic testing is unnecessary if it cannot detect the presumed mutation in their family. Assessment and discussion of psychosocial factors are essential for patients to make informed decisions about the risk information they receive.

► Women who believe that genetic testing can determine if they will or will not develop breast cancer are misguided and not well informed. Most breast cancers are sporadic and not hereditary or even familial. No test will currently "guarantee" that a woman will not develop breast cancer, and it is unlikely that such a test will become available within the foreseeable future. Furthermore, women who test "positive" for *BRCA–1* or *BRCA–2* may not ever develop breast cancer. Continuously updated information on genetic testing should be provided to concerned women.

When family history of breast cancer is a consideration, clinicians should take a 3–generation pedigree of all relatives (female and male) for breast, ovarian, colon, and prostate cancer. If an autosomal dominant genetic pattern is suggested, then *BRCA1–2* genetic testing should be considered for the patient with diagnosed invasive breast cancer. Genetic counseling for that patient (and for related family members if the woman so desires) should be provided before a decision is reached about genetic testing. Furthermore, if the woman wishes to proceed with genetic testing, further genetic counseling is indicated when the results are known.

This review by Pat Kelly, who is one of the pioneers in breast cancer genetic counseling, is a clear, concise practical overview of risk assessment and provides pragmatic guidance for clinicians.

W.H. Hindle, M.D.

Frequency of Breast Cancer Attributable to *BRCA1* in a Population-based Series of American Women

Newman B, Mu H, Butler LM, et al (Univ of North Carolina, Chapel Hill; Univ of Washington, Seattle; Yale Univ, New Haven, Conn)

JAMA 279:915–921, 1998 26–8

Background.—Genetic tests for *BRCA1* and *BRCA2* are now available, leading to debate about whether these tests should be used outside of research protocols. Most data on the prevalence of mutations of these genes are drawn from studies of high-risk groups, which do not reflect the general population of U.S. breast cancer patients. Knowing the true frequency of mutations could inform testing decisions in the general population. The prevalence of mutations in *BRCA1* was studied in a population-based sample, including possible differences by race, age at diagnosis, and family history.

Methods.—Case patients who were aged 20–74 years when their first invasive breast cancer was diagnosed were studied. They were frequency matched for age and race to control for women without breast cancer. The first 211 cases and 188 controls were entered into the study without consideration of race. The next 99 cases and 108 controls were all African-American. *BRCA1* gene testing was performed in cases, including analysis of germline variants at any site in the coding sequence, splice junctions, 5' untranslated region, or 3' untranslated region. Selected variants were analyzed in controls. Multiplex single-strand conformational analysis was performed for screening purposes, and genomic sequencing to confirm all potential variants.

Results.—Disease-related *BRCA1* variants—all protein-truncating mutations—were found in 3 of the 211 cases. The percentage of cases with disease-related variants among white women, after adjustment for sampling probabilities, was 3.3% (95% confidence interval, 0% to 7.2%). For African-American women, this percentage was 0%. Carriage of a disease-related variant was not predicted by young age at diagnosis. Twenty-three percent of white women with a family history of ovarian cancer had an inherited mutation, as did 13% of cases from families with 4 or more cases of breast cancer and 33% of cases with a family history of both breast and ovarian cancer with at least 4 members affected. However, these estimates were based on a small number of very high-risk families. Five patients were found to have rare missense mutations or single amino acid deletions. African-American cases were significantly more likely to have a variant in the 3' untranslated region, compared with African-American controls.

Conclusions.—This population-based study demonstrates a low prevalence of *BRCA1* mutations among women with breast cancer. Thus widespread *BRCA1* screening is not indicated. However, genotyping may be considered for families with a history of breast and ovarian cancer or with 4 or more cases of breast cancer. Where the *BRCA1* gene is concerned, family history, age, and genetics interact in complex ways among the population. All these factors should be accounted for when *BRCA1* testing is considered or interpreted.

▶ This article and the following publication by Malone (Abstract 26–9) highlight the fact that the original estimates of the prevalence of *BRCA1* (derived from an intensely selected high-risk group of women) resulted in artificially high estimates of the frequency of *BRCA* mutations and the subsequent risk of invasive breast and ovarian cancer. Furthermore, of the more than 400 *BRCA* cancer-related mutations that have been identified to date, the key primary mutations (and their major biological actions) correlated with invasive cancer are not yet known. In addition, some women with *BRCA* mutations do not have invasive cancer and, because of the inherent microbiology, a percentage of the known *BRCA* mutations are not identified by the currently available *BRCA* test. The more that is known about *BRCA* mutations, the more complex the results and their clinical implications become. Currently, the giving of pertinent information is appropriate for most women. After analysis of a 3-generation pedigree, a few highly selected women should be offered genetic counseling.

W.H. Hindle, M.D.

BRCA1 Mutations and Breast Cancer in the General Population: Analyses in Women Before Age 35 Years and in Women Before Age 45 Years With First-degree Family History

Malone KE, Daling JR, Thompson JD, et al (Fred Hutchinson Cancer Research Ctr, Seattle)

JAMA 279:922–929, 1998 26–9

Background.—Although studies of high-risk families with multiple early-onset breast cancers have been valuable for determining the type and spectrum of germline mutations on the *BRCA1* gene, such research does not provide guidance to women with modest family history profiles. General population studies are needed to assess the *BRCA1* mutation frequency in women perceived to be at high risk and to develop profiles of women most likely to be carriers.

Methods.—Two categories of women hypothesized to be at increased risk of carrying mutations were studied: those with breast cancer diagnosed before the age of 35 years, and those with breast cancer diagnosed before age 45 years and a first-degree family history of breast cancer. Subjects were drawn from 2 population-based, case-control studies.

Findings.—Of 193 women with breast cancer diagnosed before age 35 years (none selected on the basis of family history status), 6.2% had germline *BRCA1* mutations. Of 208 women with the cancer diagnosed before age 45 years and with a first-degree family history, 7.2% had germline *BRCA1* mutations. Both groups included variations in mutation frequency noted by age and family history. Mutation frequency declined as age at diagnosis increased. Greater proportions of mutations were seen in patients with at least 1 relative given a diagnosis of breast cancer before 45 years of age, in patients with greater numbers of affected relatives, and in patients with a family history of ovarian cancer. The frequency of mutations did not vary by bilateral breast cancer family history. Seventy-one control women with a first-degree family history had no frameshift or nonsense mutations, although missense changes of unknown significance were observed in case and control subjects.

Conclusion.—In this study, women with *BRCA1* germline mutations did not have a common family history profile. A large percentage of the women with a first-degree breast cancer family history and of women with a breast cancer diagnosis before age 35 did not have germline *BRCA1* mutations. Thus, although early-onset disease and a strong family history of breast cancer may be useful guidelines for checking *BRCA1* status, it may be difficult to develop *BRCA1* mutation screening criteria for women with modest family history profiles.

▶ Who should be tested for *BRCA1*? It is clear that the *BRCA* tests are not screening tests for the general population. Is there a subset of women for which *BRCA* testing should be routinely recommended? To date, the literature does not suggest such a group. Each woman will have to be individually evaluated as to the appropriateness of *BRCA* testing. Counseling is essential before recommending such testing. However, skilled genetic counseling is not widely available. Thus, primary care physicians will have to keep themselves informed through the medical literature as the complete *BRCA* testing story becomes clear. To date, indications and subsequent recommendations are not apparent. There is no consensus beyond recommending genetic counseling. Current estimates of the frequency of *BRCA1* mutation in the general female population are from 1:500 to 1:1,500. Criteria for selection of women for *BRCA* testing need to be identified.

W.H. Hindle, M.D.

Suggested Reading

Burke W, Daly M, Garber J, et al: Recommendations for Follow-up Care of Individuals With an Inherited Predisposition to Cancer: II. *BRCA1* and *BRCA2*. *JAMA* 277:997–1003, 1997.

▶ Primary care physicians are faced with anxious women asking, "Will I get breast cancer?" Although there is no answer, the commerical availability of genetic testing for *BRCA1* and *BRCA2* has led some to the mistaken idea that these are screening tests for breast cancer. They are not. In certain families with three generation pedigrees of women with diagnosed invasive breast cancer, *BRCA* testing may be indicated when the patient diagnosed with breast cancer understands the clinical significance of the *BRCA* test, whether reported as "positive" or "negative." Genetic counseling, both before the patient decides to be tested and after the test results are available, is recommended for women who wish to access their genetic information. Furthermore, it should be stressed that there is no agreement as to the appropriate recommendations for women tested as "*BRCA* positive." Most busy practicing clinicians would do well to refer women seeking *BRCA* testing to a multidisciplinary breast center which has an established genetic counseling capability.

W.H. Hindle, M.D.

Using Autopsy Series to Estimate the Disease "Reservoir" for Ductal Carcinoma in Situ of the Breast: How Much More Breast Cancer Can We Find?

Welch HG, Black WC (Veterans Affairs Med Ctr, White River Junction, Vt; Dartmouth Med School, Hanover, NH; Dartmouth-Hitchcock Med Ctr, Lebanon, NH)

Ann Intern Med 127:1023–1028, 1997 26–10

Background.—The ability to detect early forms of breast cancer will continue to improve. By reviewing autopsy results of women not known to have had breast cancer during life, the current study determined how many cases of breast cancer might be found if women were thoroughly assessed.

Methods and Findings.—Seven autopsy series of such women were identified in a MEDLINE search from 1966 to the present. The prevalences of invasive breast cancer in these studies ranged from 0 to 1.8%, with a median of 1.3%. The prevalences of ductal carcinoma in situ (DCIS) ranged from 0 to 14.7%, with a median of 8.9%. Prevalences were greater among women between 40 and 70 years of age—those likely to have been screened. The mean number of slides examined per breast ranged from 9 to 275. Studies reporting higher levels of scrutiny tended to report more cases of disease.

Conclusions.—A substantial number of DCIS cases go undetected during life. The number of DCIS cases diagnosed depends on how hard pathologists look for the disease and possibly their threshold for making the diagnosis, which has important implications for what it means to have this disease.

▶ The combined data from these 7 autopsy series yield a median prevalence rate for DCIS that is about 7 times greater than that for invasive breast cancer. What happens to DCIS that does not transform into invasive cancer? Is the lead-time critical? Or are there a variety of DCIS types with distinctly different biologic behaviors? Gupta et al. in Cardiff, Wales, studied 300 cases of invasive ductal carcinoma with associated DCIS and found that the differentiation by histologic/nuclear grading of the DCIS was correlated with the grade of the invasive carcinoma, the Nottingham prognostic index, and the clinical outcome. It was concluded, "well-differentiated DCIS probably gives rise to low grade invasive breast carcinoma with a better long-term clinical outcome." This recognizes the heterogeneity of DCIS but is at variance with the traditional theory that DCIS undergoes progressive malignant transformation into invasive carcinoma. Perhaps future genetic analysis will reveal distinctly different types of DCIS with different natural histories and biologic behaviors.

W.H. Hindle, M.D.

Reference

1. Gupta SK, Douglas-Jones AG, Fenn N, Morgan JM, et al. The clinical behavior of breast carcinoma is probably determined at the preinvasive stage (ductal carcinoma in situ). *Cancer* 80:1740–1745, 1997.

Ductal Carcinoma in Situ of the Breast

Fonseca R, Hartmann LC, Petersen IA, et al (Mayo Clinic and Mayo Found, Rochester, Minn)

Ann Intern Med 127:1013–1022, 1997 26–11

Background.—The management of ductal carcinoma in situ (DCIS) of the breast is challenging and controversial. The natural history of DCIS and results obtained with various treatments were reviewed.

Methods and Findings.—A computerized MEDLINE search of articles on DCIS published since 1966 was performed. All sources were reviewed critically. There were no randomized trials comparing mastectomy with breast-conserving treatment for patients with DCIS. One large randomized trial demonstrated the efficacy of lumpectomy plus radiotherapy. Though its value is debated, the presence of comedo necrosis and surgical margin status are often used to predict subsequent recurrence. The risk for in-breast recurrence 5 years after lumpectomy plus radiotherapy is about 8%.

Conclusions.—Lumpectomy followed by radiotherapy appears to be an appropriate treatment for most patients. Lumpectomy alone in selected patients is still debated. The relationship of DCIS to invasive breast cancer will become clearer with more refined molecular analysis.

▶ Prior to the widespread use of screening mammography, the incidence of ductal carcinoma in situ (DCIS) was given as < 2%. Now, mammographically diagnosed DCIS (by its clustered, irregular, dense, linear calcifications) is one of the most common malignancies detected by screening mammography, accounting for as many as 30% of all newly diagnosed breast cancers in some centers. The American Cancer Society estimates the annual incidence of newly diagnosed DCIS to be more than 36,000 cases.

Unfortunately, there is no consensus as to the optimum treatment of DCIS. It is clear that low nuclear grade and high nuclear grade DCIS are distinctly different types with different capacities to undergo malignant transformation into invasive carcinoma, different biologic behaviors, and different clinical prognoses. Except for comedo, the traditional histologic architectural types, e.g., cribriform, papillary (including micropapillary), and solid are not relevant to the clinical course, prognosis, and biologic behavior of DCIS. Future molecular genetic and cytogenetic research may provide the answers. Until a clinically meaningful differentiation of the heterogeneous types of DCIS is established, a uniform approach to treatment will not be successful and therapeutic consensus will not be reached.

This review from the Mayo Clinic, Rochester, Minnesota, serves health care providers for women as an up-to-date overview of the diagnosis and treatment of DCIS.

W.H. Hindle, M.D.

Standards for Diagnosis and Management of Ductal Carcinoma In Situ (DCIS) of the Breast

Winchester DP, Strom EA (American College of Surgeons; American College of Radiology)

CA Cancer J Clin 48:108–128, 1998 26–12

Background.—This article discusses the various diagnostic strategies and treatments used to identify and treat ductal carcinoma in situ (DCIS).

Diagnostic Methods.—Treatment of DCIS is based on clinical, mammographic, and pathologic findings. The history and physical examination

TABLE 2.—Results of Treatment of DCIS With Mastectomy

Reference	No. Patients	Follow-Up	Nonpalpable (%)	No. Recurrences
Ashikari et al	92	11 yrs (maximum)	0	0
Sunshine et al	68	10 yrs (minimum)	0	0
Farrow	181	5–20 yrs	0	2
Silverstein et al	228	7 yrs (median)	80	2
Von Rueden & Wilson	45	Not stated	7	0
Lagios et al	42	Not stated	60	0
Kinne et al	101	11.5 yrs (median)	59	1
Schuh et al	51	5.5 yrs (mean)	33	1
Arnesson et al	28	77 months	100	0

(Courtesy of Winchester DP, Strom EA: Standards for diagnosis and management of ductal carcinoma in situ (DCIS) of the breast. *CA Cancer J Clin* 48:108–128, 1998.)

TABLE 3.—1997 Update of National Surgical Adjuvant Breast and Bowel Project (NSABP) Protocol B-17

Type of Recurrence	Lumpectomy No.	Lumpectomy Cumulative IBTR	Lumpectomy plus Radiation Therapy No.	Lumpectomy plus Radiation Therapy Cumulative IBTR	P Value
Noninvasive	51	13.4%	30	8.2%	0.007
Invasive	53	13.4%	17	3.9%	< 0.000005
Total	104	26.8%	47	12.1%	< 0.000005

Abbreviation: IBTR, ipsilateral breast tumor recurrence (local recurrence).

Data from Mamounas E, Fisher B, Dingam J, et al. Effects of breast irradiation following lumpectomy in intraductal carcinoma (DCIS): Updated results from NSABP B-17. *Proc Soc Surg Oncol* 50:7, 1997. (Courtesy of Winchester DP, Strom EA: Standards for diagnosis and management of ductal carcinoma in situ (DCIS) of the breast. *CA Cancer J Clin* 48:108–128, 1998.)

TABLE 4.—National and International Prospective Trials of Conservative Surgery With or Without Radiotherapy for DCIS

Study	Dates	Actual or Planned Accrual	Coexisting LCIS Allowed?	Nonpalpable Tumors	Size Limits
NSABP B-17	1985–1990	790	Yes	83%	None
EORTC 10853	1986–1996	1,010	No	NS	≤5 cm
Swedish National DCIS Trial	1989–ongoing	1,000	NS	NS	<1 quadrant
UK-Australian-New Zealand Trial	1990–ongoing	1,000	Yes	NS	None

Abbreviations: EORTC, European Organization for Research and Treatment of Cancer; *LCIA*, lobular carcinoma in situ; *NS*, not stated; *NSABP*, National Surgical Adjuvant Breast and Bowel Project.

(Courtesy of Winchester DP, Strom EA: Standards for diagnosis and management of ductal carcinoma in situ (DCIS) of the breast. *CA Cancer J Clin* 48:108–128, 1998.)

TABLE 5.—Results of Conservative Surgery and Radiation for Clinically and Mammographically Detected DCIS

Reference	No. Patients	Breast Recurrence Crude Incidence (%)	Median Follow-up (Yrs)
McCormick et al	54	18	3.0
Haffty et al	60	7	3.6
Kurtz et al	47	4	5.0
Ray et al	56	9	5.0
Solin et al	51	10	5.7
Van Zee et al	63	10	6.2
Hiramatsu et al*	76	9	6.2
Sneige et al	49	10	7.2
Forquet et al	153	16	9.0
Solin et al†	268	17	10.3

*Ten-year cause-specific survival 96%.
†Ten-year cause-specific survival 97%.
(Courtesy of Winchester DP, Strom EA: Standards for diagnosis and management of ductal carcinoma in situ (DCIS) of the breast. *CA Cancer J Clin* 48:108–128, 1998.)

reveal the patient's general health and thus her suitability for conservative therapy. Bilateral mammography is used to determine the extent of disease and to allow biopsy. Stereotactic core-needle biopsy or guided-wire open biopsy should be used to identify the microcalcifications of DCIS. Axillary node involvement in DCIS is rare, and thus nodes usually need not be sampled. Pathology reports must include the nuclear grade of the lesion and indicate whether any necrosis is present. Lesion size is an important consideration, because conservative therapy has not proved useful for DCIS lesions of more than 4 cm. With conservative surgery, a repeat mammogram will ensure that the lesion was removed entirely, and the biopsy site must be reexcised to ensure that the margins are negative.

TABLE 6.—Results of Conservative Surgery and Radiation for DCIS Detected by Mammography

Reference	Total No. Patients	Actuarial Breast Recurrence (%)		Cause-Specific Survival (%)		Median Follow-up (Yrs)
		5 Years	10 Years	5 Years	10 Years	
NSABP B-17	399*	10	—	—	—	3.6 (mean)
Kuske et al	44	7	—	—	—	4.0
Fowble et al	110	1	15	100	100	5.3
Vicini et al	102	4	6	—	99	6.1
Hiramatsu et al	54	2	23	—	96	6.2
Sneige et al	31	0	8	—	—	7.2
Silverstein et al	33†	7	19	—	97	7.8
Solin et al	110	7	14	100	96	9.3

Abbreviation: NSABP, National Surgical Adjuvant Breast and Bowel Project; —, data not available.
*81% detected by mammography.
†89% detected by mammography.
(Courtesy of Winchester DP, Strom EA: Standards for diagnosis and management of ductal carcinoma in situ (DCIS) of the breast. *CA Cancer J Clin* 48:108–128, 1998.)

TABLE 7.—Results of Treatment of DCIS by Excision Alone

Reference	No. Patients	Follow-up (Months)	Recurrence (%)	Invasive (%)
Arnesson et al	169	80*	16/22†	36
Baird et al	30	43‡	13	25
Carpenter et al	28	38‡	18	20
Cataliotti et al	99	79‡	8/23†	38
Eusebi et al	80	210	20	69
NSABP B-17	403	90‡	27§	50
NSABP B-06	21	83‡	43	55
Lagios et al	79	130*	18¶	56
Salvadori et al	74	31‡	14	60
Schreer	102	56‡	24	42
Schwartz et al	194	53*	14/25†	18
Sibbering & Blamey	48	58*	6	33
Silverstein	130	45*	21§	33
Silverstein et al	85	45*	14§	33

Abbreviation: NSABP, National Surgical Adjuvant Breast and Bowel Project.
*Median.
†5-year actuarial/10-year actuarial.
‡Mean.
§8-year actuarial.
¶15-year actuarial.
(Courtesy of Winchester DP, Strom EA: Standards for diagnosis and management of ductal carcinoma in situ (DCIS) of the breast. *CA Cancer J Clin* 48:108–128, 1998.)

Treatment Methods.—DCIS rarely recurs after total mastectomy, with an incidence of only 1% to 2% (Table 2). However, recurrence is a concern after conservative therapy, with recurrence rates as high as 25.8% in the treated breast and as high as 26.8% in the ipsilateral breast (Table 3). The National Surgical Adjuvant Breast and Bowel Project has shown that radiation therapy after lumpectomy can significantly reduce recurrences compared with lumpectomy alone, and numerous prospective trials are in progress to see whether these findings can be confirmed (Table 4). Numerous retrospective trials have shown similar recurrence rates (up to 23%) after lumpectomy with radiation. In some studies the DCIS was detected on the basis of clinical and mammographic findings (Table 5); in others DCIS was detected on the basis of mammograms only (Table 6). Irradiation can begin within 2 to 4 weeks of surgery, and each field (rather than a bolus) should be treated each day.

Contraindications to radiation after lumpectomy include collagen vascular disease, previous radiation exposure, and pregnancy. Recurrence rates after lumpectomy without radiation have ranged up to 43% (Table 7).

Mastectomy is typically reserved for women with 2 or more primary breast tumors, when calcifications are diffuse and malignant, when margins remain positive despite repeated resections, and when the lesion is so large that lumpectomy could preserve only a small negative margin.

Follow-up Care.—Follow-up can detect recurrences or new cancers and allow treatment of any sequelae. Physical examinations should be performed twice a year up to 5 years and then yearly thereafter. Mammography should be performed at least annually and should include the ipsilateral breast.

▶ This article and the article by Winchester and Cox (Abstract 26–2) about invasive breast cancer are of equal importance and value for health care providers for women. The histologic diagnosis and treatment (less than mastectomy) of DCIS are uncertain and quite variable in diverse breast centers. The issues of extent of disease (mapping) and clear surgical margins are particularly vexing and without conformity. The lack of uniformity and consensus among major breast centers and prominent clinical researchers make the diagnosis, treatment, and prognosis of DCIS difficult to explain to patients. The inability to make specific recommendations to patients based on objective medical evidence is frustrating for clinicians. This article is a clear rendering of what is currently known (and at least partially agreed upon) about DCIS. Screening mammography has increased the frequency of diagnosis of DCIS more than tenfold. Thus, primary health care providers for women should be conversant with up-to-date information about DCIS. This overview is an excellent place to start.

W.H. Hindle, M.D.

Prevalence and Impact of Cyclic Mastalgia in a United States Clinic-based Sample

Ader DN, Browne MW (Univ of Health Sciences, Bethesda, Md; Walter Reed Army Med Ctr, Washington, DC)

Am J Obstet Gynecol 177:126–132, 1997 26–13

Introduction.—Premenstrual breast pain and tenderness, usually accompanied by swelling, occurs regularly in some women during the luteal phase of the menstrual cycle. Swelling and minor discomfort lasting 1–4 days premenstrually are considered normal, but some women have moderate-to-severe mastalgia for up to 14 days (Fig 1). Reported prevalence of benign breast pain is up to 69%. The extent that this disorder influences participation in breast screening is unknown. In the United States, it seems cyclic mastalgia is a common problem that is underresearched, underrecognized, and undertreated. In a sample of U.S. women, the prevalence of premenstrual breast symptoms was described, and it was determined whether cyclic mastalgia is associated with participation in mammography.

Methods.—There were 1,171 women younger than age 55 in an obstetrics and gynecological clinic who completed a questionnaire, which had 37 questions related to menstrual and obstetric history, demographic information, consumption of coffee and cola, smoking habits, and participation in breast screening.

Results.—Regular premenstrual discomfort was reported by 69 % of women who complained of tenderness, swelling pain, or lumpiness (Fig 2). A health care provider was consulted about the symptoms by 36% of

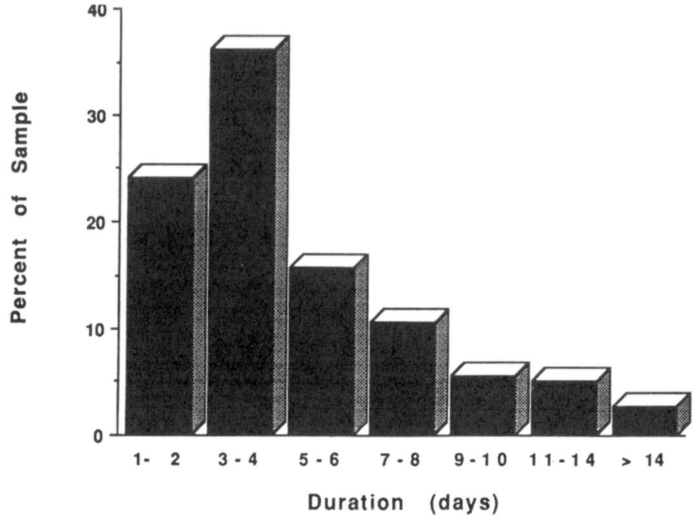

FIGURE 1.—Monthly duration of breast symptoms among women reporting recent premenstrual breast changes. (Courtesy of Ader DN, Browne MW: Prevalence and impact of cyclic mastalgia in a United States clinic-based sample. *Am J Obstet Gynecol* 177:126–132, 1997.)

patients. In 11% of women, current moderate-to-severe cyclic mastalgia was found. There was a 4.7 times likelihood that women younger than 36 who had cyclic mastalgia had undergone a mammogram when compared to asymptomatic young women. In 48% of women, mastalgia interferes with usual sexual activity; in 37% it interferes with usual physical activity;

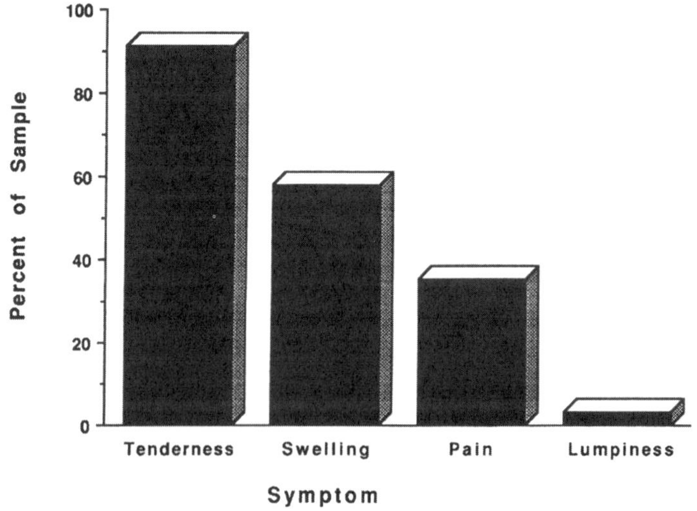

FIGURE 2.—Prevalence of various breast symptoms among women reporting recent premenstrual breast changes. (Courtesy of Ader DN, Browne MW: Prevalence and impact of cyclic mastalgia in a United States clinic-based sample. *Am J Obstet Gynecol* 177:126–132, 1997.)

in 12% it interferes with usual social activity; and in 8% it interferes with usual work or school activity.

Conclusion.—Cyclic mastalgia is associated with high use of mammography among young women and can be severe enough to interfere with usual activities. This disorder merits further biopsychosocial investigation as it is largely ignored both clinically and scientifically in the United States.

▶ Most of the English language medical literature data on benign breast diseases and symptomatology comes from Europe, particularly the United Kingdom. This descriptive study from the Walter Reed Army Medical Center is a welcome exception. As many as 40% of women will present to their health care provider with a primary complaint of mastalgia at some time during their reproductive years.[1] A 41% to 69% prevalence range of mastalgia is quoted in this current questionnaire analysis. Interestingly, of the women with cyclic mastalgia who had not reported their symptoms to their health care provider, almost 80% "thought the discomfort was normal."

Nevertheless, the profound underlying fear that women have of breast cancer magnifies their concern and anxiety that their symptoms, however mild or minimal, could be an indication of breast cancer. A woman presenting to her physician with any breast symptoms or physical signs deserves a complete breast evaluation including a detailed breast-oriented history, bilateral clinical breast examination, and a mammogram (for patients 30 or older, or of any age when the clinician suspects breast cancer). With the current emphasis on women's health and the increasing willingness of women to express their concerns to their health care providers, breast evaluation is claiming a progressively larger part of a clinical practice.

W.H. Hindle, M.D.

Reference

1. Nyirjesy I: Cyclic mastalgia. *Breast Diseases.* 4:8, 1991.

Update of Clinical and Research Issues in Cyclical Mastalgia

Ader DN, Shriver CD (Univ of the Health Sciences, Bethesda, Md; Walter Reed Med Ctr, Washington, DC)

Breast J 4:25–32, 1998 26–14

Background.—Pain, most often cyclical, is the most common clinical complaint regarding the breast. Cyclical mastalgia has not been well researched. Although widely recognized and treated in the United Kingdom, this is not the case in the United States. Current understanding of cyclical mastalgia is reviewed.

Cyclical Mastalgia.—Premenstrual breast discomfort is a common symptom, reported by more than 60% of women. Mastalgia is a monthly and clinically significant problem for about 10% to 15% of women. In this group, it may interfere with activities and may be associated with increased use of mammography. The causes of cyclical mastalgia are unclear, as is its relationship to other disorders. Circulating hormone levels are normal in women with this condition, although they may have elevated levels of saturated fatty acids. Although psychologic causes have been suggested, there are no supportive data. Evidence suggesting women with cyclical mastalgia are at elevated risk of breast cancer is limited. The relationship between cyclical mastalgia and premenstrual syndrome is unclear. Many different categories of treatment have been tried, including diet, vitamins, and diuretics; hormonal therapies; and evening primrose oil. When reassured that breast pain is not a sign of cancer, many patients request no additional treatment. Some patients gain relief from wearing a fitted support bra. Cyclical mastalgia has a placebo response rate of up to 30%, suggesting that uncontrolled trials should be interpreted with caution.

Discussion.—Cyclical mastalgia is a common problem that poses both clinical and research challenges. The authors' clinic uses a thorough evaluation protocol for this problem, which reassures patients that the problem is taken seriously, relieves anxiety, and identifies severe cases in need of treatment. With more awareness of the problem, controlled treatment trials—using a biopsychosocial, interdisciplinary research approach—may be initiated.

▶ With the current emphasis on compassionate, comprehensive women's health care, primary health care providers recognize breast pain as a significant symptom that impacts the lifestyle of many women, particularly those of reproductive age. However, few women volunteer their concern about mastalgia; they need to be asked. Questionnaires can be a non-threatening unbiased method of inquiring about breast-related symptoms. Fear of breast cancer usually underlies intense concern and apprehension, even when unspoken, of a woman with breast symptoms.

All women should be educated about breast anatomy and physiology. The myths of (1) pain as a primary sign of breast cancer and (2) the association of cyclical mastalgia with methylxanthine (caffeine) should be dispelled by giving patients factual, understandable medical data.

These authors used a retrospective screening questionnaire, visual analog pain scale (VAS), mastalgia diary, and a menstrual symptom checklist to evaluate breast symptoms in their clinic patient population. This report concisely summarizes their data and extensively reviews the pertinent medical literature. Primary care providers for women would do well to review this material and apply the information to their practices.

W.H. Hindle, M.D.

Suggested Reading

GEMB Group: Tamoxifen Therapy for Cyclical Mastalgia: Dose Randomized Trial. *Breast* 5:212–213, 1997.

▶ Tamoxifen has been used in Europe for the treatment of mastalgia (mastodynia) for many years and is effective therapy, particularly for cyclic mastalgia. This article from the Grupo de Estudio de Mastopatias Benignas, Argentina, confirms that a 10 mg daily dose of tamoxifen given from the fifteenth to the twenty-fifth day of each cycle is just as effective as a 20 mg dose. The effective response was 82% for the 10 mg regimen and 75% for the 20 mg regimen, but the difference was not statistically significant. Hot flashes, the most bothersome side effect of tamoxifen therapy, were reported in 21% of the 10 mg group and in 38% of the 20 mg group. Less than 2% of the women on the lower 10 mg dose stopped their tamoxifen therapy.

Goodwin PJ, Miller A, Del Giudice ME, et al: Breast Health and Associated Premenstrual Symptoms in Women With Severe Cyclic Mastopathy. *Am J Obstet Gynecol* 176:998–1005, 1997.

▶ Increasing societal and personal openness to discussions of breast symptoms has led to a marked increase in the perceived "incidence" of cyclic and noncyclic mastalgia. At the Breast Diagnostic Center, Women's and Children's Hospital, Los Angeles, CA, more than 30% of the women referred for evaluation present with breast pain as their chief complaint, and most of them are fearful that the pain in their breasts is a sign of breast cancer. Although a presenting complaint of breast pain is rarely associated with breast cancer, given the current availability of medical care, a compassionate and complete breast evaluation, including mammography for women 30 years of age and older, is indicated. When no significant abnormality is identified, patients can be reassured that there is no evidence of breast cancer. Most women will be satisfied by such reassurance and pharmacologic therapy will usually not be necessary. Pertinent clinical information, such as in this report and from clinical research, is slowly emerging about the true incidence and effective treatment of mastalgia. Remember, however, that the symptoms are "serious" to the patient!

W.H. Hindle, M.D.

A Review of Nipple Discharge in Chinese Women

Cheung KL, Alagaratnam TT (Univ of Hong Kong)

J R Coll Surg Edinb 42:179–181, 1997 26–15

Introduction.—In women attending a breast clinic, nipple discharge is thought to be one of the 3 most common presenting complaints with the other 2 being breast pain and finding of a lump. Nipple discharge could be 1 of the less common forms of presentation of breast cancer. A survey of the causes of nipple discharge in women was conducted retrospectively to determine the clinical features which point to nipple discharge associated with breast cancer.

Methods.—There were 104 women from a series of 7,000 who complained of nipple discharge in a breast clinic over a 13-year period with a prevalence rate of 1.5%, and 66 were available for the study. They had a mean age of 47 and ranged in age from 20 to 78 (Fig 1). Twenty-six (39%) were postmenopausal. Their records were reviewed for demographic information, characteristics of discharge, investigations performed, treatment received, and surgery performed. When the discharge was from a single duct, ductography was attempted. When women were older than 35, mammography was considered.

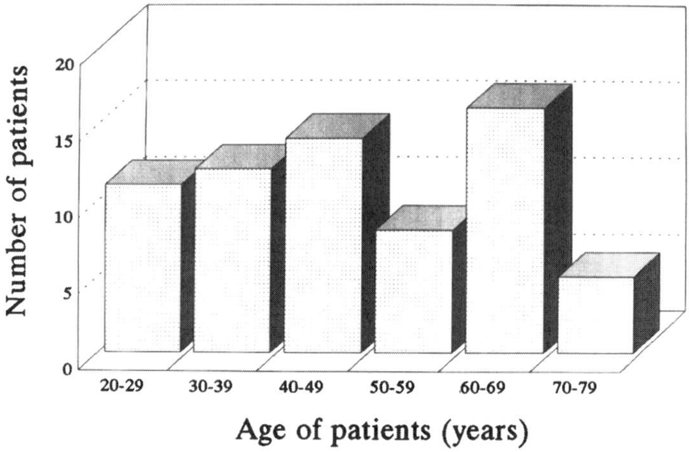

FIGURE 1.—Age distribution of patients with nipple discharge. (Courtesy of Cheung KL, Alagaratnam TT: A review of nipple discharge in Chinese women. *J R Coll Surg Edinb* 42:179–181, 1997. Blackwell Science, Ltd.)

Results.—Five women (8%) had proven breast cancer, and 17 women had benign duct papilloma. The mean duration of discharge was 24±8 weeks before the women sought treatment. In the majority of women (92%), the discharge was unilateral. There were 45.5% who had serous discharge and 54.5% who had bloody discharge. In women older than 55 and if the discharge was bloody, it was found by multivariate analysis that cancer was most likely (Table 2). In the diagnosis of duct papilloma, ductography was found to be useful. Causes of nipple discharge for those who had surgery were duct papilloma, duct ectasia, carcinoma, and fibrocystic changes (Table 1).

Conclusion.—The recommended procedure for treating women with single-duct discharge is microdochectomy. It was adequate to simply sever

TABLE 2.—Comparison Between Patients With Nipple Discharge Due to Cancer and Benign Lesions

Parameter	Patients with cancer (n = 5)	Patients without cancer (n = 61)	All patients (n = 66)
Age (years)	56±7	47±2	47±2
Age >55 (n)*	4*	20*	24
Postmenopausal (n)	4	22	26
Duration of onset (weeks)	9±3	25±9	24±8
Unilateral discharge (n)*	5*	56*	61
Bloody discharge (n)*	5*	31*	36
Single-duct discharge (n)	5	46	51
Palpable lump (n)	3	16	19
Positive mammogram (n)	1	0	1
Positive discharge cytology (n)	0	1	1
Filling defect on ductogram (n)	1	15	16

Data other than the number of patients (n) are presented as mean ± SD.
$^*P < 0.05$.
(Courtesy of Cheung KL, Alagaratnam TT: A review of nipple discharge in Chinese women. *J R Coll Surg Edinb* 42:179–181, 1997. Blackwell Science Ltd.)

TABLE 1.—Pathological Diagnoses of Patients Undergoing Surgery for Nipple Discharge

Diagnosis	Number of patients (%)
Duct papilloma	17 (47%)
Duct ectasia	4 (11%)
Carcinoma	5 (14%)
Fibrocystic changes	10 (28%)
Total	36 (100%)

(Courtesy of Cheung KL, Alagaratnam TT: A review of nipple discharge in Chinese women. *J R Coll Surg Edinb* 42:179–181, 1997, Blackwell Science Ltd.)

the ducts after microdochectomy in this series. There was an 8% incidence of cancer associated with nipple discharge in this group, which is within the range of 3% to 47% described in the literature.

▶ Traditionally, mass, pain, and nipple discharge are given as the "common" breast presenting complaints. Furthermore, mention and discussion of nipple discharge occurs frequently in the lay press and in professional literature about breast cancer from the American Cancer Society and other organizations. By contrast, the 1.5% incidence of nipple discharge as the presenting complaint to a breast clinic reported in this series does not qualify as "common." However, it is similar to our experience at the Breast Diagnostic Center (Women's and Children's Hospital, Los Angeles County and University of Southern California Medical Center, Los Angeles) where the incidence was 1% for spontaneous nipple discharge in a review of more than 12,000 patients presenting to the center. An additional 3% (for a total of 4%) of women presenting to the center complained of elicited nipple discharge, which is rarely pathologic. Women with elicited nipple discharge should be strongly urged to cease eliciting the discharge and to return if spontaneous nipple discharge occurs. Women with spontaneous nipple discharge that is not related to pregnancy or lactation should be evaluated with a ductogram (galactogram) or consultation with a breast specialist. Most intraductal lesions will be benign intraductal papillomas (single or multiple), but rare intraductal papillary carcinomas do occur. Thus, all identified intraductal lesions should be completely excised for definitive histologic diagnosis.

W.H. Hindle, M.D.

A Comparison of Accuracy Rates Between Open Biopsy, Cutting-Needle Biopsy, and Fine-Needle Aspiration Biopsy of the Breast: A 3-year Experience

Antley CM, Mooney EE, Layfield LJ (Duke Univ, Durham, NC)
Breast J 4:3–8, 1998 26–16

Purpose.—Excisional biopsy is regarded as the gold standard for diagnosis of breast nodules. Open biopsy is generally assumed to be 100% accurate in studies comparing techniques, such as fine-needle aspiration

(FNA) cytology and cutting needle biopsy. The accuracy of FNA and large-gauge core needle biopsy are well demonstrated; however, there are few comparable data for excisional biopsy. A 3-year experience with open biopsy, cutting-needle biopsy, and FNA biopsy was reviewed to compare the sensitivity and specificity of the 3 techniques.

Methods.—The analysis included specimens from 412 open breast biopsies and 17 non-image-guided Tru-cut biopsies. Histologic follow-up was available in 388 cases and at least 2 years of clinical follow-up in 25. Also studied were 450 FNA specimens, with histologic or cytologic follow-up in 215. The biopsy procedures were performed by a small number of operators and read by the same diagnostic pathology staff.

Results.—The open biopsy specimens with histologic follow-up showed a sensitivity of 99% and specificity of 99.5%, with 2 false-negatives and 1 false-positive detected on repeat biopsy or on review of the initial specimen. The cases with open biopsy and clinical follow-up showed no erroneous diagnoses. Cutting-needle biopsy had a sensitivity of 85% and specificity of 100%, with 2 false-negatives and no false-positives. FNA cytology had a sensitivity of 96.2% and a specificity of 99.6%, with 1 false-positive and 5 false-negatives.

Conclusions.—This experience suggests that FNA cytology compares favorably with open biopsy and cutting-needle biopsy for the diagnosis of breast nodules. Although its diagnostic performance is not as good as open biopsy, it is more accurate than cutting-needle biopsy. The 3 techniques have essentially identical specificity. The decision as to which biopsy technique to use should be based on accurate knowledge of its sensitivity and specificity, rather than the assumption that open biopsy is an infallible technique.

► In this day of progressively increasing numbers, both absolute and proportional, of patients covered by managed care and of increasing pressure upon health care providers to cut costs, traditional diagnostic procedures are being questioned, particularly when alternative methods have been "time tested" and can achieve nearly the same level of accuracy. FNA of a palpable breast mass is one attractive alternative to traditional open surgical biopsy. FNA, using a 22-gauge needle in a procedure that is no more painful than a venipuncture and takes about the same time to perform, is expedient and humane. The cytologic results of FNA can be obtained in a short time (minutes to hours depending on the logistics of the clinical situation). In addition, an FNA is readily performed in the office or clinic setting without the aid of expensive specialized equipment. However, a definitive diagnosis requires that FNA be in concordance with the clinical impression by history and palpation and with mammography (the Diagnostic Triad). If not, further diagnostic testing must be pursued until a definitive diagnosis is achieved.

At the Breast Diagnostic Center (Women's and Children's Hospital, LAC+USC Medical Center, Los Angeles, Calif.) our protocol for the diagnosis of a palpable dominant breast mass is to follow the history and examination with an FNA. If a specific cytologic diagnosis is not established, tissue core-needle biopsy, usually with ultrasound guidance, is the next diagnostic procedure. If that does not establish a specific histologic diagnosis, then the traditional open surgical biopsy, following NSABP lumpectomy protocol,[1] is performed as an outpatient surgical procedure (under local anesthesia). In addition, for women aged 30 or older (or at any age if the clinical impression is of malignancy) diagnostic mammography is performed, thus completing the Diagnostic Triad (triple test).

W.H. Hindle, M.D.

Reference

1. Margolese R, Poisson R, Shibata H, et al: The technique of segmental mastectomy (lumpectomy) and axillary dissection: A syllabus from the National Surgical Adjuvant Breast Project workshops. *Surgery* 102:828–834, 1987.

Clinical Examination, Mammography, and Fine-needle Aspiration Cytology in the Management of Palpable Breast Masses

Tartter PI, Samuels J, Bratton J, et al (Mount Sinai Med Ctr, New York)
Breast J 3:127–130, 1997 26–17

Background.—The "triple test"—a combination of examination, mammographic, and fine-needle aspiration cytologic findings—is increasingly used for the management of palpable breast masses. It can confirm malignancy, indicate the urgency of excisional biopsy, and identify lesions that can be safely followed without biopsy. However, each of the 3 components is known to be highly dependent on training and experience. Thus, the triple test may vary in accuracy. A 6-year experience with the triple test for investigation of palpable breast masses was reviewed.

Methods.—The experience included 198 consecutive patients with palpable breast masses who underwent clinical examination, mammography, and fine-needle aspiration cytology, followed by excisional biopsy. All were referred by a breast specialist; patients who did not undergo excisional biopsy were excluded from the analysis. Aspirations were repeated

TABLE 1.—Pathologic Findings

Benign	
Fibrocystic	57
Fibroadenoma	19
Fibrosis	5
Abscess	1
Inflammation	1
Lipoma	1
Malignant	
Infiltrating ductal carcinoma	90
Infiltrating lobular carcinoma	10
Ductal carcinoma in situ	6
Other	4

(Courtesy of Tartter PI, Samuels J, Bratton J, et al: Clinical examination, mammography, and fine-needle aspiration cytology in the management of palpable breast masses. *Breast J* 3:127–130, 1997.)

TABLE 2.—Comparison of Clinical, Mammographic, and Cytologic Findings in Benign and Malignant Lesions

	Benign	Malignant	Sensitivity	Specificity
n	88	110		
Age	44	56		
Clinical examination				
Benign	66	4		
Positive/suspicious	22	106	96%	75%
Mammography				
Benign	79	20		
Positive/suspicious	9	90	82%	90%
Cytology				
Benign	77	17		
Positive/suspicious	11	93	85%	82%

(Courtesy of Tartter PI, Samuels J, Bratton J, et al: Clinical examination, mammography, and fine-needle aspiration cytology in the management of palpable breast masses. *Breast J* 3:127–130, 1997.)

until an adequate specimen was obtained. Each of the 3 components of the triple test—alone and in combination—was assessed for sensitivity and specificity. The importance of concordant and discordant results was evaluated, with the expectation that at least 1 breast cancer with triple false negative results would be identified.

Results.—Excisional biopsy revealed malignancy in 110 patients and benign lesions in 88 (Table 1). Diagnostic sensitivity was 96% for clinical examination, 82% for mammography, and 85% for fine-needle aspiration cytology. Specificity was 75%, 90%, and 82%, respectively (Table 2). No lesion was falsely classified as malignant by all 3 tests (Table 3). Fifty percent of infiltrating lobular cancers were false negative on fine-needle aspiration. The results were interpreted as atypical or suggestive of carcinoma, never unequivocally malignant. Overall, 70% of lesions were concordant by all 3 tests. Four lesions were false positive by all 3 tests; all were fibrocystic disease.

Conclusions.—At the study center, the triple test is a valid approach to the investigation of palpable breast masses. This combination of tests will

TABLE 3.—The Value of Combining Clinical, Mammographic, and Cytologic Information

	Benign	Specificity	Malignant	Sensitivity
n	88		110	
Clinical examination				
with mammography	64	73%	108	98%
with cytology	64	73%	107	97%
with mammography and cytology	57	65%	110	100%
Mammography				
with cytology	68	83%	103	94%

(Courtesy of Tartter PI, Samuels J, Bratton J, et al: Clinical examination, mammography, and fine-needle aspiration cytology in the management of palpable breast masses. *Breast J* 3:127–130, 1997.)

vary in accuracy among physicians, and must be validated by excisional biopsy. For legal and reimbursement reasons, most benign palpable breast lesions in the United States will continue to be excised.

▶ These results add to numerous published reports validating the effectiveness and accuracy of the Diagnostic Triad (clinical examination, mammography, and fine-needle aspiration), or Triple Test. The 3 diagnostic modalities were concordant in 70% of the cases. Thus, those patients could have been evaluated and managed in the outpatient setting without resorting to the traditional open surgical (excision) biopsy. Because the intensity of the search for palpable breast cancer now results in an estimated 1,000,000 breast biopsies a year, potentially as many as 700,000 breast biopsies might be "avoided" by initiating the evaluation of a palpable breast mass with the Diagnostic Triad. A keenly significant dollar amount[1] of savings would result. Furthermore, studies[2, 3] have shown that when a preoperative diagnosis of malignancy is known beforehand, excision biopsies tend to be done following the National Surgical Adjuvant Breast and Bowel Project guidelines, resulting in clear surgical margins in most cases (as high as 90%). Otherwise, re-excision for grossly involved surgical margins may be necessary in as many as 50% of biopsy cases when biopsy was the initial procedure. Wider application of the Diagnostic Triad would seem to be both a humane and cost-effective practice for the evaluation of a persistent, palpable, dominant breast mass.

W.H. Hindle, M.D.

References

1. Silverman JF: Diagnostic accuracy, cost-effectiveness, and triage role of fine-needle-aspiration biopsy in the diagnosis of palpable breast lesions. *Breast J* 1:3–8, 1995.
2. Cox CE, Reintgen DS, Nicosia SV, et al: Analysis of residual cancer after diagnostic breast biopsy: An argument for fine-needle aspiration cytology. *Ann Surg Oncol* 2:201–206, 1995.
3. Tartter PI, Bleiweiss IJ, Levchenko S: Factors associated with clear biopsy margins and clear reexcision margins in breast cancer specimens from candidates for breast conservation. *J Am Coll Surg* 185:268–273, 1997.

The Diagnostic Impact of Aspiration Cytodiagnosis of Breast Masses in Association With Pregnancy and Lactation With an Emphasis on Clinical Decision Making

Gupta RK (Wellington Hosp, New Zealand)

Breast J 3:131–134, 1997 26–18

Purpose.—Several studies have demonstrated the effects of fine-needle aspiration (FNA) cytology on the diagnosis of breast masses. Some women are referred for evaluation of breast masses developing during pregnancy and lactation, and FNA cytology may be useful in this situation. The use of FNA cytology to investigate breast masses developing during pregnancy and lactation was reviewed.

TABLE 1.—Fine-needle Aspiration Cytodiagnosis in 331 Cases: Pregnancy and/or Lactation

Diagnosis (FNA)	Number of cases	%
Pregnancy of lactational effects (benign findings)	167	50.45
Nondiagnostic (scanty)	6	1.81
Cysts	33	9.96
Fibroadenoma	71	21.45
Lactating adenoma	3	0.90
Inflammatory	39	11.78
Highly suspicious*	2	0.60
Carcinoma†	10	3.05
	331	100.00

*On biopsy, ductal carcinoma of the breast was confirmed.

†All carcinomas were confirmed on histology. All other patients with a diagnosis other than "suspicious" or "carcinoma" were observed for a period of 1.5–2 years; in none of the patients was any evidence of carcinoma found, and the initial fine-needle aspiration-diagnosed lesion was found to regress within a few months to 2 years after delivery or discontinuation of breast feeding.

(Courtesy of Gupta RK: The diagnostic impact of aspiration cytodiagnosis of breast masses in association with pregnancy and lactation with an emphasis on clinical decision making. *Breast J* 3:131–134, 1997.)

Methods.—From 1983–1996, the study institution's cytology unit evaluated FNA specimens from 18,695 women with breast masses. Of those, 331 aspirates had developed during pregnancy and lactation. Clinical, surgical, postsurgical, and follow-up information on these patients was obtained from the physicians' charts.

Results.—The aspirates were obtained between 8 and 30 weeks' gestation, in the postpartum period, or after breast-feeding. When this occurred, aspiration was repeated up to 3 times to reduce the chances of missing a diagnosis. The rate of nondiagnostic samples was less than 2%. In 2 patients (0.6%), the FNA was deemed highly suggestive of carcinoma; both patients had features of ductal carcinoma on breast biopsy. Ten patients (3%) had an FNA diagnosis of carcinoma made in the first specimen obtained, and each case was confirmed by subsequent tissue examination. Cytologic features of specimens showing carcinoma included high cellularity and numerous malignant cells with moderate cytoplasm, hyperchromatic nuclei, pleomorphism, and mitoses. These were easily distinguished from fibroadenomas, which were diagnosed in 71 cases (21%) (Table 1).

Conclusions.—Fine-needle aspiration cytology is a very useful test for the diagnosis of breast masses developing during pregnancy and lactation. With careful follow-up, it has a significant impact on clinical decision making and reduces the number of surgical biopsies performed. Open biopsy is needed only in patients with cytologic findings highly suggestive of carcinoma on repeated aspiration samples.

► A persistent, dominant, palpable breast mass must be definitively diagnosed. Although less effective and more uncomfortable for the patient, the same rigorous evaluation of a palpable dominant breast mass is indicated when a woman is pregnant or lactating. Unlike mammography, which has decreased effectiveness (accuracy) in pregnant and lactating women, FNA is effective and efficient. However, the cytopathologist must have the information that the patient is pregnant or lactating as both conditions are associated with cellular changes that may be described as "atypical" if the patient's condition is unknown to the cytopathologist. As emphasized by the authors of this study, a repeat aspiration should be performed if the aspirate is paucicellular. Histologic diagnosis by tissue core-needle biopsy (or open surgical biopsy) should be obtained if repeated FNAs fail to result in a definite cytologic diagnosis. The Swedish experience indicates that 90% of palpable breast masses can be specifically diagnosed by FNA cytology.

W.H. Hindle, M.D.

Suggested Reading

National Cancer Institute: Final Version: The Uniform Approach to Breast Fine-Needle Aspiration Biopsy, *Breast Journal* 3:149–168, 1997.

▶ This is the final formal version of the National Cancer Institute–sponsored conference held in September 1996 and previously reported in synopsis format.[1] The emphasis is on formal organized training and supervised experience. The recommendations are fairly broad and general. With appropriate instruction and training, most interested obstetrician-gynecologists (or other primary health care physicians) could qualify. As with all techniques, ongoing audits of performance and results are essential.

Reference

1. National Cancer Institute: The uniform approach to breast fine needle aspiration biopsy. *Acta Cytologica* 10:1120–1126, 1996.

Logrono R, Kurtycz DF, Inhorn SL: Criteria for reporting fine needle aspiration on palpable and nonpalpable masses of the breast. *Acta Cytologica* 41:623–627, 1997.

▶ The formal written cytology report has often been confusing and ambiguous for clinicians performing breast fine-needle aspirations. This detailed editorial gives a logical systematic approach to such cytology reports. With this proposed format, most clinicians would be clear as to the precise diagnosis and its implications. Hopefully, these or similar criteria will be adopted and uniformly used by cytopathologists throughout the United States (and elsewhere).

Mitre BK, Kanbour AI, Mauser N: Fine Needle Aspiration Biopsy of Breast Carcinoma in Pregnancy and Lactation. *Acta Cytol* 41:1121–1130, 1997.

▶ This report from the Magee-Women's Hospital and University of Pittsburgh School of Medicine identifies cellular dyshesion; overlapping nuclei; and enlarged, pleomorphic nuclei with irregular nuclear membranes, coarse nuclear chromatin, and mitoses as distinctive cytologic features of malignancy that can be differentiated from the known cytologic changes in breast ductal epithelium which occur during pregnancy and lactation. However, since a cytopathologist could confuse the normal ductal cell pregnancy/lactational changes with well-differentiated malignancy, it is critical that the clinician performing breast fine-needle aspiration provide the cytopathologist with the date of the patient's last menstrual period and the fact that the patient is pregnant or lactating.

W.H. Hindle, M.D.

Accuracy of Mammographic Appearances After Breast Fine-needle Aspiration

Hindle WH, Chen EC (Univ of Southern California, Los Angeles)

Am J Obstet Gynecol 176:1286–1292, 1997 26–19

Background.—Fine-needle aspiration (FNA) and mammography, together with clinical examination, are used for evaluation of palpable breast masses. The FNA procedure can affect the accuracy of mammography; still, for practical reasons, the 2 tests are often scheduled for the same day. An experience with more than 1,000 palpable breast masses was analyzed to determine the effects of FNA on the subsequent mammographic findings.

Methods.—The retrospective study included 1,007 women with palpable solid breast masses evaluated over a 3-year period. All underwent FNA of the mass, followed within 2 weeks by mammography. Fine-needle aspiration was performed by a modified 22-gauge needle-alone technique. The results of FNA cytology, mammography, and breast biopsy were correlated to establish the clinical accuracy of mammography performed after FNA. The findings were analyzed for all patients and by age.

Results.—The cytologic or histologic diagnosis was malignancy in 91 patients. The mammogram was classified as "suspicious" in 79% of these cases and "nonsuspicious" in 21% (Table 2). Mammography had a positive predictive value of 58%, negative predictive value of 98%, a sensitivity of 79%, and a specificity of 94% (Table 3). There were no apparent differences by age (Table 4). Overall, 916 patients had benign results on FNA cytology; mammograms were "nonsuspicious" in 94% and "suspicious" in 6%. Women who previously underwent FNA were more likely to have "suspicious" mammograms (Table 5).

Conclusion.—For the patient with a palpable breast mass, FNA can be performed at the initial visit and followed within 2 weeks by mammography. The timing of these 2 tests causes no clinical confusion or misleading mammographic findings, while offering patient convenience and prompt diagnosis. With the technique used in this study, FNA causes no clinically significant hematomas or changes in the mammographic appearance.

TABLE 2.—Fine-Needle Aspiration Results Correlated With Corresponding Mammograms

Mammogram results	*FNA + for CA*	*FNA − for CA*
"Suspicious" (codes, 4, 5)	72	52
"Nonsuspicious" (codes 1, 2, 3, 6)	19	864

Note: $\chi^2 = 422.35$, $P < 0.005$.
Abbreviations: FNA, fine-needle aspiration; +, positive; *CA*, cancer; −, negative.
(Courtesy of Hindle WH, Chen EC: Accuracy of mammographic appearances after breast fine-needle aspiration. *Am J Obstet Gynecol* 176:1286–1292, 1997.)

TABLE 3.—True-Positive, False-Positive, and Negative Mammograms by Age Group

	Age <30 yr	*30–39 yr*	*40–49 yr*	*>50 yr*
True-positive mammograms (*n* = 72)	3	15	22	32
False-positive mammograms (*n* = 52)	19	7	14	12
False-negative mammograms (*n* = 19)	0	5	10	4
True-negative mammograms (*n* = 864)	398	197	184	85
TOTAL (N = 1007)	420	224	230	133

(Courtesy of Hindle WH, Chen EC: Accuracy of mammographic appearances after breast fine-needle aspiration. *Am J Obstet Gynecol* 176:1286–1292, 1997.)

► Ever since warnings published in 1982–1983 that "suspicious" mammographic findings (subsequently proven to be benign and probably related to hematoma formation) were being perceived on mammograms taken after FNA, the dictum has been that mammograms should be taken before or more than 2 weeks after FNA. However, following this policy could produce an anxious delay (both for the patient and for the clinician) in establishing a definitive diagnosis and could result in "loss to follow-up" of mobile, medically underserved patients.

This observational review is consistent with unpublished data from other sources showing that if the mammographer is aware that an FNA has been performed, immediate (or same day) mammography is reliable and accurate in the evaluation of a palpable breast mass. This diagnostic approach is convenient for the patient and clinically useful in a patient population that may have a high rate of failed follow-up appointments.

W.H. Hindle, M.D.

TABLE 4.—Cytologic Diagnoses of Women With False "Suspicious" Mammograms and No Fine-Needle Aspiration Evidence of Cancer, by Age Group

	Age <30 yr	*30–39 yr*	*40–49 yr*	*>50 yr*
Fibroadenoma (*n* = 19)	10	4	3	2
Benign breast tissue (*n* = 22)	6	3	6	7
Other breast conditions (*n* = 4)	3	0	0	1
Cyst (*n* = 7)	0	0	5	2
TOTAL (N = 52)	19	7	14	12

(Courtesy of Hindle WH, Chen EC: Accuracy of mammographic appearances after breast fine-needle aspiration. *Am J Obstet Gynecol* 176:1286–1292, 1997.)

TABLE 5.—Association Between Fine-Needle Aspiration and Occurrence of "Suspicious" Findings on Mammograms

	With FNA	*Without FNA*
"Suspicious" mammograms	124	277
"Nonsuspicious" mammograms	883	4293

Note: $\chi^2 = 39.30$; $P < 0.005$.
Abbreviation: FNA, fine-needle aspiration.
(Courtesy of Hindle WH, Chen EC: Accuracy of mammographic appearances after breast fine-needle aspiration. *Am J Obstet Gynecol* 176:1286–1292, 1997.)

Stereotactic Core-needle Biopsy of the Breast: A Report of the Joint Task Force of the American College of Radiology, American College of Surgeons, and College of American Pathologists

Bassett L, Winchester DP, Caplan RB, et al (Univ of California, Los Angeles; Northwestern Univ, Chicago; American Society of Breast Surgeons, Portsmouth, Va; et al)

Breast J 3:317–330, 1997 26–20

Introduction.—Stereotactic core-needle biopsy is a less invasive biopsy technique for mammographic lesions suggestive of carcinoma. A joint task force of the American College of Radiology, the American College of Surgeons, and the College of American Pathologists was formed to review important issues related to this technique. Although the technique appears to be effective, the indications for biopsy should not be altered simply because it is available. Based on a comprehensive literature review, the task force presents its recommendations for the use of stereotactic core-needle biopsy.

Stereotactic Core-needle Biopsy.—Stereotactic core-needle biopsy offers several important advantages over fine-needle aspiration cytology for the diagnosis of mammographic abnormalities. It can be interpreted without special pathology treatment, it almost always provides a sufficient specimen, it usually differentiates between intraductal and invasive carcinoma, and it provides a more complete characterization of the lesion in question. Reports disagree as to the sensitivity and specificity of stereotactic core-needle biopsy; the results are usually better when 14-gauge needles, rather than smaller needles, are used. False negative diagnoses are possible if the lesion is missed during core-needle sampling. Other reported concerns include variability according to type of lesion, lack of standardization for research purposes, and failure to identify invasion. Although stereotactic core-needle biopsy has the potential to reduce costs, this will be the case only if the threshold for biopsy is not significantly lowered.

Indications and Contraindications.—Most nonpalpable mammographic abnormalities for which open biopsy would be considered are suitable for stereotactic core-needle biopsy. Needle biopsy cannot be done until a complete imaging workup and physical examination have been done. For most patients with "probably benign" mammographic abnormalities,

6-month mammographic follow-up is appropriate. However, stereotactic core-needle biopsy may be recommended in certain situations, such as a family history of breast cancer. For patients with "suspicious" abnormalities, stereotactic core-needle biopsy is very useful in distinguishing between patients who need surgery and those who can be followed up. For patients with "highly suggestive" mammographic abnormalities, stereotactic core-needle biopsy can confirm the preoperative diagnosis and aid surgical planning and treatment. There are some relative contraindications to stereotactic core-needle biopsy, including patient size; breast thickness; and certain types of masses, such as multiple, noncalcified, and circumscribed lesions. Core biopsy may be difficult when microcalcifications are not tightly clustered or if individual microcalcifications cannot be accurately visualized, localized, and retrieved. In small lesions, the physician should use caution in removing the lesion completely, in case re-excision is necessary..

Discussion.—Radiologists, surgeons, and pathologists must coordinate their efforts to achieve the best patient outcomes with stereotactic core-needle biopsy. In addition to the performance of and indications for stereotactic core-needle biopsy, this report covers the issues of informed consent, specimen handling and reporting, communication of results, management, follow-up, equipment, quality control, quality assurance, and quality improvement. Particularly for patients with "suspicious" mammographic abnormalities, stereotactic core-needle biopsy is a useful diagnostic approach.

▶ Stereotactic tissue core-needle biopsy has become a major diagnostic procedure for nonpalpable (mammographically detected) breast abnormalities. This report is a formal consensus of the colleges of Pathologists, Surgeons, and Radiology. These groups are primarily involved in performing this technique, which has become widely utilized in the United States. The summary data cover more than 3,000 cases with a mean sensitivity of 94% and a mean specificity of 98%. The authors' review of the medical literature reveals that a definitive histopathologic diagnosis can be obtained in almost 90% (mean value) of the cases. Traditional stereotactic needle-localization surgical-excision biopsies are necessary for the remaining undiagnosed cases.

Primary health care providers for women should understand the indications for and the limitations and complications of this diagnostic procedure for nonpalpable breast abnormalities. Any physician ordering screening mammography should be familiar with this so-called "minimally invasive" technique and should be comfortable responding to patients' questions regarding stereotactic tissue core-needle breast biopsy.

W.H. Hindle, M.D.

The Gothenburg Breast Screening Trial: First Results on Mortality, Incidence, and Mode of Detection for Women Ages 39–49 Years at Randomization

Bjurstam N, Björneld L, Duffy SW, et al (Sahlgrens Univ, Gothenburg, Sweden; MRC Biostatistics Unit, Cambridge, England; Umeå Univ, Sweden)

Cancer 80:2091–2099, 1997 26–21

Introduction.—The debate continues regarding the effectiveness of mammographic screening for breast carcinomas in women younger than 50 years. The influence of mammographic screening on breast carcinoma mortality in women younger than 50 was assessed in a randomized trial of invitation to mammography screening in Gothenburg, Sweden.

Methods.—A total of 25,941 women aged 39–49 were randomized to either a study group (11,724 women) that was invited to mammographic screening every 18 months or a control group (14,217 women) that was not invited to undergo mammography until the fifth screening of the study group (6–7 years after randomization). Patients were followed up for mortality rate and the incidence of breast carcinomas diagnosed during the trial.

Results.—Compared with controls, the study group had a 45% decrease in mortality from breast carcinomas. As predicted, there was a higher rate of breast carcinomas in the study group up to the first screening of the control group. After the group's first screening, the incidence of breast carcinomas was nonsignificantly higher in the control group compared with the study group. Women with screen-detected carcinomas have a low fatality rate. The proportional incidence of breast carcinomas was low for the first 12 months but rose dramatically to more than 50% in 12–18 months. About 72% of breast carcinoma deaths in the study group and 63% of those in the control group occurred before age 50. The incidence of lymph-node–positive tumors in the study group was consistent with the effects on mortality.

Conclusion.—These findings add to earlier evidence regarding a decrease in breast carcinoma mortality in women younger than age 50 who participate in regular mammographic screening. The reduction in mortality can be substantial if high-quality mammography is used and an 18-month interscreening interval is rigorously followed.

► The addition of this scrupulously precise data from Gothenburg provides statistical significance to the relative reduction in breast cancer mortality in the age group 40–49 for all the Swedish and all the population-based screening mammography clinical trials.[1] The objection that there is no published statistically significant mortality data to support the benefit of screening mammography in this age group can no longer be raised. It is of keen interest that this trial used an 18-month interval. Because more aggressive cancers tend to become clinically manifest in this age group, it may well be that annual mammography will further decrease mortality. For those who are responsible for health care financing, the cost-effectiveness of population-based screening mammography for this age group is a critical issue. Analysis suggests that the cost-effectiveness of screening women 40–49 years of age is 5 times greater than for women 50–69 years of age.[2] However, for the personal benefit of the individual woman, I continue to recommend screening mammography every year beginning at age 40 years.

W.H. Hindle, M.D.

References

1. Tabar L, for the Organizing Committee and Collaborators: Breast cancer screening with mammography in women aged 40–49 years. *Int J Cancer* 68:693–699, 1996.
2. Salzmann P, Kerlikowske K, Phillips K: Cost-effectiveness of extending screening mammography guidelines to include women 40 to 49 years of age. *Ann Intern Med* 127:955–965, 1997.

A Clinical Algorithm for the Management of Abnormal Mammograms: A Community Hospital's Experience

Gist DL, Llorente J, Mayer J (Sharp HealthCare, San Diego, Calif; San Diego State Univ, Calif)

West J Med 166:21–28, 1997 26–22

Objective.—The value of mammography in early detection of breast cancer is well established. However, some authors have suggested that mammography prompts many unnecessary breast biopsies. A national breast cancer conference suggested that developing a comprehensive approach to mammography may help to avoid unnecessary breast biopsies while improving early detection of breast cancers. A community hospital algorithm for the management of patients with abnormal mammogram results was studied.

Methods.—The algorithm was developed on the basis of a review of scientific literature and current practice (Fig 1). After validation, study participants received educational and print materials on the algorithm. Its effectiveness was studied in 3 5-month periods: a baseline period, a postintervention period, and a follow-up period. The dependent measure for effectiveness was the positive predictive value (PPV).

Results.—The analysis included 59 patients with abnormal mammogram results in the baseline phase, 61 in the postintervention phase, and 43 in the follow-up phase. Analysis of cases with a definite or implied recommendation for biopsy by the reporting radiologist showed a PPV of 4% at baseline, 21% in the postintervention period, and 18% in the follow-up period. The preintervention and postintervention PPVs after an abnormal mammogram result with a recommendation for biopsy were significantly different. There was no evidence of a change in the mean lesion size across the 3 study periods. Analysis found a significant change in practice for surgeons exposed to continuing medical education and the algorithm, but not those involved in the development of the algorithm.

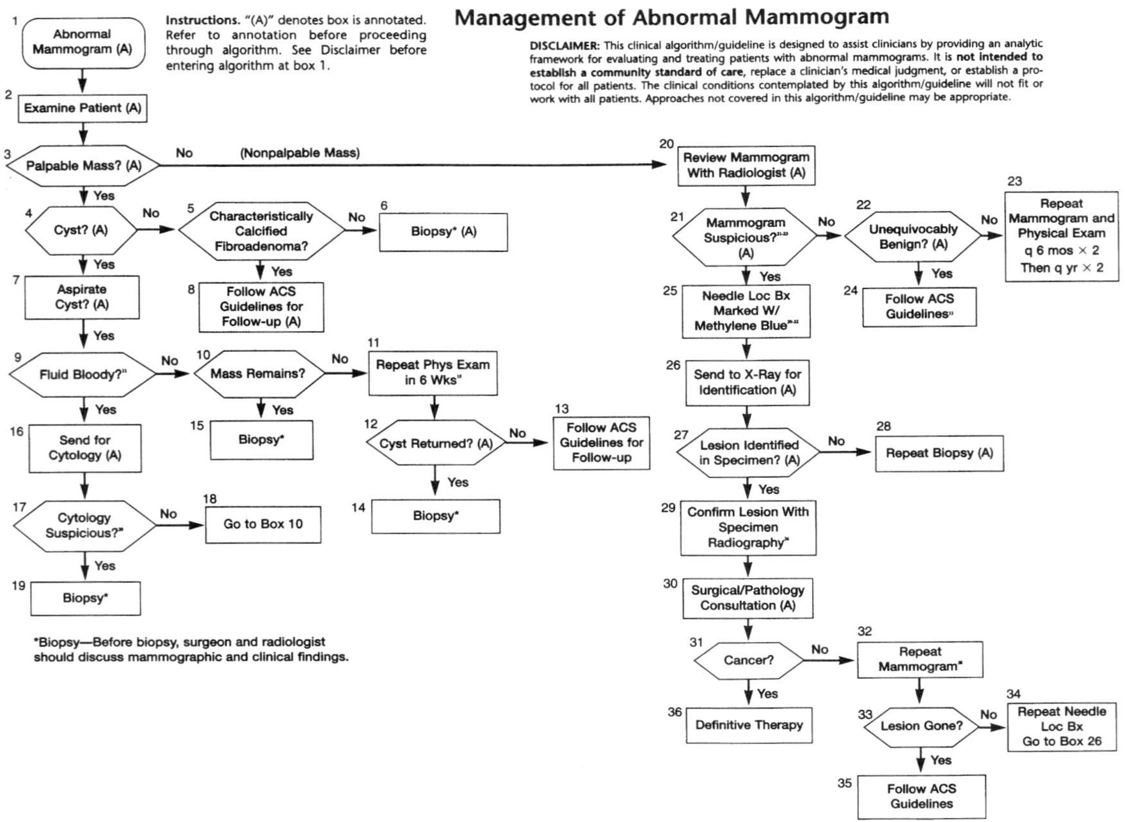

FIGURE 1.—A clinical algorithm was developed by the committee for the management of abnormal mammogram results. *Abbreviations: Loc Bx*, localization biopsy; *Phys Exam*, physical examination; *q*, every. (Courtesy of Gist DL, Llorente J, Mayer J: A clinical algorithm for the management of abnormal mammograms: A community hospital's experience. *West J Med* 166:21–28, 1997.)

Conclusions.—A clinical algorithm for the management of abnormal mammogram results effectively reduced the rate of unnecessary surgical procedures at the authors' community hospital. In cases with a radiologic recommendation for biopsy, the PPV increased from 4% to approximately 20%. The findings suggest that some surgeons may benefit from exposure to such a clinical algorithm, or that a radiologist's recommendation for breast biopsy carries more weight for some surgeons than others.

▶ In clinical practice, the goal for breast cancer screening should be to diagnose all breast cancers before the lesions become palpable. Screening mammography has proved to be effective in identifying nonpalpable lesions suggestive of malignancy. However, many nonpalpable lesions identified by mammography are perceived to be mammographically benign, probably benign, or indeterminate. What to do with lesions not suggestive of malignancy? This is a decision to be made by the mammographer. If the patient or her physician continues to be anxious or doubtful about the diagnosis or recommendations, a second opinion by another mammographer is appropriate. If doubt persists, the patient (and her films) should be referred to a multidisciplinary breast center. The algorithm presented in this article is an attempt to limit interventions while "not missing cancers." Similar clinical pathways for breast evaluation have proved useful in other centers.

W.H. Hindle, M.D.

Suggested Reading

Kerin MJ, O'Hanlon DM, Khalid AA, et al: Mammographic Assessment of the Symptomatic Nonsuspicious Breast. *Am J Surg* 173:181–184, 1997.

▶ This prospective study from the National Breast Cancer Research Institute, University College Hospital, Galway, Ireland, covers a 1-year breast clinic experience of 585 women with breast symptoms but no clinical or cytologic evidence of malignancy. Mammography led to a diagnosis of cancer in 3% of these women. Twenty-eight percent of cancers were DCIS. Most of the women presented with breast pain or nonspecific nodularity. It is of keen clinical interest that "in 8 cases a palpable abnormality was present on reexamination corresponding to the mammographic abnormality." Overall, this study re-enforces the value of the diagnostic triad (physical examination, mammography, and fine-needle aspiration of a dominant breast mass) for the evaluation of breast symptoms. The question remains: for what age should diagnostic mammography be routine in a breast clinic? At the Breast Diagnostic Center (Women's and Children's Hospital, LAC+USC Medical Center, Los Angeles, CA) our policy is to obtain mammography on all breast clinic patients 30 and older.

W.H. Hindle, M.D.

False Negative Mammography: Causes and Consequences
Given-Wilson R, Layer G, Warren M, et al (St George's Hosp, London)
Breast 6:361–366, 1997 26–23

Background.—A negative result on screening mammography can provide a false sense of security. False–negative mammograms are an important issue and can lead to delayed treatment and an increased risk of axillary lymph node involvement. Certain patient characteristics and types of breast cancer have been linked to false–negative mammography. A retrospective study was performed to identify factors associated with an increased risk of false–negative mammography and to determine if false–negatives affect the timeliness of diagnosis and clinical stage.

Methods and Results.—The 2–year review included 174 consecutive symptomatic patients attending a breast clinic who subsequently proved to have breast cancer. On review of the mammographic, clinical, and pathological findings, there were 29 negative mammograms for a false–negative rate of 17%. Mammography had an overall sensitivity of 83%, 95% confidence interval 77% to 89%. Factors associated with a negative mammography report in this group of breast cancer patients were age < 50 years, premenopausal status, dense breast parenchyma, carcinoma in situ, tumor size < 20 mm, and negative cytologic results. Definitive treatment was delayed in women with false–negative mammograms, with a median time to treatment of 7 weeks vs. 3 weeks for those with true–positive mammograms. Mean treatment times were 13 and 4 weeks, respectively. The 12 patients with negative mammograms who had a delay in treatment experienced clinical progression in the interval.

Conclusions.—False–negative mammograms are common among symptomatic women with breast cancer. Some patients will have false–negative results of both mammography and cytology. The clinician should suspect the possibility of false–negative results in patients with factors associated with false–negative mammograms, including young age, dense breasts, small tumors, and carcinoma in situ. If the clinical or cytologic findings are suspicious, a false mammogram should not delay definitive histologic diagnosis.

► Failure to diagnose breast cancer is a major allegation in medical malpractice litigation. Although mammography is a primary method of evaluating or discovering breast abnormalities, it is an imperfect technique even under optimum conditions. It is well known that as many as 10% of palpable breast cancers are not perceived in mammographic films, even with retrospective analysis. Some breast cancers do not have enough difference in tumor density vis-à-vis the background fibroadipose tissue, do not produce perceptible changes in the breast pattern, or remain unseen because of overlying "mammographic density." Thus, a "negative" mammogram does not rule out cancer. If the patient's history, physical examination, or other diagnostic procedures suggest malignancy, further diagnostic evaluation and procedures should be urgently obtained, or the patient should be expeditiously referred to a breast specialist.

W.H. Hindle, M.D.

Suggested Reading

Thurfjell EL, Holmberg LH, Persson IR: Screening Mammography: Sensitivity and Specificity in Relation to Hormone Replacement Therapy. *Radiology*: 339–341, 1997.

▶ This report from University Hospital, Uppsala, Sweden, provides larger numbers of patients and conflicting results compared to a prior publication by Laya.[1] In this current report, it is reassuring that for women currently on or with past use of hormone replacement therapy (HRT) there was no decrease in the sensitivity of screening mammography and only marginal decrease in the specificity. It has been well documented from multiple centers that HRT can increase mammographic density in estrogen-deficient women.[2–4] The increase is seen in about 25% of current estrogen replacement therapy (ERT) and HRT users. It is of keen clinical interest that the maximum increased mammographic density was seen in women on continuous combined HRT and, to a lesser extent, in women on cyclic combined HRT.[2] This makes one wonder about the effect of progesterone on mammographic density. Certainly the clinician should record the patient's history of hormone replacement therapy (current or past) on the mammogram request so that the mammographer may be aware of the therapy when interpreting the mammogram films.

W.H. Hindle, M.D.

References

1. Laya MB, Larson EB, Taplin SH, et al: Effect of estrogen replacement therapy on the specificity and sensitivity of screening mammography. *J Natl Cancer Inst* 88:643–649, 1996.
2. Persson I, Thurfjell E, Holmberg L: Effect of estrogen and estrogen-progestin replacement regimens on mammographic breast parenchymal density. *J Clin Oncol* 15:3201–3207, 1997.
3. Laya MB, Gallagher JC, Schreiman JS, et al: Effect of postmenopausal hormonal replacement therapy on mammographic density and parenchymal pattern. *Radiology* 196:433–437, 1995.
4. McNicholas MMJ, Heneghan JP, Milner MH, et al: Pain and increased mammographic density in women receiving hormonal replacement therapy. *Am J Roentgenol* 163:311–315, 1994.

Subject Index

B

C

D

E

F

G

H

K

L

M

O

Q

R

S

U

V

Author Index

S

T

U

V

W

X

Y

Z